Contents

4   Factors Related to Speech Sound Disorders 109
Nicholas W. Bankson, John E. Bernthal, and Peter Flipsen Jr.

5   Classification and Comorbidity in Speech Sound Disorders 153
Peter Flipsen Jr., John E. Bernthal, and Nicholas W. Bankson

6   Assessment: Data Collection 191
Nicholas W. Bankson, Peter Flipsen Jr., and John E. Bernthal

7   Assessment: Decision Making 233
John E. Bernthal, Nicholas W. Bankson, and Peter Flipsen Jr.

8   Using Evidence-Based Practice in Treatment 265

Peter Flipsen Jr., Nicholas W. Bankson, and John E. Bernthal

9   The Basics of Remediation 277

Nicholas W. Bankson, Peter Flipsen Jr., and John E. Bernthal

10   Motor-Based Treatment Approaches 307

John E. Bernthal, Peter Flipsen Jr., and Nicholas W. Bankson

11   Linguistically Based Treatment Approaches 343

Peter Flipsen Jr., Nicholas W. Bankson, and John E. Bernthal

About the Faculty Materials

To guide faculty in using this text in their course, an Instructor's Resource Manual and Test Bank is available online. The manual includes key points, discussion topics, and instructional ideas for each chapter, as well as a test bank of multiple choice, short answer, and essay questions. Verified faculty may access, download, and print the Instructor's Resource Manual and Test Bank for educational use.

To access the materials that come with this book:

1. Go to the Brookes Download Hub: http://downloads.brookespublishing.com

2. Register to create an account (or log in with an existing account) using your verified university (.edu) email address.

3. Filter or search for the book title *Speech Sound Disorders in Children*.

Note: These materials are for verified faculty members only. If you do not see the materials listed on the book's page and require them for your course, please contact the Brookes Publishing sales representative for your territory. (To find your sales representative, visit https://brookespublishing.com/customer-service/contact/ and select your state in the form.)

About the Authors

John Bernthal, Ph.D., is an Emeritus Professor at University of Nebraska–Lincoln. His career included positions in the public schools of Louisiana, and at Northwestern State (Louisiana), Minnesota State University–Mankato, University of Maryland, University of Northern Iowa, and University of Nebraska–Lincoln. Dr. Bernthal served for 30 years as a department chair at the latter two institutions. He has published articles, tests, and books in the area of speech sound disorders in children. Dr. Bernthal has received the Honors of the American Speech-Language-Hearing Association, the Council of Academic Programs in Communication Sciences and Disorders, and the National Student Speech-Language and Hearing Association. He has also been named 2007 Kansas University Distinguished Allied Health Alumnus and served as President of the American Speech-Language-Hearing Association.

Nicholas Bankson, Ph.D., is an Emeritus Professor at James Madison University. His career included tenured positions at the University of Maryland, Boston University, and James Madison University. Dr. Bankson served for 27 years as a department chair that included the latter two institutions. He has published articles, tests, and books in the areas of speech sound disorders in children and child language disorders. He has received the Honors of the American Speech-Language-Hearing Association, the Council of Academic Programs in Communication Sciences and Disorders, and the National Student Speech-Language and Hearing Association.

Peter Flipsen Jr., Ph.D., S-LP(C), CCC-SLP, is a Professor of Speech-Language Pathology at Pacific University, Oregon. He previously served on the faculty at Minnesota State University-Mankato, the University of Tennessee, Knoxville, and Idaho State University. Using his more than 30 years of experience in the field as a clinician, teacher, and researcher, Dr. Flipsen teaches courses in phonetics, speech sound disorders in children, and research methods. He has published more than 30 peer-reviewed journal articles in the field and presented his work nationally and internationally. His research has focused on classification of speech sound disorders, measurement of intelligibility of speech, speech and language development in children with cochlear implants, and the treatment of residual speech errors in older children.

About the Contributors

Leah Fabiano-Smith, Ph.D., CCC-SLP, is an Associate Professor and Director of the Multicultural and Bilingual Certificate program at the University of Arizona. Her research interests focus on phonological acquisition and disorders in bilingual Spanish-English speaking children and health disparities for the Latinx community due to misdiagnosis of disorder.

Gail T. Gillon, Ph.D., is Director of the Child Well-Being Research Institute at the University of Canterbury, New Zealand, and is co-director of A Better Start National Science Challenge, a 10-year program of research focused on ensuring all children's learning success and well-being. She has an extensive publication record in children's speech-language and literacy development.

Brian Goldstein, Ph.D., CCC-SLP, is the Chief Academic Officer and Executive Dean of the College of Rehabilitative Sciences at the University of St. Augustine for Health Sciences. He holds a B.A. in linguistics and cognitive science from Brandeis University and an M.A. and Ph.D. in speech-language pathology from Temple University. Dr. Goldstein is well-published in the area of communication development and disorders in Latino children. His focus is on phonological development and disorders in monolingual Spanish-speaking and Spanish-English bilingual children. He is a fellow of the American Speech-Language-Hearing Association (ASHA) and received ASHA's Certificate of Recognition for Special Contribution in Multicultural Affairs.

Aquiles Iglesias, Ph.D., is a Professor and the founding Director of the Speech-Language Pathology program at the University of Delaware. Dr. Iglesias's work focuses on language development and assessment of bilingual (Spanish/English) children. He is the author of the Bilingual/English Spanish Assessment (BESA), Systematic Analysis of Language Transcripts (SALT), Quick Interactive Language Screener (QUILS), and Quick Interactive Language Screener: English/Spanish (QUILS: ES).

Laura Justice, Ph.D., is Distinguished Professor of Educational Psychology at The Ohio State University. Dr. Justice is also Executive Director of the Crane Center for Early Childhood Research and Policy, as well as the Schoenbaum Family Center.

A certified speech-language pathologist, much of her research focuses on identifying strategies to improve the language skills of young children, including those with disabilities.

Raymond D. Kent, Ph.D., is Professor Emeritus of the Department of Communication Sciences and Disorders, University of Wisconsin–Madison. Dr. Kent's primary research interests are 1) speech intelligibility in various clinical populations, especially motor speech disorders in children and adults; 2) typical and atypical development of speech in children; and 3) the development and refinement of methods for the study of speech and its disorders. Most recently, he collaborated on an NIH-supported project that uses MR and CT imaging, along with acoustic analyses, to study the anatomic development of the vocal tract in relation to its acoustic properties. Dr. Kent has published several specialty books and is currently working on a dictionary of communication sciences and disorders.

Sharynne McLeod, Ph.D., is a speech-language pathologist and Professor of Speech and Language Acquisition at Charles Sturt University, Australia. She is an elected Fellow of the American Speech-Language-Hearing Association and life member of Speech Pathology Australia. She was named Australia's research field leader in audiology, speech and language pathology (2018, 2019, 2020) and has won editors' awards from the *Journal of Speech, Language, and Hearing: Speech* (2018) and the *American Journal of Speech-Language Pathology* (2019). She was an Australian Research Council Future Fellow, previous editor-in-chief of the *International Journal of Speech-Language Pathology*, and has coauthored 11 books and over 200 peer-reviewed journal articles and chapters focusing on children's speech acquisition, speech sound disorders, and multilingualism.

Brigid C. McNeill, Ph.D., is a speech-language therapist and Professor and Deputy Head of School of Teacher Education in the College of Education, Health and Human Development at the University of Canterbury. Dr. McNeill is an international expert on literacy development in children with childhood apraxia of speech. Her research also focuses on developing and evaluating methods to better prepare teachers to support children's early literacy development.

Carol A. Tessel, Ph.D., CCC-SLP, is an Associate Professor at Albizu University–Miami. Dr. Tessel has been a bilingual speech-language pathologist for 20 years, with clinical specialties in early intervention, bilingualism, and speech sound disorders. Her research includes issues of second language acquisition, bilingual phonology, neurophysiology of speech perception, and pedagogy in communication sciences and disorders. She currently teaches courses in disorders of articulation and phonology, evaluation and treatment of culturally and linguistically diverse populations, clinical phonetics, acoustics, and research methods in communication sciences and disorders.

Preface

We are pleased to share with you the ninth edition of our speech sound disorders text-book. We continue to hear that this text is regarded as a classic resource for providing clinicians with an expansive knowledge base in the area of speech sound disorders. The first edition was published in 1981, and since then it has been utilized as a college textbook and resource by many aspiring and practicing speech-language pathologists. As in previous editions, we continue to endeavor to provide a comprehensive and timely summary of the literature in the area of speech sound disorders. There is no doubt that certain information and knowledge are retained over the years; however, there also continue to be changes and developments in contemporary clinical practice that we seek to incorporate in each new edition, including this ninth edition. We are pleased to share with you, our reader, what we hope will be a useful resource in your professional library.

NEW TO THIS EDITION

In this ninth edition, we have retained the general organization from the previous edition, but we have also:

1. Added learning objectives to introduce every chapter.

2. Included brief cases in several chapters to illustrate some key points, which we have called Clinical Vignettes.

3. Expanded our use of boxes to highlight some important concepts.

4. Reorganized much of the content in the second half of the book, with the net result being an expansion from 12 to 15 chapters. This reorganization included:

   a. Creating separate chapters for Evidence-Based Practice (now Chapter 8) and Remediation Basics (now Chapter 9) to allow for a more in-depth discussion of each area.

   b. Expanding our discussion of Motor-Based Approaches (now Chapter 10) to include vowel remediation and modifications to traditional therapy.

c. Expanding our discussion of both childhood apraxia and treatment for older children and moved them into a separate chapter (now Chapter 12).

d. Expanding what was previously an appendix into a now complete chapter on accent modification (now Chapter 15).

As with previous editions, in all chapters, we and our guest authors have attempted to synthesize the most up-to-date research and literature in the field while maintaining our eclectic perspective relative to the nature and treatment of speech sound disorders. In the assessment and treatment chapters, you will continue to see some of our biases regarding clinical management. We continue, however, to defer to clinician judgment in deciding which assessment and treatment procedures are most useful to them and the clients they serve.

We are indebted to several professionals who have once again contributed their knowledge and expertise in specialized areas to this text: Leah Fabiano-Smith, Gail Gillon, Brian Goldstein, Aquiles Iglesias, Laura Justice, Ray Kent, Sharynne McLeod, Brigid McNeill, and Carol Tessel. We also appreciate the contributions and suggestions from several anonymous reviewers of the eighth edition of the text. Thanks to Melissa Bernhardt for her assistance with reformatting and updating the reference list. Finally, thanks also to Kelly Farquharson for once again preparing the Instructor's Resource Manual.

As authors, we assume all responsibility for errors, oversights, and misconceptions that may appear in this book. Our hope is that this edition will provide you with a comprehensive source of information on the management of individuals with speech sound disorders and that it will be a valuable resource as you learn about and practice clinical interventions for this important clinical population.

Dedicated to John E. Bernthal (1940–2021)

1

Introduction to the Study of Speech Sound Disorders

JOHN E. BERNTHAL, NICHOLAS W. BANKSON, AND PETER FLIPSEN JR.

LEARNING OBJECTIVES

This chapter introduces the reader to a major subdiscipline of the field of speech-language pathology—speech sound disorders. By the end of this chapter, the reader should be able to:

- Describe how the practice of working with individuals with speech sound disorders has evolved over time.
- Understand the basic distinction between articulation and phonological disorders, and some of the limitations of that distinction.
- Understand how common speech sound disorders are and how they arise.
- Discuss the importance of working with individuals with speech sound disorders.
- List the three main elements of evidence-based practice.

Welcome to the world of clinical intervention for individuals with speech sound disorders! You are about to learn about one of the most frequently occurring communication disorders that speech-language pathologists (SLPs) encounter. We use the term *clinical* to indicate that this book is focused on how you, as a clinician, will assess and treat disorders related to speech sound production. This is in contrast to studying production of speech sounds from the standpoint of phonetics, linguistics, or acoustics—any one of which is often a course of study in and of itself. Although knowledge from each of these areas is important background information in the study of speech sound disorders, the distinguishing characteristic of this text is that it is focused on individuals, primarily children, who have difficulty learning to produce and appropriately use the speech sounds of the language.

AN EVOLVING AREA OF PRACTICE

Concerns about speech sound production are certainly not a new area of study. An early work by Samuel Potter called *Speech and Its Defects*, for example, appeared in 1882. According to Moore and Kester (1953), formal studies of what was then called speech correction began to proliferate in the first decade of the 20th century. Organized efforts to address these problems in the public schools appear to have begun in the United States as early as 1910 in Chicago, Illinois, and 1916 in New York City. At about this same time, studies of the prevalence of speech problems in schoolchildren *and Phonological Disorders*). Some SLPs have differentiated these two terms for purposes of assessment and treatment of speech sound disorders. *Articulation disorders* refer to production-based (or motor-based) speech sound errors, and *phonological disorders* denote speech sound errors that are rule based (or linguistically based). However, in reality, it may be difficult to determine which of these concepts is most appropriate to describe a particular client's error(s) productions. We must also recognize that there may be variables beyond motor production and rule acquisition that we need to attend to when we try to understand speech sound disorders. The revised title of this latest edition of the book reflects our attempt to better encapsulate the relationships among all of these terms.

ASHA, in its clinical portal (a website designed to assist clinicians), has defined *speech sound disorders* as "an umbrella term referring to any difficulty or combination of difficulties with perception, motor production, or phonological representation of speech sounds and speech segments—including phonotactic rules governing permissible speech sound sequences in a language" (ASHA, n.d.-c). In this book we use the terms *articulation, phonology,* and *speech sound disorders* somewhat interchangeably, but will hold to the traditional differentiation we have referred to between *articulation* and *phonology* when we talk about assessment and treatment.

THE SCOPE OF THE PROBLEM

Speech sound disorders may be described as ranging from something as mild as a lisp (interdentalizing the /s/ sounds; sometimes identified as substituting /θ/ for an /s/) to a disorder as significant as that found in an individual who is completely unintelligible. The terms *delay* and *deviant* are concepts that are often used to describe the nature of the sound errors produced by children. *Delay* refers to speech sound errors that are often noted as normal errors found in young children as they learn the proper use of sounds (e.g., lisps, misarticulations of /r/ or the affricates, sound substitutions and omission of sounds) but which persist in some children. *Deviant* refers to errors not typically observed in young children's development (e.g., lateralization of sibilants, backing of alveolars, vowel errors). It should be noted that some scholars argue that the labels *delay* and *deviance* are not particularly useful because, in terms of overall language development (including speech sounds), delay often leads to deviance. This progression occurs because of the high degree of coordination involved in the development of all aspects of language (e.g., speech sounds, vocabulary, syntax). If one area is slow to develop (i.e., delayed), it may lead to difficulties across several areas of development, which results in errors that we might then describe as deviant.

Typically, speech sound disorders are seen in children, and the pediatric population is the focus of this text. As discussed earlier, there have been many estimates and studies of how common these disorders are (i.e., their prevalence). In 2003, Campbell and colleagues presented data suggesting that speech sound disorders occur in approximately 15.6% of 3-year-old children. A prevalence of 11% was reported by Dodd and colleagues (2018) in a group of 1,494 Australian 4 year olds. Findings reported by Shriberg et al. (1999) indicated that by age 6 years, up to 3.8% of that age group continues to have difficulty with speech sound production. The differences in prevalence between these three percentages indicates that many of these problems are resolved during the preschool period. Although a positive trend, it does not remove the need for intervention for some children in order to learn accurate production of speech sounds. This is seen most obviously in the report of Mullen and Schooling (2010), who reported in a national study, among prekindergarten children referred for possible communication difficulties, that approximately 75% were identified as having articulation/intelligibility difficulties (the most frequently identified disorders category). In addition, in that same study it was reported that up to 56% of the overall caseloads of school-based clinicians may involve instruction of speech sound production problems. More recently, a 2018 survey by ASHA indicated that 90% of clinicians working in the schools regularly serve children with speech sound disorders.

The nature of SLPs' work with speech sound disorders has expanded in recent decades. As mentioned previously, many of these disorders often coexist with disorders in comprehension or production of language (something we discuss in more detail later in this text). Most speech sound disorders occur in children under the age of 8 years, but speech sound production errors may persist past that point and occur in older children and adults. Working with older children and adults may require some unique considerations, and thus a major portion of a separate chapter is devoted to that group. Information contained in this book is relevant to the treatment of any client who faces difficulties producing speech sounds; however, adult speech sound disorders are often related to organic conditions, and thus you will need to review other materials when planning treatment for most adult clients. One notable exception is that of individuals acquiring English as a second language and the question of foreign accent. Thus, we conclude this text with a chapter devoted to that topic.

THE CAUSE OF THE PROBLEM

As we begin our discussion of speech sound disorders, it is important to recognize that, for many children, the cause of the disorder may be unknown. Often it is assumed that many children do not say their sounds properly because of difficulty in their language development that is also reflected in learning speech sounds. In some instances, the problem may be related to difficulty with other aspects of language (e.g., vocabulary, syntax). As will be discussed in a later chapter, a number of variables have been studied as they relate to such learning problems (e.g., familial history, motor development, speech sound discrimination). Definitive research evidence regarding the causes of speech sound disorders has been difficult to establish but studies are ongoing. Certainly, efforts to categorize or classify various types of speech sound disorders (e.g., speech delay related to otitis media with effusion, motor speech involvement, genetic factors) is a step in the direction of helping us better understand children with speech sound disorders of unknown origin. For some children, the cause of their disorder may be more obvious (e.g., hearing loss, cleft palate); however, even then, the impact of an organic condition does not necessarily determine the type of speech sound disorder a client may have, nor how they will respond to treatment.

In thinking about causes and treatment, it is also important to put speech sounds into their broader communicative context. As we have already mentioned, speech sounds are but one component of language (i.e., the phonology). Other aspects of language include semantics, which refers to meaning attached to words as reflected in vocabulary; morphology, which is defined as minimum meaningful units in the language that include words, and attachments to words such as plural markers (e.g., /s/ in *hats*) and tense markers (e.g., *ed* in *walked*, indicating past tense), or parts of words (e.g., *doghouse* has two minimum meaningful units); syntax, that is, grammatical rules for putting words together in phrases and sentences; pragmatics, which refers to using language appropriately in a social context; and discourse, the ability to string sentences together in a meaningful manner while communicating with others. Each of these areas of language is acquired gradually and simultaneously by young children. Initially, we are concerned that children learn to use meaningful utterances to express themselves, but soon thereafter, we become concerned about accurate sound usage because it is largely through correct production of speech sounds that the child is understood by the listener, or, in other words, becomes intelligible.

To recap, SLPs are initially concerned with a young child's acquisition of semantics and vocabulary, then phonology, and then grammatical rules (morphology and syntax), although these areas are being acquired all at the same time. Concern over pragmatics and discourse come later because they are based on vocabulary and syntax. Thus, it is often older children for whom pragmatics and discourse may be targeted for instruction.

THE IMPORTANCE OF THE PROBLEM

As mentioned earlier, our understanding of speech sound disorders has changed dramatically over the years. Such problems are often about more than just being able to say individual sounds. Fundamentally, the issue is about being able to connect with others through communication—to make ourselves understood. And increasingly, it is being recognized that a normal sound system is important in terms of literacy development, or, in other words, learning to read and spell. Children's phonological awareness skills (or their ability to mentally manipulate the sounds and syllables in words) have been shown to impact literacy skills, and children with speech sound disorders are at risk for inappropriate development of phonological awareness and later literacy (Tambyraja et al., 2020). For this reason, clinicians have been drawn into using their knowledge of phonology as a way to understand a child's literacy development.

Before we decide that there actually is a problem, however, we need to recall some of our earlier discussion. We must recognize that some children use different speech sounds than those found in their environment because perhaps their first language is different from English, or maybe they are a part of a regional or cultural group that uses a less common dialect of English. Certainly, the increasing cultural diversity, the number of second-language learners, and other languages spoken in the United States make us acutely aware of the fact that linguistic differences are a part of everyday communication. As SLPs, we are primarily focused on disorders that individuals may have in their speech communication. When the clinician does not speak the language or dialect of a client, it is sometimes very challenging to determine what constitutes a disorder and what is a language or dialectal difference. Although there are some guidelines to help us, the reality is that there is a growing need for clinicians who are bilingual and/or represent different language/dialect groups. All sound systems, whether they are a part of a separate language or dialect, are legitimate and deserve acceptance. In some instances, the clinician may, however, help an individual learn an alternative sound system in order to fit in with speakers of other dialects of English when a client elects to do this, often for educational, business, or social reasons.

It is also important to place the work we do in this area into its broadest context. Regardless of whether we are discussing a speech sound disorder, use of a dialect that is different from that of our own, or an individual in the process of learning a new language, it is important to remember that the desire to communicate is fundamental to who we are as human beings. A wish to support this fundamental aspect of humanity is likely why most SLPs (including the authors of this book) entered the field. This view is so pervasive that a recent issue of the *International Journal of Speech-Language Pathology* (vol. 20, no. 1, 2018) was dedicated to discussing it as a basic human right. In their foreword to that issue, McEwin and Santow (2018) remind us that communication is actually a right that was enshrined in Article 19 of the United Nations Universal Declaration of Human Rights.

> *"Everyone has the right to freedom of opinion and expression; this right includes freedom to hold opinions without interference and to* **seek, receive and impart information and ideas** *through any media and regardless of frontiers."*
>
> United Nations, 1948 (emphasis added)

As the primary vehicle for human communication, our ability to use language (of which speech sounds are an integral part) is extremely important to our ability to function in modern society. And as we have transitioned to a more knowledge-based economy and society, Ruben (2000) has argued that individuals with communication disabilities may end up even more disadvantaged than those with other types of disabilities. Those individual disadvantages end up having a cumulative impact on our entire society. In his now 20-year-old analysis, Ruben estimated that failure to address communication disabilities costs the U.S. economy between $154 and $186 billion. Given the pace of technological advancement since then, one can only imagine how much larger that impact must be today. Thus, our work with individuals with speech sound disorders is by no means a trivial endeavor.

AN EVIDENCE-BASED APPROACH

A final note in laying the groundwork for our study of speech sound disorders is to acknowledge that we are now in an era of accountability. Those who pay for our services, whether taxpayers, school or hospital administrators, insurance executives, or our clients and their families, can reasonably ask that we as a profession demonstrate that the services we provide are both effective (i.e., they actually work) and efficient (i.e., they do so in the most cost-effective way). No longer is it sufficient for us to simply say, "Trust us; we know what we're doing." We need to provide scientific evidence; put another way, we need to demonstrate that we are engaging in evidence-based practice (EBP). In her 2007 book on EBP, Christine Dollaghan suggests that EBP requires the conscientious, explicit, and judicious integration of 1) best available *external* evidence from systematic research, 2) best available evidence *internal* to clinical practice, and 3) best available evidence concerning the preferences of a fully informed patient (p. 2, italics in original).

Relative to external evidence, this book has, since its first edition, been about presenting the best of the available scientific studies related to working with children who have speech sound disorders. This edition continues and expands that effort. In addition to discussing published external evidence, we will also discuss how the conscientious clinician can and should generate their own internal evidence about whether what they are doing with each client is in fact resulting in meaningful change.

Finally, relative to patient preferences, the past 30 years have yielded a long and varied menu of treatment approaches, which we will highlight. It is no longer a matter of clinicians simply telling parents that we will "do artic therapy." Rather, parents of children with speech sound disorders may well come to us forearmed with information obtained online and/or from family and friends about various treatment options.

When they do (or even if they don't), EBP mandates that they be partners in determining which approach or instructional format may be best prescribed for their child. So, we need to be able to discuss the various options intelligently and objectively. Taken a step further, to the extent that they are able to do so, children themselves should be given a say in the goals and approaches to be used in working with them. Such a person-centered approach also means that our goals may not always be for a 100% perfect match to the adult normal model; in some cases, we may want to work primarily on improving functional communication (the ability to effectively accomplish the intended communication objectives in everyday activities).

Each of the chapters that follow was developed with the thought of providing the latest information and research relative to speech sound disorders. The breadth and depth of information presented is designed to provide a broad-based perspective of how SLPs can go about helping children who face difficulties producing the sounds of the language.

2

Normal Aspects of Articulation

RAY KENT

LEARNING OBJECTIVES

This chapter discusses the normal aspects of speech production; that is, the way that speech is produced by individuals who do not have a communication disorder. This information is essential background to the understanding of speech sound disorders. By the end of this chapter, the reader should be able to:

- Identify the basic components that are used in analyzing the structure of language.
- Explain how vowel articulation is specified using both traditional phonetic description and distinctive features.
- Explain how consonant articulation is specified using both traditional phonetic description and distinctive features.
- Discuss what is meant by the suprasegmental features of speech.
- Define coarticulation and explain why it occurs.
- Discuss how aerodynamics is used to understand speech production.
- Discuss how acoustic analysis is used to understand speech production.
- Explain how sensory information plays a role in the production of speech.
- Discuss how speech production can be analyzed in different levels of organization and information.

This book is focused on the ability of humans to produce sounds that are used to convey a message. The act of producing such sounds is identified as *articulation,* and this activity is a major component of speech, as distinguished from the term language. *Speech* consists of an organized set or system of sounds that are used to convey meaning. Meaning itself is based in *language,* which includes the collection of words that are used in phrases and sentences, and the grammar or rules of the language that we use to create those phrases and sentences. More formally, language may be described as an arbitrary system of signs or symbols used according to prescribed rules to convey meaning within a linguistic community. Of course, once an arbitrary association of symbol with meaning has been developed, the users of that language must learn and use this association of symbols if they want to communicate with one another. The word *dog* has a certain meaning in the English language, and this word can be communicated to other users of English through speaking, writing, or signing it with symbols used by people who are deaf.

Speech is but one modality for the expression of language; however, speech has special importance because it is the primary, first-learned modality for hearing language users. Speech is a system in the sense that it consistently and usefully relates the meanings of a language with the sounds by which the language is communicated.

Not all sound variations in speech are related to meaning. When a person suffers from a cold, they have a different way of talking, but so long as the cold is not so severe as to make speech unintelligible, the relation of sound to meaning is basically the same as when the person is healthy. The acoustic signal of speech; that is, the vibrations of air molecules in response to the energy source of human speech, carries more information than just the expression of meaning. As we listen to a speaker, we often make judgments not only about the intended meaning but also about the speaker's age and sex (if the speaker isn't visible), the speaker's mood, the speaker's state of health, and perhaps even the speaker's dialectal background. Thus, on hearing a simple question—"Could you tell me the time, please?"—we might deduce that the speaker is a young southern woman in a hurry, an elderly British gentleman in a cheerful mood, or a young boy quite out of breath.

STRUCTURE OF LANGUAGE

Speech sounds, then, may be viewed from two perspectives: 1) as motor production (speech) and 2) as units that facilitate the expression of meaning (language). When sounds are studied as part of the language system, they are called *phonemes.*

To derive a speaker's meaning, the listener is basically concerned with the phonemes in the speech message. From a linguistic perspective, phonemes are sound units related to decisions about meaning. In the list *cat hat mat bat sat fat that chat,* each word rhymes with every other word because they all end with the same sounds (the vowel /æ/ and the consonant /t/). However, the words differ in their initial sounds, and these differences can change the meaning of the syllables. In fact, the linguist identifies the phonemes in a given language by assembling lists of words and then determining the sound differences that form units of meaning. The layperson usually thinks of words as the units of meaning, but the linguist recognizes a smaller form called the *morpheme.* For example, the linguist describes the words *walked* and *books* as having two morphemes: *walk + past tense for walked,* and *book + plural for books.* If two sounds can be interchanged without changing word meaning, or if they never occur in exactly the same combination with other sounds, then they are not different phonemes. Hence, phonemes are the minimal sound elements that represent and distinguish language units (words or morphemes).

A *phonemic transcription* (which is always enclosed in virgules / /) is less detailed than a *phonetic transcription* (which is enclosed in brackets [ ]). A phonetic transcription is sensitive to sound variations within a phoneme class. An individual variant of this kind is called an *allophone.* Thus, a phoneme is a family of allophones. Phonemes are the minimal set of sound classes needed to specify the meaningful units (words or morphemes) of the language. Allophones are a more numerous set of distinct sounds, some of which may belong to the same phoneme family. As a very simple example, the word *pop* begins and ends with the same phoneme but often begins and ends with a different allophone. If the final /p/ is produced by holding the lips together after they close, then this sound is the unreleased allophone of the /p/ phoneme. However, the initial /p/ must be released before the vowel is formed, so this sound is the released allophone of the /p/ phoneme. The /p/ phoneme also includes a number of other allophones, though perhaps not as obvious as these two.

To understand more clearly the difference between phonemes and allophones, say the following word pairs to yourself as you try to detect a difference in the production of the italicized sounds.

*k*eep – *c*oop	(phoneme /k/)
m*a*n – b*a*t	(phoneme /æ/)
te*n* – te*n*th	(phoneme /n/)

In the first pair of words, the phoneme /k/ is articulated toward the front of the mouth in the first word and toward the back of the mouth in the second. Despite the differences in the place of tongue contact, the two sounds are heard by speakers of English to be the same phoneme. Speakers of other languages, such as Arabic, may hear the two sounds as different phonemes. The tongue-front and tongue-back versions are allophones of the /k/ phoneme in English.

In the next pair of words, *man* and *bat,* the pertinent difference might be more easily heard than felt through articulation. In the word *man,* the vowel is nasalized (produced with sound transmission through the nose) owing to the influence of the surrounding nasal consonants. But in the word *bat,* the vowel /æ/ is not normally nasalized. The phonetic environment of the vowel, that is, its surrounding sounds, determines whether the vowel is nasalized. The nasal and nonnasal versions of the vowel are allophones of the /æ/ phoneme.

Finally, in comparing /n/ in the words *ten* and *tenth,* you might notice that your tongue is more toward the front (just behind the upper front teeth) in the word *tenth.* The final *th* sound exerts an articulatory influence on the preceding /n/, causing it to be dentalized or produced at the teeth. Again, the two types of /n/ are simply allophones of the /n/ phoneme.

Allophonic variation is of two types: complementary distribution and free variation. In *complementary distribution,* two (or more) allophones never occur in exactly the same phonetic environment, so the occurrence of one is complementary (nonoverlapping) to the occurrence of the other. For example, the front and back /k/ discussed previously are in complementary distribution. The front /k/ occurs in the environment of vowels made in the front of the mouth, and the back /k/ occurs in the environment of vowels made in the back of the mouth. Similarly, the nasal and nonnasal allophones of /æ/ are in complementary distribution, determined by the presence or absence of nasals in the phonetic environment. The nasalized /æ/ occurs only when this vowel is preceded or followed by nasal sounds. Allophones are said to be in *free variation* when they can occur in the same phonetic context. For example, the released /p/ and the unreleased /p/ are in free variation in word-final position in words like *pop* or *map.* As previously indicated, the final /p/ can be released audibly with a small burst as the lips open, or it can be unreleased if the lip closure is maintained.

The discipline of linguistics is concerned primarily with the structure of language. The disciplines of psychology and speech-language pathology are concerned primarily with the processing of language—with its formulation and its reception. The linguistic study of language structure has influenced the study of language processing and, to some degree, the reverse is true as well. Descriptions of language processing often use terms such as *syntax, semantics, phonology*, and *phonetics* that denote traditional areas of linguistic study. These terms have come to have a dual usage, one referring to structure and another to processing.

To briefly round out our discussion of the structure of language, we need to say a little more about how phonemes are used to build larger units, such as morphemes and words, and how these in turn are used to make phrases and sentences. Phonemes are combined to produce meaningful units, called morphemes, which we usually identify as words. But as mentioned earlier, it should be recognized that a given word, such as *walked,* may actually be composed of two or more morphemes. In the case of *walked,* the morphemes are the verb *walk* and the past tense marker *ed* (i.e., past tense carries meaning). Morphemes and words are combined into phrases and sentences according to the grammatical rules of the language, and these combinations are referred to as the *syntax* of the language. Thus, language includes a set of phonemes and morphemes that are combined according to certain rules to reflect the syntax of the language. Meaning that is ascribed to individual words is identified as the *semantics* of the language. In a sense, the components of language (phonology, morphology, syntax) are one side of the coin, with semantics being the other side. Much of the knowledge that children have about the language they are learning is implicit; that is, they can understand and produce constructions such as sentences without being able to express the rules or processes that underlie this ability.

Figure 2.1 is a diagram of an information-processing model of verbal formulation and utterance production. The diagram attempts to show how different types of information are processed in the act of speaking. The cognitive level is where a thought is initiated. This is a prelinguistic, propositional level that involves decisions such as the

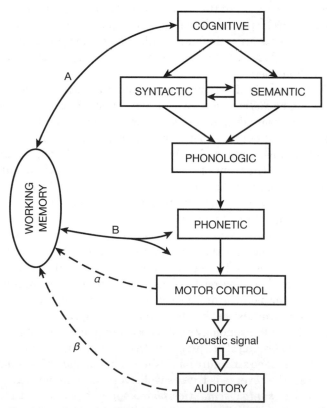

Figure 2.1. Information-processing model of verbal formulation production. *Source:* Bock (1982).

identification of participants and actions. For example, the cognitive processing that preceded formulation of the sentence, *The dog chased the cat,* involved the identification of a dog and a cat as participants and chasing or pursuit as an action. However, the specific words *dog, cat,* and *chased* were not actually selected. Rather, concepts that later lead to the identification of these words at the semantic level are established.

Information from the cognitive level is used to make decisions at the syntactic and semantic levels. Syntax involves the ordering of words in a sentence, and semantics involves the selection of words. Research on verbal formulation indicates that syntactic and semantic processing is interactive (hence, the arrows between them in the diagram). Deciding on a particular syntactic structure for a sentence can influence word selection, and selection of particular words can limit or direct syntactic decisions. The semantic level is sometimes called *lexicalization,* or the choice of lexical units. Lexicalization appears to be a two-stage process. The first stage is selection of a lexical concept, not a phonologically complete word. Phonologic specification, that is, specification of the word's sound pattern, is accomplished in the second stage of the process. The phonologic level in Figure 2.1 is the level at which the evolving sentence comes to have phonologic structure. Various decisions are made at this level to ensure that a sound pattern accurately represents the syntactic and semantic decisions made earlier. The phonologic information then directs decisions at the phonetic level, where the details of the sound pattern are worked out. We might think of the phonetic level as producing a detailed phonetic representation of the utterance.

The output of the phonetic level is sufficient to specify the phonetic goals to be satisfied in speech production. Actual motor instructions are determined by a motor control level. This level selects the muscles to be activated and controls the timing and strength of the muscle contractions. This is no small task. Speech requires rapid changes in the activation of about 100 muscles, which are controlled to meet exacting spatiotemporal goals. Once the muscles have done their work, the acoustic speech signal is produced. This signal is then processed by the speaker and the listener(s) as auditory information. For the speaker, the auditory processing completes a feedback loop.

One component that remains to be explained in Figure 2.1 is working memory and its connections to other parts of the diagram. Working memory is a speaker's operational memory—the memory that is used to keep track of the information involved in sentence production. But this memory is limited, so it is in the interest of efficient processing to minimize demands on it. Therefore, the theory goes, two kinds of processing are involved in utterance production. One is *controlled processing,* which makes demands on working memory. The other is *automatic processing,* which does not require allocation of working memory. Verbal formulation is performed with both controlled processing and automatic processing. Controlled processing can be identified in Figure 2.1 by the arrows labeled A and B. Note that syntactic, semantic, and phonologic processing are automatic; that is, the speaker does not have direct access to these operations. It is for this reason that slips of the tongue are not detected until they are actually spoken.

Feedback is provided by two channels, labeled α and β in Figure 2.1. Channel α represents information from touch and movement. Channel β represents auditory feedback.

Researchers have concluded that when a person ordinarily produces a sentence, they don't make all of the syntactic, semantic, and phonologic decisions before beginning to speak. Rather, it is likely that the individual will utter a few words and then formulate the remainder of the utterance.

According to this view of verbal formulation, producing a sentence involves highly interactive levels of processing and a complex time pattern for this processing. It would not be surprising, then, to discover that articulation is affected by syntactic, semantic, and phonologic variables.

FUNDAMENTALS OF ARTICULATORY PHONETICS

The following discussion of articulatory phonetics presents basic information on speech sound production. For the student who has had a course in phonetics, this chapter will serve as a summary review. The student without such background should be able to acquire at least the basics of articulatory phonetics. The topics to be discussed are as follows:

The Speech Mechanism

Vowels
    Monophthongs (single vowels)
    Diphthongs

Consonants
    Stops
    Nasals
    Fricatives
    Affricates
    Liquids
    Glides

Suprasegmentals

Coarticulation

Aerodynamics

Acoustics

Sensory Information

Levels of Organization

The Speech Mechanism

The anatomy of the speech production system is not within the scope of this chapter, but some general anatomical descriptions are needed to discuss the fundamentals of articulatory phonetics. The basic aspects of speech production can be understood by an examination of six principal organs or subsystems, illustrated in Figure 2.2. The *respiratory system,* consisting of the lungs, airway, rib cage, diaphragm, and associated structures, provides the basic air supply for generating sound. The *larynx,* composed of various cartilages and muscles, generates the voiced sounds of speech by vibration of the vocal folds, or it allows air to pass from lungs to the vocal tract (the oral and nasal cavities) for voiceless sounds. The *velopharynx*—the soft palate (or velum) and associated structures of the velopharyngeal port—joins or separates the oral and nasal cavities so that air passes through the oral cavity, the nasal cavity, or both. The *tongue,* primarily a complex of muscles, is the principal articulator of the oral cavity; it is capable of assuming a variety of shapes and positions in vowel and consonant

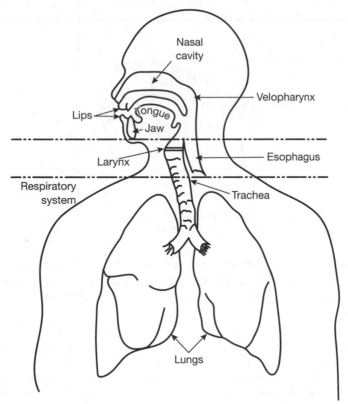

Figure 2.2. Organs of speech production.

articulation. For articulatory purposes, the tongue is divided into five major parts: tip or apex, blade, back or dorsum, root, and body. These divisions are illustrated in Figure 2.3. The *lips,* along with the jaw, are the most visible of the articulators; they are involved in the production of vowels and consonants. The *jaw,* the massive bony structure and its associated muscles, supports the soft tissues of both tongue and lower lip. It participates in speech production by aiding tongue and lip movements and by providing skeletal support for these organs. Other anatomical features shown in Figure 2.2 provide general orientation or are relevant in a significant way to the processes of speech and hearing.

The respiratory system and larynx work together to provide the upper airway with two major types of air flow: a series of pulses of air created by the action of the vibrating vocal folds (for voiced sounds like the sounds in the word *buzz*) and a continuous flow of air that can be used to generate noise energy in the vocal tract (for voiceless sounds like the *s* in *see*). The basic function of the respiratory system in speech is to push air into the airway composed of the larynx and the oral and nasal cavities. The basic function of the larynx is to regulate the airflow from the lungs to create both voiced and voiceless segments. The upper airway, often called the *vocal tract,* runs from the larynx to the mouth or nose and is the site of what is commonly called *speech articulation.* For the most part, this process is accomplished by movements of the *articulators,* which are those structures that move to create the sounds during the production of speech: tongue, lips, jaw, and velopharynx. The vocal tract may be viewed as a flexible tube that can be lengthened or shortened (by moving the larynx up

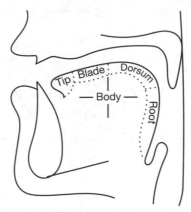

Figure 2.3. Divisions of tongue into five functional parts for speech articulation.

and down in the neck or by protruding and retracting the lips) and constricted at many points along its length by actions of the tongue, velopharynx, and lips. Speech articulation is thus a matter of lengthening, shortening, and constricting the tube known as the vocal tract.

This entire process is controlled by the nervous system, which must translate the message to be communicated into a pattern of signals that run to the various muscles of the speech mechanism. As these muscles contract, a variety of things can happen: air may be pushed out of the lungs, the vocal folds may start to vibrate, the velopharynx may close, the jaw may lower, or the lips may protrude. The brain has the task of coordinating all the different muscles so that they contract in the proper sequence to produce the required phonetic result. The margin for error is small; sometimes an error of just a few milliseconds in the timing of a muscle contraction can result in a misarticulation.

It is appealing to suppose that speech production is controlled at some relatively high level of the brain by discrete units, such as phonemes. However, a major problem in the description of speech articulation is to relate the discrete linguistic units that operate at a high level of the brain to the muscle contractions that result in articulatory movements. For example, to say the word stop, a speaker's brain must send nerve instructions, in the proper sequence, to the muscles of the respiratory system, larynx, tongue, lips, and velopharynx. The full understanding of speech production therefore involves a knowledge of *phonology* (the study of how sounds are put together to form words and other linguistic units), *articulatory phonetics* (the study of how the articulators make individual sounds), *acoustic phonetics* (the study of the relationship between articulation and the acoustic signal of speech), and *speech perception* (the study of how phonetic decisions are made from the acoustic signal).

Vowel Articulation: Traditional Phonetic Description

A vowel sound is usually formed as sound energy from the vibrating vocal folds escapes through a relatively open vocal tract of a particular shape. Because a syllable must contain a vowel or vowel-like sound, vowels sometimes are called *syllable nuclei*. Each vowel has a characteristic vocal tract shape that is determined by the position of the tongue, jaw, and lips. Although other parts of the vocal tract, like the velum, pharyngeal walls, and cheeks, may vary somewhat with different vowels, the positions

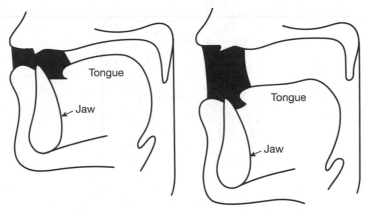

Figure 2.4. Variations in mouth opening (shaded area) related to lowering of jaw and tongue.

of the tongue, jaw, and lips are of primary consequence. Therefore, individual vowels can be described by specifying the articulatory positions of tongue, jaw, and lips. Furthermore, because the jaw and tongue usually work together to increase or reduce the mouth opening (Figure 2.4), for general phonetic purposes, vowel production can be described by specifying the positions of just two articulators, tongue and lips. Usually the vocal folds vibrate to produce voicing for vowels, but exceptions, such as whispered speech, do occur.

The two basic lip articulations can be demonstrated with the vowels in the words *he* and *who.* Press your finger against your lips as you say first *he* and then *who.* You should feel the lips push against your finger as you say who. The vowel in this word is a rounded vowel, meaning that the lips assume a rounded, protruded posture. Vowels in English are described as being either rounded, like the vowel in *who,* or unrounded, like the vowel in *he.* Figure 2.5 illustrates the lip configuration for these two vowels.

The tongue moves in essentially two dimensions within the oral cavity, as shown in Figure 2.6. One dimension, front-back, is represented by the motion the tongue makes as you alternately say *he, who* or *map, mop.* The other dimension, high-low, is represented by the motion the tongue makes as you say *heave, have* or *who, ha.* With these two dimensions of tongue movement, we can define four extreme positions of the

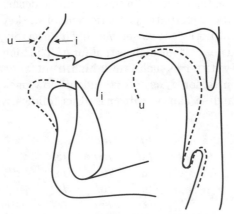

Figure 2.5. Vocal tract configurations for /i/ and /u/. Note lip rounding for /u/.

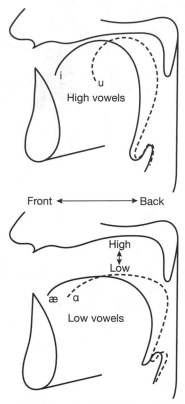

Figure 2.6. The two major dimensions of tongue position, front-back and high-low.

tongue within the oral cavity, as shown in Figure 2.7. The phonetic symbols for these four vowels also are shown in the illustration. With the tongue high and forward in the mouth, the high-front vowel /i/ as in *he* is produced. When the tongue is low and forward in the mouth, the low-front vowel /æ/ as in *have* is produced. A tongue position that is high and back in the mouth yields the high-back vowel /u/. Finally, when the tongue is low and back in the mouth, the vowel is the low-back /ɑ/. The four vowels, /i/, /æ/, /u/, and /ɑ/, define four points that establish the *vowel quadrilateral,* a four-sided figure against which tongue position for vowels can be described. In Figure 2.8, the vowels of English have been plotted by phonetic symbol and key word within the quadrilateral. As an example, notice the vowel /ɪ/ as in *bit* has a tongue position that is forward in the mouth and not quite as high as that for /i/. The tongue position for any one vowel can be specified with terms such as mid-high, front for /ɪ/ as in *bit;* mid-low, front for /ɛ/ as in *bet;* mid-central for /ɝ/ as in *Bert;* and mid-low, back for /ɔ/ as in *bought.*

The vowels of English can be categorized as follows with respect to tongue position:

Front vowels:	/i/	/ɪ/	/e/	/ɛ/	/æ/		
Central vowels:	/ɝ/	/ʌ/	/ɚ/	/ə/			
Back vowels:	/u/	/ʊ/	/o/	/ɔ/	/ɑ/		
High vowels:	/i/	/ɪ/	/u/	/ʊ/			
Mid vowels:	/e/	/ɛ/	/ɝ/	/ʌ/	/ɚ/	/ə/	/o/	/ɔ/
Low vowels:	/æ/	/ɑ/					

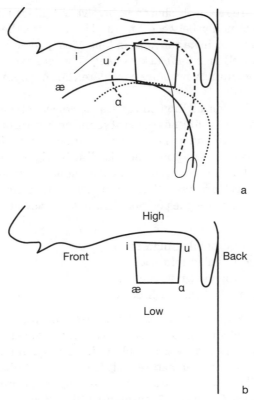

Figure 2.7. The four corner vowels /i/, /u/, /ɑ/, and /æ/ are shown (a) as tongue positions in the oral cavity and (b) as points of a quadrilateral.

The vowels can also be categorized with respect to lip rounding, with the following being rounded: /u/, /ʊ/, /o/, /ɔ/, and /ɝ/. All other vowels are unrounded. Notice that, in English, the rounded vowels are either back or central vowels; front rounded vowels do not occur.

Vowel production is also commonly described as *tense* (long) or *lax* (short). Tense vowels are longer in duration and supposedly involve a greater degree of muscular

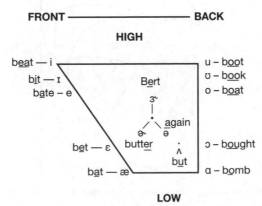

Figure 2.8. English vowels identified by phonetic symbol and key word and plotted within vowel quadrilateral.

tension. Lax vowels are relatively short and involve less muscular effort. One way of demonstrating the distinction between tense and lax is to feel the fleshy undersurface of your jaw as you say /i/ as in *he* and /ɪ/ as in *him*. Most people can feel a greater tension for /i/ (a tense vowel) than for /ɪ/ (a lax vowel). The tense vowels are /i/, /e/, /ɝ/, /u/, /o/, /ɔ/, and /ɑ/. The remaining vowels are considered lax, but opinion is divided for the vowel /æ/ as in *bat*.

In standard production, all English vowels are voiced (associated with vibrating vocal folds) and nonnasal (having no escape of sound energy through the nose). Therefore, the descriptors *voiced* and *nonnasal* usually are omitted. However, it should be remembered that vowels are sometimes devoiced, as in whispering, and nasalized, as when they precede or follow nasal consonants. For phonetic purposes, it is usually sufficient to describe a vowel in terms of the three major characteristics of tenseness: laxness, lip configuration, and tongue position. Examples of vowel description are given as follows:

/i/   tense, unrounded, high, front
/o/   tense, rounded, mid, back
/ɝ/   tense, rounded, mid, central
/ʊ/   lax, rounded, mid-high, back

In traditional phonetic description, vowels are considered to have an articulatory position that is unchanging during production of the vowel; that is, they are truly *monophthongs,* or single sounds with a stable articulation. But recent research shows that vowels are more dynamic in nature and that their articulation changes during the vowel segment. The acoustic consequence of this dynamic property is called *vowel inherent spectral change* (Morrison & Assmann, 2012). Recognition of this aspect of vowel production has attracted considerable interest and represents a new chapter in the understanding of vowels.

Closely related to the vowels are the *diphthongs*, which, like vowels, are produced with an open vocal tract and serve as the nuclei for syllables. But unlike vowels, diphthongs have long been recognized as having an articulation that gradually and markedly changes during production of the sound. Diphthongs are dynamic sounds because they involve a progressive change in vocal tract shape. An example of the articulation of /ɑɪ/ is shown in Figure 2.9. Many phoneticians regard diphthongs as combinations

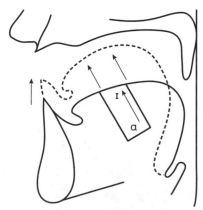

Figure 2.9. Articulation of diphthong /ɑɪ/ (as in *eye*), represented as onglide (/ɑ/) and offglide (/ɪ/) configurations.

of two vowels, one called the *onglide* portion and the other called the *offglide* portion. This vowel + vowel description underlies the phonetic symbols for the diphthongs, which have the *digraph* (two-element) symbols /aɪ /, /aʊ/, /ɔɪ/, /eɪ/, and /oʊ/. Key words for these sounds are as follows:

/aɪ/	*I, buy, why, ice, night*
/aʊ/	*ow, bough, trout, down, owl*
/ɔɪ/	*boy, oil, loin, hoist*
/eɪ/	*bay, daze, rain, stay*
/oʊ/	*bow, no, load, bone*

While the diphthongs /aɪ/, /aʊ/, and /ɔɪ/ are truly phonemic diphthongs, /eɪ/ and /oʊ/ are not; they are variants of the vowels /e/ and /o/, respectively. The diphthongal forms /eɪ/ and /oʊ/ occur in strongly stressed syllables, while the monophthongal (single-vowel) forms /e/ and /o/ tend to occur in weakly stressed syllables. For example, in the word *vacation,* the first syllable (weakly stressed) is produced with /e/ and the second syllable (strongly stressed) is produced with /eɪ/. Stressed syllables tend to be long in duration and, therefore, allow time for the articulatory movement of the diphthong. The diphthongs /aɪ/, /aʊ/, and /ɔɪ/ do not alternate with monophthongal forms. To produce a recognizable /aɪ/, /aʊ/, or /ɔɪ/, a speaker must use a diphthongal movement.

As shown in Figure 2.10, the onglide and offglide segments of the diphthongs are roughly located by the positions of the digraph symbols on the vowel quadrilateral. For example, in diphthong /aɪ/, the tongue moves from a low-back to nearly a high-front position. However, it should be noted that these onglide and offglide positions are only approximate and that substantial variation occurs across speakers and speaking conditions.

Vowel Articulation: Description by Distinctive Features

The phonetic descriptions considered to this point are one method of classifying vowel sounds. An alternative is a method relying on *distinctive features,* as defined by the linguists Noam Chomsky and Morris Hallé (1968). The distinctive features are a set of binary (two-valued) features designed to describe the phonemes in all languages of the world. A convenient example of a binary feature is nasality. In general terms, a given speech sound is either nasal or nonnasal, meaning that sound energy is transmitted through the nose (nasal) or is not (nonnasal). If nasality is described as

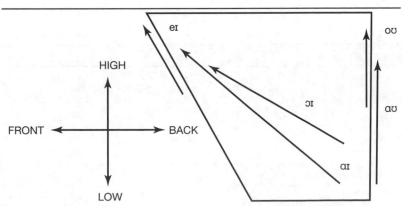

Figure 2.10. Diphthong articulation shown as onglide to offglide arrows in the vowel quadrilateral.

a binary feature, then sounds can be classified as +nasal (indicating the nasal trans-mission of sound) or –nasal (indicating the absence of nasal transmission). Hence, a positive value (+nasal) means that the property is present or is relevant to description of the sound. In some ways, distinctive feature analysis is similar to the guessing game Twenty Questions, in which the participants have to identify an object by asking ques-tions that can be answered with only yes or no. Chomsky and Hallé proposed a set of 13 binary features, which, given the appropriate yes (+) or no (–) answers, can describe all phonemes used in the languages of the world.

In the Chomsky-Hallé system, the voiced vowels are specified primarily with the features shown in Table 2.1. First, notice the three major class features of sonorant, vocalic, and consonantal. A *sonorant sound* is produced with a vocal cavity configura-tion in which spontaneous voicing is possible. Essentially, the vocal tract above the larynx is sufficiently open so that no special laryngeal adjustments are needed to ini-tiate voicing. For nonsonorants, or *obstruents,* the cavity configuration does not allow spontaneous voicing. Special mechanisms must be used to produce voicing during the nonsonorant sounds. *Vocalic sounds* are produced with an oral cavity shape in which the greatest constriction does not exceed that associated with the high vowels /i/ and /u/ and with vocal folds that are adjusted so as to allow spontaneous voicing. This fea-ture, then, describes the degree of opening of the oral cavity together with the vocal fold adjustment. Finally, *consonantal sounds* have a definite constriction in the *mid-sagittal,* or midline, region of the vocal tract; nonconsonantal sounds do not. Vowels are described as +sonorant, +vocalic, and –consonantal. Taken together, these three features indicate that vowels are produced with a relatively open oral cavity, with no severe constriction in the midsagittal plane and with a vocal fold adjustment that allows for spontaneous vocal fold vibration.

Vowels are also described with respect to cavity features and manner of articula-tion features, some of which are shown in Table 2.1 (the others will be discussed with respect to consonants later in this chapter). The features of primary concern in vowel description include those related to the size and configuration of the resonating cavity.

Table 2.1. Distinctive features for selected vowel sounds (the class features distinguish vowels from various consonants; therefore, all vowels have the same values for these features)

Class features	i	ɪ	ɛ	æ	ʌ	ɝ	u	ʊ	ɔ	ɑ
Sonorant	+	+	+	+	+	+	+	+	+	+
Vocalic	+	+	+	+	+	+	+	+	+	+
Consonantal	–	–	–	–	–	–	–	–	–	–
Cavity features										
High	+	+	–	–	–	–	+	+	–	–
Low	–	–	–	+	–	–	–	–	+	+
Back	–	–	–	–	–	–	+	+	+	+
Rounded	–	–	–	–	–	+	+	+	+	–
Nasal	–	–	–	–	–	–	–	–	–	–
Manner of articulation feature										
Tense	+	–	–	+	–	+	+	–	+	+

Tongue Body Features: High-Nonhigh; Low-Nonlow; Back-Nonback (see Figure 2.11a, b, c)

High sounds are produced by raising the body of the tongue above the level that it occupies in the neutral (or resting) position, as shown in Figure 2.11a. *Low* sounds are produced by lowering the body of the tongue below the level that it occupies in the neutral position, as shown in Figure 2.11b. *Back* sounds are produced by retracting the body of the tongue from the neutral position, as shown in Figure 2.11c.

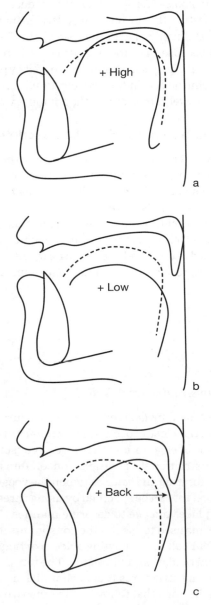

Figure 2.11. Vocal tract drawings illustrating the tongue body features (a) high, (b) low, and (c) back relative to the neutral tongue position (broken line).

Other cavity features include:

Rounded-Nonrounded. Rounded sounds have a narrowing or protrusion of the lips.

Nasal-Nonnasal. Nasal sounds are produced with a lowered velum so that sound energy escapes through the nose.

Table 2.1 shows that most vowels can be distinguished using the cavity features. For example, /i/ and /u/ differ in the back and rounded features, and /æ/ and /i/ differ in the high and low features. Most other distinctions can be made by referring to a manner of articulation called *tense-nontense.* Tense sounds are produced with a deliberate, accurate, maximally distinct gesture that involves considerable muscular effort. The tense-nontense distinction is best illustrated with the vowel pairs /i/-/ɪ/ and /u/-/ʊ/. Vowels /i/ and /u/ are tense vowels because they are lengthened and are produced with marked muscular effort. The difference in muscular effort can be felt by placing your fingers in the fleshy area just under the chin and saying alternately /i/-/ɪ/. A greater tension occurs during production of the tense vowel /i/ than during the nontense vowel /ɪ/.

Consonant Articulation: Traditional Phonetic Description

The consonants generally differ from the vowels in terms of the relative openness of the vocal tract and the function they play within the syllable. Vowels are produced with an open vocal tract; most consonants are made with a complete or partially constricted vocal tract. Within a syllable, vowels serve as a nucleus, meaning that a syllable must contain one and only one vowel (the only exceptions to this rule are the diphthongs, which are like vowels plus vowel glides, and certain syllabic consonants to be discussed later). Consonants are added to the vowel nucleus to form different syllable shapes, such as the following, where V represents a vowel and C represents a consonant:

VC shape: *on, add, in*

CV shape: *do, be, too*

CVC shape: *dog, cat, man*

CCVC shape: *truck, skin, clap*

CCCVCC shape: *screams, squint, scratched*

Consonants are described by degree or type of closure and by the location at which the complete or partial closure occurs. The *manner* of consonant articulation refers to the degree or type of closure, and the *place* of consonant articulation refers to the location of the constriction. In addition, consonants are described as *voiced* when the vocal folds are vibrating and *voiceless* when the vocal folds are not vibrating. Thus, an individual consonant can be specified by using three terms: one to describe voicing, one to describe place, and one to describe manner. Tables 2.2 and 2.3 show combinations of these terms used to specify the consonants of English.

Table 2.2 contains four columns, showing place of articulation, phonetic symbol and key word, manner of articulation, and voicing. The terms for place of articulation usually signify two opposing structures that accomplish a localized constriction of the vocal tract. In the definitions that follow, notice the two structures involved for the place terms:

Bilabial: two lips (*bi* = *two* and *labia* = *lip*)

Labial/velar: lips, and a constriction between the dorsum or back of the tongue and the velum

Table 2.2. Classification of consonants by manner and voicing within place

Place of articulation	Phonetic symbol and key word	Manner of articulation	Voicing
Bilabial	/p/ (pay)	Stop	–
	/b/ (bay)	Stop	+
	/m/ (may)	Nasal	+
Labial/velar	/ʍ/ (which)	Glide (semivowel)	–
	/w/ (witch)	Glide (semivowel)	+
Labiodental	/f/ (fan)	Fricative	–
	/v/ (van)	Fricative	+
Linguadental (interdental)	/θ/ (thin)	Fricative	–
	/ð/ (this)	Fricative	+
Linguaalveolar	/t/ (two)	Stop	–
	/d/ (do)	Stop	+
	/s/ (sue)	Fricative	–
	/z/ (zoo)	Fricative	+
	/n/ (new)	Nasal	+
	/l/ (Lou)	Lateral	+
	/ɾ/ (butter)	Flap	+
Linguapalatal	/ʃ/ (shoe)	Fricative	–
	/ʒ/ (rouge)	Fricative	+
	/tʃ/ (chin)	Affricate	–
	/dʒ/ (gin)	Affricate	+
	/j/ (you)	Glide (semivowel)	+
	/r/ (rue)	Rhotic	+
Linguavelar	/k/ (back)	Stop	-
	/g/ (bag)	Stop	+
	/ŋ/ (bang)	Nasal	+
Glottal (laryngeal)	/h/ (who)	Fricative	–
	/ʔ/	Stop	+(–)

Table 2.3. Classification of consonants by place and voicing within manner

Manner	Place	Voiced	Voiceless
Stop	Bilabial	b	p
	Linguaalveolar	d	t
	Linguavelar	g	k
	Glottal		ʔ
Fricative	Labiodental	v	f
	Linguadental	ð	θ
	Linguaalveolar	z	s
	Linguapalatal	ʒ	ʃ
	Glottal		h
Affricate	Linguapalatal	dʒ	tʃ
Nasal	Bilabial	m	
	Linguaalveolar	n	
	Linguavelar	ŋ	
Lateral	Linguaalveolar	l	
Rhotic	Linguapalatal	r	
Glide	Linguapalatal	j	
	Labial/Velar	w	ʍ

Labiodental: lower lip and upper teeth

Linguadental or interdental: tip of tongue and upper teeth (*lingua = tongue*)

Linguaalveolar: tip of tongue and the alveolar ridge

Linguapalatal: blade of tongue and palatal area behind the alveolar ridge

Linguavelar: dorsum or back of tongue and roof of mouth in the velar area

Glottal: the two vocal folds

Each of these places of articulation is discussed more fully on the next several pages. To get a feeling for these different places of consonant articulation, concentrate on the first sounds in each word as you say the sequence *pie, why, vie, thigh, tie, shy, guy, hi.* Notice in Figure 2.12 that the initial sounds constitute a progression from front to back in place of articulation.

Table 2.3 provides a breakdown of English consonants by place and voicing within manner classes. The manner of production associated with complete closure is the *stop,* which is formed when two structures completely block the passage of air from the vocal tract, building up air pressure behind the closure. Usually, when the closure is released, the air pressure built up behind the constriction causes a burst of escaping air. The burst is audible in words like pie and two.

Fricatives, like the initial sounds in *sue* and *zoo,* are made with a narrow constriction so that the air creates a noisy sound as it rushes through the narrowed passage.

Affricates, as in *church* and *judge,* are combinations of stop and fricative segments; that is, a period of complete closure is followed by a brief fricative segment. The stop + fricative nature of the affricates explains why these sounds are represented by the digraph symbols /tʃ/ and /dʒ/.

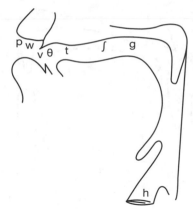

Figure 2.12. Places of articulation are marked by location of the phonetic symbols for the initial sounds in *pie*, *why*, *vie*, *thigh*, *tie*, *shy*, *guy*, and *hi*.

Nasals, as in the word *meaning* /minɪŋ/, are like stops in having a complete oral closure (bilabial, linguaalveolar, or linguavelar), but are unlike stops in having an open velopharyngeal port so that sound energy passes through the nose rather than the mouth.

The *lateral* /l/ as in *lay* is formed by making a linguaalveolar closure in the midline but with no closure at the sides of the tongue. Therefore, the sound energy from the vibrating folds escapes laterally, or through the sides of the mouth cavity.

The *rhotic* (or *rhotacized*) /r/ as in *ray* is a complex phoneme sometimes called retroflex in the phonetic literature. *Retroflex* literally means turning or turned back and refers to the appearance of the tongue tip, as viewed in x-ray films, for some /r/ productions. But in other productions of /r/, the tongue has a bunched appearance in the center or near the front of the mouth cavity. Because /r/ is produced in at least these two basic ways, the general term rhotic (Ladefoged, 1975) is preferable to the narrower term retroflex. This issue is discussed in more detail later in this chapter.

The /ʍ/, /w/, and /j/ sounds are said to have a *glide* (semivowel) manner of production. These sounds are characterized by a gliding, or gradually changing, articulatory shape. For example, in /ʍ/ and its voiced counterpart /w/, the lips gradually move from a rounded and narrowed configuration to the lip shape required by the following vowel simultaneously with a change in tongue position from high-back (like that for /u/) to the position for the following vowel. The glides are always followed by vowels.

In the following summary, manner of articulation is discussed for different places of articulation, proceeding from front to back.

Bilabial Sounds

In American English, the only consonant phonemes produced with a complete or partial closure (bilabial production) are the voiceless and voiced stops /p/ as in *pay* and /b/ as in *bay,* the nasal /m/ as in *may,* and the voiced and voiceless glides /w/ as in *witch* and /ʍ/ as in *which.* The vocal tract configurations for /p/, /b/, and /m/ are shown in Figure 2.13. These three sounds share a bilabial closure but differ in voicing and nasality. The stops /p/ and /b/ are called voiced and voiceless *cognates,* which means that they differ only in voicing. The production of these bilabial sounds is usually marked

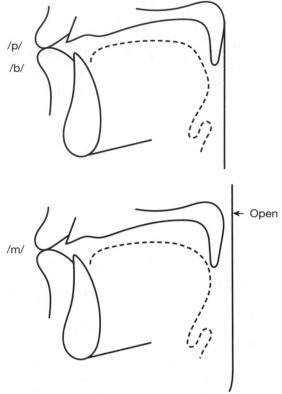

Figure 2.13. Vocal tract configurations for /p/, /b/, and /m/. Note labial closure for all three sounds and the open velopharynx for /m/.

by a closed jaw position because the jaw closes somewhat to assist the constriction at the lips. The tongue is virtually unconstrained for /p/, /b/, and /m/ so that these bilabial sounds often are made simultaneously with the tongue position for preceding or following vowels. In other words, when we say words like *bee, pa,* and *moo,* the tongue is free to assume the required shape for the vowel during the closure for the bilabial, as illustrated in Figure 2.14.

The glides /w/ and /ʍ/ have a specified tongue position, roughly like that for the high-back vowel /u/, so these sounds cannot interact as freely with preceding or following sounds. Students (and even some practicing clinicians) sometimes fail to appreciate the importance of tongue articulation for /w/ and /ʍ/. For these sounds, both the tongue and lips execute gliding movements, as shown for the word *we* in Figure 2.15.

Labiodental Sounds

The voiceless and voiced fricatives /f/ as in *fan* and /v/ as in *van* are the only labiodental sounds in American English. The articulation is illustrated in Figure 2.16. Frication noise is generated by forcing air through the constriction formed by the lower lip and the upper teeth, principally the incisors. The noise is quite weak, very nearly the weakest of the fricatives. Like the labial sounds /p/, /b/, and /m/, the labiodentals allow the tongue to assume its position for preceding or following sounds. The jaw tends to close to aid the lower lip in its constricting gesture.

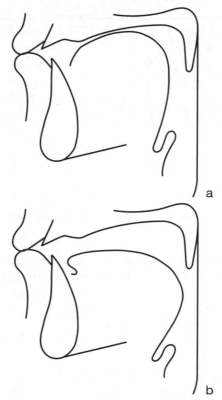

Figure 2.14. Variation in tongue position during a bilabial closure: (a) tongue position during *pea*; (b) tongue position for *pa*.

Interdental Sounds

There are only two interdentals, both fricatives: the voiceless /θ/ (e.g., *thaw*) and voiced /ð/ (e.g., *the*), which are illustrated in Figure 2.17. The frication noise is generated as air flows through the narrow constriction created by the tongue tip and the edge of the incisors. The weak frication noise is not much different from that for /f/ or /v/. The

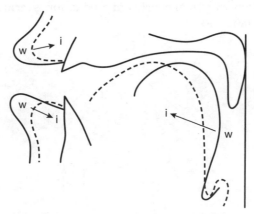

Figure 2.15. Illustration of gliding motion of tongue and lips for the word *we* (/wi/).

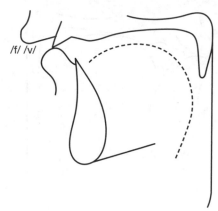

Figure 2.16. Vocal tract configuration for /f/ and /v/. Note labiodental constriction.

weak intensity of these sounds should be remembered in articulation testing, and the clinician should include both visual and auditory information in evaluating this pair of sounds. Jaw position for /θ/ and /ð/ usually is closed to aid the tongue in making its constriction. These sounds may be produced with either an interdental projection of the tongue or tongue contact behind the teeth.

Alveolar Sounds

The alveolar place of production is used for two stops: the voiceless /t/ (e.g., *too*) and the voiced /d/ (e.g., *do*); a nasal: /n/ (e.g., *new*); a lateral: /l/ (e.g., *Lou*); and two fricatives: the voiceless /s/ (e.g., *sue*) and the voiced /z/ (e.g., *zoo*). Not surprisingly, given the frequent and diverse movements of the tongue tip in the alveolar region, motions of the tongue tip are among the fastest articulatory movements. For example, the major closing and release movement for the stops /t/ and /d/ is made within about 50 milliseconds, or a 20th of a second. For /t/ and /d/, an airtight chamber is created as the tongue tip closes firmly against the alveolar ridge and the sides of the tongue seal against the lateral oral regions. The site of tongue tip closure actually varies to a limited degree with phonetic context. When /t/ or /d/ are produced before the dental fricatives /θ/ and /ð/, the stop closure is made in the dental region. This context-dependent modification of alveolar consonant production is termed *dentalization* and is illustrated for /t/ in Figure 2.18.

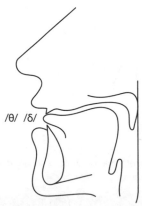

Figure 2.17. Vocal tract configuration for /θ/ and /ð/. Note linguadental (interdental) constriction.

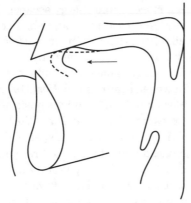

Figure 2.18. Dentalization of /t/. The normal alveolar closure is shown by the solid line, and the dental closure is shown by the broken line.

The nasal /n/ is similar in basic tongue shape and movement to the stops /t/ and /d/. But /n/ differs from both /t/ and /d/ in having an open velopharyngeal port, making /n/ nasalized. But /n/ further differs from /t/ in that /n/ is voiced; /t/ is not. Because /n/ and /d/ are very similar in lingual articulation and voicing, failure to close the velopharyngeal port for /d/, as might happen with some speech disorders, results in /n/. Like /t/ and /d/, /n/ is dentalized when produced in the same syllable and adjacent to a dental sound like /θ/; compare, for example, the second /n/ in *nine* /naɪn/ with the second /n/ in *ninth* /naɪnθ/.

The lateral /l/ is a *liquid* formed with midline closure and a lateral opening, usually at both sides of the mouth (see Figure 2.19). Because of the midline closure made by

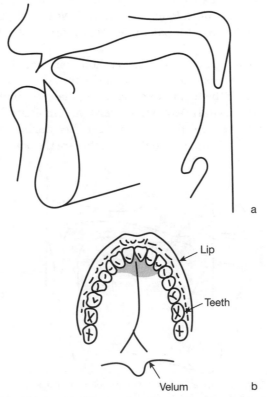

Figure 2.19. Articulation of /l/, shown in side view of a midline section (a) and as regions of tongue closure (shaded areas in b) against roof of mouth.

the tongue tip against the alveolar ridge, sound energy escapes through the sides of the oral cavity. Although /l/ is the only lateral sound in English, there are at least two major allophones. Historically, these allophones have been termed *light* and *dark,* but phoneticians have disagreed as to exactly how these allophones are formed. Wise (1957a, 1957b) explained that the light /l/ is made with linguadental contact, while the dark /l/ is made with a linguaalveolar contact. However, Kantner and West (1960) contend that the light /l/ has a greater lip spread and a lower and flatter tongue position than the dark /l/.

An important feature of /l/, presumably, is a raising of the tongue toward the velum or palate. Giles (1971) concluded from x-ray pictures of speech that for allophonic variations of /l/, the position of the tongue dorsum falls into three general groups regardless of phonetic context: prevocalic, postvocalic, and syllabic (with syllabic being similar to postvocalic /l/). The postvocalic allophones had a more posterior dorsal position than the prevocalic allophones. Tongue tip contact occasionally was not achieved for the postvocalic allophones in words like *Paul*. Otherwise, the only variation in tongue tip articulation was dentalization influenced by a following dental sound. Apparently, then, /l/ can be produced with either a relatively front (light /l/) or back (dark /l/) dorsal position, but the light and dark variants are perhaps just as well termed prevocalic and postvocalic. Linguaalveolar contact is not essential at least for /l/ in postvocalic position, which explains why postvocalic /l/ in words like *seal* may sound like /o/ or /ʊ/. The fricatives /s/ and /z/ are made with a narrow constriction between the tongue tip and the alveolar ridge (see Figure 2.20).

Palatal Sounds

The palatal sounds include the voiceless and voiced fricatives /ʃ/ (e.g., *shoe*) and /ʒ/ (e.g., *rouge*), the voiceless and voiced affricates /tʃ/ (e.g., *chin*) and /dʒ/ (e.g., *gin*), the glide /j/ (e.g., *you*), and the rhotic or retroflex /r/ (e.g., *rue*). For these sounds, the blade or tip of the tongue makes a constriction in the palatal region, the area just behind the alveolar ridge (see Figure 2.21).

The fricatives /ʃ/ and /ʒ/, like /s/ and /z/, are sibilants associated with intense noisy energy. For /ʃ/ and /ʒ/, this noise is generated as air moves rapidly through a constriction formed between the blade of the tongue and the front palate. Similarly, the affricates /tʃ/ and /dʒ/ are made in the palatal area as stop + fricative combinations. The airstream is first interrupted during the stop phase and then released during the fricative phase that immediately follows. In English, the only affricates are the palatal /tʃ/ and /dʒ/.

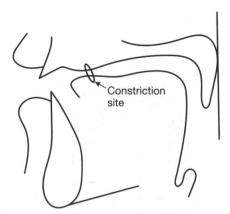

Figure 2.20. Vocal tract configuration or /s/ and /z/. Note linguaalveolar constriction.

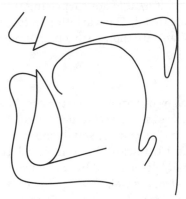

Figure 2.21. Vocal tract configuration for /ʃ/ and /ʒ/. Note linguapalatal constriction.

The glide /j/ is similar to the high-front vowel /i/ (as in *he*). The tongue is initially far forward and high in the mouth, and subsequently moves toward the position for the following vowel. The similarity between /j/ and /i/ can be demonstrated by saying the biblical pronoun *ye* while noting the tongue position. Because the glide /j/ must be followed by a vowel, its articulation involves a gliding motion from the high-front position to some other vowel shape. The gliding motion can be felt during articulation of the words *you, yea,* and *ya*.

As mentioned previously, the articulation of /r/ is highly variable. It sometimes is produced as a retroflexed consonant, in which case the tongue tip points upward and slightly backward in the oral cavity. But /r/ also can be produced with a bunching of the tongue, either in the middle of the mouth or near the front of the mouth. These basic articulations are illustrated in Figure 2.22. Some speakers also round their lips for /r/, and some constrict the lower pharynx by pulling the root of the tongue backward. Because /r/ is variably produced, it seems advisable to use rhotic or rhotacized (Ladefoged, 1975) rather than retroflex as a general articulatory descriptor. It is not yet clear what factors govern the selection of one type of /r/ articulation over another, but it has been observed that the bunched articulation may be favored in the postvocalic (following the vowel) position by some speakers (Mielke et al., 2016). Given

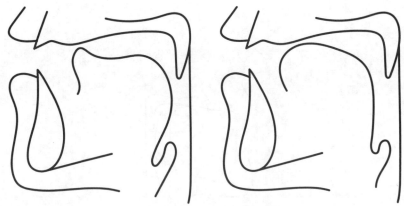

Figure 2.22. The two major articulations of /r/: (left) the retroflexed articulation; (right) the bunched articulation.

the complicated articulation of /r/, it is not surprising that it should present a major problem to children learning to talk. The variation in tongue shape and position also complicates a speech clinician's attempts to teach /r/ articulations to a child who mis-articulates the sound.

Velar Sounds

A velar constriction, formed by elevation of the tongue dorsum toward the roof of the mouth, occurs for the voiceless and voiced stops /k/ and /g/ and for the nasal /ŋ/. This articulation is illustrated in Figure 2.23, which shows that the constriction can be made with the tongue relatively toward the front or relatively toward the back. The tongue placement is generally determined by the vowel context, with a front place-ment for velars adjacent to front vowels (e.g., /g/ in *geese*) and a back placement for velars adjacent to back vowels (e.g., /g/ in *goose*). The nasal /ŋ/ has a tongue constric-tion similar to that for /k/ and /g/ but has an open velopharyngeal port for nasaliza-tion. The velar and bilabial places of speech sound are similar in that both are used in English only for stops and nasals.

Glottal Sounds

The glottis, or chink between the vocal folds, is primarily involved with only two sounds, the voiceless fricative /h/ and the stop /ʔ/ (a stoppage of air at the vocal folds). The fricative is produced with an opening of the vocal folds so that a fricative noise is generated as air moves at high speed through the glottis. A similar vocal fold adjust-ment is used in whisper.

It can be seen from Tables 2.2 and 2.3 that more types of sounds are made at some places of articulation than at others. Moreover, some sounds occur more frequently in the English language than others, contributing to a further imbalance in the use of places of articulation. Actual data on the frequency of occurrence of English conso-nants, grouped by place of articulation, are shown in Figure 2.24. In this circle graph, based on data from Dewey (1923), the relative frequencies of occurrence of different places of articulation are shown by the relative sizes of the pieces of the graph. Notice that alveolar sounds account for almost 50% of the sounds in English.

The rank order of frequency of occurrence for place of articulation, from most to least frequent, is alveolar, palatal, bilabial, velar, labiodental, interdental, and glottal. Within each place-of-articulation segment in Figure 2.24, the individual consonants

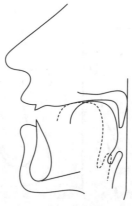

Figure 2.23. Vocal tract configurations for velar consonants. Note variation in site of closure.

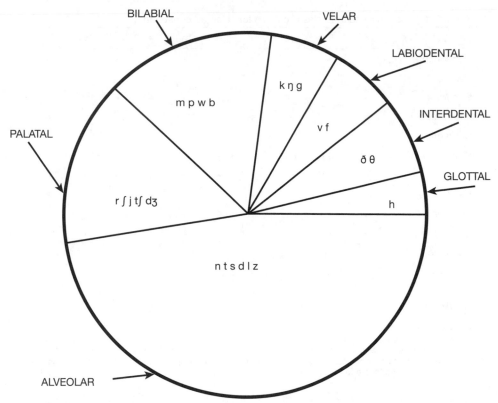

Figure 2.24. Circle graph showing relative frequency of occurrence of consonants made at different places of articulation. *Source:* Dewey (1923).

are listed in rank order of frequency of occurrence. For example, /n/ is the most frequently occurring alveolar consonant (in fact, it is the most frequently occurring of all consonants). Because of the differences in frequency of occurrence of consonants, a misarticulation affecting one place of articulation can be far more conspicuous than a misarticulation affecting another place. Therefore, statistical properties of the language are one consideration in the assessment and management of speech sound disorders.

Consonant Articulation: Description by Distinctive Features

Distinctive features, discussed earlier with respect to vowels, can be used as an alternative to the place-manner chart to describe consonants. One simple example is the feature of voiced. All voiced consonants can be assigned the feature value of +voiced, and all voiceless consonants can be assigned the value of –voiced. Some important features for consonants are defined briefly following and are used for consonant classification in Table 2.4. The definitions that follow are based on Chomsky and Hallé (1968):

> *Consonantal* sounds have a radical or marked constriction in the midsagittal region of the vocal tract. This feature distinguishes the true consonants from vowels and glides.

> *Vocalic* sounds do not have a radical or marked constriction of the vocal tract and are associated with spontaneous voicing. The voiced vowels and liquids are vocalic; the voiceless vowels and liquids, glides, nasal consonants, and obstruents (stops, fricatives, and affricates) are *nonvocalic* (i.e., –vocalic).

Table 2.4.   Distinctive feature classifications for selected consonants

Feature	p	b	m	t	d	n	s	l	θ	k
Consonantal	+	+	+	+	+	+	+	+	+	+
Vocalic	−	−	−	−	−	−	−	−	−	−
Sonorant	−	−	+	−	−	+	−	+	−	−
Interrupted	+	+	−	+	+					+
Strident	−	−	−	−	−	−	+	−	−	−
High	(−)	(−)	(−)ᵃ	−	−	−	−	−	−	+
Low	(−)	(−)	(−)	−	−	−	−	−	−	−
Back	(−)	(−)	(−)	−	−	−	−	−	−	+
Anterior	+	+	+	+	+	+	+	+	+	−
Coronal	−	−	−	+	+	+	+	+	+	−
Rounded	−	−	−	−	−	−	−	−	−	−
Distributed	+	+	+	−	−	−	−	−	+	−
Lateral	−	−	−	−	−	−	−	+	−	−
Nasal	−	−	+	−	−	+	−	−	−	−
Voiced	−	+	+	−	+	+	−	+	−	−

ᵃFeature values enclosed in parentheses indicate that the feature in question may not be specified for this sound. For example, tongue position for /p/, /b/, and /m/ is not really specified because it is free to assume the position required for the following vowel.

Sonorant sounds have a vocal configuration that permits spontaneous voicing, which means that the airstream can pass virtually unimpeded through the oral or nasal cavity. This feature distinguishes the vowels, glides, nasal consonants, and lateral and rhotacized consonants from the stops, fricatives, and affricates (the class of obstruents).

Interrupted sounds have a complete blockage of the airstream during a part of their articulation. Stops and affricates are +interrupted, which distinguishes them from fricatives, nasals, liquids, and glides. Sometimes the feature *continuant* is used rather than interrupted, with opposite values assigned; that is, +continuant sounds are −interrupted and vice versa.

Strident sounds are those fricatives and affricates produced with intense noise: /s/, /z/, /ʃ/, /ʒ/, /tʃ/, /dʒ/. The amount of noise produced depends on characteristics of the constriction, including roughness of the articulatory surface, rate of air flow over it, and angle of incidence between the articulatory surfaces.

High sounds are made with the tongue elevated above its neutral (resting) position (see Figure 2.11a).

Low sounds are made with the tongue lowered below its neutral position (see Figure 2.11b).

Back sounds are made with the tongue retracted from its neutral position (see Figure 2.11c).

Anterior sounds have an obstruction that is farther forward than that for the palatal /ʃ/. Anterior sounds include the bilabials, labiodentals, linguadentals, and linguaalveolars.

Coronal sounds have a tongue blade position above the neutral state. In general, consonants made with an elevated tongue tip or blade are +coronal.

Rounded sounds have narrowed or protruded lip configuration.

Distributed sounds have a constriction extending over a relatively long portion of the vocal tract (from back to front). For English, this feature is particularly important to distinguish the dental fricatives /θ/ and /ð/ from the alveolars /s/ and /z/.

Lateral sounds are coronal consonants made with midline closure and lateral opening.

Nasal sounds have an open velopharynx, allowing air to pass through the nose.

Voiced sounds are produced with vibrating vocal folds.

The feature assignments in Table 2.4 are for general illustration of the use of features. The features should be viewed with some skepticism because several different feature systems have been proposed, and any one system is subject to modification. It should be understood that distinctive features are one type of classification system. It should also be realized that distinctive features have an intended linguistic function that may not always be compatible with their application to the study of articulation disorders. The issue is beyond the scope of this chapter, but the interested reader is referred to Walsh (1974) and Parker (1976).

The relationship between the traditional place terms of phonetic description and the distinctive features is summarized in the chart that follows. For each traditional place term, the associated features are listed. As an example, a bilabial stop is +anterior, –coronal, and +distributed. (The placement of both features within brackets indicates that they are considered together in sound description.)

Bilabial	+anterior
	–coronal
	+distributed
Labiodental	+anterior
	–coronal
	–distributed
Interdental	+anterior
	+coronal
	+αdistributed*
Alveolar	+anterior
	+coronal
	–αdistributed*
Palatal	–anterior
	+high
	–back
Velar	–coronal
	+high
	+back

*The symbol α is a dummy variable and is used here to indicate that the Chomsky-Hallé features can distinguish the interdental and alveolar consonants only if they differ with respect to the feature *distributed*. Thus, if interdentals are regarded as –distributed, then alveolars must be +distributed. (See Ladefoged [1971] for development of this issue.)

Suprasegmentals

The phonetic characteristics discussed to this point are *segmental,* which means that the units involved in the description are the size of phonemes or phonetic segments. *Suprasegmentals* are characteristics of speech that involve larger units, such as syllables, words, phrases, or sentences. Among the suprasegmentals are stress, intonation, loudness, pitch level, juncture, and speaking rate. Briefly defined, the suprasegmentals, also called *prosodies,* or *prosodic features,* are properties of speech that have a domain larger than a single segment. This definition does not mean that a single segment cannot, at times, carry the bulk of information for a given suprasegmental; on occasion, a segment, like a vowel, can convey most of the relevant information. Most suprasegmental information in speech can be described by the basic physical quantities of amplitude (or intensity), duration, and fundamental frequency (f0) of the voice. Stated briefly, *amplitude* refers to the perceptual attribute of loudness; *duration,* to the perceptual attribute of length; and *fundamental frequency,* to the perceptual attribute of vocal pitch. The segmental and suprasegmental components of an utterance are woven together so that an utterance carries not only the meaning imparted by its morphemic content but also the information signaled by its suprasegmental features. We now examine what these features are.

Stress

Stress refers to the degree of effort, prominence, or importance given to some part of an utterance. For example, if a speaker wishes to emphasize that someone should take the *red* car (as opposed to a blue or green one), the speaker might say, "Be sure to take the *red* car," stressing the word red to signify the emphasis. There are several varieties of stress, but all generally involve something akin to the graphic underline or boldface used to denote emphasis in writing. Although underlining is seldom used in writing, stress is almost continually used in speech. In fact, any utterance of two or more syllables may be described in terms of its stress pattern. Because it has influences that extend beyond the segment, stress usually is discussed with respect to syllables. The pronouncing guide of a dictionary places special marks after individual syllables to indicate stress. For example, the word *ionosphere* is rendered as (ɑɪ-ɑn'ə-sfir'), with the marks' and' signifying the primary and secondary stress for the syllables.

The International Phonetic Alphabet (IPA) uses a different stress notation from that commonly found in dictionaries. In the IPA, the stress mark precedes the syllable to which it refers, and the degree of stress is indicated by whether any stress mark is used and by the location of the stress mark in the vertical dimension. The strongest degree of stress is indicated by a mark above the symbol line: 'ɑn (like a superscript); the second degree of stress is indicated by a mark below the symbol line: ,ɑɪ (like a subscript); and the third degree of stress is simply unmarked: ə. The word *ionosphere* is rendered as /ɑɪɑn ə ,sfir/, with three degrees of stress marked.

Acoustically, stress is carried primarily by the vowel segment within a syllable. The acoustic correlates, roughly in order of importance, are fundamental frequency (especially with a rise in fundamental frequency on or near the stressed syllable); vowel duration (greater duration with increased stress); relative intensity (greater intensity with increased stress); sound quality (reduction of a vowel to a weaker, unstressed form, like /ɑ/ to /ə/, vowel substitution, and consonant changes); and disjuncture (pauses or intervals of silence) (Rabiner et al., 1969).

Another form of unstressed (or weakly stressed) syllable is the syllabic consonant. This type of consonant, usually /l/, /m/, or /n/ (but infrequently /r/), acts like
a vowel in forming a syllable nucleus. Examples of syllabic consonants are the final
sounds in the words *bottle* /bɑtl/, *something* /sʌmʔm/, and *button* /bʌtn/. The syllabic function of a consonant is designated by a small vertical mark placed under the
phonetic symbol. Syllabic consonants are most likely to occur when the consonant is
homorganic (shares place of articulation) with a preceding consonant because it is
economical or efficient simply to maintain the articulatory contact for both sounds.
Additional information on stress will be provided following some basic definitions of
related terms.

Intonation

Intonation is the vocal pitch contour of an utterance, that is, the way in which the fundamental frequency changes from syllable to syllable and even from segment to segment. Fundamental frequency can be affected by several factors, including the stress
pattern of an utterance, tongue position of a vowel (high vowels have a higher f0), and
the speaker's emotional state. As discussed later, intonation often involves an overall pattern of f0 change known as declination. Intonation is sometimes defined as the
melody of speech, that is, the rhythmic pattern of pitch changes during an utterance.

Loudness

Loudness is related to sound intensity or to the amount of vocal effort that a speaker
uses. Although loudness is ordinarily thought to be related to the amplitude or intensity of a sound, some evidence suggests that a listener's judgments of loudness of
speech are related more directly to the perceived vocal effort, essentially the amount
of work that a speaker does (Cavagna & Margaria, 1968). There is some evidence
(Hixon, 1971; MacNeilage, 1972) that intensity variations in speech result mostly
from respiratory activity, but variations of f0 are easily accomplished at the level of
the vocal folds.

Pitch Level

Pitch level is the average pitch of a speaker's voice and relates to the mean f0 of an
utterance. A speaker may be described as having a high, low, or medium pitch. Habitual pitch level is the pitch that a speaker typically uses.

Juncture

Juncture, sometimes called *vocal punctuation,* is a combination of intonation, pausing,
and other suprasegmentals to mark special distinctions in speech or to express certain grammatical divisions. For example, the written sentence, "Let's eat, Grandma,"
has a much different meaning than the same sentence without the comma, "Let's eat
Grandma!" A speaker can mark a comma vocally with a short pause and an adjustment in intonation. Juncture is also used to make distinctions between similar articulations, such as between the word *nitrate* and the phrase *night rate.* Intonation and
pausing enable a speaker to indicate which alternative they want to express.

Speaking Rate

Speaking rate is usually measured in words per second, syllables per second, or phonemes per second. As speaking rate increases, segment durations generally become

shorter, with some segments affected more than others. The segments most vulner-able to contraction as a speaker talks more rapidly are pauses, vowels, and consonant segments involving a sustained articulation (like fricatives). Apparently, most speak-ers do not really increase the rate of individual articulatory movement as they increase their rate of speaking. Rather, they reduce the duration of some segments and reduce the overall range of articulatory movement (Lindblom, 1963). As a result, the articu-latory positions normally assumed during a slow rate of speaking may be missed at a faster rate. The missing of articulatory positions as speaking rate increases is called *undershoot*. This is why a speaker's words are apt to sound less distinct to you as the rate of speaking increases. The speaking rate of ordinary conversational speech in adults averages about 175 words per minute (about five or six syllables per second, or 10 to 12 phonemes per second). By comparison, fast keyboarding has a rate of about 90 words per minute. Speech may be the fastest discrete motor performance in humans, which makes speech an efficient mode of communication. The linguistic use of speak-ing rate is called tempo.

Vowel Reduction

Vowels are particularly susceptible to articulatory change as speaking rate is increased or stress is decreased. Such articulatory alterations are termed *vowel reduction* and are schematized in Figure 2.25. The arrows between pairs of vowels show directions of reduction; for example, /i/ reduces first to /ɪ/ and then to /ə/, the ultimate reduced vowel. The scheme shows that, with reduction, all vowels tend toward /ə/ or /ʌ/.

Clear Versus Conversational Speech

There is considerable evidence to show that speakers alter their patterns of speech production depending on situation and listener. One variation is clear versus con-versational speech. *Clear speech* is what speakers use when they are trying to be as intelligible as possible. Compared to more casual *conversational speech,* clear speech is 1) slower (with longer pauses between words and a lengthening of some speech sounds), 2) more likely to avoid modified or reduced forms of consonant and vowel segments (such as the vowel reduction described earlier), and 3) characterized by a greater intensity of obstruent sounds, particularly stop consonants (Picheny

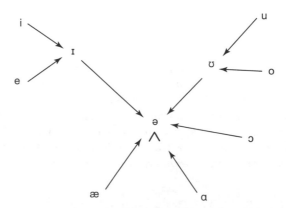

Figure 2.25.   A scheme of vowel reduction. The arrows between vowel symbols show vowel changes resulting from reduction. For example, /i/ and /e/ reduce to /ɪ/, and /ɪ/ reduces to /ə/, which is the ultimate reduced vowel. Note that these changes occur within the quadrilateral defined by the corner vowels /i/, /æ/, /ɑ/, and /u/.

et al., 1986). When talkers want to be easily understood, they usually modify their speech to make it slower and more acoustically distinctive. However, clear speech can be produced even at relatively fast speaking rates. While vowels in conversational speech often are modified or reduced, therefore losing some of their acoustic distinctiveness, these sounds in clear speech are produced in distinctive forms. Similarly, word-final stops in conversational speech frequently are not released, so the burst cue for their perception is eliminated. But in clear speech, stop consonants (and consonants in general) tend to be released, and this feature enhances their perception.

These differences are central to a hypothesis proposed by Lindblom (1990) that speakers vary their speech output along a continuum from *hypospeech* to *hyperspeech* (the H&H hypothesis). The basic idea is that speakers adapt to the various circumstances of communication to match their production patterns to communicative and situational factors. When a speaker believes that special care is required to be understood, they alter articulation accordingly. In Lindblom's view, clear speech (hyperspeech in his H&H hypothesis) is not simply loud speech but reflects an articulatory reorganization (Moon & Lindblom, 1989). Adams (1990), however, reported contrary evidence. He concluded from an x-ray microbeam study of speech movements that changes in speech clarity did not seem to reflect a reorganization of speech motor control. Adams observed that in clear speech, articulatory movements tended to be both larger and faster, but there was no general indication that the speech patterns were organized differently than in conversational speech. The important point for clinical purposes is that speech articulation can be controlled by a speaker to enhance intelligibility when conditions warrant such deliberate effort. The primary articulatory change appears to be in the magnitude and speed of movement.

New Versus Given Information

New information in a discourse is information that the listener would not be expected to know from the previous conversation or from the situation. Given information is predictable, either from the previous discourse or from the general situation. New information often is highlighted prosodically. For example, Behne (1989) studied prosody in a mini-discourse such as the following:

"Someone painted the fence."

"Who painted the fence?"

"Pete painted the fence."

In this exchange, the new information ("Pete") is lengthened and produced with a higher fundamental frequency. In effect, the speaker uses prosody to highlight the new information.

Contrastive Stress in Discourse

Another discourse-related prosodic effect is *contrastive stress*. Such stress can be given to almost any word, phrase, or clause that the speaker considers to contradict or contrast with one that was previously expressed or implied. For instance, a speaker who wants to emphasize that she took the red ball rather than the green or blue one, might say, "I took the *red* ball" (where the italicized word receives contrastive stress). Contrastive stress is sometimes used clinically to give prosodic variation to an utterance or to elicit a stressed form of a target element.

Phrase-Final Lengthening

At the syntactic level, juncture and pause phenomena are used to mark multiword units. For example, in English, *phrase-final lengthening* operates to lengthen the last stressable syllable in a major syntactic phrase or clause. For example, contrast the following two sentences:

1. Red, green, and blue are my favorite colors.

2. Green, blue, and red are my favorite colors.

The word *blue* will be longer in the first sentence than in the second because in the former this word is at the end of the subject-noun phrase and is therefore subject to phrase-final lengthening. This regularity can be exploited clinically to obtain durational adjustments for a target word. In addition, Read and Schreiber (1982) showed that phrase-final lengthening is helpful to listeners in parsing (i.e., recognizing the structure of) spoken sentences. They also suggested that children rely more on this cue than adults do and, moreover, that prosody assists the language learner by providing structural guides to the complex syntactic structures of language.

Declination

Another effect at the syntactic level is *declination,* or the effect in which the vocal fundamental frequency contour typically declines across clauses or comparable units. Why this tilt in the overall fundamental frequency pattern occurs is a matter of debate (Cohen et al., 1982), but it is a robust feature of prosody at the sentence or clause level. This pattern is helpful to listeners in recognizing the structure of discourse, such as in identifying sentence units.

Lexical Stress Effects

These effects operate at the level of the word. For example, English has many noun-verb pairs like *'import* versus *im'port,* or *'contrast* versus *con'trast,* in which the difference between the members of a pair is signaled primarily by stress pattern. Another common effect at the word level occurs with a distinction between compounds and phrases. For example, the compound noun *'blackbird* (a particular type of bird) contrasts with the noun phrase *black 'bird* (any bird that is black).

Although the lay listener often thinks stress in English is just a matter of giving greater intensity to part of an utterance, laboratory studies have shown that stress is signaled by duration, intensity, fundamental frequency, and various phonetic effects (Fry, 1955). It is important to remember that stress affects segmental properties, such as the articulation of vowels and consonants (de Jong, 1991; Kent & Netsell, 1972). Segments in stressed syllables tend to have larger and faster articulatory movements than similar segments in unstressed syllables. For this reason, stressed syllables often are favored in some phases of articulation therapy.

Summary of Suprasegmentals

In this section, we have seen that speech is richly invested with a variety of suprasegmental information. Because suprasegmentals like stress and speaking rate influence the nature of segmental articulation, some care should be taken to control suprasegmental variables in articulation tests and speech materials used in treatment. Vowels carry much of the suprasegmental information in speech, but stress, speaking rate, and other suprasegmentals can influence consonant articulation as well. The suprasegmental features of speech have been discussed by Crystal (1973), Lehiste (1970), and Lieberman (1967), and the reader is referred to these accounts for a more detailed consideration of this complex area. The development of prosody in a first language is covered in detail in a recently published book by Prieto and Esteve-Gibert (2018).

COARTICULATION: INTERACTIONS AMONG SOUNDS IN CONTEXT

Convenient though it might be to consider phonemes as independent, invariant units that are simply linked together to produce speech, this simplistic approach does not really fit the facts. When sounds are put together to form syllables, words, phrases, and sentences, they interact in complex ways and sometimes appear to lose their separate identity. The influence that sounds exert on one another is called *coarticulation,* which means that the articulation of any one sound is influenced by a preceding or following sound. Coarticulation makes it impossible to divide the speech stream into neat segments that correspond to phonemes. Coarticulation implies nonsegmentation or, at least, interaction of the presumed linguistic segments. Hockett (1955) provided a famous and colorful illustration of the transformation from phoneme to articulation:

> Imagine a row of Easter eggs carried along a moving belt; the eggs are of various sizes, and variously colored, but not boiled. At a certain point, the belt carries the row of eggs between the two rollers of a wringer, which quite effectively smashes them and rubs them more or less into each other. The flow of eggs before the wringer represents the series of impulses from the phoneme source. The mess that emerges from the wringer represents the output of the speech transmitter. (p. 210)

Although this analogy makes the process of articulation sound completely disorganized, in fact, the process must be quite well organized if it is to be used for communication. Phoneme-sized segments may not be carried intact into the various contractions of the speech muscles, but some highly systematic links between articulation and phonemes are maintained. Research on speech articulation has provided a clearer understanding of what the links are, although the total process is far from being completely understood.

It often is possible to describe coarticulation in terms of articulatory characteristics that spread from one segment to another. Examine the following examples of coarticulation:

1a. He sneezed /h i s n i z d/ (unrounded /s/ and /n/)

1b. He snoozed /h i s n u z d/ (rounded /s/ and /n/)

2a. He asked /h i æ s k t/ (nonnasal /æ/)

2b. He answered /h i æ n s ɚ d/ (nasal /æ/)

The only phonemic difference between the first two items is the appearance of the unrounded vowel /i/ in 1a and the appearance of the rounded vowel /u/ in 1b. The lip rounding for /u/ in *He snoozed* usually begins to form during the articulation of the /s/. You might be able to feel this anticipatory lip rounding as you alternately say *sneeze* and *snooze* with your finger lightly touching your lips. In articulatory terms, the feature of lip rounding for the vowel is assumed during the /sn/ consonant cluster as the consequence of anticipating the rounding. The contrast between *sneeze* and *snooze* shows that the /sn/ cluster acquires lip rounding only if it is followed by a rounded vowel. This example of sound interaction is termed *anticipatory lip rounding* because the articulatory feature of rounding is evident before the rounded vowel /u/ is fully articulated as a segment.

Another form of anticipatory coarticulation occurs in 2b. Perhaps you can detect a difference in the quality of the /æ/ vowel in the phrases *He asked* and *He answered.* You should be able to detect a nasal quality in the latter because the vowel tends to assume the nasal resonance required for the following nasal consonant /n/. In this case, we can say that the articulatory feature of velopharyngeal opening (required for nasal resonance) is anticipated during the vowel /æ/. Normally, of course, this vowel is not nasalized. The contrasts between 1a and 1b and between 2a and 2b illustrate a type of coarticulation called *anticipatory.* Another type, *retentive,* applies to situations in which an articulatory feature is retained after its required appearance. For example, in the word me, the vowel /i/ tends to be nasalized because of a carryover velopharyngeal opening from the nasal consonant /m/. The essential lesson to be learned is that coarticulation occurs frequently in speech—so frequently, in fact, that the study of articulation is largely a study of coarticulation.

Phonetic context is highly important in understanding allophonic variation. For example, you should be able to detect a difference in the location of linguavelar closure for the /k/ sounds in the two columns of words shown here:

Keen	*Coon*
Kin	*Cone*
Can	*Con*

The point of closure tends to be more to the front of the oral cavity for the words in the first column than it is for the words in the second column. This variation occurs because, in English, the velar stops /k/ and /g/ do not have a narrowly defined place of articulation; all that is required is that the dorsum, or back, of the tongue touch the ceiling of the mouth. Therefore, the tongue is simply elevated at the position needed for the following vowel. When the tongue is in the front of the mouth (note that the vowels in the left column are front vowels), the dorsal closure is made in the front of the mouth, and when the tongue is in the back of the mouth (as it would be for the vowels in the right column), the point of closure is to the back of the velar surface.

Coarticulation arises for different reasons, some having to do with the phonology of a particular language, some with the basic mechanical or physiological constraints of the speech apparatus. Hence, some coarticulations are learned, and others are the inevitable consequences of muscles, ligaments, and bones of the speech apparatus that are linked together and unable to move with infinite speed. Consider, for example, the closing and opening of the velopharyngeal port. This articulatory gesture is rather sluggish (compared to movements of the tongue tip), so it is not surprising that the velopharyngeal opening for a nasal consonant carries over to a following vowel, as in the word *no.* The extent of this carryover nasalization, however, varies with the phonologic characteristics of a particular language. In French, vowel nasalization is phonemic (i.e., it can make a difference in meaning), but in English, vowel nasalization is only allophonic. Some aspects of coarticulation reflect universal properties of the human speech mechanism and, hence, affect all languages. Other coarticulations are governed by the phonemic structure of a particular language and are therefore learned with that language. Many coarticulatory effects are assimilatory in that a feature from one segment is adopted by an adjacent segment. For example, the nasalization of vowels by neighboring nasal consonants is nasal assimilation. Such effects may make speech production easier and faster because articulatory movements can be adapted to a particular phonetic and motor sequence. Assimilation is a general process in spoken language.

Another aspect of coarticulation is the overlapping of articulations for consonants in clusters. Quite often, the articulation for one consonant is made before the release of a preceding consonant in any two-consonant cluster. For example, in the word *spy* /spaɪ/, the bilabial closure for /p/ is accomplished shortly (about 10 to 20 msec) before the release of the constriction for /s/. This overlapping of consonant articulations makes the overall duration of the cluster shorter than the sum of the consonant durations as they occur singly; that is, the duration of /sp/ in *spy* is shorter than the sum of the durations of /s/ in *sigh* /s aɪ/ and /p/ in *pie* /p aɪ/. The overlapping of articulation contributes to the articulatory flow of speech by eliminating interruptions. The temporal structure of a /spr/ cluster, as in the word *spray,* is pictured schematically in Figure 2.26. Notice that the constrictions for /s/ and /p/ overlap by 10 to 20 milliseconds and that the closure for /p/ overlaps with the tongue position for /r/ by a similar amount. Because consonants in clusters frequently present special difficulties to children (and adults) with articulation disorders, clinicians must know how such clusters are formed. Because clusters have overlapping articulations of the constituent consonants, in general, the cluster is a tightly organized sequence of articulatory gestures. The articulation of clusters is further complicated by allophonic variations, such as those listed in Table 2.5. In English, unaspirated released stops occur only when stops follow /s/, as in the words *spy, stay,* and *ski.* Otherwise, released stops are aspirated, meaning that the release is followed by a brief interval of glottal frication (/h/-like noise). Similarly, the devoiced /l/ and /r/ normally occur only after voiceless consonants, as in the words *play* and *try.*

The examples of context-dependent articulatory modifications in Table 2.5 show the variety of influences that sounds exert on adjacent sounds. For a given sound, place of articulation, duration, voicing, nasalization, and rounding may vary with phonetic context, and these variations are noted with the special marks shown in Table 2.5.

Some aspects of coarticulation can be understood by knowing the extent to which individual sounds restrict the positions of the various articulators. Table 2.6 summarizes degrees of restriction on lips, jaw, and parts of the tongue for the different places of consonant articulation. A strong restriction is indicated by an X, a slight to moderate restriction by a —, and a minimal restriction by an O. Because this table shows

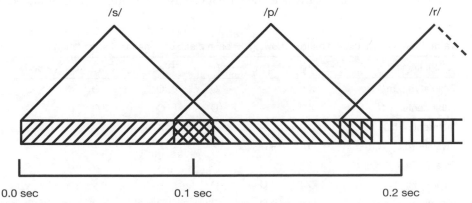

Figure 2.26. Schematic drawing of the articulatory organization of a /spr/ consonant cluster (as in the word *spray*), showing overlapping of consonantal articulations. *Source:* Kent and Moll (1975).

Table 2.5. Examples of context-dependent modifications of phonetic segments

Modification	Context description
Nasalization of vowel	Vowel is preceded or followed by a nasal, e.g., [ɔ̃n]—*on* and [mæ̃n]—*man*
Rounding of consonant	Consonant precedes a rounded sound, e.g., [k̫win]—*queen* and [t̫ru]—*true*
Palatalization of consonant	Consonant precedes a palatal sound, e.g., [kɪʃ ju]—*kiss you*
Devoicing of obstruent	Word-final position of voiced consonant, e.g., [dɔg̊]—*dog* and [liv̥]—*leave*
Devoicing of liquid	Liquid follows word-initial voiceless sound, e.g., [pl̥eɪ]—*play* and [tr̥i]—*tree*
Dentalization of coronal	Normally alveolar sound precedes a dental sound, e.g., [wɪd̪θ]—*width* and [naɪn̪θ]—*ninth*
Retroflexion of fricative	Fricative occurs in context of retroflex sounds, e.g., [harʂɚ]—*harsher* and [pɝʂɚ]—*purser*
Devoicing of sound	Consonant or vowel in voiceless context, e.g., [sɪ̥stɚ]—*sister*
Lengthening of vowel	Vowel preceding voiced sound, especially in stressed syllable, e.g., [ni: d]—*need*
Reduction of vowel	Vowel in unstressed (weak) syllable, e.g., [tæbjuleɪt] [tæbjəleɪt]—*tabulate*
Voicing of sound	Voiceless in voiced context, e.g., [æbsɝd]—*absurd*
Deaspiration of stop	Stop follows /s/, e.g., [sp⁼aɪ]—*spy* vs. [pʰaɪ]—*pie*

which parts of the vocal tract are free to vary during articulation of a given consonant, it can be used to predict certain aspects of coarticulation. For example, because
bilabial sounds (e.g., /p, b/) do not restrict the tongue as long as it does not close off
the tract, Os are indicated for all parts of the tongue. Jaw position is shown as moderately restricted for most places of articulation because some degree of jaw closing
usually aids consonant formation. The ability of jaw movement to aid tongue movement declines as place of articulation moves back in the mouth, so a velar consonant
(e.g., /k, g/) may not restrict jaw position as much as more frontal articulation (Kent
& Moll, 1972). The only sound that allows essentially unrestricted coarticulation is
the glottal /h/. Thus, /h/ usually is made with a vocal-tract configuration adjusted to

Table 2.6. Coarticulation matrix, showing for each place of consonant articulation

Articulation place	Lip	Jaw	Tip	Blade	Dorsum	Body
Bilabial /b,p,m/	X	—	O	O	O	O
Labiodental /v,f/	X	—	O	O	O	O
Interdental /ð,θ/	O	—	X	X	—	—
Alveolar /d,t,z,s,l,n/	O	—	X	X	—	—
Palatal /ʃ,ʒ, dʒ, tʃ, j, r/	O	—	—	X	X	X
Velar /g,k,ŋ/	O	O	O	—	X	X
Glottal /h/	O	O	O	O	O	O

Articulators that have strong restrictions on position are marked with X, those that have some restriction on position are marked with —, and those that are minimally restricted are marked with O.

an adjacent sound, such as the following vowel in the words *he* /hi/, *who* /hu/, *ham* /hæm/, and *hop* /hɑp/. Note that the glides /w/ and /ʍ/ are not included as they involve secondary articulations.

Investigators of speech articulation (Daniloff & Moll, 1968; Kent & Minifie, 1977; Moll & Daniloff, 1971) have shown extensive overlapping of articulatory gestures across phoneme-sized segments, causing debate about the size of unit that governs behavior. Some investigators propose that the decision unit is an allophone, others argue for the phoneme, and still others for the syllable. A popular syllable-unit hypothesis is one based on CV (consonant-vowel) syllables, with allowance for consonant clustering (CCV, CCCV, etc.). This hypothesis states that articulatory movements are organized in sequences of the form CV, CCV, CCCV, and the like so that a word like *construct* would be organized as the articulatory syllables /kɑ/ + /nstrʌkt/. Notice the odd assembly of the second syllable. This issue is of more than academic importance. Discovery of the basic decision unit would have implications for speech remediation; for example, enabling a speech clinician to choose the most efficient training and practice items for correcting an error sound. In addition, syllabic structures may explain certain features of speech and language development, as discussed by Branigan (1976).

Coarticulation also has clinical relevance, in that a sound might be more easily learned or more easily produced correctly in one context than in others. In other words, the phonetic context of a sound can facilitate or even interfere with correct production of the sound. A relevant concept is that of coarticulatory resistance, or the degree to which a given phonetic segment resists the potential interference of neighboring phonetic segments. A segment with high coarticulation resistance has articulatory characteristics that are affected very little by changes in phonetic context. The effect of phonetic context could explain why misarticulations are often inconsistent, with correct production on certain occasions and incorrect productions on others. By judiciously selecting the phonetic context where an error sound is initially corrected, the clinician can sometimes enhance the efficiency of speech remediation. Such examples show why a thorough knowledge of articulatory phonetics is important to decisions in the management of articulation disorders.

AERODYNAMIC CONSIDERATIONS IN SPEECH PRODUCTION

Because the production of speech depends on the supply and valving of air, a knowledge of air pressure, flow, and volume is essential to an understanding of both normal and disordered speech. Many abnormalities of speech production are caused by irregularities or deficiencies in the supply and valving of air, and a number of clinical assessment techniques rely on measures of air pressure, flow, or volume. To understand the regulation of air pressures and flows in speech, it is important to recognize that 1) air flows only in one direction—from a region of greater pressure to one of lesser pressure—and 2) whenever the vocal tract is closed at some point, the potential exists for the buildup of air pressure behind the closure.

English speech sounds are normally *egressive,* meaning that, in sound production, air flows from the inside (usually the lungs) to the outside (the air around us). The basic energy needed to produce sound is developed in the lungs. After air is inspired by enlargement of the lung cavity, the muscle activation changes so that the lung cavity returns to a smaller size. If the airway above is closed, the same volume of air is enclosed in a smaller space. Because the same amount of air is contained in a smaller cavity, the air pressure within the lungs increases. This overpressure (relative to atmosphere) in the lungs is the source of the egressive air flow for all speech sounds. It is a fact of clinical importance that the air flow requirements for speech are not much greater than the requirements for ordinary breathing; that is, the volume of air inspired and expired in speaking is not much different from that in quiet respiration.

The regulation of air pressure and flow for speech is diagrammed in Figure 2.27, a simple model of the vocal tract. This model, in the form of the letter F, shows the three general areas where constriction (narrowing or closure) can occur: the laryngeal, oral, and nasal sections. The first site of constriction for egressive air is in the larynx. If the vocal folds close tightly, no air can escape from the lungs. If the folds are maximally open, then air passes through the larynx readily. If the folds are closed with a moderate tension, then the buildup of air pressure beneath them eventually blows them apart, releasing a pulse of air. After the folds are blown apart, they quickly come together again through the action of various physical restoring forces. This alternation of closed and open states, occurring many times per second, is called *voicing*. Successive pulses of air from the vocal folds are a source of acoustic energy for all voiced sounds, such as vowels.

The F-shaped vocal tract model shown in Figure 2.27a illustrates the air flow for vowel sounds. The vocal folds are shown as being partly closed to represent the vibratory pattern of opening and closing. The nasal tube is tightly closed because vowels in English are nonnasal unless they precede or follow nasal consonants. The oral tube is widely open to represent the open oral cavity in vowel articulation. Because the nasal tube is closed, the acoustic energy from the vibrating vocal folds passes through the oral tube.

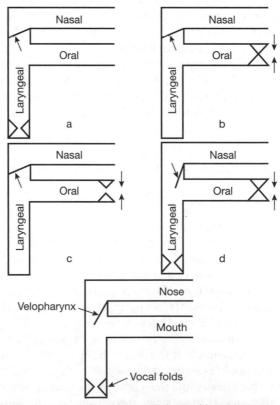

Figure 2.27. Simple models of vocal tract for major sound classes: (a) vowels, liquids, and glides; (b) voiceless stops; (c) voiceless fricatives; (d) nasals. The major parts of the model are shown at the bottom of the figure.

The configuration of the vocal tract for a voiceless stop like /p/, /t/, or /k/ is diagrammed in Figure 2.27b. The constriction at the larynx is shown as completely open because air from the lungs passes readily through the larynx and into the oral cavity. The constriction at the velopharynx is shown as closed to indicate that no air flows through the nasal tube. The oral constriction is closed to represent the period of stop closure. After this period, the oral constriction opens rapidly to allow a burst of air to escape from the oral pressure chamber. Assuming a stop closure of suitable duration, the air pressure developed within the oral cavity can be nearly equal to that in the lungs because the open vocal folds permit an equalization of air pressure in the airway reaching from the lungs up to the oral cavity. Therefore, voiceless stops have high intraoral air pressures. Also, it should be noted that children may use greater intraoral air pressures than adults (Bernthal & Beukelman, 1978; Netsell et al., 1994; Subtelny et al., 1966).

The model for voiceless fricatives in Figure 2.27c is like that for voiceless stops, but instead of a complete oral constriction, the model has a very narrow constriction, required for fricative noise. Because the velopharyngeal constriction is tightly closed and the laryngeal constriction is open, voiceless fricatives like /s/ and /ʃ/ have high intraoral air pressures. The voiceless stops and fricatives are sometimes called *pressure consonants*.

Voiced stops and fricatives differ from voiceless stops and fricatives in having vibrating vocal folds. Therefore, the models in Figure 2.27b and c would have a partial laryngeal constriction to represent voicing of these sounds. Because a certain amount of air pressure is lost in keeping the vocal folds vibrating (i.e., pressure across the glottis drops), the voiced stops and fricatives have smaller intraoral air pressures than their voiceless cognates.

Finally, the model for nasal consonants is depicted in Figure 2.27d. A partial constriction at the larynx represents the vibrating vocal folds, and a complete oral constriction represents the stoplike closure in the oral section of the vocal tract. For nasal consonants, the acoustic energy of voicing is directed through the nasal cavity. Very little air pressure builds up within the oral chamber.

Liquids and glides can be modeled in essentially the same way as vowels (Figure 2.27a). Because the oral constriction for these sounds is only slightly greater than that for vowels, there is very little intraoral air pressure buildup.

Pressures and flows can be used to describe the function of many parts of the speech system. For example, a normal efficient operation of the larynx can often be distinguished from inefficient pathological states by the excessive air flow in the latter conditions. This excessive flow, or air wastage, may be heard as breathiness or hoarseness. Velopharyngeal incompetence can be identified by recording air flow from the nose during normally nonnasal segments. Frequently, velopharyngeal incompetence is signaled both by inappropriate nasal air flow (e.g., air flow during stops or fricatives) and by reduced levels of intraoral air pressure. Sometimes, more than one pressure or flow must be recorded to identify the problem. For example, reduced levels of intraoral air pressure for consonants can be related to at least three factors: 1) respiratory weakness, resulting in insufficient air pressure; 2) velopharyngeal dysfunction, resulting in a loss of air through the nose; or 3) an inadequacy of the oral constriction, allowing excessive air to escape.

Clinically, aerodynamic assessment is especially important when dealing with a structural problem (such as cleft palate) or a physically based control problem (as in cerebral palsy, vocal fold paralysis, and other neurologic disorders). Young children may use greater intraoral air pressure than adults for consonant production, so normative pressure data obtained from adults should be used with caution in clinical evaluation of children. Moreover, the higher pressures in children's speech mean that children must close the velopharyngeal port even more tightly than adults to prevent nasal loss of air during stop or fricative consonants. Speech and language clinicians who do not possess equipment for aerodynamic recordings of speech should nonetheless be aware of the pressure and flow requirements in speech production. These requirements have important implications for the diagnosis and evaluation of communicative problems and for the design of remediation programs.

ACOUSTIC CONSIDERATIONS OF SPEECH

It is far beyond the scope of this chapter to consider in any detail the acoustic structure of speech sounds, but it is possible to draw here a few major conclusions about the acoustic signal of speech. Acoustic signals can be described in terms of three fundamental physical variables: frequency, amplitude, and duration. *Frequency* refers to the rate of vibration of a sound. Generally, the faster the rate of vibration, the higher the pitch heard. In other words, frequency is the most direct physical correlate of pitch. *Amplitude* refers to the strength or magnitude of vibration of a sound. The higher the magnitude of vibration, the louder the sound heard. Amplitude is the most direct physical correlate of loudness. Because the actual amplitude of vibration is minute and, therefore, difficult to measure, sound intensity or sound pressure level is used instead when making actual speech measurements. *Duration* refers to the total time over which a vibration continues. Duration is the most direct physical correlate of perceived length.

Virtually all naturally occurring sounds, speech included, have energy at more than a single frequency. A tuning fork is designed to vibrate at a single frequency and is one of the very few sound sources with this property. The human voice, musical instruments, and animal sounds all have energy at several frequencies. The particular pattern of energy over a frequency range is the *spectrum* of a sound. Speech sounds differ in their spectra, and these differences allow us to distinguish sounds perceptually.

Table 2.7 is a summary of the major acoustic properties of several phonetic classes. The table shows the relative sound intensity, the dominant energy region in the spectrum, and the relative sound duration for each class. Vowels are the most intense speech sounds, have most of their energy in the low to mid frequencies, and are longer in duration than other sounds (although the actual duration of vowel sounds

Table 2.7. Summary of acoustic features for six phonetic classes

Sound class	Intensity	Spectrum	Duration
Vowels	Very strong	Low-frequency dominance	Moderate to long
Glides and liquids	Strong	Low-frequency dominance	Short to moderate
Strident fricatives and affricates	Moderate	High-frequency dominance	Moderate
Nasals	Moderate	Very low-frequency dominance	Short to moderate
Stops	Weak	Varies with place of articulation	Short
Nonstrident fricatives	Weak	Flat	Short to moderate

may range from about 50 msec to half a second). Because vowels are the most intense sounds, they typically determine the overall loudness of speech. The most intense vowels are the low vowels and the least intense, the high vowels.

The glides and liquids are somewhat less intense than the vowels and have most of their energy in the low to mid frequencies. The duration of the glides /w/ and /j/ tends to be longer than that of the liquids /l/ and /r/.

The strident fricatives and affricates (/s, z, ʃ, ʒ, tʃ, dʒ/) are more intense than other consonants but considerably weaker than vowels. The stridents have energy primarily at the high frequencies and, therefore, are vulnerable to high-frequency hearing loss. A good recording of the stridents requires a wide frequency response. Stridents tend to be relatively long in duration, especially compared to other consonants, and fricatives typically are longer than affricates.

The nasals are sounds of moderate intensity, low-frequency energy, and brief to moderate duration. The nasals have more energy at very low frequencies than do other sounds.

The stops are relatively weak sounds of brief duration. The burst that results from release of a stop closure can be as short as 10 milliseconds. The primary energy for stops varies over a wide range of frequencies—from low to high; bilabials have relatively low-frequency energy, while velars and alveolars have most of their energy in, respectively, the mid and mid-to-high frequencies.

The nonsibilant fricatives /f, v, θ, ð/ are weak sounds of typically moderate duration. They tend to have a flat spectrum, meaning that the noise energy is distributed fairly uniformly over the frequency range. Of all sounds, /θ/ usually is the weakest—so weak that it can barely be heard when produced in isolation at any distance from a listener.

Finally, two points should be made concerning acoustic implications for clinical assessment and management. First, the absolute frequency location of energy for speech sounds varies with speaker age and sex. Men have the lowest overall frequencies of sound energy, women somewhat higher frequencies, and young children the highest frequencies. This relationship follows from the acoustic principle that an object's resonance frequency is inversely related to its length. The longest pipe in a pipe organ has a low frequency (or low pitch) and the shortest pipe a high frequency (high pitch); similarly, the adult male vocal tract is longer than a woman's or a child's and, therefore, has resonances of lower frequency. This difference has practical implications. Historically, most acoustic data were reported for men's speech, but more recent studies have provided substantial datasets for women's and children's speech, so acoustic data are now available for speakers of both sexes and of many different ages, including infants. Modern methods of acoustic analysis make it easier to adjust measurement parameters to make them optimal for different speakers. For example, because the speech of women and children has a wider range of frequencies than men's speech, it is usually advisable to extend the range of frequencies when analyzing speech patterns for women and children, especially for fricatives and affricates.

Second, because speech sounds vary widely in intensity, dominant energy region, and duration, they are not equally discriminable under different listening situations. The acoustic differences summarized in Table 2.7 should be kept in mind when testing articulation or auditory discrimination. These variations in acoustic properties become even more important in providing clinical services for individuals with hearing loss.

SENSORY INFORMATION IN SPEECH PRODUCTION

As speech is produced, several different kinds of sensory information are generated. The types of information include tactile (touch and pressure), proprioceptive (position sense), kinesthetic (movement sense), and auditory. The total sensory information is genuinely plurimodal; that is, available in several modalities. Most authorities agree that the rich sensory information associated with speech production is particularly important in speech development and in the management of some speech disorders, as when a child must learn a new articulatory pattern. A clinician therefore should be knowledgeable about the kinds and characteristics of sensory, or afferent, information.

The major characteristics of the sensory systems in speech were reviewed by Hardcastle (1976) and later by Kent and colleagues (1990). Tactile receptors, which consist of free nerve endings and complex endings (e.g., Krause end-bulbs and Meissner corpuscles), supply information to the central nervous system on the nature of contact (including localization, pressure, and onset time) and direction of movement. Remarkably, the oral structures are among the most sensitive regions of the body. The tongue tip is particularly sensitive and can therefore supply detailed sensory information. Tactile receptors belong to a more general class of receptors called *mechanoreceptors* (which respond to mechanical stimulation). These receptors respond not only to physical contacts of articulatory structures but also to air pressures generated during speech.

The proprioceptive and kinesthetic receptors include the muscle spindles, Golgi tendon organs, and joint receptors. Muscle spindles provide rich information on the length of muscle fibers, the degree and velocity of stretch, and the direction of movement of a muscle. Golgi receptors relay information on the change of stretch on a tendon caused by muscular contraction or by other influences, including passive movement. Joint receptors, located in the capsules of joints, inform the central nervous system on the rate, direction, and extent of joint movement. Even a relatively simple movement, such as closing the jaw and raising the tongue, supplies a variety of afference to the central nervous system.

The auditory system supplies information on the acoustic consequences of articulation. Because the purpose of speech is to produce an intelligible acoustic signal, auditory feedback is of particular importance in regulating the processes of articulation. Interestingly, when an adult suffers a sudden and severe loss of hearing, speech articulation usually does not deteriorate immediately, but only gradually. The other types of sensory information are probably sufficient to maintain the accuracy of articulation for some time.

Many tactile receptors are comparatively slow acting because the neural signals travel along relatively small fibers in a multisynaptic pathway (a pathway composed of several neurons). Much of the tactile information is available to the central nervous system after the event to which it pertains. This information is particularly important to articulations that involve contact between articulatory surfaces, such as stops and fricatives. Obviously, prolonging an articulation helps to reinforce its sensory accompaniment. When the mucosal surfaces of the articulators are anesthetized, one of the most disturbed class of sounds is the fricatives.

Computational models of speech (Guenther, 1995; Houde & Nagarajan, 2011) often use sensory-motor maps to represent the coordination of information between a sensory modality and motor control. For example, an auditory-motor map represents the relationship between auditory and motor information. If this approach is used to model speech development in children, then we can imagine the construction of different maps that consolidate a child's growing proficiency with speech. For example, a child may establish auditory-motor and somatosensory-motor maps that establish and maintain the integrity of speech production. Some maps pertain to both self-produced and other-produced information. In the case of the auditory-motor map, auditory information can be derived from a speaker's own vocalizations or from the vocalizations of others. Similarly, we can imagine a visual-motor map that represents the visual information from a speaker's face related to the motor commands that produce the facial movements. Once these maps are in place, a speaker can shift from one kind of map to another as the need arises and can thereby compensate for a temporary loss of information in any particular sensory modality.

SUMMARY OF LEVELS OF ORGANIZATION OF SPEECH

Various levels of organization of speech are shown in Table 2.8, beginning with the syllable and working down to the acoustic sequence that might be seen on a spectrogram or visual representation of sounds. Although syllabic integrity is the highest level shown, the table could have begun with an even higher level, such as a phrase or a sentence. However, for our purposes here, it is sufficient to consider only the levels presented in the table. The syllable is an organizational unit that consists of one or more phonemes; in this case, the syllable /pɑ/ includes the phonemes /p/ and /ɑ/. Because phonemes are abstract, a phonemic description does not touch on a number of details of phonetic organization and speech behavior. Some of these details are shown in the level of phonetic properties. The phoneme /p/ has as its phonetic representation the aspirated [pʰ], and the phoneme /ɑ/ has as its phonetic representation the lengthened [ɑː]. These phonetic representations are, of course, allophones of the /p/ and /ɑ/ phonemes. The English phoneme /p/ is always aspirated in syllable-initial position, and the phoneme /ɑ/ frequently is lengthened when uttered in an open monosyllable (i.e., a CV syllable).

Segmental features comprise the next level of the table. These features are phonetic dimensions or attributes by which sounds may be described. For example, the consonant [p] is defined by its inclusion in the classes of stops, labials, and consonantals, and by its exclusion from the classes of nasals and voiced sounds. These features are similar to the distinctive features discussed earlier in this chapter, but they are intended to be more phonetic in character. Even without rigorous definitions of the features suggested, it should be clear that each feature defines an articulatory property of the sound in question; for example, vowel [ɑ] is a syllable nucleus, is not a consonant, is low back and unrounded, and is a voiced nonnasal sound.

The features are less abstract than phonemes but still must be interpreted by the motor control system of the brain to provide proper neural instructions to the speech muscles; that is, the features listed for [p] and [ɑ] must be translated into a pattern of muscle contractions that yields the articulatory sequence shown in the next-to-last level of the table. The –nasal feature of [p] requires that the velopharynx be closed, and the –voice feature of the same segment requires that the vocal folds be abducted (open). In this way, each feature requirement is given an articulatory interpretation, accomplished by the contraction of muscles.

Finally, as the consequence of muscle contractions, a series of speech sounds is uttered. In this acoustic sequence, the last level of the table, one can see acoustic segments of the kind visible on a spectrogram. Notice that one acoustic segment does not necessarily correspond to a single phoneme. The phoneme /p/ is associated with at

Table 2.8.   Levels of organization of speech

Syllabic integrity	/p ɑ/
Phonemic composition	/p/ + /ɑ/
Phonetic properties	[pʰɑː]
Note: Stop /p/ is aspirated, and vowel /ɑ/ is lengthened	
Segmental features	[p] — +Stop
	+Labial
	+Consonantal
	–Nasal
	–Voice
	[ɑ] — +Syllabic
	–Consonantal
	–Front
	+Low
	–Round
	–Nasal
	+Voice
Articulatory sequence	Closure of velopharynx
	Abduction of vocal folds
	Adjustment of tongue for /ɑ/
	Closure of lips
	Opening of lips and jaw
	Adduction of vocal folds
	Final abduction of vocal folds
Acoustic sequence	Silent period during /p/ closure
	Noise burst for /p/ release
	Aspiration period as folds close
	Voiced period after folds close, with distinct resonant shaping

least three acoustic segments: a silent period corresponding to the bilabial closure, a noise burst produced as the lips are rapidly opened, and an aspiration interval related to a gradual closure of the vocal folds in preparation for voicing the following vowel.

Although Table 2.8 is fairly detailed, it represents only part of the complexity of speech. In the linguistic-phonetic organization of speech behavior, we need to consider three major components: the segmental (or phonetic) component, the suprasegmental (prosodic) component, and the paralinguistic component. The first two have already been discussed in this chapter. The *paralinguistic component* is similar to the prosodic component in that it might be called nonsegmental. This component includes those aspects of speech represented by terms such as emotion and attitude. A speaker who plans an utterance must decide not only about phonetic sequencing but also about prosodic structure and emotional and attitudinal content (i.e., tone of voice). The segmental component includes words, syllables, phonemes, and features. The supra-segmental or prosodic component includes stress, intonation, juncture, rate, loudness, and pitch level. The paralinguistic component is made up of tension, voice quality, and voice qualifications (Crystal, 1969).

It might seem, then, that a child learning speech is faced with a daunting task. Fortunately, most children meet the challenge and are able to produce intelligible speech that is nuanced with emotion and attitude. But some do not, and that is why this book is needed. The next chapter discusses the process of speech acquisition.

QUESTIONS FOR CHAPTER 2

1. Discuss the relationship among the following concepts: *morpheme, phoneme*, and *allophone*. For example, explain why a morpheme is relevant to identifying phonemes and why phonemes are relevant to identifying allophones.

2. This chapter summarized two ways of describing vowel articulation: traditional phonetic description and distinctive features. Discuss the similarities and differences between these two approaches.

3. Using Table 2.2 as a guide, classify all of the consonants in the phrase *Good morning, take a ticket, and get in line* according to place of articulation, manner of articulation, and voicing. Note that in all of the words containing two or more consonants, the consonants share a phonetic feature. What is this feature for each word?

4. What is coarticulation, and why does it occur?

3

Speech Sound Acquisition

SHARYNNE McLEOD

LEARNING OBJECTIVES

This chapter discusses typically developing children's acquisition of speech. By the end of this chapter, the reader should be able to:

- Describe how knowledge of children's acquisition of speech sounds can be useful to clinicians working with children evidencing speech sound disorders.
- Identify the major characteristics of models used to describe the process of speech sound acquisition.
- Summarize how speech acquisition data are obtained.
- Explain the advantages and disadvantages of diary studies, cross-sectional studies, and longitudinal studies.
- Outline the overall sequence of speech sound acquisition.
- Describe the development of the structure and function of the oral mechanism.
- Outline infants' development of speech perception and production.
- Describe the current state of knowledge regarding how children transition from words to speech.
- Summarize children's speech acquisition between the ages of 2 and 5 years.
- Discuss the relationship between speech and literacy for children aged 5 years and older.
- Describe factors influencing typical acquisition of speech and the range of evidence.

From the moment children are born, they vocalize. Refinement of this vocalization into intelligible speech takes many years, while children's body structures develop and their perception and production systems become more sophisticated and attuned to their ambient (native) language. This chapter explores typical or normal speech sound acquisition. At the beginning of the chapter, we consider the reasons it is important for speech-language pathologists (SLPs) to understand typical speech sound acquisition, models of speech sound acquisition, and the research methods that have been employed to understand how children learn to produce speech sounds. The remainder of the chapter examines children's speech sound acquisition of English from infancy to the school years. Because this chapter addresses only the acquisition of English speech sounds, the symbol /r/ is used to indicate /ɹ/, following the convention of Ladefoged (2005).

RELEVANCE OF UNDERSTANDING TYPICAL SPEECH
SOUND ACQUISITION FOR SPEECH-LANGUAGE PATHOLOGISTS

An understanding of typical speech sound acquisition is akin to having solid foundations under a house. In pediatric SLP practice, judgments about whether a child's speech is typical occurs daily. This decision making is guided by knowledge of research data as well as clinicians' experience. Studies of children's typical speech sound acquisition are the primary research data used by SLPs to make these decisions.

Seven main areas of SLP practice are informed by a comprehensive understanding of speech sound acquisition:

1. *Referral.* Providing advice to parents, educators, and health professionals regarding whether a child should be referred for a speech assessment.

2. *Assessment.* Deciding which assessment tools are appropriate to examine speech behaviors that are relevant for the age of the child. For example, if the child is 1;6, an inventory of consonants, vowels, and syllable shapes should be determined. If the child is 7;0, polysyllabic words and phonological awareness skills also should be assessed.

3. *Analysis.* Analyzing the speech sample in order to decide whether the child's speech is age appropriate on a range of measures.

4. *Diagnosis.* Determining whether a child has a delay or disorder and whether their areas of difficulty warrant speech sound intervention.

5. *Selecting intervention targets.* There are two major schools of thought regarding how to use knowledge of typical speech sound acquisition to select intervention targets. Proponents of the *traditional developmental approach* suggest that intervention targets should focus on errors on the production of early developing sounds (Rvachew & Nowak, 2001; Shriberg & Kwiatkowski, 1982b). Proponents of the *complexity approach* (also called *nontraditional approach* and *least knowledge approach*) select later-developing sounds; the aim of such an approach is to produce a system-wide change (Gierut, 2007; Gierut et al., 1996).

6. *Intervention.* Adapting teaching and feedback to an age-appropriate level and determining that a child has achieved their goals to the expected level.

7. *Dismissal/discharge.* Deciding whether a child's speech is within normal limits for their age (Tyler, 2005) and whether their speech sound intervention should be concluded for other reasons; for example, the child has progressed as far as they are going to and are no longer making progress, or the child lacks motivation for continued therapy.

The goal of this chapter is to assist SLPs in all these areas by providing basic or foundational knowledge for working with children with speech sound disorders.

MODELS OF SPEECH ACQUISITION

The acquisition of speech and language is a complex process whose precise nature is not known. Many models of acquisition have been proposed. Each model provides a different insight into how the process might work. Thus, it is useful for SLPs working with children to have knowledge of a range of models. Barlow and Gierut (1999, p. 1482) recommend that when considering models of speech acquisition, an adequate model must account for "(a) the actual facts of children's productions and the mismatches between a child's output and the adult input forms; (b) the generalities that span children's sound systems, as well as associated variability within and across developing systems; and (c) the changes that occur in children's grammars over time." They also indicated that an adequate model must be testable and falsifiable. With these premises in mind, a range of models of speech acquisition will be presented. For a comprehensive account, see Ball and Kent (1997).

Traditionally, SLPs used a behaviorist model to explain how children learn the sounds of the language. More recently, linguistic-based models have evolved based on theories of generative phonology, natural phonology, nonlinear theory, optimality theory, and sonority. Such approaches not only provided SLPs with insight into children's developing speech systems but also extended and enhanced guidelines for assessment, analysis, and intervention. Most linguistic theories maintain that innate or natural mechanisms govern a child's phonological system. These are expressed as distinctive features in generative phonology, phonological processes (or patterns) in natural phonology, multi-tiered representations in nonlinear phonology, and constraints in optimality theory. However, although linguistic-based models provided descriptions of children's phonology, they failed to provide explanations of the underlying cognitive mechanisms involved in the perception and production of speech. Consequently, the most recent explanations are psycholinguistic models of speech development.

Traditional Models of Speech Acquisition: Behaviorist Models

Behaviorism focused on describing overt and observable behaviors. Behaviorism was proposed by Watson (1913/1994, p. 248) in his article "Psychology as a Behaviorist Views It" and was described as an "objective experimental branch of natural science that can be studied without references to consciousness." The most influential proponent of behaviorism was B. F. Skinner. Skinner's operant conditioning can be traced back to the stimulus-response psychology of the Russian physiologist Pavlov, who trained a dog to respond by salivating when hearing the stimulus of a bell ringing. Skinner created the concept of operant or instrumental conditioning to focus on controlling acts by changing the consequences that occur immediately following the act (Skinner, 1972; Thomas, 2000). In a behaviorist approach, consequences can be described either as positive or negative, reinforcement or punishment. Skinner's behaviorism has been applied to a wide range of ages, cultures, and behaviors (including physical, social, and emotional). Behaviorist principles have been applied throughout SLP practice, particularly from the 1950s to the 1970s.

Application to Typically Developing Children When behaviorist models have been applied to speech acquisition, the focus has been on observing environmental conditions (stimuli) that co-occur and predict overt verbal behaviors (responses). For example, Olmsted (1971) suggested that sounds that were easy to discriminate would be learned first; however, his order has not been supported by subsequent research. Behaviorist researchers documented normative behaviors of large groups of children during the speech acquisition period. SLPs described speech development as correct pronunciation of speech sounds. Age-of-acquisition data were collected to provide descriptive normative information (e.g., Templin, 1957).

A major criticism of the application of behaviorism to children's speech acquisition is that children master speech and language acquisition more quickly than they could if they had to depend on stimulus-response mechanisms to learn each element. That is, there is no capacity for parental/environmental reinforcement of all speech behaviors, leading to mastery of such a complex skill as speech and language. Another criticism is that acquisition of speech and language is too complex to be explained solely by reinforcement.

Application to Speech-Language Pathology Practice   Although behaviorism as an explanation for sound acquisition has not been supported, behavioral principles have had a significant impact on speech-language pathology practice for children with speech sound disorders. Speech production for many years was considered a motor activity, and analysis of speech was conducted using segmental error analysis. Speech was analyzed as a series of sounds, and the function of different sounds to signal meaning differences was not taken into consideration (e.g., Van Riper & Irwin, 1958). The stimulus-response paradigm was the basis of traditional articulation intervention. Using this behavioral approach, a child was presented with a sound or word that they were required to say and then received positive reinforcement in the form of praise, a sticker, or a token on a set schedule (Winitz, 1969).

Linguistic Models of Speech Acquisition

In the traditional models of speech acquisition, there was limited consideration of the patterns, structures, and contexts of misarticulations (with some exceptions, such as McDonald, 1964b) or of the cognitive dimension of linguistic knowledge. This gave rise to the linguistic models of speech acquisition.

Generative Phonology

Generative phonology is a theory of the sound structure of human languages and was developed by Noam Chomsky. The term *generative* refers to the belief that speech sounds are generated by transforming the underlying representation into a surface form using a language-specific rule. The key principles of generative phonology were illustrated in the landmark study of English phonology presented in Chomsky and Hallé's (1968) book, *The Sound Pattern of English*. Generative phonology moved away from the traditional phonemic analysis and introduced two major concepts:

1. Phonological rules map underlying representations onto surface pronunciations.

2. Phonological descriptions depend on information from other linguistic levels.

Although generative phonology incorporates consideration of semantic and syntactical aspects of language (concept 2), most phonology texts focus on concept 1. The area of generative phonology that has received the most attention is the description of phonological relationships that are expressed by proposing an abstract underlying representation and a set of phonological rules. To provide an example, generative phonology can be used to explain the way that English-speaking adults nasalize vowels before nasal consonants. In generative phonology, this concept is written as the following rule:

$$\begin{bmatrix} +\text{Vowel} \\ -\text{Consonant} \end{bmatrix} \rightarrow \textit{Nasal}/ - \begin{bmatrix} +Consonant \\ +Nasal \end{bmatrix}$$

The information to the left of the arrow indicates the segments that conform to the rule. The arrow means "is realized as." Only the relevant rules are included to the right of the arrow. Other features are assumed to remain as they were. The diagonal slash means "in the context of." The dash and information that follow provide the context of the segment described by the rule. Thus, this generative phonology rule reads: Vowels are realized as nasal in the context of (in this case, specifically just before) nasal consonants.

Application to Typically Developing Children   Generative phonology has been applied to the understanding of children's speech acquisition as it enabled description of the relationship of children's productions to adult pronunciation in terms of phonological rules (Grunwell, 1987, pp. 176–197). Grunwell indicated that generative phonology has been readily applied to children's speech because generative phonological rules can explain substitutions, distortions, omissions, additions, metathesis, and coalescence.

Some of the premises of generative phonology have received criticism in subsequent research. For example, there has been criticism of the premise that the child's underlying representation of the sound is adultlike (this viewpoint will be discussed later when we consider psycholinguistic theories). Additionally, there has been criticism of the premise that the rules that were applied had a corresponding reality to the processing and production systems of the child (i.e., it is not clear that we actually apply such rules in our heads when we comprehend and produce speech).

Application to Speech-Language Pathology Practice   As a theory, generative phonology has not seen broad application in the field of speech-language pathology. Hodson (2010b) describes generative phonology as the "first steps into phonologically based clinical analysis" (p. 55); however, additional knowledge gained from the theory of natural phonology (discussed next) led to the identification of patterns in phonological analysis procedures.

Natural Phonology

The theory of natural phonology (Stampe, 1969, 1979) formed the basis of the phonological process approach to assessment and treatment of speech sound disorders and is regarded as the phonological model that has had the greatest impact on the field of speech-language pathology (Edwards, 2007). *Natural processes* (or *patterns*) are those that are preferred or frequently used in phonological systems and are identified in two ways: those that are universal across languages and those that are frequently used by young children. According to Stampe, a phonological process is a "mental operation that applies in speech to substitute for a class of sounds or sound sequences presenting a common difficulty to the speech capacity of the individual, an alternative class identical but lacking the difficult property" (1979, p. 1), and phonological processes merge "a potential opposition into that member of the opposition which least tries the restrictions of the human speech capacity" (1969, p. 443).

In Stampe's view, the child's underlying representations are akin to adult forms. Natural (or innate) phonological processes apply to these underlying representations, resulting in the child's productions (or surface forms). For example, it is assumed that children have the adult form of a word, such as *tree* /tri/, in their underlying representation. However, natural processes such as cluster reduction are applied because the child (at least temporarily) has some limitation to produce a particular sound or group of sounds. In this case, the surface form (child's production) would most likely be [ti]. Later, in the discussion of psycholinguistic models, we will critique the notion that children's underlying representations are akin to the adult form. A shortcoming of this theory is that some errors may fit into more than one category. For example, if a child attempted to say *dance* /dæns/ and said [dæn] instead, it is not clear if this is an example of final consonant deletion, cluster reduction, stridency deletion, or some combination of these.

Application to Typically Developing Children   Natural phonology has provided insight to the understanding of typical speech acquisition. Natural processes are described as innate rules that are systematically applied to speech production until children learn to suppress them. Because these rules are universal, they are meant to apply to all children speaking all languages. Thus, speech acquisition is a progression from these innate speech patterns to the pronunciation system of the language(s) learned by the child. By applying natural phonology to English speech acquisition, Grunwell (1987) presented a table of the ages of suppression of phonological processes by typically developing children, such as cluster reduction, fronting, and stopping. Other researchers have also provided lists of natural phonological processes (e.g., Ingram, 1976; Shriberg & Kwiatkowski, 1980). Shriberg and Kwiatkowski advocated the clinical use of eight natural processes: 1) final consonant deletion, 2) velar fronting, 3) stopping, 4) palatal fronting, 5) liquid simplification, 6) cluster reduction, 7) assimilation, and 8) unstressed-syllable deletion.

Application to Speech-Language Pathology Practice   The phonological pattern/process approach to assessment and intervention based on natural phonology transformed the way that SLPs viewed children's speech sound errors. Since Ingram's (1976, 1989a) seminal work on phonological impairments in children, SLPs increasingly have applied descriptive linguistic-based models to their clinical activities. Ingram's application of natural phonology was widely accepted by SLPs in the 1970s and 1980s and remains popular for directing the assessment, analysis, and intervention of children with speech sound disorders (Bankson & Bernthal, 1990, 2020; Khan, 1982; Shriberg & Kwiatkowski, 1980; Weiner, 1979). Assessment approaches were developed to specifically assess subgroups of sounds within a given phonological pattern (e.g., Bankson-Bernthal Test of Phonology [BBTOP-2], Bankson & Bernthal, 2020). Phonological processes were also described as part of a broader analysis procedure for several speech-sampling tools (e.g., Phonological Assessment of Child Speech [PACS], Grunwell, 1985) and as stand-alone analyses to be applied to conversational speech (e.g., Natural Process Analysis, Shriberg & Kwiatkowski, 1980). One of the goals of intervention based on natural phonology is "to teach children to suppress innate simplification processes" (Hodson, 2010b, p. 55).

Limitations of the application of natural phonology to speech-language pathology practice have been identified. First, although most SLPs can readily describe children's nonadult productions using phonological process terms such as *cluster reduction* and *fronting,* SLPs' use of phonological processes are descriptive rather than an application of the theoretical tenets of natural phonology. Shriberg (1991, p. 270) described this as an "atheoretical use of process terminology." Second, natural phonology does not account for nonnatural simplifications in children's speech (Hodson, 2010a). Many children with highly unintelligible speech produce speech sounds in a way that cannot be classified using natural phonology. Terms such as *backing* and *initial consonant deletion* are in the literature to describe phonological processes that are not seen in children during typical speech sound acquisition (Dodd, 1995b).

One question that remains unresolved with natural phonology is whether the process labels being applied actually represent mental operations going on inside the head of the child. However, because such labels do capture patterns of errors being observed, the term *phonological patterns* is frequently used in place of *phonological processes*. For example, the title of a popular assessment tool in this area is the Hodson Assessment of Phonological Patterns–3 (Hodson, 2004).

Nonlinear Phonology

Nonlinear phonology refers to a collection of theories that focus on the hierarchical nature of the relationships between phonological units. Goldsmith introduced nonlinear phonology in his doctoral dissertation (1979) and later expanded upon it (Goldsmith, 1990). These theories include autosegmental theory, metrical theory, moraic theory, feature geometry theory, and underspecification theory. Nonlinear phonology attempts to account for the idea that production of speech involves more than just production of a sequence of phonemes; it takes into account many elements (features, segments, syllables, feet, words, and phrases) both independently and in relation to one another; hence, the term *nonlinear*. There are two main tiers in nonlinear phonology:

1. The *prosodic tier* focuses on words and the structure of words and includes a number of levels: word tier, foot tier, syllable tier, onset-rime tier, skeletal tier, and segmental tier (see Figure 3.1).

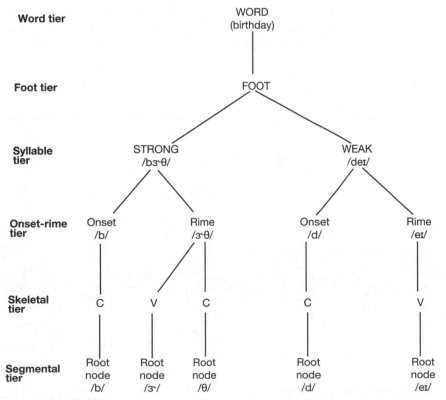

Figure 3.1. An example of the prosodic tier representation for the word *birthday*.

2. The *segmental tier* focuses on the segments or speech sounds and the features
    that make up those sounds (see Figure 3.2).

In the prosodic tier, the *word tier* simply denotes words. Immediately below the
word tier is the *foot tier,* which refers to grouping of syllables, and syllables may be
either strong (S) or weak (w). A foot can contain only one strong syllable (but can also
contain other weak syllables). A foot that includes a weak syllable can be either Sw
(left prominent, or trochaic), or wS (right prominent, or iambic). Below the foot tier
is the *syllable tier.* A syllable consists of one prominent phoneme (the peak), which is
usually a vowel and less prominent phonemes (generally consonants) that can appear
before or after the peak. Consonants that appear before the vowel are known as *onsets,*
and consonants that appear after the vowel are *codas.* The peak and the coda together
make up the *rime.* All languages allow syllables without a coda, which are sometimes
called *open syllables* (e.g., CV). Some languages do not allow for *closed syllables* that
have a coda (e.g., CVC). Across the world's languages, open syllables occur more often
than closed. Below the onset-rime tier is the *skeletal tier,* which includes slots for the
individual speech sounds.

In the *segmental tier,* features are described according to three nodes: the root
node, the laryngeal node, and the place node (see Figure 3.2). The root node [sonorant]
and [consonantal] defines the segment as a vowel/glide or a consonant. The features
[continuant] and [nasal] define the classes of stops, fricatives, and nasals. The laryngeal node includes the features of [voice] and [spread glottis] and differentiates vowels as well as voiced from voiceless consonants. The place node designates the oral
cavity characteristics of the segment and includes labial [round], coronal [anterior],
[distributed], and dorsal [high], [low], [back]. Default nodes are generally the most
frequent features (unmarked) and the easiest features for a child to use. In English,
the default consonant is /t/ because it is coronal but not continuant, not lateral, not
nasal, and not voiced.

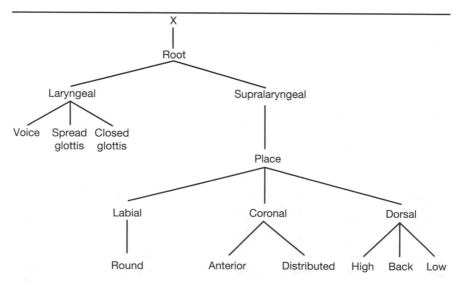

Figure 3.2.   Hierarchical tree structure (segmental tier).

Application to Typically Developing Children   Two of the major benefits of non-linear phonology to the understanding of typical phonological development are 1) the concept of links between the segmental and suprasegmental tiers and prosodic variables that highlight the interaction between speech sounds and other speech-language domains and 2) the view that development is progressive or additive, which is in contrast to the negative progression suggested by a phonological process approach whereby children learn to undelete deleted final consonants (Bernhardt & Stoel-Gammon, 1994). Bernhardt (1992a) discussed these developmental implications of nonlinear phonology and highlighted the importance of considering children's representations instead of the negative progression of rules of generative grammar. Bernhardt suggested that children's representations (or simple syllable templates such as CV units and stop consonants) account for a large proportion of young children's speech production and that children add to these representations as they mature. Nonlinear phonology also enables consideration beyond the acquisition of consonants, as it also addresses vowels, syllable shapes, words, and stress.

Application to Speech-Language Pathology Practice   Bernhardt, Stemberger, and their colleagues have been major proponents of the use of nonlinear phonology in speech-language pathology practice. Bernhardt and Stoel-Gammon (1994) presented an excellent overview of the benefits of nonlinear phonology to SLPs. Bernhardt and Stemberger developed a theoretical text (1998), a workbook for clinicians (2000), and online assessment and analysis tools in many languages (Cross-Linguistic Phonology Project, https://phonodevelopment.sites.olt.ubc.ca). Additionally, Bernhardt and Stemberger have applied principles of nonlinear phonology to goal setting and intervention for children with speech sound disorders (Bernhardt, 1992b; Bernhardt et al., 2010). In the assessment of children's speech using nonlinear phonology, attention is paid to production of consonants as well as vowels, syllables, word shapes, and stress patterns. Nonlinear intervention goals focus on utilizing established sounds in new syllable shapes and new sounds in established syllable shapes.

Optimality Theory

Optimality theory was first described by Prince and Smolensky (1993) in their report "Optimality Theory: Constraint Interaction in Generative Grammar." Optimality theory originally was developed to describe adult languages. Its basic units are constraints, which are of two major types:

1. *Markedness constraints* (also called *output constraints*) capture limitations on what can be produced (or the output). Output is simplified by markedness constraints that are motivated by the frequency and distribution of sounds in the ambient language as well as perceptual and articulatory characteristics of the sounds. Sounds that are difficult to pronounce or perceive are marked.

2. *Faithfulness constraints* capture the features to be preserved, prohibiting addition and deletion that violate the ambient language.

Constraints are assumed to be universal to all languages (Barlow & Gierut, 1999). There is a reciprocal relationship between faithfulness and markedness constraints (Kager, 1999). Faithfulness can result in the inclusion of phonological features, whereas markedness can result in their exclusion.

Application to Typically Developing Children and Speech-Language Pathology Practice   Optimality theory has been applied to the understanding of the typical development of children's speech (see Barlow & Gierut, 1999, for an overview). The aim during development is for the output to match the adult target, which is achieved by promoting faithfulness constraints and demoting markedness constraints. One example of the application of optimality theory has been to develop a model of children's acquisition of polysyllabic words (James et al., 2008). The model proposes five stages, each of which elucidates relevant faithfulness constraints. In Stage 1 (ages 1;0 to 2;3), children are faithful to the stressed syllable and the duration of the whole word. Stage 2 (ages 2;4 to 3;11) focuses on faithfulness to the number of syllables in a word. That is, during this stage, children reduce the occurrence of weak syllable deletion, cluster reduction, and final consonant deletion. Stage 3 (ages 4;0 to 6;11) highlights faithfulness to all the phonemes in the words and can co-occur with a period of dysprosody (e.g., word rhythm is disrupted). Stage 4 (ages 7;0 to 10;11) emphasizes faithfulness to word rhythm with accurate delineation between stressed and unstressed syllables. The final stage (age 11;0 and older) represents adultlike production of polysyllabic words.

Optimality theory also has been applied to SLP practice with children with speech sound disorders (Barlow & Gierut, 1999). Children's possible productions of words are placed into a constraint table, and violations of constraints are identified. Fatal violations (involving a highly ranked constraint) are also identified. The optimal constraint (the form most likely to be produced by the child) is the one that violates the least number of constraints, or the lowest-ranking constraints. As children's speech systems mature, they rerank constraints until eventually their productions match the adult form (Edwards, 2007).

Sonority Hypothesis

Sonority, first described in 1865 (see Clements, 1990), refers to the relative loudness of a sound relative to other sounds with the same pitch, stress, and length (Ladefoged, 1993). The sonority of a sound depends on the degree of voicing and the amount of opening (stricture) involved in producing the sound. Voiced sounds are more sonorous than voiceless sounds. Sounds with open articulation (e.g., vowels and liquids) are highly sonorous, whereas sounds with closed articulation (e.g., stops and fricatives) are less sonorous. Phonemes are allocated a numerical value to represent their degree of sonority. A number of different value hierarchies have been proposed, with the one by Steriade (1990) being the one most commonly used within speech-language pathology (e.g., Gierut, 1999; Ohala, 1999). Steriade proposed that voiceless stops (value of 7) are the least sonorous phonemes, and vowels (value of 0) are the most sonorous sounds.

The Sonority Sequencing Principle (SSP) is a "presumed universal which governs the permissible sequence of consonants within syllables" (Gierut, 1999, p. 708). Thus, phonemes with low sonority values are found at the syllable margins, and sounds with high sonority values are located toward the center of the syllable (Clements, 1990; Roca & Johnson, 1999). In the word *drink,* for example, the vowel /ɪ/ has high sonority; therefore, it is found in the middle of the syllable. The next most sonorous sounds are liquids (such as /r/) and nasals (such as /n/); hence, they are found on either side of the vowel. The least sonorous sounds are stops (such as /d/ and /k/). These are found at the syllable margins.

Application to Typically Developing Children   In accordance with the SSP, it has been proposed that children reduce word-initial consonant clusters in a manner that produces a maximal rise in sonority and that word-final consonant clusters are reduced to produce a minimal fall in sonority. This pattern of reduction is termed the *sonority hypothesis*. Ohala (1999) considered the application of the sonority hypothesis when he described the productions of consonant clusters in nonsense words produced by 16 typically developing children aged 1;9 to 3;2. When the children reduced word-initial fricative + stop clusters (e.g., /sp/) and word-initial fricative + nasal clusters (e.g., /sn/), the remaining consonant was consistently the least sonorous element. Additionally, when the children reduced word-final fricative + stop consonant clusters (e.g., /st/), the remaining consonant was consistently the most sonorous element. Wyllie-Smith and colleagues (2006) analyzed the production of word-initial consonant clusters of 16 typically developing 2-year-old children over two occasions for each child. Overall, the sonority hypothesis was adhered to when the children reduced a consonant cluster by producing one of the target elements; however, reductions to nontarget consonants were inconsistent (some adhered to and some violated the sonority hypothesis). Yavaş (2006) led an international study to examine children's use of the sonority hypothesis. The hypothesis was upheld across children with typical speech acquisition who spoke languages as diverse as Turkish, Norwegian, and Israeli Hebrew.

Application to Speech-Language Pathology Practice   Sonority has been used as a theoretical basis for making clinical decisions regarding target selection with children who have a speech sound disorder (Anderson, 2000; Baker, 2000; Ball & Müller, 2002; Gierut, 1998, 1999; Gierut & Champion, 2001). It has been used to analyze children's phonemic awareness skills (Yavaş, 2000; Yavaş & Core, 2001; Yavaş & Gogate, 1999) and productions of consonant clusters of children with speech sound disorders (Anderson, 2000; Baker, 2000; Chin, 1996; Gierut, 1998, 1999; Gierut & Champion, 2001; Wyllie-Smith et al., 2006; Yavaş & McLeod, 2010).

Psycholinguistic Models

Although linguistic applications are useful for the description of children's phonological systems, psycholinguistic applications provide the potential for the explanation of children's phonology. A *psycholinguistic model* draws on the fields of psychology and linguistics and attempts to account for psychological processes or mental mechanisms involved in the "perception, storage, planning and production of speech as it is produced in real time in real utterances" (McCormack, 1997, p. 4). At the simplest level, a psycholinguistic model describes the distinction between underlying representations of words and their production (Fee, 1995). It is used to map interactions between auditory input, underlying cognitive-linguistic processes, and speech production output (Dodd, 1995a). In doing so, psycholinguistic models attempt to provide explanations for the descriptive or symptomatic information derived from linguistic-based assessments (Stackhouse & Wells, 1993). An example of such a model is presented in Chapter 5 (Figure 5.1).

Application to Typically Developing Children   Numerous authors have been involved in the construction of psycholinguistic models of speech development. These include N.V. Smith (1973); Menn and colleagues (Kiparsky & Menn, 1977; Menn, 1971, 1978; Menn & Matthei, 1992; Menn et al., 1993); Macken (1980a, 1980b); Spencer (1986,

1988); Hewlett and colleagues (Hewlett, 1990; Hewlett et al., 1998); and Stackhouse and colleagues (Pascoe et al., 2006; Stackhouse & Wells, 1993, 1997). A number of useful historical accounts and critiques of psycholinguistic models exist (e.g., Bernhardt & Stemberger, 1998; Maxwell, 1984; Menn & Matthei, 1992; Vihman, 1996).

In a psycholinguistic model, the first point of the speech process is the *input*, which is the speech signal that the child hears. The final point of the speech process is the *output*, which is the speech signal (usually words) actually produced/spoken by the child. The possible events that occur between input and output are the focus of psycholinguistic models. Menn (1994) describes psycholinguistic modeling as a black box approach, whereby input and output are examined to construct a mechanism, which can explain the effects seen:

> input ──► black box ──► output

Within the black box, different levels of representation of knowledge are hypothesized. *Underlying representation* refers to "the basic unaltered pronunciation before any processes have had a chance to operate" (Spencer, 1996, p. 50). Thus, the underlying representation is the phonological information that is stored in the speaker's mind about the words known and used:

> input ──► underlying representation ──► output

The child's underlying representation is stored in the *lexicon* or mental dictionary (Maxwell, 1984, p. 18). Depending on the theoretical model being considered, the lexicon may contain semantic or meaning-based information (Bernhardt & Stemberger, 1998) and/or phonological information (e.g., Menn, 1978; N.V. Smith, 1973). Stackhouse and Wells (1997) suggest the lexicon contains phonological, semantic, grammatical, orthographic, and motor programming information. Definitions of the storage, nature, and number of underlying representations differ among researchers.

Initially, *single-lexicon models* of the speech process were posited, whereby children were considered to have an adultlike underlying representation of speech (e.g., N.V. Smith, 1973). The lexicon was synonymous with the underlying representation and contained information about the adult pronunciation of words. Development of single-lexicon models continued through the 1970s (Braine, 1979; Macken, 1980a; N.V. Smith, 1978). However, this was subsequently revised because evidence did not support N.V. Smith's (1973) original assumption that the child's perception was always adultlike. Consequently, N.V. Smith (1978) revised his model by adding a perceptual filter to account for the possibility that the child may have inaccurate perception.

Early single-lexicon models could not account for variable pronunciations, in particular, for instances when different tokens of a word could be pronounced in different ways, and when one phoneme could be pronounced differently in different words (Bernhardt & Stemberger, 1998). Consequently, *two-lexicon models* in which two levels of underlying representation exist—the input and output lexicons—were proposed. The *input lexicon* refers to the perceptually based phonological representations that enable the child to perceive speech, or "all the child's knowledge that permits him or her to recognize a word" (Menn & Matthei, 1992, p. 214). The *output lexicon* refers to the articulatorily based phonological representations that enable the child to produce speech. Menn (1983) described the output lexicon as "ways-to-say-words." If it exists independently, the input lexicon is almost certain to be richer in contrasts than the output lexicon (Hewlett, 1990), and some suggest that the input lexicon contains the same information as the adult surface representations (Spencer, 1988).

input ⟶ input lexicon ⟶ output lexicon ⟶ output

Two-lexicon models allowed for the notion that young children may have underlying representations that are unique to their own system. That is, the output (production) lexicon was able to hold underlying representations that were not adultlike (for a complete discussion, see Maxwell, 1984).

In a two-lexicon account, the child stores underlying adultlike perceptual representations in the input lexicon. These perceptual representations are then modified off-line through the application of rules or processes to create underlying production representations in the output lexicon. Once a child has stored a word in the output lexicon, subsequent productions are accessed from the output lexicon rather than from the input lexicon and modified on-line.

Although two-lexicon models provided a way of accounting for the variability in children's speech, there are three primary criticisms of the two-lexicon accounts (Bernhardt & Stemberger, 1998; Chiat, 1994; Menn & Matthei, 1992; Vihman, 1996). First, with the potential for duplication of lexical items, particularly in the output lexicon, the models fail to explain how children select one representation over another or how representations change to being more adultlike; that is, the models do not explain when and how old forms are deleted (Bernhardt & Stemberger, 1998; Dinnsen et al., 1997; Vihman, 1996). A second criticism concerns the continuity hypothesis (Bernhardt & Stemberger, 1998; Menn, 1994). Developmentalists argue that there should not be one model that applies to children and another for adults because accounting for the shift between the two models is difficult. It has been suggested that a child's output lexicon will eventually match their input lexicon because the forms within the output lexicon will become adultlike; thus, adults may have only a single lexicon. The third major criticism is that both single- and two-lexicon models were designed to describe single-word production and do not take into account constraints that occur between words in connected speech (Hewlett, 1990; Vihman, 1996).

The hard-walled boxes of the two-lexicon accounts are now being represented by connectionist models (Bernhardt & Stemberger, 1998; Menn & Matthei, 1992; see Baker et al., 2001, for a description). Connectionist models use computer modeling to test a cognitive task, such as speech production. Networks of nodes connect the input and output, and during computer simulations, the probability of the activation of each node is tested. Connectionist models can be run many times to provide the probability of a specific output occurring, thus enabling testing of hypotheses of speech and language acquisition.

Application to Speech-Language Pathology Practice   The earliest authors in the field of speech-language pathology to suggest consideration of children's underlying representation were Shriberg and Kwiatkowski (1980) and Edwards (1983). Since then, consideration of underlying representation has been presented in speech-language pathology intervention case studies (e.g., Bryan & Howard, 1992; McGregor & Schwartz, 1992; Stackhouse et al., 2006). Baker and colleagues (2001) provide a tutorial of the application of psycholinguistic models to SLP practice, and an important series of books has been written for SLPs on assessment and intervention for speech and literacy within a psycholinguistic framework (Pascoe et al., 2006; Stackhouse & Wells, 1997, 2001; Stackhouse et al., 2007).

The first part of this chapter included several models of speech sound acquisition that we related to clinical practice. As stated earlier, each model has its strengths, with some perhaps being more helpful than others to one's understanding of how sounds are acquired. In the section that follows, we shift our attention from theories to how to gather data to inform us about how speech sound acquisition has been observed, recorded, and analyzed.

HOW SPEECH SOUND ACQUISITION DATA ARE OBTAINED

It is important for SLPs to be well acquainted with typical speech sound development. Later in this chapter, a wide range of speech acquisition data important to clinical practice is presented. Before getting to the actual developmental data, it is beneficial to understand how these speech acquisition data were obtained, because some are based on small samples of children taken over a long period of time, whereas other data are based on large groups of children seen during a relatively short period of time. Three major techniques have been used for collecting speech acquisition data: diary studies, large-group cross-sectional studies, and longitudinal studies.

Historically, research into typical speech sound acquisition was conducted using diary studies. Famous historical diary studies include descriptions of the speech of children such as Amahl (N.V. Smith, 1973), Hildegarde (Leopold, 1947), and Joan (Velten, 1943). With the influence of behaviorism, large cross-sectional group studies became prevalent. Wellman and colleagues (1931), Poole (1934), and Templin (1957) conducted the earliest cross-sectional group studies relating to English-speaking children's speech sound acquisition. Next, longitudinal studies comprising a smaller group of participants have complemented the large-scale cross-sectional studies to enhance the understanding of speech acquisition (e.g., Carroll et al., 2003; Dodd, 1995a; McLeod et al., 2001b; Walker & Archibald, 2006; Watson & Scukanec, 1997a, 1997b). Each of these methodologies has strengths and weaknesses. A primary difference is in the trade-off between the extent of data analyzed and reported versus the number of participants.

To summarize the discussion of research methods of typical English speech sound acquisition, an overview of key studies is presented later in this chapter. You are encouraged to access the original sources in order to utilize the full range of information offered by these researchers. For a wide-ranging overview of speech acquisition in a range of English dialects and languages other than English, see *The International Guide to Speech Acquisition* (McLeod, 2007a), a summary of consonant acquisition for 27 languages in McLeod and Crowe (2018), and the Multilingual Children's Speech website (https://www.csu.edu.au/research/multilingual-speech/speech-acquisition). Note that most speech acquisition studies have used either cross-sectional or longitudinal data collection methods. Those that used a cross-sectional design typically used single-word sampling. Those that used a longitudinal design typically used connected speech sampling. Each of these research techniques is described in detail next.

Diary Studies of Typical Speech Sound Acquisition

Diary studies were the initial major source of data about children's speech and language development. Typically, a parent who was a linguist or psychologist kept a comprehensive diary of their child's speech and/or language development over a period of time. An early diary study of a child's language development was that of Humphreys (1880). Famous diary studies that have focused on speech development include Leopold's (1939–1949) four-volume account of his daughter Hildegarde, Velten's (1943) study of his daughter Joan, and N.V. Smith's (1973) extensive analysis of his son Amahl's speech.

The parental diary study has continued to be used as a method for data collection, but more specifically to collect data on a specific issue rather than general speech and language development. For example, Berg (1995) collected data from his German-speaking daughter on a daily basis from the age of 3;4 to 4;3. He presented data on interword variation in the development of velars. Other examples of diary studies of typical phonological development include Menn's (1971) report on her son's early constraints on sound sequences, the account by Elbers and Ton (1985) of Elbers's son's words and babbling within the first-word period, Stemberger's (1988) account of his eldest daughter's between-word processes and his (1989) account of both daughters' nonsystemic errors within and across phrases, French's (1989) account of her son's acquisition of word forms in the first 50-word stage, and Lleó's (1990) report of her daughter's use of reduplication and homonymy as phonological strategies. The diary study methodology also has been used to study typical speech acquisition of children where the researchers are not the parents (e.g., Bernstein-Ratner, 1993; Fey & Gandour, 1982).

An extension of diary studies is the single case study methodology that has been particularly beneficial for the documentation of intervention effects on children with speech sound disorder (e.g., Camarata, 1989; Camarata & Gandour, 1985; Crosbie et al., 2006; Crystal, 1987; Grunwell & Yavaş, 1988; Leonard & Leonard, 1985; McGregor & Schwartz, 1992; Pascoe et al., 2005).

Advantages and Disadvantages of Diary Studies

The primary advantage of diary studies is that they contain some of the most detailed accounts of speech acquisition. The depth and breadth of detail enables examination of descriptive, exploratory, and explanatory intent. The detail places change into context because diary studies allow for the retention of the holistic and meaningful characteristics of the child's real-life events (Yin, 1989).

Although general trends about speech acquisition cannot be derived from diary study data, the rich source of data (often contained in appendices) has been used to test and retest statements and hypotheses long after the original reason for collecting the data has been superseded. For example, the extensive data N.V. Smith (1973) provided in his appendices have been reexamined by Braine (1979) and Macken (1980a) to find evidence against N.V. Smith's earlier conclusion that the child's underlying representations must be adultlike. Similarly, Greenlee (1974) reexamined data from a number of cross-linguistic diary studies to describe a sequence of development for consonant clusters.

Using diary studies as the only means to understand children's speech acquisition has a number of disadvantages. First, it is easy to assume that the single child under study is typical unless reference is made to other normative studies. An example can be seen with Leopold's daughter Hildegarde, who replaced word-initial /f/ with a [w] or [v] (Leopold, 1947). These substitutions are atypical according to Ingram and colleagues (1980), who did not find a single such instance in their study of the typical acquisition of fricatives in 73 children. Second, the fact that the children studied are primarily those of linguists suggests that these children may be precocious or at least different in their acquisition from the general population, whether as a result of genetic endowment or environment. Thus, being the child of a linguist may mean either inheriting genes that code for faster language learning or being exposed to more diverse lexical input. This latter point is supported by a study by B. L. Smith and colleagues (2006), who demonstrated that 2-year-old children's phonological performance was more closely related to lexical size than chronological age. Other disadvantages of using diary studies include potential randomness and lack of structure in data collection, and potential observer bias because the parent is often the researcher (Ingram, 1989b). Until recently, many diary studies relied on on-line transcription, making it impossible to determine transcription reliability. Some of these problems were overcome with the introduction of the large-group cross-sectional study and the longitudinal study.

Large-Group Cross-Sectional Studies of Typical Speech Sound Acquisition

From the 1950s to 1970s, behaviorism was a major theoretical paradigm for considering speech sound acquisition, and the emphasis in data collection in the fields of psychology, linguistics, and speech-language pathology moved from diary studies to *large-group cross-sectional studies*. Using this methodology, researchers attempted to describe typical behavior by establishing developmental norms through the observation of large numbers of children. Commonly, children were placed into selected age groupings, and each child underwent the same testing procedure. Possible confounding influences such as gender, socioeconomic status, language background, and intelligence were controlled. The results of these experiments were presented as proportions and percentages, often in large tables indicating the age of acquisition of phonemes or the age of decline of certain phonological processes or patterns.

The majority of research describing the typical acquisition of English speech sounds uses large-group cross-sectional methodology (Anthony et al., 1971; Arlt & Goodban, 1976; Bankson & Bernthal, 1990, 2020; Chirlian & Sharpley, 1982; Dodd et al., 2002; Flipsen, 2006a; Haelsig & Madison, 1986; Ingram et al., 1985; Irwin & Wong, 1983; James, 2001; Kilminster & Laird, 1978; Lowe et al., 1985; McLeod & Arciuli, 2009; Olmsted, 1971; Paynter & Petty, 1974; Poole, 1934; Prather et al., 1975; Preisser et al., 1988; Smit, 1993a, 1993b; Smit et al., 1990; Templin, 1957; Wellman et al., 1931).

Wellman and colleagues (1931) and Poole (1934) conducted the pioneering large-group cross-sectional studies of typical speech acquisition. However, the most famous study was conducted in 1957 when Templin undertook an extensive study of the speech development of 480 children aged 3;0 to 8;0. She provided comprehensive text, 71 tables, and 9 figures to explain children's acquisition of articulation, speech sound discrimination, sentence development, and vocabulary as well as academic performance. Templin presented the age of acquisition at which 75% of children could produce each speech sound in initial-, medial-, and final-word positions. Templin's classic study has been quoted as an authoritative source on speech development by researchers (e.g., Powell & Elbert, 1984; Smit, 1986; Stockman & Stephenson, 1981; Young, 1987) and SLPs (e.g., Stewart & Weybright, 1980) for many years. Templin's study was considered to need updating in 1976 by Arlt and Goodban, who noted "expanding effects of television, earlier schooling ... the accelerating effects of developments in education" and suggested that "for purposes of revalidation it seems appropriate to update or examine such norms at 10-year intervals"

(Arlt & Goodban, 1976, p. 173). Their suspicions possibly were confirmed when they found that "33% of the sounds tested in this investigation were produced correctly by 75% of the children at least 1 year earlier than would be expected from previously established norms" (p. 176).

The largest and most currently cited large-group cross-sectional study of American English was undertaken by Smit and colleagues (1990), who studied 997 children's productions of consonants and consonant clusters. They not only reported age of acquisition of phonemes but also presented graphical data (Sander, 1972) that indicated the progression of development from age 3;0 to 9;0. These graphs described the trajectory for boys' and girls' speech acquisition. Other large-group cross-sectional studies of speech acquisition include those by Kilminster and Laird (1978), who studied the speech acquisition of 1,756 Australian English-speaking children; Nagy (1980), who studied the speech acquisition of 7,602 Hungarian children; and Nakanishi and colleagues (1972), who studied the speech acquisition of 1,689 Japanese children. The largest studies of Spanish-speaking children were conducted by Acevedo (1993) and Jimenez (1987), who each studied 120 Mexican children.

Recently, two review papers have been published that summarize consonant acquisition data from large-group cross-sectional studies of more than 10 children. First, McLeod and Crowe (2018) summarized consonant acquisition data from 64 studies reporting on a total of 26,007 children speaking 27 languages across 31 countries. Their analysis also included summaries of English consonant acquisition data from 15 studies of 7,369 children who spoke English in Australia, the Republic of Ireland, Malaysia, South Africa, the United Kingdom, and the United States. Second, Crowe and McLeod (2020) summarized English consonant acquisition data from 15 studies of 18,907 children from the United States. Similar findings for the acquisition of English were identified across both studies (see Table 3.3); specifically, that most consonants are acquired by the age of 5 years.

Advantages and Disadvantages of Large-Group Cross-Sectional Studies

The primary advantage of large-group cross-sectional studies is that they provide normative information by which to compare children. Such norms are beneficial to SLPs in the identification of impairment. It is assumed that if enough participants are selected for each age group, then typical behavior is observed. Consequently, general trends are ascertained from summary tables provided by such studies. Another advantage of large-group cross-sectional studies is that the emphasis on methodology encourages systematic observation of behavior (Ingram, 1989b). All participants are studied for the same amount of time for the same behaviors. The third advantage of large-group cross-sectional studies is that there is an emphasis on standardized measurement tools so that studies can be replicated.

Disadvantages of such studies include the facts that 1) they typically are collected using single-word, not connected, speech samples; 2) they often use imitated (rather than spontaneous) productions; 3) they collect data in specific geographical regions that may have dialectical variants; and 4) the experience and reliability of examiners is not always reported (Smit, 1986). Additionally, Peña and colleagues (2006) questioned the assumptions behind the selection of children for participation in large-group cross-sectional studies. They argued that, traditionally, children were excluded from cross-sectional studies if they were not experiencing typical development. However, Peña and colleagues indicated that this strategy was akin to "shooting ourselves in the foot." They concluded that if the purpose of a normative study is to identify children who are not developing typically, then the normative sample should include children who are not developing typically. Although their study addressed the area of children's language, their claims are likely to also be true for children's speech.

To conclude, the major strengths of the large-group cross-sectional studies are also a weakness. The grouping of data for statistical analyses means that the data collected for individual children are not reported. The only glimpse of individual variation can be found in the standard deviations from the mean. Longitudinal studies, a third approach, can elucidate individual variability and provide additional insights into children's speech acquisition.

Longitudinal Studies of Typical Speech Sound Acquisition

The possibility that children follow different paths and strategies in typical speech and language acquisition prompted a shift in focus from the large-group studies to *longitudinal studies* of smaller groups of children. Ingram (1989b) expressed the concern that many of the diary and large-group studies considered only superficial issues, such as the timing of the occurrence of particular features in children's speech. Quotes such as the following from Khan (1982, p. 78) occur commonly within the literature expressing the need for "controlled, longitudinal examination of large numbers of children."

Longitudinal studies of speech sound acquisition are characterized by the study of groups of children at repeated intervals. These studies are usually conducted for specific purposes that are beyond describing the age of acquisition of phonemes, such as writing rules and explaining the acquisition process. Longitudinal studies share a number of characteristics with diary case studies, in that they study the same children over time; however, they have three primary differences. First, the researcher is independent (recall that diary studies often were conducted by the parent of the child). Second, instead of only one or two children, a small group typically is studied. Third, children in longitudinal studies usually are studied for a set period of time each week or month instead of daily or at random intervals. Thus, longitudinal studies have the potential to capitalize on the strengths of both diary and large-group studies.

Ferguson and Farwell (1975) conducted one of the earliest and most influential longitudinal studies of speech development. They studied the emergence of words and sounds in early language development, plotting the progress of three young children and the point of 50 words in the children's vocabularies. The data for one of the children were extracted from the diary of Leopold's (1947) daughter Hildegarde; Ferguson and Farwell personally studied the other two children and presented phone trees of data to demonstrate individual learning strategies undertaken by these children.

Since Ferguson and Farwell's original work, a number of longitudinal studies considering different aspects of the development of young children's phonology have been conducted (e.g., Anderson, 2004; Dodd, 1995b; Dyson, 1986, 1988; Dyson & Paden, 1983; Fee & Ingram, 1982; McLeod et al., 2001b; Otomo & Stoel-Gammon, 1992; Robb & Bleile, 1994; Schwartz et al., 1980; Stoel-Gammon, 1985; Vihman & Greenlee, 1987; Walker & Archibald, 2006; Watson & Scukanec, 1997a, 1997b). For example, Robb and Bleile (1994) conducted a comprehensive longitudinal study of the consonant inventories of seven children aged 8–25 months and were able to present valuable individualized data on the sequence of development over time. Similarly, Selby and colleagues (2000) studied the development of vowels in five children aged 15, 18, 21, 24, and 36 months of age.

Advantages and Disadvantages of Longitudinal Studies

There are two major advantages of conducting longitudinal studies of a select group of children. First, studying a small group of children allows researchers to capture individual variations in approaches to learning that may be masked by a large-group study. Knowing about these individual differences increases the likelihood of creating successful individualized teaching and learning experiences for SLP clients. Second, longitudinal studies allow for the reporting of developmental trends (Macken, 1995). For example, Lleó and Prinz (1996) reported that German- and Spanish-speaking children produced word shapes in the following developmental sequence: CV → CVC → CVCC → CCVCC. Knowing about typical developmental sequences enhances the ability of SLPs to assess whether their clients are delayed or disordered and may yield a more accurate understanding of the learning process, which could be replicated in intervention strategies.

Interestingly, despite the unique data that result from longitudinal studies, not all such studies report individual developmental information. For example, Dyson and Paden (1983) conducted a longitudinal study of 40 children and reported grouped findings from the first and eighth observations; however, they did use their data to propose sequences of development.

Longitudinal studies have three major disadvantages. First, longitudinal studies frequently use small numbers of children. As a result, the findings may not be representative of the general population. Second, longitudinal studies generally have regularly scheduled intervals of weeks or months between visits. Such scheduling may allow the child to show considerable change between observations. On the other hand, possible crucial periods of change may occur over a day or two, and a flexible schedule may be more appropriate to allow emergency visits when alerted by parental reports of change (Ingram, 1989b). Finally, researchers using longitudinal methodology often prepare stimulus materials for elicitation; thus, a picture of the child's natural speech may not be obtained (French, 1989).

Combined Data-Collection Procedures

To obtain the advantages of both cross-sectional and longitudinal methodologies, a number of researchers have developed combined methodologies. Some fundamentally cross-sectional studies have assessed children more than once, thus gaining some longitudinal continuity in their data. For example, Roberts and colleagues (1990) used a combination of cross-sectional and longitudinal methodologies in their examination of 145 children between the ages of 2;6 and 8;0. Over the 6-year period, 13 of these children were examined six times, 24 were tested five times, and so on, with 32 being tested only once. Similarly, Stoel-Gammon (1985) studied 33 children's development of phonetic inventories; 7 children were studied at age 15 months, 19 children at age 18 months, 32 children at age 21 months, and 33 children at age 24 months. Neither of these studies presented individualized longitudinal results.

Another approach is to undertake a longitudinal study in which children are studied over time, but different cohorts of children are studied at different ages (e.g., Chervela, 1981; Dyson, 1988). For example, Chervela conducted a longitudinal and cross-sectional study (p. 63) of the development of medial consonant clusters in four children aged 1;6 to 3;0. He selected one child at each of the ages of 1;6, 2;0, 2;6, and 3;0. The data were collected for each child once a month for 6 months. A combination of data-collection methodologies enables researchers to manipulate the advantages and disadvantages of each methodology to provide more comprehensive findings about the typical developmental sequence. As Stokes and colleagues (2005, p. 828) recommend: "Large-scale longitudinal studies, combined with statistical analyses, would provide the best possible view of the nature of phonemic development." With this understanding of data-collection procedures, we next explore data that have been collected on children's speech acquisition.

OVERALL SEQUENCE OF SPEECH SOUND ACQUISITION

It takes a child many years to progress from the first cries at birth to intelligible speech incorporating adultlike production of vowels, consonants, syllable structures, and prosody (including tones, if applicable). The four phases of speech acquisition (adapted from Bleile, 2004) are:

Phase 1.   Laying the foundations for speech (birth–1 year)

Phase 2.   Transitioning from words to speech (1–2 years)

Phase 3.   The growth of the inventory (2–5 years)

Phase 4.   Mastery of speech and literacy (5+ years)

During the first year, the child produces sounds, first reflexively and then more purposefully. Children cry, coo, and babble during their first year, and toward the end of this time, they produce their first words. Within Phase 2, children's communicative focus is on transitioning from words to speech. During their second year, they can produce a small vocabulary with a simplified phonological structure. During Phase 3, from 2 to 5 years of age, children learn to produce the majority of speech sounds and syllable structures as well as grammatical and syntactical structures. Finally, Phase 4 is a period of mastery that includes the sophistication of timing, prosody, and accurate production of polysyllabic words and consonant clusters. Additionally, sounds are conveyed through writing (reading and spelling) and are no longer only in the spoken domain. Each phase of speech acquisition is described further in the sections that follow.

PHASE 1: LAYING THE FOUNDATIONS FOR SPEECH

Development of the Structure and Function of the Oral Mechanism

An interrelationship exists between the ability to produce intelligible speech and the development of a child's oromotor, neurological, respiratory, and laryngeal systems (Kent, 1976). Children learn to speak in the context of a changing vocal tract. The development of oral structure and function begins in the fetus, starts to approximate the adult configuration at age 6 years, and is finished at approximately 18 years of age (Kent & Tilkens, 2007). The development of the anatomical structures and functions that support speech acquisition are described next.

Anatomical Structures Supporting Speech Acquisition

The vocal tract of the newborn differs both in size and shape from that of an adult. It is three times smaller than that of the adult and is considered to be similar to a single tube to facilitate coordination between breathing, sucking, and swallowing (Kent & Tilkens, 2007; Vorperian et al., 1999). The adult vocal tract is considered to be akin to two tubes, with the oral tube enabling a wide variety of articulations and the laryngeal tube facilitating coordination between breathing and swallowing. The newborn's larynx is located between the first and fourth cervical vertebrae; however, by 6 years of age, it has descended to the adultlike position between the fourth and seventh vertebrae (Kent & Tilkens, 2007). Vorperian and colleagues (2005) indicated that children's tongues reach 70% of the adult size by 6 years of age, with no sex differences noted. From puberty onward, there is a significant sex difference in the overall vocal tract length and the proportions of the pharyngeal and oral cavities (Fitch & Giedd, 1999).

In infancy, the respiratory system consists of a "bellows-like displacement of the diaphragm" (Kent & Tilkens, 2007, p. 9), and infants' breathing rate at rest is between 30 and 80 breaths per minute. By age 6 months, the infant's rib cage is horizontal, and by 1 year of age, respiration for speech and breathing is differentiated (Parham et al., 2011). Respiration matures at approximately 7 years of age, when the lung architecture is similar to that of an adult (Kent & Tilkens, 2007). However, during speaking tasks, children still have greater subglottal air pressure than adults. Low birth weight is a major factor in poor adult respiratory function, as identified in a large prospective longitudinal birth cohort study conducted by Canoy and associates (2007).

Neurological development is also important for speech acquisition, and significant neurological development occurs over the life span (Sowell et al., 2004). The central auditory system appears to be particularly sensitive to phonology during the last trimester of pregnancy through to the end of the first year of life (Ruben, 1997). Between infancy and adolescence, brain weight and intracranial space grows by approximately 25% and then declines in late adulthood to brain volumes similar to those of young children (Courchesne et al., 2000). In a longitudinal study, Sowell, Thompson, Leonard, and colleagues (2004) studied children between the ages of 5 and 11 years and found that brain growth progressed at a rate of 0.4 to 1.5 millimeter per year. They also found that significant thickening was restricted to left Broca's and Wernicke's areas; gray matter thickness was correlated with changing cognitive abilities. Additionally, rapid myelination occurs during the first year of life (Barkovich et al., 1988) and is important for gross- and fine-motor movements, including speech (Bleile, 2007).

Anatomical Functions Supporting Speech Acquisition

Mastery of precision of articulatory movements of the lip, jaw, and tongue commences in infancy and continues to develop well into adolescence (Walsh & Smith, 2002). Green and colleagues (2002) examined vertical movements of the upper lip, lower lip, and jaw during speech for children and adults. They found that jaw movements matured before lip movements, with 1- and 2-year-old children's jaw movements being similar to adults' jaw movements. However, the upper and lower lip movements were more variable and became more adultlike with maturation. Steeve and colleagues (2008) found that different mandibular control for sucking, chewing, and babbling matured as children progressed from 9 months to 12 months to 15 months of age. Cheng and colleagues used electropalatography (EPG) and electromagnetic articulography (EMA) to conduct a number of studies of the maturation of tongue control for speech in children, adolescents, and adults (Cheng et al., 2007; Cheng et al., 2007a, 2007b). Using EPG, Cheng and colleagues (2007a) found that children's tongue/palate contact for the sounds /t/, /l/, /s/, and /k/ largely resembled those of adults; however, the children aged 6–11 years displayed increased palatal contact and an excessively posterior tongue placement compared with adults. The researchers also indicated that the maturation of the speech motor system was nonuniform and that significant changes in the maturation of tongue control occurred until 11 years of age. During adolescence, tongue control was continually refined. Cheng and associates (2007b) used EMA to consider the coordination of tongue and jaw. They found that maturation continued until 8–11 years of age with continual refinement into adolescence. The relationship between the tongue-tip and tongue-body movement with the jaw differed. The tongue-tip became increasingly synchronized with jaw movement, but the tongue-body retained movement independence with the jaw.

Speech and articulation rates also have been studied in children (Flipsen, 2002a; Ozanne, 1992; Robb et al., 2003; Robb & Gillon, 2007; Robbins & Klee, 1987; P. Williams & Stackhouse, 1998, 2000) and are relevant to our consideration of the maturation of oral functioning. Increasing rate may serve as an indicator of improving control over the articulators. P. Williams and Stackhouse (1998) suggested that typically developing children aged 3–5 years increased their accuracy and consistency but not rate of production during diadochokinetic (DDK) tasks. P. Williams and Stackhouse (2000) suggested that rate was not as useful a predictor as accuracy and consistency of response. Similarly, Walker and Archibald (2006) conducted a longitudinal study of articulation rates in children 4, 5, and 6 years old. They found that articulation rate did not increase significantly with age. However, Flipsen (2002a) reviewed a series of studies of articulation rate and concluded that rate does increase across the developmental period.

Infant Perception

Another important foundation of speech acquisition is infant perception.

Infant Auditory Perception

Humans are able to perceive sound well before birth (Lasky & Williams, 2005). For example, in a study of 400 fetuses at 16 weeks' gestation, it was found that they were able to respond to pure tone auditory stimuli at 500 Hz (Shahidullah & Hepper, 1992). In a follow-up study, Hepper and Shahidullah (1994) described the progression of the fetuses' responses to different sound frequencies:

- 19 weeks' gestation. Fetuses responded to 500 Hz.

- 27 weeks' gestation. Fetuses responded to 250 and 500 Hz (but not 1,000 and 3,000 Hz).

- 33 to 35 weeks' gestation. Fetuses responded to 250, 500, 1,000, and 3,000 Hz.

As the fetuses matured, they required a lower intensity of sound (20 to 30 dB) in order to respond. Hepper and Shahidullah (1994, p. F81) concluded that "the sensitivity of the fetus to sounds in the low frequency range may promote language acquisition." Another study demonstrated that fetuses demonstrate the ability not only to hear but also to perceive differences in sounds. DeCasper and colleagues (1994) asked mothers to recite a nursery rhyme to their fetus three times a day for 4 weeks between 33 and 37 weeks' gestation. They found that the fetuses responded with a change in heart rate when presented with a recorded version of the nursery rhyme but not when presented with an alternative rhyme. They concluded that by the third trimester, "fetuses become familiar with recurrent, maternal speech sounds" (DeCasper et al., 1994, p. 159).

After birth, infants demonstrate sophisticated perceptual skills. Traditionally, the main experimental technique that has been used to ascertain infants' ability to discriminate sounds is the *high-amplitude sucking technique* developed by Siqueland and Delucia (1969). Using this technique, infants sucked on a nonnutritive nipple that was equipped to detect changes in pressure. Experimenters found that infants sucked vigorously when a new sound was played, but as they became familiar with it, their sucking decreased in frequency and intensity. When a new sound was played, their sucking again became vigorous and then diminished with familiarity with the signal. More recently, *event-related potentials (ERPs)* have been used to determine infants' ability to discriminate aspects of communication (e.g., Shafer et al., 1998). Event-related potentials are low-amplitude neurophysiological responses that follow presentation of a stimulus and are typically recorded via electrophysiological instrumentation such as electroencephalograms (EEGs) or electromyograms (EMGs). ERPs are suitable for studying infants' perceptions because they are noninvasive and require no overt response. Using both of these techniques (high-amplitude sucking, ERPs), researchers have discovered that infants prefer voices rather than other sound stimuli and have the ability to discriminate speech sounds.

The fact that infants demonstrate a preference for voices, particularly their mothers' voices, has been shown by a number of researchers (e.g., Augustyn & Zuckerman, 2007). For example, DeCasper and Fifer (1980) demonstrated that by 3 days of age, children can distinguish their mothers' voices from a stranger's voice and show a preference for their mothers' voices. Infants appear to prefer child-directed speech (also called motherese) to adult-directed speech. Cooper and Aslin (1990) found that this held true for children as young as 2 days old and was still apparent in children who were 1 month old.

Infants also have been shown to be able to discriminate both place and voicing features of consonants. For example, Eimas (1974) showed that children who were 2 months old could discriminate between the place contrast of /d/ and /g/. Similarly, Aslin and colleagues (1983) showed that children could discriminate between /f/ and /θ/ (which also differ by place). A number of authors have demonstrated that infants can discriminate between voiced and voiceless consonants. Eimas and colleagues (1971) showed that infants who were 1 and 4 months old could discriminate between synthesized voiced and voiceless contrasts such as in the stimuli /pa/ and /ba/. Similarly, Eilers and associates (1977) demonstrated that 6-month-old infants could discriminate /sa/ and /za/.

As children are exposed to their native language and reach the end of their first year, some authors suggest that their ability to discriminate nonnative sounds diminishes. It has been reported that by as early as 2 days of age, the neonate can discriminate acoustic distinctions that are language specific. By age 12 months children have the ability to categorize only phonemes in their native language (Ruben, 1997). However, more research is needed prior to confirming this view (Rvachew, 2007a) because we do not know whether all infants can discriminate all phonetic inputs, nor do we know that all infants lose the ability to discriminate language-specific inputs. Some research indicates that infants may retain the ability to discriminate vowels without supporting input (Polka & Bohn, 2003), whereas other children may lose the ability to perceive contrasts despite receiving supporting input (Nittrouer, 2001). A significant relationship exists between infants' speech perception and subsequent language skills at 2–3 years (Tsao et al., 2004) and vocabulary and receptive language skills in older children (Edwards et al., 2002; Vance et al., 2009).

Infant Visual Perception

In addition to auditory perception, visual speech perception plays a critical role in infants' learning of language. It has long been known that infants prefer looking at faces compared with objects and are even able to discriminate and imitate facial expressions (Field et al., 1982). However, it also has been discovered that infants are able to distinguish between familiar and unfamiliar languages using only visual cues (Weikum et al., 2007). Weikum and colleagues found that infants of 4 and 6 months of age were able to distinguish between English (familiar) and French (unfamiliar) using a video (without auditory input) of an adult; however, by 8 months of age, this ability had been lost.

Infant Production

Infants enter the world being able to vocalize through crying. Throughout their first months, the repertoire of sounds and prosodic features increases. Two developmental summaries of early speech production follow, one based on work by Stark and colleagues and the other based on work by Oller and colleagues.

Stark's Typology of Infant Phonations

The *Stark Assessment of Early Vocal Development–Revised* (hereafter referred to as *Stark Assessment*) is based on work by Stark and colleagues (Nathani et al., 2006; Stark et al., 1983). This typology includes five levels of development of infant vocalizations (see Box 3.1). Level 1 comprises *reflexive* sounds, including *quasi-resonant nuclei (Q)*, defined as "faint low-pitched grunt-like sounds with muffled resonance" (Nathani et al., 2006, p. 367). Reflexive vocalizations are common between 0 and 6 weeks of age (Stark et al., 1983) and include fussing and crying. McGlaughlin and Grayson (2003) indicated that the mean amount of crying within a 24-hour period fell from 90 minutes when children were from 1 to 3 months of age, to 60–65 minutes from 4 to 9 months of age, and then went back to 86 minutes from 10 to 12 months of age. However, McGlaughlin and Grayson reported that other studies show a decrease in crying after 10 months of age.

Level 2 of the *Stark Assessment* is called *control of phonation*. During this level, *fully resonant nuclei (F)* occur and are defined as "vowel-like sounds . . . that have energy across a wide range of frequencies (not restricted to low frequencies like Q)" (Q refers to the quasi-resonant nuclei as defined previously) (Nathani et al., 2006, p. 367). Additionally, both *closants* (consonant-like segments such as a raspberry, click, or isolated consonant) and *vocants* (vowel-like segments) are produced during Level 2. During Level 3, *expansion,* infants produce isolated vowels, two or more vowels in a row, vowel glide combinations, ingressive sounds, squeals, and marginal babbling. Marginal babbling comprises a series of closant and vocant segments. Additionally, Gratier and Devouche (2011) reported that 3-month-old infants and their mothers selectively imitated a variety of prosodic contours during vocalization. Level 4, *basic canonical syllables,* occurs between 5 and 10 months of age. Infants during this level produce canonical babbling, single consonant-vowel syllables, whispered productions, disyllables (CVCV), and a consonant-vowel combination followed by a consonant (CV-C). Canonical babbling is seen as an important stage in the transition from babbling to speech. Nathani and associates (2006) define *canonical babbling* as including both reduplicated babbling (e.g., [baba]) and nonreduplicated babbling (e.g., [badu]). It is important for SLPs to pay attention to infants' babbling because late

---

BOX 3.1   Two typologies of infants' vocalizations

Typology 1: *Stark Assessment of Early Vocal Development–Revised* (Nathani et al., 2006)

1. *Reflexive* (0–2 months). Vegetative sounds, sustained crying/fussing, quasi-resonant nuclei (Q) ("faint low-pitched grunt-like sounds with muffled resonance" [p. 367])

2. *Control of phonation* (1–4 months). Fully resonant nuclei (F), two or more Fs, closants (consonant-like segments: raspberry, click, isolated consonant), vocants (vowel-like segments), closant-vocant combinations, chuckles, or sustained laughter

3. *Expansion* (3–8 months). Isolated vowels, two or more vowels in a row, vowel glide, ingressive sounds, squeals, marginal babbling

4. *Basic canonical syllables* (5–10 months). Single consonant-vowel syllable, canonical babbling, whispered productions, consonant-vowel combination followed by a consonant (CV-C), disyllables (CVCV)

5. *Advanced forms* (9–18 months). Complex syllables (e.g., VC, CCV, CCVC), jargon, diphthongs

Typology 2: Oller's typology of infant phonations (Oller, 2000; Oller et al., 2006)

1. Non-speechlike vocalizations

   a. *Vegetative sounds.* Burps, hiccups

   b. *Fixed vocal signal.* Crying, laughing, groaning

2. Speechlike vocalizations (protophones)

   a. *Quasi-vowels* (0–2 months). Vowel-like productions without shaping of the articulators

   b. *Primitive articulation stage* (2–3 months). Vowel-like productions produced by shaping the articulators

   c. *Expansion stage* (3–6 months). Marginal babbling comprising a consonant-like and a vowel-like sound

   d. *Canonical babbling* (6+ months). Well-formed syllables such as [baba]

---

onset of canonical babbling may be a predictor of later speech sound disorders. For example, Oller and colleagues (1999) found children who had late onset of canonical babbling had smaller production vocabularies at 1;6, 2;0, and 3;0 years of age.

The final level (Level 5) of the *Stark Assessment* is titled *advanced forms*. This level typically occurs between 9 and 18 months of age. During this time, children produce complex syllables (e.g., VC, CCV, CCVC), jargon, and diphthongs. Nathani and colleagues (2006) applied the *Stark Assessment* to 30 infants in a mixed cross-sectional and longitudinal design spanning five age ranges from 0 to 20 months of age. They found that as the children increased in age, speechlike utterances increased in frequency, whereas non-speechlike utterances decreased in frequency. Productions typically associated with Levels 1 and 2 decreased with age, whereas productions associated with Level 4 were rarely produced before 9 months of age. Level 5 vocalizations occurred only 10% from 0 to 15 months but jumped to 20% by 16 to 20 months of age.

Oller's Typology of Infant Phonations

Oller and colleagues (Oller, 2000; Oller et al., 2006) indicated that infants' vocalizations can be classified as being non-speechlike and speechlike (see Box 3.1). Non-speechlike vocalizations include *vegetative sounds,* such as burps and hiccups, and *fixed vocal signals,* such as crying, laughing, and groaning. Speechlike vocalizations are then classified into four stages of development: quasi-vowels, primitive articulation stage, expansion stage, and canonical babbling. From 0 to 2 months of age, children phonate and produce quasi-vowels (vowel-like productions) and glottals (Oller et al., 1999). The phase between 2 and 3 months of age (the primitive articulation stage) is where children begin to produce vowel-like sounds that are sometimes called *gooing* (Oller et al., 1999) or *cooing* (Stark et al., 1983). From 3 to 6 months of age (the expansion stage), children expand their repertoires, producing full vowels and raspberries (Oller et al., 1999). They also begin to produce syllablelike vocalizations (Stark et al., 1983) or marginal babbling (Oller et al., 1999). From 6 months of age onward, infants produce canonical babbling; that is, well-formed canonical syllables (e.g., [babababa]) (Oller et al., 1999).

Babbling and Speech

The developmental typologies mentioned earlier indicate that children's babble consists of a series of consonants and vowels. However, over the years, there have been differing views on the importance of babbling to children's speech acquisition. Some time ago, Jakobson (1968, p. 24) described babbling as "purposeless egocentric soliloquy" and "biologically orientated tongue delirium.'" More recent researchers have opposed Jakobson's extreme views that babbling and speech are discontinuous. Indeed, most researchers now believe that there is continuity between babbling and early speech (Davis & MacNeilage, 1995; Storkel & Morrisette, 2002) and suggest that babbling and early words share consonants (such as /m, n, p, b, t, d/) and vowels.

It has been proposed that babbling leads to independent control of the articulators. For example, Davis and MacNeilage (1995) have suggested that as children develop control of their jaw movements, using "rhythmic mandibular oscillation" (p. 1199), their babbling increases and becomes refined. The frame-content theory proposed by MacNeilage and Davis (1993) states that the frames (syllablelike structures) and content (segmentlike structures) emerge in infants as a result of this rhythmic opening and closing of the jaw accompanied by vocalization.

There are differences between the babbling of children who are typically developing and those who have additional learning needs. For example, researchers compared the babbling of children with hearing loss to children who were typically developing (Oller & Eilers, 1988; Stoel-Gammon & Otomo, 1986). They found that babies with hearing loss babbled later, babbled less frequently, used fewer syllables, were more likely to use single syllables than repeated syllable combinations, and used a disproportionate number of glides and glottal sequences. Morris (2010) reviewed studies of the babbling of 207 infants and found that late talking (defined as talking that begins at 24 months) could be predicted by a lower-than-expected mean babbling level. The babbling of late talkers has also been found to be different from typically developing children. Stoel-Gammon (1989) indicated that less canonical babbling was produced by late talkers from 9 to 21 months than for typically developing children.

As children near their first birthdays, they utter their first words. These words are to be distinguished from babbling and from phonetically consistent forms (PCFs). Owens (1994) suggested two indicators that designate production of true words:

1. The child's utterance must have a phonetic relationship to an adult word (i.e., it sounds somewhat similar).

2. The child must use the word consistently in the presence of a particular situation or object.

Therefore, if a child babbled mama but their mother was not present, this would not qualify as a word because there was no referent. Similarly, phonetically consistent forms that children regularly produce that do not have a relationship to an adult word (e.g., taka for *dog*) are not true words because they do not meet the first indicator.

PHASE 2: TRANSITIONING FROM WORDS TO SPEECH

Children's First 50 Words

Children's pronunciation in the first 50-word stage appears to be constrained by their physiology, ambient language, and child-specific factors (Vihman, 1992). There is much individual and phonetic variability during this stage (Grunwell, 1982). First words typically consist of one or sometimes two syllables and are of the following shapes: CV, VC, CVCV. Consonants produced at the front of the mouth predominate (e.g., /p, b, d, t, m, n/) (Robb & Bleile, 1994). Final consonants are typically omitted or followed by a vowel (e.g., *dog* may be produced as *do* or *doggy*). Young children also produce a limited repertoire of vowels. According to Donegan (2002), children favor low, nonrounded vowels during their first year and produce height differences in vowels before they produce front-back differences. Common phonological processes (or patterns) produced by young children include reduplication, final consonant deletion, and cluster reduction.

It has been suggested that young children use selection (preferences) and avoidance strategies in the words they produce. Possible selection patterns are the size and complexity of syllables and the sound types included (Ferguson, 1978). As well, early words are thought to be initially learned as whole word patterns or unanalyzed wholes rather than a sequence of individual sounds. Homonyms are common in children's early words (e.g., *tap* for *tap, cap, clap; no* for *no, snow, nose*). Researchers suggest that children can approach homonyms in two ways: Sometimes, they use them to increase their lexicon; at other times, they appear to limit the number of homonyms to be intelligible. As children mature, the number of homonyms decreases (McLeod et al., 1998, 2001a).

Two different learning styles have been suggested for children learning to speak. Vihman and Greenlee (1987) conducted a comprehensive longitudinal study comparing the speech development of 10 typically developing children between 9 and 17 months of age and then examined them again at age 3. They reported wide individual variation, particularly for specific segment substitutions and cluster reductions. They described two differing learning styles that were evident in their children at 1 year and remained at 3 years of age. They proposed a continuum of tolerance for variability on which they could place the children as being either systematic (and stable) or exploratory (and variable) (Vihman & Greenlee, 1987, p. 519). These two learning styles are reminiscent of the research into the learning styles used by young children in language acquisition (Bates et al., 1995). Bates and associates described children with learning style 1 as being word oriented and having high intelligibility, a segmental emphasis, and consistent pronunciation across word tokens. In contrast, children with learning style 2 were described as intonation oriented, having low intelligibility, a suprasegmental emphasis, and variable pronunciation across word tokens.

Young Children's Consonant Inventories

Children's early consonant inventories have nasal, plosive, fricative, approximant, labial, and lingual phonemes (Grunwell, 1981). As children grow older, the number of consonants in their inventories increases. In a large study of more than 1,700 children, Ttofari-Eecen and colleagues (2007) reported that by age 1;0, children had an average of 4.4 consonants in their inventories (median = 4; range = 0–16), and typically these were /m, d, b, n/. Robb and Bleile (1994) conducted a longitudinal study of seven children, examining phonetic inventories from ages 0;8 to 2;1. The most frequent manner of articulation was stops, and the most frequent places of articulation were toward the front of the mouth: labials and alveolars. Their findings, summarized in Table 3.1, demonstrate the broader range of consonants produced in syllable-initial compared with syllable-final position. For example, at 8 months of age, the children produced five syllable-initial consonants (typically /d, t, k, m, h/) and three syllable-final consonants (typically /t, m, h/). By age 2;1, children produced 15 syllable-initial consonants and 11 syllable-final consonants.

Table 3.1. Summary of studies of English-speaking children's consonant inventories

Age	Number of syllable-initial consonants	Number of syllable-final consonants
0;8	5	3
0;9	5	2
0;10	6	4
0;11	4	2
1;0	5	2
1;1	6	2
1;2	10	2
1;3	6	2
1;4	6	2
1;5	9	3
1;6	6	3
1;7	11	6
1;8	10	5
1;9	9	4
1;10	11	3
1;11	12	5
2;0	10	4
2;1	15	11

Phonological Knowledge and Vocabulary Acquisition

A close relationship appears to exist between young children's phonological knowledge and their acquisition of vocabulary (Stoel-Gammon, 2011; Storkel, 2006). According to Storkel, phonological knowledge can be defined in terms of three phonotactic constraints:

1. *Inventory constraints.* Inventory of sounds that are produced by the child

2. *Positional constraints.* Sounds that are produced in different syllable positions

3. *Sequence constraints.* Restrictions on the co-occurrence of sounds

During the first year of life, children learn words that are consistent with phonotactic constraints within their babbling. According to Locke (2002, p. 249), "The sounds babbled most frequently are produced more accurately by English-learning 2-year-olds, and appear more often in the languages of the world, than other sounds."

Sounds within a child's inventory are sometimes described as IN sounds, and those not used within their inventories are described as OUT sounds. Much research has been conducted on the perception and production of IN and OUT sounds for infants who have learned fewer than 50 words. These young children appear to have opposite preferences for perception and production. Infants tend to listen to OUT sounds longer than to IN sounds (Vihman & Nakai, 2003, cited in Storkel, 2006). However, when infants are taught to produce new words, they tend to learn words containing IN sounds more quickly than those with OUT sounds (Schwartz & Leonard, 1982). Storkel (2005, 2006) extended this work by considering the role of IN and OUT sounds in word learning for preschool children beyond the 50-word stage. She found that these older children were more accurate in learning words containing OUT sounds than they were in learning words containing IN sounds. This finding held for both typically developing children and children with speech impairment and was counter to the finding for the younger children in the first 50-word stage.

PHASE 3: THE GROWTH OF THE INVENTORY

This section discusses the third phase of speech acquisition and focuses on typical acquisition of aspects of speech sound production beyond approximately 2–5 years of age. Traditionally, many SLPs' understanding of typical speech sound acquisition has been informed by normative data on the age of acquisition of phonemes (e.g., Smit et al., 1990) and the age at which phonological processes disappear (e.g., Grunwell, 1981). These measures typically address the final product; that is, the age of mastery of certain phonemes and phonological processes. In addition to such data, however, many other data on typical speech sound acquisition are available and should be used in clinical decision making. For example, data on the route of development include typical range of errors of phonemic, phonetic, and syllable inventories. This shift in emphasis to include both the end-point and the route of development equips SLPs with information to identify children with impaired speech at a younger age than we have historically been able to.

A comprehensive overview of typical speech sound acquisition includes many facets (see Box 3.2). Each of these areas is described, and speech sound acquisition data are summarized according to children's ages. Additionally, under each heading in the next section, a table highlights findings from the available research studies. Data from a range of studies are presented in the columns to enable comparison of findings

---

BOX 3.2   Components of a comprehensive overview of typical English speech acquisition

1. Intelligibility
2. Comparison of the child's speech sounds with the adult target

    a. *Acquired sounds.* Consonants, consonant clusters, vowels

    b. *Percentage of correct productions (percentage of error productions).* Consonants, consonant clusters, vowels

    c. *Common mismatches.* Consonants, consonant clusters, vowels

    d. *Phonological patterns/processes*

3. Abilities of the child (without comparison to the adult target)

    a. *Phonetic inventory.* Consonants, consonant clusters, vowels

    b. *Syllable structure*

4. Prosody
5. Metalinguistic/phonological awareness skills

---

and encourage consideration of diversity and individuality across studies and children. However, rates of development vary among typically developing children.

Intelligibility

Intelligibility has been described as "the single most practical measurement of oral communication competence" (Metz et al., 1985). A speaker's intelligibility can be affected by articulatory, phonological, suprasegmental, and other linguistic features. For example, Vihman (1988) indicated that at 3 years of age, children who used more complex sentences were more difficult to understand. Additionally, intelligibility is affected by the speaker's relationship with the listener; for example, differences occur according to whether the listener is the child's parent, a stranger, or a person trained in phonetic transcription (e.g., Flipsen, 1995; McLeod et al., 2012; McLeod, 2020).

Kent and colleagues (1994) provide a comprehensive review of procedures for the evaluation of intelligibility, including a range of commercially available instruments. Flipsen (2006b) has discussed several variations of the Intelligibility Index (II) (Shriberg et al., 1997a). The II is "the percentage of words in an entire sample that the transcriber could reliably understand" (Flipsen, 2006b, p. 306).

The results reported in several studies of children's intelligibility demonstrate that as children grow older, the percentage of intelligible words increases. The extent of intelligibility is also influenced by the children's relationship with the person to whom they are speaking. Roulstone and associates (2002) conducted the largest study of 2-year-old children's intelligibility. As a result of their study of 1,127 children who were 25 months of age, the researchers reported that "children were mostly intelligible to their parents, with 12.7% of parents finding their child difficult to understand and only 2.1% of parents reporting that they could rarely understand their child" (p. 264). In contrast, studies that considered children's intelligibility to strangers demonstrated that 2-year-old children's speech was 50% intelligible to strangers (Coplan & Gleason, 1988; Vihman, 1988), and by 3 years of age, children's speech was around 75% intelligible to strangers (Coplan & Gleason, 1988; Vihman, 1988). Bernthal and Bankson (1998, p. 272) concluded that "a client 3 years of age or older who is unintelligible is a candidate for treatment." Flipsen (2006b) reported data from 320 children regarding the percentage of words that could be reliably understood by a transcriber and found intelligibility gradually increased across this age range from an average of 95.68% for 3-year-old children, to 99.01% for 8-year-old children. Between 4 and 5 years of age, typically developing children are usually to always intelligible, and their speech is considered to be most intelligible to their parents; followed by their immediate family, friends, and teachers; and least intelligible to strangers (McLeod, 2020; McLeod et al., 2015).

Age of Acquisition of Speech Sounds

One of the major techniques for considering speech sound acquisition has been to compare children's development with the adult target. *Age of acquisition* refers to the age at which a certain percentage of children have acquired a speech sound. Large-group cross-sectional studies have predominantly been used for this purpose. Consonants have been the primary focus of these studies; however, some studies have examined consonant clusters and vowels. Age-of-acquisition data have had a long history of credence within the SLP profession. Well-known U.S. studies include those by Templin (1957) and, more recently, Smit and colleagues (1990). However, studies examining age of acquisition of speech sounds have been published for English dialects beyond American English and many languages around the world, including Arabic, Cantonese, Dutch, Finnish, German, Greek, Hungarian, Hebrew, Japanese, Korean, Maltese, Norwegian, Portuguese, Putonghua, Spanish, Thai, Turkish, and Welsh (McLeod, 2007a; McLeod & Crowe, 2018), and the age of acquisition may vary by language.

When considering the age-of-acquisition reports for consonants, consonant clusters, and vowels, it is important to remember the methodological constraints of the data. The samples in these studies typically have been elicited from single words (not conversation) and often only one word has been elicited for each speech sound in each word position. Thus, the samples may not be representative of typical speaking situations, and variability in production not considered. Some studies have scored productions as either correct or incorrect and have not considered phonological development (hence, readers also need to consider additional data such as phonological processes, mismatches, etc.).

Another issue with these studies is that they vary in terms of the criterion for determining age of acquisition. For example, Templin (1957) indicated that a sound had to be acquired in the initial-, medial-, and final-word positions, whereas others have used only initial- and final-word positions (e.g., Prather et al., 1975; Smit et al., 1990). Studies have shown that children's productions of consonants can differ in the onset and coda positions (e.g., Lin & Demuth, 2015). In addition, a range of standards (e.g., 50%, 75%, 90%, and 100% correct) have been used as criteria for age of acquisition (Crowe & McLeod, 2020; McLeod & Crowe, 2018). Tables 3.3 to 3.5 provide the criterion adopted by each researcher. In 1972, Sander emphasized the importance of presenting age-of-acquisition data using a continuum rather than a definite age at which phonemes are acquired. Consequently, a number of authors (e.g., Smit et al., 1990) have adopted this approach and have presented graphical displays of acquisition for each speech sound across the different ages.

Consonants

Table 3.2 provides a summary of studies of English-speaking children's age of acquisition of consonants based on the review by Crowe and McLeod (2020) and Table 3.3 provides the raw data for some of the English consonant acquisition studies included in the review. It includes studies of English dialects spoken in the United States, England, Scotland, and Australia. As the table indicates, the majority of English consonants are acquired by the age of 3–4 years. As Porter and Hodson (2001, p. 165) indicated, "3-year-olds had acquired all major phoneme classes, except liquids . . . sibilant lisps were still common until the age of 7 years." However, the findings in Table 3.3 suggest that acquisition of all singleton consonants in English does not conclude until 8–9 years of age. It should be noted as well that in each study, the youngest and oldest ages of acquisition are affected by the age range that has been studied. For example, only three studies included in Table 3.3 assessed the speech of children who were 2 years old (Chirlian & Sharpley, 1982; Paynter & Petty, 1974; Prather et al., 1975). Thus, it could be that children acquire some sounds even earlier, as evidenced by studies of languages other than English (e.g., Cantonese and Vietnamese) (Phạm & McLeod, 2019; So & Dodd, 1995; To et al., 2013).

While considering Table 3.3, notice the differences in the age of acquisition of consonants provided from these studies. Dodd, Holm, and colleagues (2003), for example, reported a higher number of consonants acquired by age 3;0 than most of the other studies. This finding was probably influenced by their inclusion of children's spontaneous and imitated productions of speech sounds in defining age-appropriate production, whereas many other studies have been based on only spontaneous productions. The age of acquisition for the fricatives /s/ and /z/ appears to vary more than any other speech sounds. For example, some authors suggest that /z/ is acquired at age 3 years (Dodd, Holm et al., 2003), others at 4 years (Arlt & Goodban, 1976), others at 5 years (Kilminster & Laird, 1978; Anthony et al., 1971; Smit et al., 1990 [females]), others at 6 years (Smit et al., 1990 [males]), others at 7 years (Templin, 1957), and others after 9 years (Chirlian & Sharpley, 1982). Similarly, the age range for the acquisition of /s/ extends from age 3 (Dodd, Holm et al., 2003; Prather et al., 1975) to age 7 (Poole, 1934). There are at least three possible reasons for the variability in the age of acquisition of

Table 3.2. Summary of age of consonant acquisition for English-speaking children across the globe (McLeod & Crowe, 2018) and within the United States (Crowe & McLeod, 2020)

	Global[a, b]	United States[a]
Criteria	90%–100%	90%
No. of studies at each criterion	8	10
2;0 to 3;11 (Early)	/p, b, m, d, n, h, t, k, g, w, ŋ, f, j/	/b, n, m, p, h, w, d, g, k, f, t, ŋ, j/
4;0 to 4;11 (Middle)	/l, dʒ, tʃ, s, v, ʃ, z/	/v, dʒ, s, tʃ, l, ʃ, z/
5;0 to 6;11 (Late)	/r, ʒ, ð, θ/	/r, ð, ʒ, θ/

Note: The total United States sample is based on 15 studies of 18,907 children analyzed in Crowe and McLeod (2020). Global sample is based on 15 studies of 7,369 analyzed in McLeod and Crowe (2018).

[a] The order of consonants within age groups was based on the average age of acquisition. Six papers were analyzed in both McLeod and Crowe (2018) and Crowe and McLeod (2020).

[b] English-speaking children in the global sample lived in Australia, the Republic of Ireland, Malaysia, South Africa, the United Kingdom, and the United States.

Table 3.3. Summary of studies of English-speaking children's age of acquisition of consonants (ordered chronologically)

	Dodd, Holm, et al. (2003)	Smit et al. (1990) (females)	Smit et al. (1990) (males)	Chirlian and Sharpley (1982)	Kilminster and Laird (1978)	Aritt and Goodban (1976)	Prather et al. (1975)	Paynter and Petty (1974)	Anthony et al. (1971)	Templin (1957)
Age range tested	3;0 to 6;11	3;0 to 9;0	3;0 to 9;0	2;0 to 9;0	3;0 to 9;0	3;0 to 6;0	2;0 to 4;0	2;0 to 2;6	3;0 to 6;0	3;0 to 8;0
Criterion	90%	75%	75%	75%	75%	75%	75%	90%	90%	75%
Country	England and Australia	United States	United States	Australia	Australia	United States	United States	United States	Scotland	United States
2;0				m, n, h			m, n, ŋ, h, p	h, w		
2;4							j, d, k, f			
2;6				p, ŋ, w, d, g				p, b, t, m		
2;8							w, b, t			
3;0	p, b, t, d, k, g, m, n, ŋ, f, s, z, h, w, l, j	m, n, h, w, p, b, t, d, k, g, f, s[a]	m, n, h, w, p, b, t, d, k, g	j, k, f, ʃ	p, b, m, n, ŋ, h, w, j, t, d, k, g, ʒ[a]	p, b, t, d, k, g, m, n, ŋ, h, f, w	g, s		p, b, m, t, d, n, w, j	m, n, ŋ, p, f, h, w
3;4							l, r			
3;6	ʧ	j	f, j	b, t, ʧ, ʤ	f	v			k, g, ŋ, f, v, h	j
3;8				ʃ, ʧ						

(continued)

Table 3.3. *(continued)*

	Dodd, Holm, et al. (2003)	Smit et al. (1990) (females)	Smit et al. (1990) (males)	Chirlian and Sharpley (1982)	Kilminster and Laird (1978)	Arlt and Goodban (1976)	Prather et al. (1975)	Paynter and Petty (1974)	Anthony et al. (1971)	Templin (1957)
Age range tested	3;0 to 6;11	3;0 to 9;0 (females)	3;0 to 9;0 (males)	2;0 to 9;0	3;0 to 9;0	3;0 to 6;0	2;0 to 4;0	2;0 to 2;6	3;0 to 6;0	3;0 to 8;0
Criterion	90%	75%	75%	75%	75%	75%	75%	90%	90%	75%
Country	England and Australia	United States	United States	Australia	Australia	United States	United States	United States	Scotland	United States
4;0	ʒ, ʤ	v, ð, ʃ, ʧ	ʤ	l, ʒ, s	l, ʃ, ʧ	s, z, ʒ, ʧ, ʤ, l	ð, ʒ			k, b, d, g, r
4;6		ʤ, l[a]	v		ʤ, s[a], z[a]	ʃ	v, θ, z		l	s, ʃ, ʧ
5;0	ʃ	z[a]	s[a], ʃ, ʧ	r	r	θ, ð, r	ʤ			
5;6		ŋ, θ	ð, r						s, z, ʃ, ʒ	
6;0	r	r	ŋ, θ, z, l		v					t, θ, v, l
6;6									θ, ð, ʧ	
7;0	θ, ð								ʤ, r	ð, z, ʒ, ʤ
7;6				ð, θ						
8;0					ð					
8;6				v	θ					
9;0										
9;0+				z						
Not tested					j					

[a] Reversal occurs at a later age group.

/s/ and /z/. The first concerns whether children who had lost their central incisor teeth but had not yet acquired their adult dentition were included. Such an absence of teeth might well affect their ability to produce a correct /s/. The second possibility concerns differences in the definition of an adultlike /s/, particularly whether dentalized /s/ sounds are considered to be correct (Smit et al., 1990). The final possibility relates to the methodology employed within the studies, including the complexity of the words elicited and the criterion for acquisition associated with such data.

Another approach to the consideration of the age of acquisition is that taken by Shriberg (1993), who created a profile of consonant mastery based on the average percentage correct in continuous conversational speech. Using data from 64 children aged 3–6 years with speech delays, Shriberg suggested that there were three stages of phoneme acquisition:

1. Early 8 [m, b, j, n, w, d, p, h]

2. Middle 8 [t, ŋ, k, g, f, v, ʧ, ʤ]

3. Late 8 [ʃ, θ, s, z, ð, l, r, ʒ]

Shriberg (1993) tested the validity of these three stages against four studies of speech sound acquisition (Shriberg, 1993, Table 8; Sander, 1972; Prather et al., 1975; Hoffmann, 1982 [articulation and connected speech samples]; Smit et al., 1990). Shriberg reported that there were a number of differences between studies of typical development and his speech-delay data. For example, in the comparison with the Sander (1972) report, 15 of the 24 consonant ranks fell within their assumed groups on the consonant mastery profile. However, overall, Shriberg (p. 122) concluded, "Thus, as a cross-sectional estimate of the rank-order of consonant mastery in speech-delayed children, the reference consonant mastery profile agrees quite well with estimates of the developmental order of consonant acquisition." Shriberg's profile of consonant mastery has received a large amount of attention within the SLP profession (e.g., Bleile, 2013), but it should be remembered that its basis is the mastery of phonemes by children with speech delay.

Recently, Crowe and McLeod (2020) reviewed data from 10 studies of typically developing children in the United States and suggested the three stages of phoneme acquisition were slightly different from those of Shriberg (1993):

1. Early 13 (2;0 to 3;11) = /b, n, m, p, h, w, d, g, k, f, t, ŋ, j/ (all plosives, nasals, and glides)

2. Middle 7 (4;0 to 4;11) = /v, ʤ, s, ʧ, l, ʃ, z/

3. Late 4 (5;0 to 6;11) = /r, ð, ʒ, θ/

Consonant Clusters

The age of acquisition of consonant clusters for English-speaking children is summarized in Table 3.4, which includes four comprehensive studies (Anthony et al., 1971; McLeod & Arciuli, 2009; Smit et al., 1990; Templin, 1957) and one more narrowly focused study that considered the acquisition of three /s/ clusters (Higgs, 1968). Olmsted (1971) also has data on the acquisition of consonant clusters; however, his data were not included because the definition of initial and final positions related to the sentence rather than a word. McLeod and colleagues (2001a) presented an extensive literature review of the acquisition of consonant clusters. They indicated that

Table 3.4. Summary of studies of English-speaking children's age of acquisition of consonant clusters

	Smit et al. (1990) (females)	Smit et al. (1990) (males)	McLeod and Arciuli (2009)	Templin (1957)	Higgs (1968)	Anthony et al. (1971)	Templin (1957)	Anthony et al. (1971)
Age range tested	3;0 to 9;0	3;0 to 9;0	5;0 to 12;11	3;0 to 8;0	2;6 to 5;6	3;0 to 5;6	3;0 to 8;0	3;0 to 5;6
Criterion Word position	90% word initial	90% word initial	90% word initial	75% word initial	75% word initial	75% word initial	75% word final	75% word final
3;0							ŋk	nt
3;6	tw, kw	tw, kw					rk, ks, mp, pt, rm, mr, nr, pr, kr, br, dr, gr, sm	
4;0	pl, bl, kl			pl, pr, tr, tw, kl, kr, kw, bl, br, dr, gl, sk, sm, sn, sp, st		kw	lp, rt, ft, lt, fr	
4;6	sp, st, sk, sw˙, gl, fl, kr˙, skwᵃ	gl	br, tr, dr, kr, gr, fr, sp, st, sk, sm, sn, sl, sw, skw, skr, str	gr, fr	sp, st, sk	kr, fl	lf	
5;0	sm, sn	sp, st, snᵃ, bl, dr˙		fl, str		glᵃ, tr, kl, br	rp, lb, rd, rf, rn, ʃr, mbr	
5;6		pl, kl, fl, pr, tr, kr, gr, fr				sl		dz, mps, ŋgz
6;0	sl, pr, br, tr, dr, gr, fr, spl	sk, sw, br		skw		θr, sm, st, str, sp	lk, rb, rg, rθ, nt, nd, ðr, pl, kl, bl, gl, fl, sl, str, rst, ŋkl, ŋgl, rdʒ, ntθ, rʃ	sk
7;0	θr	sm, sl, θr, skw, spl	spl	θr, ʃr, sl, sw, skr, spl, spr			lz, zm, tθ, sk, st, skr, kst, dʒd	
8;0	spr, str, skr	spr, str, skr					kt, tr, sp	
>8;0			pr, θr, spr, skr				lfθ, tl	

ᵃ A reversal occurs in older age groups.

2-year-old children are able to produce at least some consonant clusters correctly; however, complete mastery may take until 9 years of age. Typically, two-element consonant clusters (e.g., /sp, st, sk/) are mastered before three-element consonant clusters (e.g., /spr, str, skr/). Clusters containing fricatives (e.g., /fl/) usually are more difficult than clusters containing stops (e.g., /kl/). To date, Templin (1957) and Anthony and associates (1971) are the only researchers to study the acquisition of word-final consonant clusters in English (see Table 3.4). It is important to consider the influence of morphological structures on the acquisition of word-final consonant clusters. For example, Templin reported that /kt/ was acquired at 8 years of age; however, this consonant cluster occurs both in monomorphemic contexts such as *act* and morphophonemic contexts such as *lacked* created by the past tense morpheme. Morphophonemic clusters may be acquired later due to their complexity (Howland et al., 2019).

Vowels

The description of the age of acquisition of vowels has received much less attention than that for consonants. One reason for this is that vowels are influenced by the accent or dialect spoken by the child. For example, general American English has either 18 or 19 vowels (depending on whether /ɔ/ is included) and three or four diphthongs (depending on whether /ju/ is included) (Smit, 2007). In contrast, there are 12 vowels and 8 diphthongs in English spoken in England (Howard, 2007), Australia (McLeod, 2007b), and New Zealand (Maclagan & Gillon, 2007), although there are differences between the exact vowels produced in each dialect. Scottish English has 10 vowels and 3 diphthongs (Scobbie et al., 2007). Howard and Heselwood (2002) provide a discussion of the sociophonetic variation between vowel productions for speakers of different dialects.

There are two aspects of acquisition of vowels: paradigmatic and syntagmatic acquisition (James et al., 2001). The *paradigmatic* aspect to mastering vowel production refers to learning to produce vowels in isolation or in simple monosyllabic words. Typically developing children attempt the paradigmatic aspects of vowel production at a very young age. In the first year, low, nonrounded vowels are favored, and height differences appear before front-back vowel differences (Donegan, 2002). Otomo and Stoel-Gammon (1992) conducted a longitudinal study of six children's acquisition of the unrounded vowels between 22 and 30 months of age and found that /ɪ/ and /ɛ/ were mastered early, then /e/ and /æ/, whereas /ɪ/ and /ɛ/ were least accurate. Children master the paradigmatic aspects of vowels by the age of 3 (Donegan, 2002; Selby et al., 2000; Vihman, 1992) or 4 years (Dodd, Holm et al., 2003). Statements such as the following are plentiful throughout the literature on typical speech acquisition:

- "By the age of 3 years, all normal children have evolved a stabilized vowel system" (Anthony et al., 1971, p. 12).

- "The literature on vowel development suggests that vowels are acquired early, both in production and perception. There is considerable variability in their production, but most studies suggest that vowel production is reasonably accurate by age 3, although some studies call this into question" (Donegan, 2002, p. 12).

However, these comments refer to the mastery of vowels in a paradigmatic context.

The second aspect of acquisition of vowels is called the *syntagmatic* acquisition (James et al., 2001). It refers to the ability to produce sequences of vowels within syllables and words in conjunction with other phonological variables such as stress.

Knowledge of the syntagmatic aspect of vowel production is particularly apparent in the ability to produce schwa correctly in polysyllabic words. According to James and colleagues (2001), children acquire at least some of the syntagmatic aspects of vowels between 3 and 5 years of age; however, mastery of vowels in polysyllabic words and stressed syllables extends beyond 3 years of age (Allen & Hawkins, 1980; James et al., 2001; Masso, Baker et al., 2017; Selby et al., 2000; Stoel-Gammon & Herrington, 1990). For example, Allen and Hawkins (1980) found that children mastered vowels in stressed syllables by 3 years of age but did not master vowels in unstressed syllables until they were 4–5 years old.

Percentage of Sounds Correct/Percentage of Sounds in Error

Consonants

Another index of speech sound acquisition is percentage of consonants correct (PCC), which considers the number of consonants produced correctly divided by the total number of consonants. Table 3.5 summarizes data from a range of studies detailing PCC at different ages. As can be seen, when children reach 2 years of age, it is typical for around 70% of their consonants to be produced correctly. For example, Watson and Scukanec (1997b) described longitudinal PCC data for 12 U.S. children. The mean PCC for the children at age 2;0 was 69.2%, and by age 3;0 it had climbed to 86.2%. As children age, their PCC increases. For example, Dodd, Holm, and associates (2003) found that children aged 5;6 to 6;6 produced 95.9% of consonants correctly. McLeod and Crowe (2018) examined PCC in 15 studies of children's speech acquisition across

Table 3.5. Summary of studies of English-speaking children's percentage of consonants correct (PCC)

Age	Pollock (2002)	Stoel-Gammon (1987)	Watson and Scukanec (1997b)	Dodd, Holm, et al. (2003)	James et al. (2002)	Waring et al. (2001)
1;6	53%					
2;0	70%	70%	69.2% (53–91)			
2;3			69.9% (51–91)			
2;6	81%		75.1% (61–94)			
2;9	92%		82.1% (63–96)			
3;0			86.2% (73–99)	82.11%	76.77% (MSW)	
3;6	93%				76.41% (PSW)	85.2%
4;0	93%			90.37%	83.97% (MSW)	88.5%
4;6	94%				82.45% (PSW)	
5;0	93%				89.54% (MSW)	93.4%
5;6	96%			95.86%	88.36% (PSW)	
6;0	97%				93.74% (MSW)	95.1%
6;6	93%				90.76% (PSW)	
7;0					93.93% (MSW)	98.4%
7;6					90.99% (PSW)	

Key: MSW, monosyllabic words; PSW, polysyllabic words.

12 languages (Arabic, Danish, English, French, German, Hungarian, Malay, Portuguese, Setswana, Swahili, Turkish, and Xhosa). They found that children achieved an
average PCC of 63.50 at 2;0 and 93.80 by 5;0.

Although Shriberg and Kwiatkowski's (1982a) original recommendations for
computing PCC refers to connected speech samples, different sampling techniques
have been applied to this metric. James and colleagues (2002) demonstrated that there
are significant differences between PCC scores depending on the speech-sampling
task. Significantly higher PCCs were found for children's productions of monosyllabic
versus polysyllabic words (see Table 3.5). The PCC will be discussed in Chapter 7 as a
data analysis procedure employed in speech sound assessment.

Consonant Clusters

A few researchers have described children's percentage of consonant clusters correct at different ages (see Table 3.6). Roulstone and colleagues (2002) indicated that
1,127 children who were 25 months of age had an error rate of 78% (22% correct) for
production of consonant clusters. In a longitudinal study of Australian 2-year-olds,
McLeod and colleagues (2002) reported that overall, 31.5% of consonant clusters were
produced correctly in connected speech. Word-final consonant clusters (e.g., /nd/ in
hand) were more likely to be correct (48.9% of the time), followed by word-initial fricative clusters (e.g., /sn/ in *snail*) (38.5%) and word-initial stop clusters (e.g., /bl/ in *blue*)
(24.3%). Waring and associates (2001) presented cross-sectional data on Australian
children's productions of consonant clusters in single words. They found that children
aged 3;5 to 3;11 were able to produce 51 of a total of 59 (86%) consonant clusters correctly. By ages 7;0 to 7;11, most consonant clusters were produced correctly (58/59 to
98%). McLeod and Arciuli (2009) studied consonant cluster production by 74 children
between the ages of 5 and 12 years. They found that two-element /s/ clusters were produced correctly 96.8% of the time, followed by two-element /r/ clusters at 94.0% of the

Table 3.6. Summary of studies of English-speaking
children's percentage of consonant clusters correct (PCCC)

Age	Roulstone et al. (2002)	McLeod et al. (2002)	Waring et al. (2001)
2;0	22%[a]		
2;6		31.5%	
3;0			86.4%
3;6			
4;0			88.4%
4;6			
5;0			94.9%
5;6			
6;0			96.6%
6;6			
7;0			98.3%
7;6			

[a] Conversion from mean error rate of 78%.

time, and three-element /s/ clusters at 92.0% of the time. The children's ability to produce consonant clusters changed from 92.4% at 5–6 years to 98.8% at 11–12 years.

Vowels

A summary of studies of the percentage of vowels produced correctly by children at
different ages is provided in Table 3.7. Pollock and colleagues (Pollock, 2002; Pollock &
Berni, 2003) have conducted the most extensive study of U.S. children's acquisition of
rhotic (vowels with r-coloring such as /ɝ/) and nonrhotic vowels. They demonstrated
that the nonrhotic vowels are more likely to be correct than rhotic vowels for a child of
the same age. The studies by Dodd, Holm, and colleagues (2003) and James and associates (2001) were conducted on nonrhotic vowels because rhotic vowels are not present
in English produced in England and Australia. The data from Australian and English
children are similar to those reported by Pollock and Berni (2003) regarding nonrhotic
vowels. James and associates (2001) indicated that the accuracy of vowel production
decreased with an increase in the number of syllables in the word; there was higher
accuracy for vowels in monosyllabic words compared with polysyllabic words.

Phonological Patterns/Processes

Bankson and Bernthal (1990, p. 16) defined *phonological processes* as "simplification
of a sound class in which target sounds are systematically deleted and/or substituted." As mentioned in the section on natural phonology, the notion of systematic-
ity was introduced to the field of linguistics by Stampe (1969) and then adapted and
called phonological processes by authors such as Ingram (1976). Since that time, many
authors have provided differing lists of phonological processes. Table 3.8 provides a

Table 3.7. Summary of studies of English-speaking children's percentage of
vowels correct (PVC)

Age	Pollock (2002) Rhotic	Pollock and Berni (2003) Nonrhotic	Dodd, Holm et al. (2003) Nonrhotic	James et al. (2001) Nonrhotic
1;6	23.52%	82.19%		
2;0	37.54%	92.39%		
2;6	62.52%	93.90%		
3;0	79.24%	97.29%	97.39%	94.90% (MSW)
3;6	76.50%	97.19%		88.28% (PSW)
4;0	90.11%	98.06%	98.93%	95.20% (MSW)
4;6	86.80%	98.20%		92.08% (PSW)
5;0	88.21%	99.21%		94.80% (MSW)
5;6	80.31%	99.38%	99.19%	94.30% (PSW)
6;0	77.20%	98.5%		95.39% (MSW)
6;6		99.19%		94.86% (PSW)
7;0				95.10% (MSW)
7;6				95.44% (PSW)

Key: MSW, monosyllabic words; PSW, polysyllabic words.

Table 3.8.   Definitions and examples of commonly occurring phonological processes/patterns

Overarching description	Phonological process	Definition	Example
Assimilation processes: When one sound in the word becomes similar to another sound in the word	Assimilation (consonant harmony)	One sound is replaced by another that is the same or similar to another sound within the word	*dod* instead of *dog*
Substitution processes: When one sound is substituted by another sound in a systematic fashion	Fronting	Velars are realized as sounds produced further forward in the oral cavity (typically alveolars)	*tar* instead of *car*
	Gliding	Liquids /l, r/ are replaced by a glide /w, j/ or another liquid	*wabbit* instead of *rabbit*
	Stopping	Fricatives and/or affricates are realized as stops	*tun* instead of *sun*
	Depalatization	Palatal sounds are realized as sounds produced further forward in the oral cavity (typically alveolars)	*fis* instead of *fish*
	Deaffrication	Affricates are realized as fricatives	*shursh* instead of *church*
Syllable structure processes: Phonological processes that affect the syllable structure	Final consonant deletion	Deletion of the final consonant in the word	*do* instead of *dog*
	Cluster simplification/ reduction	Deletion of one element of the cluster	*pane* instead of *plane*
	Weak syllable deletion	Deletion of the unstressed syllable	*nana* instead of *banana*

Source: Adapted from Bankson and Bernthal (1990), pp. 16–19.

summary of definitions and examples of commonly occurring phonological processes. Recall, as mentioned earlier, that the term *pattern* is now more typically used than the term *process.*

In 1981, Grunwell presented a graphical display of the chronology of phonological processes that has been used widely as a means for identifying the age at which phonological processes are typically suppressed. Since that time, a number of other researchers have presented the age of suppression of phonological processes (e.g., Dodd, 1995a; Haelsig & Madison, 1986; James, 2001; Pressier et al., 1988; Roberts et al., 1990). A summary of these studies is presented in Table 3.9. Some of the findings from these studies indicate that the most prevalent processes for young children (18–29 months) were cluster reduction (e.g., *spoon* – [pun]) and liquid deviation (e.g., *leaf* – [wif]) (Pressier et al., 1998). According to Roberts and colleagues (1990), there was a marked decline in the usage of phonological processes between 2;6 and 4;0 years, with the most prevalent processes during these years being final consonant deletion, cluster reduction, fronting, stopping, and liquid gliding.

In 1999, James and colleagues presented data on 240 children's (aged 5;0 to 7;11) use of phonological processes. Among other findings, they reported four clusters of

Table 3.9. A summary of studies of children's use of phonological processes/patterns

Age	Dodd, Holm et al. (2003)	Grunwell (1981, 1987)	Preisser et al. (1988)	Watson and Scukanec (1997b)	Lowe et al. (1985)	James (2001)	Haelsig and Madison (1986)
2;0		Present: Weak syllable deletion; final consonant deletion, cluster reduction, fronting of velars, stopping, gliding, context-sensitive voicing Declining: Reduplication, consonant harmony	Most prevalent: Cluster reduction, liquid deviations (gliding)	Present: Final consonant deletion, liquid simplification, later stopping, cluster reduction, vowelization			
2;6		Present: Weak syllable deletion; cluster reduction, fronting of velars, fronting /ʃ/, stopping /v, θ, ð, tʃ, dʒ/, gliding, context-sensitive voicing Declining: Final consonant deletion			23% fronting	Declining: Affrication, depalatalization, gliding, metathesis, prevocalic voicing, vowel changes	
3;0	Present: Gliding, deaffrication, cluster reduction, fronting,[a] weak syllable deletion, stopping	Present: Weak syllable deletion; stopping /v, θ, ð/, fronting /ʃ, tʃ, dʒ/, gliding Declining: Cluster reduction		Later stopping, cluster simplification		Declining: Backing, cluster reduction, deaffrication, final consonant deletion, final devoicing, initial consonant deletion, labial assimilation, palatalization, stopping, unstressed syllable deletion, fricative simplification	Gliding of liquids, weak syllable deletion, glottal replacement, alveolar and labial assimilation, cluster reduction, stopping, vocalization,[b] final consonant deletion

3;6	Present: Gliding, deaffrication, cluster reduction, fronting,[c] weak syllable deletion	Present: Stopping /θ, ð/ Declining: Weak syllable deletion, cluster reduction, gliding	Weak syllable deletion, vocalization[b], gliding of liquids (20% criterion)
4;0	Present: Gliding, deaffrication, cluster reduction (three-element clusters)	Present: /θ/ → [ð], /ð/ → [d, v], depalatization of /ʃ, tʃ, dʒ/, gliding Declining: Cluster reduction	Declining: Depalatalization, gliding, glottal replacement
4;6	Present: Gliding, deaffrication	Declining: Stopping /θ, ð/, gliding /r/	
5;0	Present: Gliding	Declining: Stopping /θ, ð/, gliding /r/	Declining: Deaffrication, epenthesis, metathesis, fricative simplification (v/ð)
5;6	Present: Gliding		

[a] Voicing pattern not present at any age.
[b] Sometimes called vowelization.
[c] Fronting of /k, g/ ended at age 3;11, whereas fronting of /ŋ/ continued until 5;0 in the word *fishing*.

phonological process use from those that were rarely present (Cluster 1) to those that were present in a majority of possible occurrences (Cluster 4):

Cluster 1. Context-sensitive voicing, early stopping, final consonant deletion, nasal assimilation

Cluster 2. Later stopping, velar assimilation, velar fronting

Cluster 3. Deaffrication and palatal fronting

Cluster 4. Cluster reduction, cluster simplification, fricative simplification, liquid simplification, and liquid deletion

James (2001) presented further data on the use of phonological processes by 365 children aged 2;0 to 7;11 years. She found that the major decline in the use of phonological processes was between the ages of 3 and 4 years; however, some processes had fluctuating distributions. For example, gliding declined by 50% or more between 2 and 3 years and then again between 4 and 5 years.

Common Mismatches

As well as the identification of the age at which children generally learn to produce sounds, it is useful to have data to describe the typical errors, or mismatches, children make in their attempts to produce the adult form of sounds. Phonological processes provide typical patterns of errors, but Smit (1993a, 1993b) has taken this further by presenting errors children make when attempting individual speech sounds. Smit reanalyzed the data from Smit and associates (1990) and provided tables of data containing frequent to rare errors children make in their attempts to produce consonants (Smit, 1993a) and consonant clusters (Smit, 1993b) (for a summary, see Table 3.10). Readers are encouraged to consult Smit (1993a, 1993b) to use the exhaustive information provided.

In Smit's analysis, two sounds warranted extra attention: /s/ and /r/. Smit (1993a) indicated that when children were aged 2;0 and 2;6, they were more likely to produce word-initial /s/ as [t] or [d]; however, for children from 3;0 to 9;0 years, the most common error in the word-final context was dentalization. Lateralized [ɬ] productions were rare, which suggests that SLPs should consider that lateral production of /s/ warrants intervention regardless of the child's age. Smit (1993a) also indicated that the most common error production for word-initial /r/ was [w]. Less commonly, children used derhotacized and labialized productions.

Perception

Earlier in this chapter, we considered infants' perceptual capabilities. As children's speech develops, so does the link between their production and perceptual capabilities. This link was described in our consideration of the psycholinguistic models of speech acquisition. Although some authors believe that perception for speech is achieved in infancy, Rvachew (2007a, p. 28) suggests that there are three stages of development of "adult-like acoustic, phonological and articulatory representations" and that these stages are clinically relevant:

1. The child is unaware of the phonological contrast and can produce realizations that are acoustically and perceptually similar.

2. The child is aware of the phonological contrast and may produce acoustically different realizations that are not perceptible to adult listeners.

Table 3.10. Children's common errors in producing consonants and consonant clusters (errors occurred >15%)

Age	Smit (1993a) Consonants	Smit (1993b) Two-element consonant clusters	Smit (1993b) Three-element consonant clusters
2;0	ŋ → n	pr → p, pw	skw → k, t, kw, gw
	j → θ	br → b, bw	spl → p, b, pl, pw
	l → w	tr → t, tw	spr → p, pw, pr, sp
	r → w	dr → d, dw	str → t, d, st, tw, sw
	v → b	kr → k, kw	skr → k, w, kw, gw, fw
	θ → f	gr → g, gw	
	ð → d	fr → f, fw	
	s → dentalized[a]	θr → f, θw	
	z → d	sw → w	
	ʃ → s	sm → m	
	tʃ → t/d	sn → n	
	ʒ → d	sp → p, b	
		st → t, d	
		sk → k	
3;0	ŋ → n	pr → pw	skw → θkw
	r → w	br → bw	spl → θpl, spw
	v → b	tr → tw	spr → θpr, spw
	θ → f	dr → dw	str → θtr, stw
	ð → d	kr → kw	skr → θkr, skw
	s → dentalized	gr → gw	
		fr → fw	
		θr → fr	
		st → θt	
4;0	θ → f	pr → pw	skw → θkw
	s → dentalized	br → bw	spl → θpl, spw
		tr → tw	spr → θpr, spw
		dr → dw	str → θtr, stw
		kr → kw	skr → θkr, skw
		gr → gw	
		fr → fw	
		θr → fr	
		st → θt	
5;0		pr → pw	
5;6		br → bw	skw → θkw
		tr → tw	spl → θpl, spw

(continued)

Table 3.10.   *(continued)*

	Smit (1993a)	Smit (1993b)	Smit (1993b)
Age	Consonants	Two-element consonant clusters	Three-element consonant clusters
		dr → dw	spr → θpr, spw
		kr → kw	str → θtr, stw
		gr → gw	skr → θkr, skw
6;0		tr → tw	skw → θkw
			spl → θpl
			spr → θpr, spw
			str → θtr, stw
			skr → θkr, skw

[a] Smit (1993b) used dentalized (dnt), whereas /θ/ is used in the present table.

3. The child is aware of the phonological contrast and can produce different realizations that are acoustically and perceptually accurate.

Rvachew suggests that children's perceptual capabilities continue to develop into late childhood. For example, Hazan and Barrett (2000) found that children from 6 to 12 years of age showed increasing mastery in the ability to discriminate synthesized differences in place, manner, and voicing, but had not yet achieved adultlike accuracy.

Suprasegmentals/Prosody

Prosody refers to the suprasegmental aspects of speech production, including stress, intonation, and rhythm. Gerken and McGregor (1998) present a helpful overview of prosody and its development in children, and Wells and Peppé (2003) provide a helpful overview of prosody in children with speech and language impairment. There appears to be a close interaction between suprasegmentals, motherese, and early language development.

Intonation develops before stress. For example, Snow (1994) found that young children acquire skills that control intonation earlier than final-syllable timing skills. At 6 months of age, children use intonation, rhythm, and pausing in their speech (Crystal, 1986). By 1–2 years of age, children use intonation and stress to reduce homonyms and to differentiate between commands, requests, and calling (Dore, 1975).

Kehoe (1997) studied the ability of 18 children, aged 22, 28, and 34 months, to produce three- and four-syllable words. She found that there was a significantly higher number of stress errors in SwS words (S = strong, w = weak) and a tendency for a higher number of stress errors in SwSw words. Stress errors were more frequent in imitated than in spontaneous productions. She suggested that stress errors may be associated with articulatory and phonetic-control factors. Omission of unstressed and nonfinal syllables is common in young children, while stressed and final syllables are usually preserved (Kehoe, 2001; James, 2007). Gerken and McGregor (1998) suggest that children leave an acoustic trace of the omitted syllable; that is, although changes cannot be detected by the human ear, spectrographic analysis can reveal changes in factors such as voice onset time and vowel length.

PHASE 4: MASTERY OF SPEECH AND LITERACY

During the school years, refinement of children's speech production and perception skills continues until eventually they reach adultlike mastery. This refinement occurs in a number of domains, including prosody, phonotactics, and their production of speech segments. As illustrated in the tables of speech sound acquisition previously presented in this chapter, studies show continued growth in skill until 8–9 years of age. A major area of attention during the school years is the development of literacy—specifically, reading and spelling. In the psycholinguistic model discussed earlier in this chapter, authors such as Stackhouse and Wells (1993) closely link speech and literacy in input–storage–output pathways. Phonological awareness is a skill that is closely associated with speech and literacy and will be discussed in detail in Chapter 13.

Phonological Awareness

Phonological awareness is "the ability to reflect on and manipulate the structure of an utterance as distinct from its meaning" (Stackhouse & Wells, 1997, p. 53) and is essential for the development of reading and spelling (Gillon, 2004). Children's phonological awareness skills also affect their perception of salient auditory cues (Mayo et al., 2003). Phonological awareness includes phonemic awareness, onset-rime awareness, and syllable awareness, and can be assessed via detection, deletion, and blending and segmentation of phonemes, syllables, and consonant clusters (Masso et al., 2014). For example, during blending tasks, children are presented with elements of a word and are asked to put them together to produce a word. Thus, an example of syllable blending is *com-put-er = computer* and an example of phoneme blending is *f-i-sh = fish*. Segmentation tasks are the reverse; a child is asked to segment a word into either syllables or phonemes.

Children with speech sound disorders typically find phonological awareness tasks difficult. Severity and type of speech sound disorder have both been suggested as significant predictors of performance of phonological awareness tasks (Holm et al., 2007; Leitão & Fletcher, 2004; Masso, Baker et al., 2017; Rvachew, 2007b; Stackhouse & Wells, 1997; Sutherland & Gillon, 2007). Phonological awareness skills (particularly phoneme isolation) were improved during a randomized controlled trial for children with speech sound disorders (Hesketh et al., 2007).

Acquisition of Phonological Awareness

Children's acquisition of phonological awareness is said to consist of three stages. Goswami and Bryant (1990) proposed that the three stages are: 1) awareness of syllables and words, 2) awareness of onsets and rimes, and 3) awareness of phonemes. Carroll and associates (2003) conducted a longitudinal study of 67 preschool-age children and assessed them at the following average ages: 3;10, 4;2, and 4;9 years. They recommended a revised series of stages: 1) early implicit large-segment sensitivity (associated with vocabulary knowledge), 2) sound similarity, and 3) explicit awareness of phonemes.

A number of researchers have considered English-speaking children's acquisition of phonological awareness skills, and their results are summarized in Table 3.11. The results listed in this table demonstrate that children have emerging skills from 3 to 4 years of age. As Dodd and Gillon (2001, p. 142) reported, "The majority of 4-year-old children . . . will not exhibit phonological awareness other than syllable segmentation and the emergence of rhyme awareness." By 5 years of age, the following skills

Table 3.11. Summary of studies of English-speaking children's acquisition of phonological awareness

Age	Lonigan et al. (1998) United States	Burt et al. (1999) United Kingdom	Dodd and Gillon (2001) United Kingdom and Australia	Gillon and Schwarz (2001) New Zealand	Carroll et al. (2003) United Kingdom
2;0	Wide variability; some children could perform above the level of chance on rhyme oddity detection, alliteration oddity detection, blending, and elision				
3;0			Emerging skills		Easiest to most difficult: 1. Rime matching 2. Syllable matching 3. Initial phoneme matching
4;0		Awareness of the concepts of syllable, onset, and rime but not awareness of individual phonemes	Awareness of syllable segmentation and rhyme awareness	Easiest to most difficult: 1. Generation of rhyming words 2. Phoneme blending 3. Phoneme segmentation	Easiest to most difficult: 1. Rime matching 2. Syllable matching 3. Initial phoneme matching
4;6					Easiest to most difficult: 1. Rime matching 2. Initial phoneme matching 3. Phoneme completion 4. Phoneme deletion
5;0	Syllable blending established for middle-income but not lower-income children		Established skills: syllable segmentation, rhyme awareness, phoneme isolation, letter knowledge		
5;6			Established skills: phoneme segmentation		
6;0			Australia 6;0–6;5 Established skills: syllable segmentation, rhyme awareness, alliteration awareness, phoneme isolation Australia 6;6–6;11 Established skills: phoneme segmentation, syllable segmentation, rhyme awareness, alliteration awareness, phoneme isolation, letter knowledge, phoneme segmentation		

are established: syllable segmentation, rhyme awareness, alliteration awareness, phoneme isolation, and letter knowledge. Phoneme segmentation is one of the latest skills to be established when children are 6–7 years old.

FACTORS INFLUENCING TYPICAL ACQUISITION OF SPEECH

Many factors influence typical acquisition of speech. The tables in this chapter clearly indicate that one of the major influences is the age of the child. As children mature, so does their accuracy of all aspects of speech production. However, within the literature, there is discussion of other aspects that may influence speech acquisition. These include gender, socioeconomic status, and concomitant language development.

Gender

There is a range of differing evidence regarding the effect of gender (sex) on the age of acquisition of speech sounds. Some normative studies present separate norms, some have separate norms at earlier ages, and some never separate by gender (sex). However, one generalization can be made: If separate norms are reported, girls acquire speech earlier than boys. Kenney and Prather (1986) found that boys made significantly more speech sound errors than girls at ages 3;0, 3;6, 4;0, 4;6, and 5;0, but not at 2;6. Smit and colleagues (1990) reported that boys and girls had different ages of acquisition for 11 sounds with significant differences between genders at ages 4;0, 4;6, and 6;0. All consonants except for /ʤ/ were acquired earlier by the girls. Dodd, Holm, and colleagues (2003) found no gender differences in speech acquisition for children aged 3;0 to 5;5; however, girls outperformed the boys at ages 5;6 to 6;11 in areas such as production of interdental fricatives and consonant clusters. Similarly, Poole (1934) indicated that girls acquired sounds earlier than boys after 5;6 years, while their development was similar at younger ages. In a study of the occurrence of phonological processes, McCormack and Knighton (1996) reported that boys age 2;6 had more final consonant deletion, weak syllable deletion, and cluster reduction than girls. In a study of phonological awareness, Gillon and Schwarz (2001) found that 6-year-old girls performed significantly better than boys. The suggestion that boys differ from girls in speech acquisition is consistent with the reports of more boys than girls being identified as having a speech sound disorder (Campbell et al., 2003; Law et al., 1998; McKinnon et al., 2007) and with the results of a meta-analysis that girls surpassed boys in a wide range of verbal behaviors (Hyde & Linn, 1988).

Socioeconomic Status

The effect of socioeconomic status (SES) on speech sound acquisition is not straightforward because of the different ways that SES can be measured (income, education, occupation, urban/suburban/rural, etc.) and the level of inference that is made about factors such as home language environment (Dodd, Holm et al., 2003). In some large-scale studies, SES has not been found to affect age of acquisition of speech (Dodd, Holm et al.; Smit et al., 1990); however, in others, children from a high SES background performed better than those from a low one (Templin, 1957). SES background has been found to have a significant effect on the acquisition of phonological awareness skills with children from mid- to high-SES backgrounds outperforming children from low-SES backgrounds (Burt et al., 1999; Gillon & Schwarz, 2001; Lonigan et al., 1998). For example, Lonigan and associates (1998) found that at 5 years of age, 89%

of children from a middle-income background performed above chance on syllable blending tasks, whereas only 27% of children from a lower-income background performed above chance on the same task.

Language Development

Speech and language acquisition are intimately connected during the early stages of language acquisition (Paul & Jennings, 1992; Roulstone et al., 2002; Stoel-Gammon, 1991). For example, Roulstone and colleagues (2002) reported an interrelationship between speech and language for 1,127 children age 25 months. Although these children were of the same age, they had differing levels of expressive language. The number of phonological errors decreased as the level of language increased. For instance, for the production of velar consonants, children at the single-word stage had 57% errors, children at the two-word utterance stage had 37% errors, and children at the three- to four-word utterance stage had only 24% errors. This pattern was repeated for fricatives (single-word, 61%; two-word, 48%; three- to four-word, 30%); liquids (75%, 66%, and 51%, respectively); postvocalic consonants (48%, 33%, and 15%, respectively); and consonant clusters (88%, 80%, and 66%, respectively).

B. L. Smith and colleagues (2006) also studied the interaction between language and speech for 2-year-old children. Their study compared the phonological development in lexically precocious (advanced vocabulary) 2-year-olds with age-matched and language-matched (2 1/2-year-old) peers. They found that the phonological skills of the lexically precocious 2-year-olds were similar to the language-matched peers and superior to the age-matched peers, again supporting the correlation between speech and language learning in the early years.

Individual Variability

Within the literature, variability is generally used in two ways: between individuals and within individuals. First, we examine *variability between individuals;* that is, variability in individuals' rates and/or sequences of development. Variability between individuals is also referred to as individual differences (e.g., Bleile, 1991; Ferguson & Farwell, 1975) and occurs when different children of the same age or stage of development have different realizations for speech sounds for the same words. Variability between individuals also describes different rates of development, different patterns of consistency in repetitions of words, and different styles of learning. Most researchers agree that no two children follow identical paths of development. Progress beyond the first 50 words has been understood as a period of significant transition for children developing language. For example, Vihman and Greenlee (1987) studied 10 typically developing children at 1 and 3 years of age. Significant differences were reported between the children's rate of vocabulary acquisition, phonological maturity, and general approach to learning.

Alternatively, variability is sometimes used to describe differences *within individuals* (e.g., Barlow, 1996; Berg, 1995; Bernhardt & Stemberger, 1998; French, 1989; Leonard et al., 1982; Sosa, 2015) and occurs in two different forms. First, variability occurs when a child has different realizations of a particular speech sound for different lexical items. For example, /s/ may be realized as [s] in *sea,* but [t] in *seat.* Second, variability occurs when a child has different realizations for multiple productions of the same lexical item. For example, a child with variable repeated productions of *sleep* may realize /sl/ as [sl] in [sliː], simplify /sl/ by substituting [sw] in [swip], reduce /sl/ to

[s] in [sip], and omit /sl/ entirely in [ip]. Leonard and colleagues (1982) described some of the reasons for variable productions of words: "Variable words are most often those which have more advanced canonical forms or sounds" and "Word shape as well as consonant composition may play a role in intra-word variability" (p. 56).

There are numerous examples of variability within the production of speech sounds by typically developing children. Ferguson and Farwell (1975) described a child age 1;3 who produced the word *pen* in 10 different ways. Vogel Sosa and Stoel-Gammon (2006) conducted a longitudinal study of four typically developing children between 1 and 2 years of age. They found high overall variability as well as a peak in variability that corresponded to the onset of two-word utterances. Stoel-Gammon (2004) conducted a longitudinal study examining the speech of five children aged 21 to 33 months and found high rates of variability, even in CVC words. Dyson and Paden (1983) conducted a longitudinal study over a 7-month period to consider phonological acquisition strategies used by 2-year-olds. Comparisons of each child's productions of target words across time led them to comment, "This period of roughly two to three-and-one-half years of age seems to be one of extreme variability with subjects 'trying out' a variety of strategies to approximate the adult model" (p. 16). Menn and Stoel-Gammon (1995, pp. 340–341) indicated that early words are "extremely variable in pronunciation." Similarly, in a longitudinal study of typically developing 2- to 3-year-old children, McLeod and Hewett (2008) examined variability in the production of words containing consonant clusters produced in spontaneous speech. Half (53.7%, range = 42.4%–77.6%) of all repeated words were produced variably. As the children reached age 3, they increased the accuracy and decreased the variability of their productions; however, variability between and within individuals continued to occur. Sosa (2015) reported similar findings for 33, 2- to 3-year-old children's productions of 25 target words. She found that children commonly produced each word differently and had more variability for longer words. Holm and colleagues (2007) considered the variability of the speech of 405 typically developing children aged 3;0 and 6;11 on a single-word task that contained many polysyllabic words. The younger children demonstrated the highest levels of variability (13%), and their variable productions predominantly reflected maturational influences.

As will be noted in later chapters, variability has been considered a diagnostic marker of speech sound disorder (see the discussion in Chapter 5 on Childhood Apraxia of Speech; also see Holm et al., 2007). However, the presence of high degrees of variability in typically developing children's speech should be taken into account (Stoel-Gammon, 2007). If the speech of typically developing children is highly variable, then the extent and nature of variability must be defined when it is used as a diagnostic marker of speech impairment (McLeod & Hewett, 2008). From the studies examined here, there is much variability between children in the acquisition of speech. Additionally, there is variability within the speech of individuals. Variability within individuals is more likely to occur with younger children and in spontaneous speech contexts.

CONCLUSION: UNDERSTANDING AND APPLYING TYPICAL SPEECH ACQUISITION

As SLPs, we use information on typical speech acquisition as the foundation of our clinical decision making. Thomas (2000) suggests that there are two ways of understanding normal speech acquisition: 1) knowledge of statistical similarity (typical acquisition) and 2) understanding of attitudes and desirability within the child's speech and language culture (acceptable acquisition). The majority of this chapter has examined the literature on typical speech acquisition and has described ages of attainment of a wide range of measures. The tables presented will be useful as a resource in your SLP practice. However, you are also encouraged to think as an anthropologist in terms of the communities and clients with whom you are working. Such understanding underlies notions of correctness and acceptability appropriate to a given child's speech and language behaviors. Chapter 14 discusses these understandings in more detail.

QUESTIONS FOR CHAPTER 3

1. Describe how the following models of speech acquisition add to our overall picture of how children acquire speech: behaviorism, generative phonology, natural phonology, nonlinear phonology, sonority, optimality theory, and psycholinguistic theory.

2. Describe the advantages and disadvantages of the three major research methods employed to examine speech acquisition.

3. Delineate the stages of infant vocal production from birth to age 1.

4. How do perception and production interact in infants?

5. Describe the characteristics and accomplishments of the transition stage of speech acquisition.

6. Review the large-scale normative data for English and identify early, mid, and late developing sounds.

7. What are phonological patterns/processes? Describe young children's use of phonological patterns.

8. How would a child at age 2 years and a child at age 5 years with typical speech say *cheese, hat, spoon, caterpillar, running,* and *three*? To answer this question, consider:

   a. What phonemes are in the words? When are they normally mastered?

   b. Which word position are they in?

   c. What syllable shapes are represented? Would a child of this age typically produce these syllable shapes?

   d. What phonological patterns normally operate at this age?

   e. What are normal mismatches for a child of this age?

9. What is the importance of the acquisition of phonological awareness in school-age children?

10. How are children similar and different in speech acquisition?

4

Factors Related to Speech Sound Disorders

NICHOLAS W. BANKSON, JOHN E. BERNTHAL, AND PETER FLIPSEN JR.

LEARNING OBJECTIVES

This chapter discusses the speech and hearing mechanism, cognitive-linguistic, and psychosocial factors that have been associated with speech sound disorders (SSDs). By the end of this chapter, the reader should be able to:

- Describe the possible role of otitis media in SSDs.

- Describe speech sound perception and its relationship to SSDs in terms of testing and its role in treatment.

- Outline the potential impact of various minor structural deviations of the speech mechanism on SSDs.

- Summarize the role of oral sensory skills in speech and SSDs.

- Discuss the relative value of various measures of speech motor skill relative to SSDs.

- Describe the current state of knowledge of oral myofunctional disorders and their possible relationship to SSDs.

- Discuss the potential impact of pacifier use on speech acquisition and SSDs.

- Discuss the relationship between cognitive status and SSDs.

- Describe the role of phonological memory in both speech and reading.

- Outline top-down, bottom-up, and synergistic perspectives on the interplay of the speech sound system and other aspects of language.

- Discuss the potential impact of SSDs on academic achievement.

- Describe how SSDs might be manifest across different ages and genders.

- Summarize the association between SSDs and socioeconomic status.

- Discuss familial tendencies in the population of children with SSDs.

- Discuss the relationship of siblings and SSDs.

- Describe the possible relationship between personality and SSDs.

A longstanding interest of clinicians and researchers who are focused on SSDs is that of causality of this type of speech impairment. Over the years, attempts have been made to identify various factors or characteristics that are possibly related to the presence of these disorders. Although no single characteristic or set of characteristics that might describe causality of SSDs in these children has yet been identified, it appears that certain factors may be associated and/or co-occur with some of them. An appreciation of these factors is important because they may offer insight into the nature of the problem for specific children. It also provides useful information for the discussion of the various attempts at classification of SSDs found in Chapter 5.

At the present time, the largest group of associated or causal factors that has been identified is in the area of structure and function of the speech and hearing mechanism. These are presented first in this chapter. Next, the chapter discusses motor abilities, followed by cognitive-linguistic factors, and in the final section, psychosocial factors.

Before diving into the topics to be covered in this chapter, it is important to note that many of the research studies reviewed in this chapter consist of relatively small samples of children. This creates at least two serious challenges for both researchers and clinicians. First, it makes it difficult to generalize any findings obtained in a study with a small sample of children to the entire population of children with SSDs. Second, it makes it difficult to obtain statistically significant results because of limited statistical power. The obvious solution would be to only conduct studies with large samples. As easy as that might sound, researchers are often hard pressed to find enough research participants (i.e., children) living in the same area who meet the subject inclusion criteria required in a study. That is why wherever possible this chapter presents findings from multiple studies to look for what is called converging evidence.

Another point to be made at the beginning of this chapter relates to the terminology used to identify disorders in the production of the sounds of the language. As pointed out earlier in this text, historically the term *articulation* was the accepted term to identify this type of speech disorder, and some years later the term *phonology* was often employed. Presently, the accepted term is *speech sound disorder*, which encompasses both articulation (motor aspects of production) and phonology (linguistic rules aspect of productions). These three terms are used interchangeably in this chapter, as research and writings in the field reflect each of these as time has evolved, and thus in keeping with sources cited, we have retained the terminology used by various researchers and authors.

STRUCTURE AND FUNCTION OF THE SPEECH AND HEARING MECHANISM

An obvious consideration when evaluating an individual's speech sound production skills relates to the potential for problems that may be manifested in the structure and function of the speech and hearing mechanism. Problems of this nature may require at least consultation with other medically related professionals. An example of this is a child with a history of cleft palate who is experiencing difficulty with correct production of stops, fricatives, and affricates, possibly due to inadequate velopharyngeal closure. Assessment followed by either surgical or prosthetic management coordinated by a cleft palate or craniofacial team would be the typical approach. On the other hand, surgical intervention for lesser problems, such as a mild case of relative macroglossia (a normal-sized tongue in a small oral cavity) sometimes observed in individuals with Down syndrome, might be more difficult to justify (see the study by Parsons et al., 1987, which showed that such procedures appear to offer little improvement in speech production). A more typical approach in such cases would be to teach specific compensatory strategies such as controlling speaking rate (i.e., slowing down). It should be noted, however, that final decisions about intervention approaches for many individuals who exhibit deficiencies in structure and/or function of the speech and hearing mechanisms will not be made by the speech-language pathologist (SLP) alone. An SLP's input to a team decision is often essential. An appreciation of the impact of speech and hearing mechanism issues on SSDs is vital to what we do as SLPs.

Otitis Media With Effusion (OME)

It has long been inferred that frequent episodes of middle ear disease in children, which are accompanied by a buildup of liquid in the middle ear space, may result in a delay in speech sound development. This condition is called *otitis media with effusion (OME)*. The assumption is that the accumulating liquid blocks the transmission of sound, resulting in a mild to moderate hearing loss, which may then impact speech sound acquisition. Although otitis media invariably resolves and hearing usually returns to normal at about 6–7 years of age, frequent episodes may result in a history of inconsistent and distorted auditory input, which creates the potential for subsequent delays in speech sound development. A significant amount of research has examined this issue with mixed research findings. In one of the more comprehensive reviews of research concerning the effects of OME on speech development, Shriberg, Flipsen, and colleagues (2000) identified 27 studies conducted on possible speech delay associated with frequent episodes of OME. Of the 27 studies, 17 (63%) suggested no impact, whereas 21 (78%) suggested some impact. (Some studies included comparisons using multiple measurement approaches and reported both impacts and no impacts.) Many factors likely contribute to these seemingly conflicting results and are highlighted in Box 4.1.

BOX 4.1   The Challenge of Determining the Effect of Otitis Media on Speech Development

1. Most children experience at least one middle ear infection before age 5 years, but most have only one (see Adams & Benson, 1991).

2. A subset of children (perhaps 30%) seem more susceptible and have many episodes, but researchers have defined *many* in different ways.

3. Some children experience episodes but show no outward symptoms (a condition called silent otitis; see Marchant et al., 1984). Such children may have ended up in the no otitis group by mistake.

4. Timing of the OME episodes may be critical. Most studies did not consider when episodes occurred. Episodes occurring between 18 and 24 months of age may be especially detrimental (see Shriberg, Friel-Patti et al., 2000).

5. Some children receive immediate treatment, while it may be delayed for others. The studies typically didn't document the timing or extent of treatment.

6. Studies differed on the standard for deciding if otitis media was present; parent report versus visual inspection of the eardrums versus tympanometry.

7. Not every episode results in any level of hearing loss. Few studies actually measured hearing level directly.

8. Even when hearing loss is present it is at most a moderate loss. Unlike severe or profound hearing loss, OME effects are unlikely to be extreme.

9. Different speech outcome measures have been used.

10. Socioeconomic status (SES) may play a role both in susceptibility and in access to treatment. Most studies failed to document SES or differ widely in how they did so.

One proposal to deal with the complexity of OME and its possible effect on speech development has been to use longitudinal studies in which children are recruited in the first year of life and monitored for several years. Roberts and colleagues (2004) surveyed 14 such prospective studies using a statistical technique known as a *meta-analysis* and concluded that there were "no to very small associations of OM to speech and language development in most children" (p. 247). Roberts and colleagues did note that such a conclusion assumes an optimal learning environment, which may not always be present.

Another concern about research examining the relationship of OME to speech development is the search for a significant difference approach used in most studies assumes an all-or-nothing effect. It may be more productive to assume that particular children may be at higher risk for delayed speech development associated with OME. A study by Shriberg, Flipsen, and colleagues (2000) took a relative risk approach and their findings support such a conclusion. Using two different groups, these authors reported that having frequent OME resulted in no increased risk of delayed speech in a group of children from a university-affiliated, general pediatric clinic group, but a significantly increased risk of approximately 4.6 times for a group of Native American children living on a reservation. Children in the latter group were from a lower SES background and had poorer access to good-quality medical care. Thus, under one set of circumstances frequent OME made no difference, but under a different set of circumstances it made a significant difference.

Speech Sound Perception/Discrimination

Being able to hear is clearly important to speaking. We need to hear what others are saying in a communicative context to make a connection between words and the meaning they represent. In addition, we need to be able to monitor our own output to make sure we have produced what we have intended and, if not, correct it. The vast majority of children with SSDs have normal hearing acuity (i.e., they pass a basic hearing screening). Those who do not may qualify as hearing impaired and this group of children will be discussed in Chapter 5.

However, passing a basic hearing screening test does not always mean having normal speech perception (often referred to as *speech discrimination*) skills (see also Box 4.2). According to Rvachew and Grawburg (2006), "Speech perception is the process of transforming a continuously changing acoustic signal into discrete linguistic units" (speech sounds) (p. 76). These speech perception skills allow the child to 1) make the association between the sounds of the native language and the meaning that can be expressed with those sounds, 2) make the association between the sounds the child generates and the movements of the vocal tract, 3) make the association between the sounds the child produces and the meaningful units of the language, and 4) adapt their productions to changes to their own vocal tract (i.e., adjust for their own growth). Given the importance of speech perception, it should not be surprising that SLPs have long been interested in the relationship between the perception and production of speech sounds in individuals with SSDs.

In the early days of the profession, many clinicians assumed that a major reason children produced speech sounds in error was because they didn't properly discriminate or perceive one sound from another (e.g., /s/ in *some* from /θ/ in *thumb*). The possibility of such a relationship was first investigated in the 1930s. This early perceptual research, referred to as *speech sound discrimination research*, relied primarily on general measures of speech sound discrimination (tests comparing a wide

---

BOX 4.2   It's Not Just About Hearing!

Being able to understand speech, as well as being able to use what we know to generate meaningful speech, requires a complex set of skills, including the ability to hear. That's why a basic hearing test is part of most speech assessment protocols. But a basic hearing test only measures the ability to detect or notice if any sound is present. This is called *speech detection.*

But not all sound around us is speech. Listeners also must be able to distinguish between speech and other types of sound. This is called *speech recognition.*

Even speech recognition is not enough. Listeners also need to be able to separate the continuous stream of speech into its smallest linguistic units. This means being able to discriminate among the individual speech sounds (phonemes and allophones) of a language. This is called *speech perception* (sometimes called speech discrimination).

Speech perception is particularly important for the developing child who is learning speech and language for the first time. Once children sort out the individual speech sounds they then can start to associate how variations in each sound are used to create different meanings within the language (i.e., they learn the sound system or the phonology of the language).

---

variety of sound contrasts; e.g., boat/goat; Sue/zoo), which required the participant to judge whether word or nonsense pairs verbally presented by the examiner were the same or different. In such tests, the assumption was that any deficit found would be an overall problem with distinguishing among many speech sounds. There was no attempt to determine whether the problem was more specific to certain sound pairs (i.e., whether the individual was only making perceptual errors on the same sounds that they had difficulty producing). These early studies yielded mixed findings. Some (e.g., Clark, 1959; Kronvall & Diehl, 1954; Travis & Rasmus, 1931) found that typical speakers had significantly better discrimination skills than speakers who produced speech sound errors, and several investigators found a positive correlation between performance on articulation tests and performance on tests of speech sound discrimination (Carrell & Pendergast, 1954; Reid, 1947a). Other studies, however, found no such relationship (Garrett, 1969; Hall, 1938; Mase, 1946; Prins, 1962b; Veatch, 1970).

General Versus Phoneme-Specific Measures

Although there were differences across studies in terms of how groups were selected (e.g., Sherman & Geith, 1967) or differences in the discrimination task being used (e.g., Schwartz & Goldman, 1974) in the late 1970s, a consensus emerged that children with SSDs did not have a general problem with speech perception. The general tests of discrimination being used became viewed as being of limited value. Researchers such as Locke (1980a) pointed out that in children with SSDs, the critical issue is their ability to discriminate the particular sound or segments that they misarticulate. Locke recommended that measures of speech sound perception should be not only phoneme specific but also context specific. He argued that perceptual tasks should reflect the child's production errors and reflect those phonetic environments (words) in which error productions occur and include both the error productions and the target productions. Locke (1980b) studied a group of 131 children aged 3.1–9.9 years who performed a perceptual task in which the examiner produced imitations of the participants' error productions. The participants were then required to judge whether the examiner's productions were correct productions of the target word. Locke reported that 70% of the children correctly perceived the correct and incorrect forms of the target words, thus indicating that many children could correctly discriminate sounds made by an adult that had been produced in error. About one-third of the participants still misperceived the contrasts that had been produced in error.

Locke's notion of a direct connection between perceptual errors and errors in the production of the same sounds is also supported by a more recent study by Hitchcock and colleagues (2020). That study examined the ability of 15 children aged 7–14 years with /r/ errors to ". . . perceive small acoustic contrasts in synthetic speech stimuli." (p. 1). Findings indicated that the children performed as well as their same-age peers who had no errors in their speech on most speech contrasts. The one exception was their ability to discriminate the /rɑ/ - /wɑ/ contrast. Thus, their production error appeared to be linked to perceptual problems with the same sound.

The specificity of perceptual errors may also reflect inherent differences in how easy or how hard it is for particular sounds to be perceived either by all listeners or for children with SSDs in particular. A study by Hearnshaw and colleagues (2018) used a similar judgment task to Locke's and examined perception of four commonly misarticulated sounds /k, r, s, ʃ/ in word-initial position. Stimuli were both correct and incorrect productions produced by both children and adults. Participants included 12 children with SSDs (aged 48–60 months) who misarticulated one or more of those sounds. Their performance was contrasted with 13 age- and gender-matched typically developing preschool children. Results indicated that the children with SSDs had poorer speech perception skill overall than the typically developing children. Perhaps more importantly, both groups perceived /s/ and /r/ less accurately than /k/ or /ʃ/.

The notion that speech perception plays a role in production errors for only certain sounds was also demonstrated in a study of 14 children of 2 years of age. Eilers and Oller (1976) found some perceptual confusion in word and nonsense pairs when production of one segment was substituted for another. Yet, other common production errors were discriminated by most of their participants. The researchers concluded that some production errors may be related to perceptual difficulties and others to motor (or physical production) constraints.

External and Internal Discrimination

Recall the four aspects of speech sound acquisition mentioned earlier that are relevant to speech perception skills. The first of these (making the association between the sounds of the language in the environment and meaning) involves monitoring the speech of others. This is termed *external discrimination*, or monitoring. External discrimination can also include *external self-discrimination*, which involves listening to and making judgments of tape-recorded samples of one's own speech. In both cases, the listener uses air conduction auditory cues.

The other three aspects of speech sound acquisition mentioned earlier involve evaluating one's own ongoing speech sound productions, which is called *internal discrimination* or *internal monitoring*. During internal discrimination, the speaker has available both air- and bone-conducted auditory cues. Unfortunately, there is currently no unambiguous way to test internal discrimination, as bone-conduction auditory cues are only available inside a person's own head. The difference is highlighted by recalling that unless we listen to them regularly, most of us don't recognize our own voices from recordings. The closest available method is similar to testing external self-discrimination mentioned previously. It involves asking the child to judge the accuracy of their own productions of words or sounds immediately after they are produced.

A classic example of the difference between external and internal discrimination was reported by Berko and Brown (1960), who described what has come to be known as the /fɪs/ *phenomenon*. A child attempted to say a word (e.g., *fish*) but produced an error (e.g., /fɪs/). The examiner then asked, "Did you say /fɪs/?", to which the child responded, "No, /fɪs/." The child recognized the error in the examiner's speech but not in their own. Thus, they had good external discrimination skills but poor internal discrimination skills. Another example of this phenomenon is presented in Clinical Vignette 4.1.

Despite the previously documented cases of the /fɪs/ phenomenon, discrimination difficulty of this nature is relatively uncommon. Studies of speech sound discrimination skills of young children with delayed speech sound development have indicated that children frequently are able to make external judgments of sound contrasts involving their error sounds (Chaney & Menyuk, 1975; Eilers & Oller, 1976; Locke, 1980a; Locke & Kutz, 1975). A study by Aungst and Frick (1964) looked at the relationship between external and internal discrimination of /r/ productions in 27 children age 8–10 years. Each participant was asked to 1) make an immediate right–wrong judgment of their /r/ production after speaking each word, 2) make right–wrong judgments of their /r/ productions from audio recordings, and 3) make same–different judgments of their /r/ productions as they followed the examiner's correct productions presented via audiotape recording. Moderate correlation coefficients of .69, .66, and .59 were obtained between each of the three phoneme-specific discrimination tasks and scores for production of /r/ on the Deep Test of Articulation, which looks at production across a wide range of phonetic contexts. In contrast, scores on a general test of auditory discrimination did not correlate well with the articulation measure. Lapko and Bankson (1975) conducted a similar study using a group of 25 kindergarten and first-grade children exhibiting misarticulations of /s/ and reported similar findings, as did both Stelcik (1972) and Wolfe and Irwin (1973).

But the results of other investigations (Shelton et al., 1977; Woolf & Pilberg, 1971) have indicated that the findings in such studies may be influenced by factors such as the consistency of the misarticulations, the type of discrimination task used to test internal monitoring, and the nature of the stimulus items.

Clinical Vignette 4.1

Example of the /fɪs/ Phenomenon

The third author of this book, Peter Flipsen, Jr., vividly recalls an example of the /fɪs/ phenomenon very much like that in Berko and Brown (1960). A former client, Priscilla (a pseudonym), entered therapy at age 4 years with speech that was extremely difficult to understand. In addition to some other errors, she tended to substitute the palatal glide /j/ for many other sounds in prevocalic position. At one point in a therapy session, Priscilla was attempting to produce the word *rope* but instead said /joʊp/. Wanting to see if she recognized the error she had just made in her production, Dr. Flipsen repeated it back to her in question form, along with a puzzled look, "/joʊp/?"

Priscilla immediately stopped. She stood up from her chair and came around to Dr. Flipsen's side of the table. She brought her face to within a few inches of his, put her hands on her hips, and said, rather indignantly, in a firm voice, "No! /joʊp/!"

Dr. Flipsen recalls having some difficulty maintaining his composure but was able to limit his reaction to just a tight smile. Priscilla's mother, on the other hand, who had been watching from the adjoining observation room through a two-way mirror, could be heard roaring with laughter.

Neither Dr. Flipsen nor Priscilla's mother were deliberately wanting to make light of Priscilla's difficulty. Clearly, she was not, at that moment, able to notice her own production error. The humor lay solely in the extremely serious reaction coming from an otherwise highly social, extremely lovable, young child.

The Perception–Production Relationship

Historically, clinicians routinely conducted some type of discrimination training, or ear training, as it was thought to be a necessary precursor to production training. Such training is no longer a routine part of treatment. Indeed, even speech perception testing has also become less common than in the past. This change appears to be the result of the mixed findings for studies of the relationship between general perceptual skills and production errors. However, if at least some speech errors are likely perceptually based, a logical question is whether a functional relationship exists between speech sound production and speech discrimination/perception. A number of investigators have considered this question. They have asked both whether discrimination training affects production of speech sounds and if learning to correctly produce sounds enhances discrimination.

Sonderman (1971) asked both questions by administering two different speech sound discrimination training programs in alternate sequence to two matched groups of 10 children between 6 and 8 years old, all of whom produced frontal lisps. Improvement in both discrimination and articulation scores was obtained from both discrimination training and articulation training, regardless of the sequence in which the two types of training were conducted. A caveat here is that articulatory improvement did not necessarily mean that speech sound errors were fully corrected. Rather, shifts from one type of error to another (e.g., omission to substitution; substitution to distortion) were regarded as evidence of improvement.

G. Williams and McReynolds (1975) explored these same questions with four participants aged 5–6 years (two received production training first; two received discrimination training first). Findings indicated that production training was effective in changing both production and discrimination; in contrast to Sonderman (1971), however, discrimination training did not generalize to production.

Shelton and associates (1977) specifically explored the influence of articulation training on discrimination performance. One group of participants received production training on /r/ and a second group on /s/. Results from pre- and post-discrimination probes, specifically related to the error sound, indicated that both groups of participants improved in articulation performance; however, no improvement was noted in discrimination performance.

Rvachew (1994) studied the influence of speech perception training that was administered along with traditional speech sound therapy. Twenty-seven preschoolers with SSDs who misarticulated /ʃ/ were randomly assigned to three training groups: 1) listening to a variety of correctly and incorrectly produced versions of the word *shoe*, 2) listening to the words *shoe* and *moo*, and 3) listening to the words *cat* and *Pete*. Following six weekly treatment sessions, groups 1 and 2 showed superior ability to articulate the target sound in comparison to group 3. Rvachew then suggested that "speech perception training should probably be provided concurrently with speech production training" (p. 355). Later reports from Rvachew and colleagues (1999) and Rvachew and associates (2004) further supported this conclusion.

Another factor worth considering here is the concept of stimulability, which will be discussed later in this book. *Stimulability* represents the ability to correctly produce/imitate a speech sound (that is not currently being produced correctly) following presentation of a correctly produced model. If a child can correctly produce an error sound after hearing a model of the sound, the child is said to be stimulable for the error. Such ability is often seen by clinicians as a form of readiness for change. If children are stimulable following a simple model, it also suggests the ability to at least externally discriminate their error from the target and that they have the motor skill required to produce the sound. But it doesn't necessarily mean that these children have good internal discrimination skill. This is supported by the occurrence of the /fɪs/ phenomenon discussed previously and suggests that discrimination ability alone cannot explain the production skills of some children with SSDs.

Through two complementary studies, Rvachew and colleagues (1999) explored the relationship among stimulability, speech perception ability, and phonological learning. In the first study, participants were treated individually using a cycles approach as prescribed by Hodson (1989). The researchers reported that children who were stimulable for a target sound and who demonstrated good pretreatment perceptual ability for that sound made more progress in therapy than those who were stimulable for the target sound but had poor speech sound perception for that sound. Children who were not stimulable did not make progress regardless of their perceptual skills. A second study included both individual and group instruction for the participants. Lessons involved phonetically based production activities and a computer-based program of perceptual training. Results from the second study indicated that all children, regardless of pretreatment stimulability and/or speech perception skills, made progress in production. The authors concluded that "despite the independence of stimulability and speech perception ability before training, there is reason to believe that speech perception training may facilitate the acquisition of stimulability if both production and perception training are provided concurrently to children who demonstrate unstimulability and poor speech perception for the target sound" (Rvachew et al., 1999, p. 40).

Self-Monitoring

The ability to identify errors in one's own speech (referred to earlier in the chapter as internal discrimination) has long been suggested as being important to therapy progress. The ability to hear the differences in another person's speech or one's own taped productions does not, however, guarantee that a particular child will actively listen for and pay attention to those differences (i.e., that they will self-monitor). Although formal study of internal discrimination has been limited, some investigators (Koegel et al., 1986, 1988) have examined the relationship between self-monitoring skills and response generalization into the natural environment. School-age children were provided specific training in self-monitoring of their speech productions. These investigators reported that generalization of correct articulatory responses of the target sounds did not occur until a self-monitoring task was initiated in the treatment program. They concluded that such self-monitoring was required for generalization of the target sounds in the natural environment to occur. Using slightly different procedures, Gray and Shelton (1992) failed to replicate these findings. The authors indicated that different participants, treatment procedures, and environmental variables may have accounted for the different outcomes.

Kwiatkowski and Shriberg (1993, 1998) suggested that self-monitoring may actually result from the complex interaction of both 1) capability (linguistic and motor skills, physiological and cognitive limitations, psychosocial factors) and 2) focus (attention, motivation, effort). This might account for the mixed findings from studies of the role of self-monitoring in treatment outcomes. Reliable, objective measures of either self-monitoring or focus have not been developed. As such, the role of self-monitoring in the remediation of SSDs is still to be refined.

Summary

Speech sound production errors are clearly not all based in problems of speech perception. However, a meta-analysis by Hearnshaw and colleagues (2019) suggests poor perceptual skills may be part of the problem for at least some children with SSDs. Data from individual studies suggest this may include perhaps as many as 30% to 40% of this population (Locke, 1980a; Rvachew & Grawburg, 2006). Perceptual testing is therefore justified in this population, particularly testing that is focused on speech sounds that the child misarticulates (Lof & Synan, 1997). Self-monitoring of error productions would appear to be an important skill for normalization of speech sounds in spontaneous speech, but instruments to assess such skill are lacking. The efficacy of speech sound perception training as a precursor to production training has often been questioned. However, when perceptual deficiencies are present, perceptual training prior to or concurrent with direct instruction would seem appropriate. This is supported by findings from Wolfe and colleagues (2003) who compared production-only training against production training combined with perception training. They reported that adding perception training appeared to help production accuracy only for those sounds that were perceived poorly prior to therapy.

Minor Structural Variations of the Speech Mechanism

As part of an oral mechanism examination, speech clinicians are required to make judgments about the structure and/or function of the lips, teeth, tongue, and palate. These oral structures can vary significantly, even among normal speakers. Investigators have attempted to identify relationships between SSDs and structural variations of the oral mechanism.

Major structural variations will be discussed in Chapter 5 regarding organically based disorders. The following sections highlight lesser variations and their potential impact on speech sound production. Although a strict cause–effect relationship has not been established, such variations may contribute to the difficulty in speech sound production that some children experience.

Lips

Approximation of the lips is required for the formation of the English bilabial phonemes /b/, /p/, and /m/; lip rounding is required for various vowels and the consonants /w/ and /ʍ/. An impairment that would inhibit lip approximation or rounding might result in misarticulation of these sounds. Fairbanks and Green (1950) examined measurements of various dimensions of the lips in 30 adult speakers with superior consonant production and 30 with inferior consonant production and reported no differences between the two groups.

Certain anomalies of the lips, such as the enlarged lips in Ackerman syndrome (Ackerman et al., 1973) or congenital double lips (Eski et al., 2007), may interfere with speech production, but not in every case. Most such cases can be corrected surgically. These findings suggest that only major deviations in lip structure or function are likely to impact speech sound production.

Teeth

Many English consonants require intact dentition for correct production. Labiodental phonemes (/f/ and /v/) require contact between the teeth and lower lip for their production, and linguadental phonemes require tongue placement just behind or between the teeth for /ð/ and /θ/ productions. The tongue tip alveolars (/s/, /z/) require that the airstream pass over the cutting edge of the incisors.

Researchers investigating the relationship between deviant dentition and consonant production have examined the presence or absence of teeth, position of teeth (dental arch shape), and dental occlusion. *Occlusion* refers to the alignment of the first molar teeth when the jaws are closed and *malocclusion* refers to the imperfect or irregular position of those teeth when the jaws are closed. In normal occlusion (also called Class I), the upper first molar is positioned half a tooth behind the lower first molar. In a Class II malocclusion, the positions of the upper and lower first molars are reversed (i.e., the upper is half a tooth ahead). In a Class III malocclusion, the upper first molar is more than half a tooth behind the lower first molar.

Malocclusions may also affect the relative positions of the upper and lower front teeth or incisors. Often in a Class II malocclusion, the upper incisors are too far forward relative to the lower incisors, resulting in what is called an *overjet*; conversely, in a Class III malocclusion, the upper incisors are often positioned behind the lower incisors, and the result is called an *underjet* (see Figure 4.1 for examples of different types of occlusions).

A number of investigators have examined the relationship between different types of occlusion and SSDs. Bernstein (1954) identified malocclusions in children

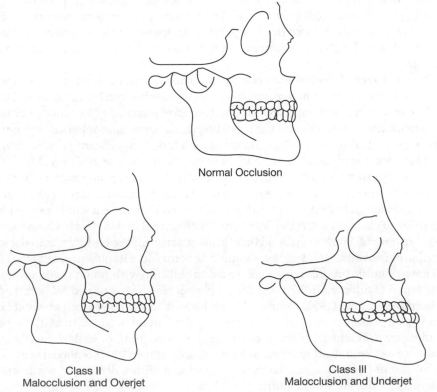

Normal Occlusion

Class II
Malocclusion and Overjet

Class III
Malocclusion and Underjet

Figure 4.1. Examples of types of occlusions.

with normal and defective speech but did not find a higher incidence of malocclusion in children with speech sound problems than in children with normal speech sound production. Fairbanks and Lintner (1951) examined molar occlusion, occlusion of the anterior teeth, and anterior spaces in 60 adults, 30 of whom were judged to have superior speech sound skills and 30 with inferior skills. The authors found that marked dental deviations occurred significantly more frequently in the inferior speakers than in the superior ones. In a report on 451 college-age students in Finland, Laine and associates (1987) reported a significantly higher number of horizontal overjet or vertical overbites in participants with audibly clear /s/ distortions compared to their peers with no speech errors. The relationship may not be strictly causal, however, as Subtelny and colleagues (1964) found malocclusion to coexist with both normal and defective speech. During /s/ production, some of their normal speakers with malocclusion (distocclusion) tended to position the tongue tip slightly to the rear of the lower incisors (i.e., using what some have called a *tongue-tip down /s/*, which is perceived by most listeners as a normal /s/) when compared to normal speakers with normal occlusion. This suggests that although speakers with normal articulatory skills tend to have a lower incidence of malocclusion than speakers with articulatory errors, malocclusion itself does not preclude normal production, as accommodation is possible.

Some connection between SSDs in children and relative tooth position has also been noted in studies of the shape of the dental arch. Starr (1972) reported that a speech sound problem is highly probable in individuals with a short or narrow maxillary (upper) arch and a normal mandibular (lower) arch. The consonants likely to be affected by such conditions are /s, z, ʃ, tʃ, f, v, t, d/. He further noted that rotated teeth and supernumerary (extra) teeth do not generally present significant speech problems. A study by Heliövaara (2011) found shorter (but not necessarily narrower) maxillary arches in 52 Finnish children (mean age 6;4) with speech errors compared to 52 age-matched children with normal speech. Mandibular arch data were not examined by Heliövaara.

Another area of interest has been the influence of missing teeth on speech sound production. In a study of kindergarten and first-grade children by Bankson and Byrne (1962), participants with intact teeth were identified who had either correct or incorrect articulation. After 4 months, articulation skills were reassessed and the number of missing central or lateral incisors was tabulated. A significant relationship was found between the presence or absence of teeth and correct production of /s/, but not of /f/, /ʃ/, or /z/. However, some children maintained correct production of /s/ despite the loss of their incisors. Snow (1961) examined the influence of missing teeth on consonant production in first-grade children. Although there was a significantly higher proportion of children with missing or grossly abnormal incisor teeth who misarticulated consonants, Snow also found that three-quarters of the children with defective dentition did not misarticulate these sounds. In contrast to Bankson and Byrne (1962), who noted significant differences compared to children with intact teeth only for /s/, Snow found significant differences for all phonemes she examined (/f, v, s, z, ð, θ/. Gable and colleagues (1995) examined 26 children whose incisor teeth were extracted before age 5 years. By age 8–10 years, their speech sound production skills were not significantly different from those of an age-matched group of children without the premature extractions. However, Pahkala and colleagues (1991) reported that earlier appearance of the permanent teeth was associated with a decreased occurrence of SSDs in a group of children acquiring Finnish.

Overall, although dental status may be a crucial factor in speech sound productions for some children, it does not appear to be significant for most. This is consistent with conclusions from reviews by Johnson and Sandy (1999) and Hassan and associates (2007). Many children appear to be able to adapt to abnormal dental relationships or atypical dental development.

Tongue

The tongue is generally considered to be the most important articulator for speech production. Tongue movements during speech production include tip elevation, grooving, and protrusion. The tongue is relatively short at birth and grows longer and thinner at the tip with age.

Ankyloglossia, or *tongue-tie*, is a term used to describe a restricted lingual frenum (sometimes called the *frenulum*). According to Hong and colleagues (2010), there is no consensus as to the precise definition of the term. Recently, specific protocols for evaluating it have been proposed (Marchesan, 2012; Martinelli et al., 2012). Kummer (2009) noted that, clinically, it is usually defined as the inability to protrude the tip of the tongue past the front teeth. A review by Segal and colleagues (2007) indicated that prevalence estimates for ankyloglossia range from 4.2% to 10.7% of the population, with the variability in these estimates likely related to differences in definitions of ankyloglossia.

At one time, it was commonly assumed that an infant or child with ankyloglossia should have their frenum clipped to allow greater freedom of tongue movement and better articulation of tongue tip sounds, and frenectomies (clipping of the frenum of the tongue) were performed relatively often. However, an early study by McEnery and Gaines (1941) recommended against surgery for ankyloglossia because of the possibility of hemorrhages, infections, and scar tissue. Advances in surgical procedures have likely reduced such risks in recent years (Mettias et al., 2013). This might partly account for findings from two recent studies indicating that the frequency of surgical correction of ankyloglossia has greatly increased in recent years (Kapoor et al., 2018; Walsh et al., 2017).

Fletcher and Meldrum (1968) studied 20 sixth-grade children with uncorrected tongue-tie. Those participants with restricted lingual movement tended to have more articulation errors than a similar group with greater lingual movement. The possibility of some relationship between frenum length and speech sound problems is supported by a study of 200 children aged 6–12 years. Ruffoli and colleagues (2005) classified the severity of ankyloglossia based on frenum length and reported "a relationship between the presence of speech anomalies and a decreased mobility of the tongue, but only for those subjects whose frenulum length resulted in moderate or severe levels of ankyloglossia" (p. 174).

Concerns about the possible impact of ankyloglossia on speech are typically based on limited tongue mobility impacting the learning of the movements for speech sounds. More indirect associations might also be possible. A study by Yoon and colleagues (2017) involved 302 patients ranging in age from 6 to 67 years (mean = 18 years) referred for orthodontia. Findings indicated significant associations between tongue mobility and both size of the maxilla and length of the soft palate (i.e., less mobility was associated with smaller maxilla and shorter soft palates). The implication is that a less mobile tongue might lead to a restricted oral cavity size, which impedes speech sound learning. Clearly further study of this possibility is needed.

Clipping of the frenum still occurs. There is limited evidence that it can be of benefit to assist with issues surrounding breastfeeding (Francis et al., 2015; O'Shea et al., 2017). Relative to speech sounds a number of small studies have been carried out. Messner and Lalakea (2002) reported results from a group of children aged 1–12 years, and formal speech evaluations indicated that 9 of 11 (82%) of the children with preoperative speech errors had improved their speech. A similar study by Heller and associates (2005) reported improvement in 10 of 11 (91%) cases. An Israeli study by Dollberg and associates (2011) compared eight children whose tongue-tie was treated in infancy against seven children with untreated tongue-tie and eight children without tongue tie. Follow-up testing at an average age of about 6 years revealed no significant differences in speech performance across the groups; there were, however, clear trends suggesting the treated children (i.e., those whose tongue-tie was surgically corrected) performed better than those who were untreated but not as well as those with no tongue-tie.

A study by Walls and colleagues (2014) found that parents of 71 children whose tongue-tie was surgically corrected rated their children's speech as significantly better compared to ratings by parents of 15 age-matched children whose tongue-tie had not been corrected. A 2019 survey by Daggumati and associates involved 77 children who had been diagnosed with ankyloglossia at a mean age of about 3½ years. When the children were an average age of 6 years, parents reported that 46 children had undergone surgical correction and 31 had not. The two groups did not differ in terms of the proportion of children who had or were receiving speech therapy (65% vs. 71% for surgery and nonsurgery, respectively). Finally, a study by Salt and colleagues (2020) compared speech production outcomes in three groups of children: those with tongue-tie treated in infancy, those with untreated tongue-tie, and those without tongue tie. Findings indicated no significant differences among the groups for tongue mobility, speech sound accuracy, or intelligibility of speech. Together, these findings suggest a somewhat mixed picture. It is not fully clear whether frenum clipping makes a positive difference in the speech of individuals with ankyloglossia. From the perspective of speech production, the inability of the tongue tip to reach the alveolar ridge (where so many speech sounds are produced) is likely the most important factor in making recommendations for clipping.

Another potential problem with the tongue relative to SSDs is *macroglossia* (a tongue that is too large). Whether it is true macroglossia or relative macroglossia (a normal-size tongue in a small oral cavity), the presumption is that the tongue has insufficient room to maneuver to perform good speech. However, the tongue is a muscular structure capable of considerable change in length and width and thus, regardless of size, is generally capable of the mobility necessary for correct sound productions. Put another way, it seems likely that individuals with mild cases of macroglossia should be able to compensate to at least some extent.

At the other end of the spectrum are those who have undergone partial glossectomy (removal of part of the tongue). In most cases these individuals appear to be able to compensate to at least some extent. Investigators have suggested that the quality of the speech outcomes becomes poorer as the amount of tissue removed becomes greater (Pauloski et al., 1998) and the degree of mobility of the remaining tissue is less than an intact tongue (Bressmann et al., 2004).

Hard Palate

Variations in hard palate dimensions relative to speech have also received some study. Brunner and colleagues (2009) examined palatal shapes and acoustic output from 32 adult speakers with normal speech representing five different languages and found that those with flat-shaped palates showed less variability in tongue height than those with dome-shaped palates. Despite this finding, both groups showed similar acoustic variability in their production of vowels, suggesting that compensation for different palatal shapes is quite possible for normal speakers. Whether the same is true of those with SSDs is unclear. Fairbanks and Lintner (1951) measured the hard palates of a group of young adults with superior consonant articulation and a group with poor consonant articulation. They reported no significant differences in cuspid width, molar width, palatal height, and maximum mouth opening. On the other hand, differences were noted in a study of Arabic speakers by Alfwaress and colleagues (2015). They compared 30 individuals aged 15–20 years with a consistent substitution of /j/ for the Arabic trilled /r/ against an age-matched control group of 30 speakers with no errors. The experimental group had significantly shorter maxillary length and dental arch lengths, as well as narrower intercanine widths compared to the control group.

Removal of any part of the maxilla has the potential to create a serious problem for the speaker because it may result in a situation similar to a congenital cleft of the palate where air escapes through the nose. This may lead to excessive nasality during speech, as well as difficulty with the production of obstruent consonants (stops, fricatives, and affricates). Medical or orthodontic intervention is often quite successful in terms of speech improvement. In a review of 96 patients who underwent surgical reconstruction, Cordeiro and Chen (2012) reported that 84% had normal or near normal speech outcomes. Likewise, the use of prostheses such as obturators to fill in the missing structure has been shown to significantly improve overall intelligibility to near normal in many cases (Sullivan et al., 2002).

Soft Palate (Velum)

The soft palate, or velum, is the backward extension of the hard palate. It, along with the lateral pharyngeal walls, serves as a valve to direct airflow and sound. It remains in a low position, allowing airflow into the nose during normal breathing and during the production of nasal sounds. For oral sounds the soft palate rises and, along with the lateral pharyngeal walls, seals off the velopharyngeal port. Deficiencies in the soft palate would manifest themselves similarly to clefts of the hard palate (difficulty with production of obstruent consonants and atypical nasality).

Specific structural issues with the soft palate are usually put into one of four categories: 1) overt clefts or holes, 2) covert or submucous clefts, 3) a soft palate that is too short (a condition termed *velopharyngeal insufficiency*), or 4) a soft palate that, while long enough, fails to function as needed (a condition termed *velopharyngeal incompetence*). The solution is almost always referral to a cleft palate or craniofacial team and medical management (either prosthetic or surgical). This is true even for velopharyngeal incompetence where, despite the fact that the soft palate operates via the action of muscles, it is generally accepted that therapy will not rectify a soft palate that is not functioning properly.

The one possible exception to the need for medical management relates to a condition called *phoneme-specific* or *context-specific nasal emission* in which air escapes through the nose during the production of one or two speech sounds (most commonly /s/ but it may include other sibilant phonemes). Therapy may be effective in such cases because the mechanism clearly works as needed for most speech sounds; thus, its failure to work for one or two sounds likely represents a learned problem (Ruscello, Shuster et al., 1991).

Tonsils

The term *tonsils* refers to at least two different structures. What most people think of as the tonsils are technically the *palatine tonsils*, which sit along each side of the oral cavity along the lateral edges of the back of the tongue. We also have *lingual tonsils*, which sit near the root of the tongue in the pharynx (i.e., not visible by looking in the mouth). Related to both of these are the *adenoids* (technically the nasopharyngeal tonsils), which sit above the level of the velum at the back of the nasal cavity. All three structures are part of the immune system. They vary in size throughout the life span, typically reaching maximum size near puberty and then becoming relatively small, and are almost invisible most of the time in adults. In both children and adults they may become hypertrophied (enlarged beyond their expected size) at various times in response to upper airway infections. There have long been concerns by SLPs about whether prolonged hypertrophy of the palatine tonsils in particular, or the adenoids, might interfere with speech acquisition. The concern is that chronically enlarged palatine tonsils might limit tongue movement or alter tongue-resting position (inhibiting speech motor learning), or that enlarged adenoids might affect velopharyngeal closure (altering nasal resonance).

Although removal of the tonsils and adenoids is no longer as common as it once was, they may still be removed to help address chronic infections (tonsillitis). Of specific concern for SLPs is whether and/or when to recommend tonsillectomy because of concerns about speech and resonance. Related to this concern is whether there might be negative impacts (i.e., unintended consequences) from such surgeries. Although no definitive guidance is possible at this time, findings from the related research in this area may be informative. Note that although adults appear to be able to adjust to the presence of enlarged tonsils (Hori et al., 1996), studies of children are our focus here.

Most studies in this area have focused on the balance between oral and nasal resonance. Kummer and colleagues (1993) noted that enlarged tonsils and adenoids can lead to nasal blockage, resulting in hyponasal speech, which may make speech more difficult to understand. In their study of 15 children with a mean age of 6.84 years, prior to surgery seven children were rated as being hyponasal, seven were rated as having normal resonance, and one was rated as being hypernasal. Following removal of the tonsils and adenoids there was a resonance rating change for 6/15 children (five changed from hyponasal to normal and one changed from hyponasal to hypernasal).

The opposite case of nasal blockage is where tonsils become so enlarged that they prevent velopharyngeal closure, leading to hypernasal speech. Hypernasality can have an especially negative impact on how understandable speech might be. Shprintzen and colleagues (1987) studied 20 such children (aged 4–19 years), and following removal of the tonsils resonance was rated as normal in 16/20 cases without any other treatment. A brief period of speech therapy following surgery (along with some temporary prosthetic management in one case) appeared to resolve the other four cases. A similar study involved 74 children aged 5–14 years (Abdel-Aziz et al., 2019). Following removal of the tonsils, although perceptually there was not a significant change in nasality, nasalance scores (a measure of the relative acoustic energy coming out of the nose and mouth) improved significantly. As well, when viewed from inside the nasal cavity, velopharyngeal closure patterns improved significantly with only a mild gap remaining in six patients.

There appears to have been very little research documenting whether the presence of enlarged tonsils might impact speech sound acquisition. The previously mentioned study by Shprintzen and colleagues (1987) mentions "Articulation difficulties, especially with phonemes requiring posterior tongue placement" (p. 48) but no specific data were presented. D'Antonioi and associates (1996) present some data on 15 children aged 4–10 years who underwent tonsillectomy. Findings revealed that perceptual ratings of articulation, resonance, and voice quality did not change significantly after surgery (see also Clinical Vignette 4.2).

Taken together, findings here suggest that enlarged tonsils may alter nasal resonance, potentially leading to both hypo- and hypernasality. Their removal appears to result in improved resonance. It is not clear, however, whether their presence would specifically alter either articulation or mastery of the motor skills involved in articulation. Further study is needed.

As noted previously, removal of tonsils and adenoids is less common than it once was. This is partly because of the recognition that as part of the immune system, their removal should not be undertaken lightly. A second reason may be the possible negative changes in nasal resonance (i.e., making the patient permanently hypernasal) documented in a number of studies (e.g., Haapanen et al., 1994; Wachtel et al., 2000; Witzel et al., 1986). This suggests that in some individuals the adenoids and/or tonsils actually assist the soft palate in closing off the velopharyngeal port.

Summary

Many minor structural deviations have the potential to impact speech but, in many cases, speakers are able to compensate for such deviations. The challenge for SLPs comes in identifying those cases where compensation does not occur; decisions about management may require consultation with medical professionals.

Clinical Vignette 4.2

Tonsils and Speech

Ryan (a pseudonym), a 9-year-old boy, was referred to an SLP with concerns about his ability to produce /r/. Testing revealed speech that was very intelligible but included pervasive distortion errors for /r/ in all word positions. Language skills and hearing were within normal limits. The oral mechanism examination revealed normal structure and function, except for very large palatine tonsils bilaterally.

A brief trial of therapy revealed that Ryan could produce a correct version of /r/ using sound shaping (see Chapter 10). However, Ryan complained that when he managed to produce a correct /r/ he felt a strong urge to vomit. Visualization with a flashlight suggested that as his tongue moved back to create /r/, the sides of his tongue were contacting his tonsils; this may have pushed them against his posterior faucial pillars, evoking a gag reflex.

A referral to an otolaryngologist for possible tonsillectomy was recommended. However, Ryan's family lived in a remote village in northern Canada without easy access to medical services. Given Ryan's otherwise normal speech and his above-average academic achievement, his parents declined the recommendation. Therapy was contraindicated and (with his parents' approval) his file was closed.

Oral Sensory Function

Oral sensory feedback plays a role in the development and ongoing monitoring of articulatory gestures and, thus, the relationship between oral sensory function and speech sound productions has been of interest. Some treatment approaches include the practice of specifically calling the client's attention to sensory cues. Bordon (1984) indicated the need for awareness of *kinesthesis* (sense of movement) and *proprioception* (position) during therapy. Almost any phonetic placement technique used to teach speech sounds (to be discussed in Chapter 10 and Appendix A) typically includes a description of articulatory contacts and movements necessary for the production of the target speech sound(s). Thus, they focus the client's attention on what is happening with the articulators, potentially increasing awareness.

The investigation of *somesthesis* (sense of movement, position, touch, and awareness of muscle tension) has focused on 1) overall oral sensitivity, 2) temporary sensory deprivation during oral sensory anesthetization (nerve block anesthesia) to determine the effect of sensory deprivation on speech production, and 3) assessment of oral sensory perception, such as two-point discrimination or oral form discrimination, to see whether such sensory perception may be related to articulatory skill. Netsell (1986) has suggested that most adults are not consciously aware of specific speech movements during running speech. It may be helpful for the reader to recall how novel the details of speech movements were to them during their introductory phonetics class. Netsell also speculated that children may not be aware of articulatory movements during the acquisition period. If this is true, asking a child to monitor running speech may be asking them to use information that is not readily available at a conscious level without instruction.

Oral Tactile Sensitivity

Early investigators of oral sensory function attempted to explore the sensitivity or threshold of awareness of oral structures to various stimuli. Ringel and Ewanowski (1965) studied this in normal-speaking individuals using measurement of awareness of two-point versus one-point discrimination. They found such ability appears to vary across different structures, with greatest to least sensitivity ranging across the tongue tip, fingertip, lip, soft palate, and alveolar ridge. They also found that midline of structures tended to be more sensitive than the lateral edges.

At least two studies (Arnst & Fucci, 1975; Fucci, 1972) examined this by measuring the threshold of vibrotactile stimulation of structures in the oral cavity. These studies found that participants with misarticulations tended to have poorer oral sensory abilities than normal-speaking participants. More specifically, at least three studies (Jordan et al., 1978; McNutt, 1977; Weinberg et al., 1970) have suggested that children with /r/ errors may have reduced oral tactile sensitivity compared to both typically speaking children and those with other speech production errors.

Oral Anesthetization

Another approach to studying the role of oral sensation during speech has involved inducing temporary states of oral sensory deprivation using oral nerve-block and topical anesthetization (similar to what occurs prior to dental work). This was followed by an examination of a variety of speech outcome variables.

Gammon and colleagues (1971) studied eight adult participants reading 30 sentences. They noted few vowel distortions, but there was a 20% rate of consonant misarticulation (especially on fricatives and affricates) under anesthesia and under anesthesia with noise. Scott and Ringel (1971) studied two adult males producing lists of 24 bisyllabic words under normal and anesthetized conditions. They noted that articulatory changes under anesthesia were largely nonphonemic and included loss of retroflexion and lip-rounding gestures, less tight fricative constrictions, and retracted points of articulation contacts.

Prosek and House (1975) studied four adult speakers reading 20 bisyllabic words in isolation and in sentences. Although intelligibility was maintained under anesthetized conditions, speech rate was slowed, and minor imprecisions of articulation were noted. When anesthetized, speakers produced consonants with slightly more intra-oral air pressure and longer duration.

A Finnish study by Niemi and colleagues (2002) examined vowels produced by seven normal-speaking adult males with and without anesthesia applied to the right lingual nerve. Significant differences in the acoustic characteristics (formant frequencies, fundamental frequency, duration) were noted for at least some of the vowels for all of the participants. Some (but not all) of the differences were large enough to qualify as just noticeable. It is noteworthy that there was considerable variability across the participants in terms of how many and which vowels were affected. This suggested that speakers may vary in their ability to compensate for anesthesia.

More recently, De Letter and colleagues (2020) examined the effects of oral anesthesia on 24 young, typically speaking Dutch adults. Speech sound accuracy was significantly reduced; consonants were affected more than vowels. Nonsense syllable repetition rates (diadochokinetic [DDK]; to be discussed later under Motor Abilities) were significantly reduced. No significant difference was observed in the frequency of the second formant (F2) of the vowel /a/.

In summary, studies involving anesthetization have found that speech remained intelligible, although participants did not speak as accurately as they did under normal conditions. However, the participants in these studies were adult speakers with normal articulation skills. It is unclear whether reduced oral sensory feedback might interfere with the acquisition of speech in children or affect remediation.

Oral Form Recognition (Oral Stereognosis)

Oral sensory function has also been investigated extensively through form recognition tasks. Ringel and associates (1970) speculated that form identification (*oral stereognosis*) may provide information on nervous system integrity because the recognition of forms placed in the mouth was assumed to require integrity of peripheral receptors for touch and kinesthesis, as well as central integrating processes. Most of these tasks require the participant to match forms placed in the oral cavity with drawings of the forms or to make same–different judgments. Stimuli are typically small, plastic, three-dimensional forms of varying degrees of similarity, such as triangles, rectangles, ovals, and circles. Participants tend to improve on such tasks as they grow older, achieving maximum performance at adolescence.

Studies in this area have yielded inconsistent results. Arndt and colleagues (1970) did not find a significant relationship between oral form recognition and articulation performance in a third-grade population. But studies by Ringel, House, and associates (1970), Hetrick and Sommers (1988), and Speirs and Maktabi (1990) reported significant differences. Relative to severity of involvement, Ringel and associates noted that children with severe misarticulations made more form recognition errors than children with mild articulation problems, although Hetrick and Sommers failed to find such differences.

Some researchers have investigated the relationship between production of specific phonemes and oral sensory function. McNutt (1977) found that children who misarticulated /r/ did not perform as well as typical speakers on oral form perception tasks; there were, however, no significant differences between the typical speakers and the children who misarticulated /s/.

Bishop and associates (1973) compared oral form recognition skills of deaf high school students who were orally trained (taught to use speech) with those who were taught to use sign language. The authors noted skill differences that favored the orally trained students and postulated that "while a failure in oroperceptual functioning may lead to disorders of articulation a failure to use the oral mechanism for speech activities, even in persons with normal orosensory capabilities, may result in poor performance on oropercepeptual tasks" (p. 257).

Oral Sensory Function and Speech Sound Learning

Jordan and colleagues (1978) studied the influence of tactile sensation as a feedback mechanism in speech sound learning. Their participants were first-grade boys, nine with good articulation skills and nine with poor articulation skills. Participants were fitted with palatal plates equipped with touch-sensitive electrodes and taught to replicate four positions of linguapalatal contact with and without topical anesthesia. Children with poor articulation performed less well on tasks of precise tongue placement than children with good articulation. Participants with poor articulation were able to improve their initially poor performance when given specific training on the tongue placement tasks.

Wilhelm (1971) and Shelton and colleagues (1973) used oral form recognition materials to teach form recognition to misarticulating children. Findings were inconsistent. Wilhelm reported articulation improved as oral form recognition improved, but Shelton and colleagues found no such effect. Ruscello (1972) reported that form recognition scores improved in children undergoing treatment for articulation errors.

Summary

The role of normal oral sensory function or somesthetic feedback in the development and maintenance of speech production is complex. Despite efforts to identify the relationship between oral sensory status and articulatory performance, conclusive findings are lacking. This review of the research suggests the following:

1. Oral form recognition improves with age through adolescence.

2. The role of oral sensory feedback in the acquisition of speech sounds is unclear.

3. During anesthesia, intelligibility is generally maintained, but articulation tends to become less accurate.

4. Individuals with poor articulation tend to achieve slightly lower scores on form perception tasks than their normal-speaking peers; however, some individuals with poor form identification skills have good articulation skills.

5. Although some individuals with SSDs may also have oral sensory deficits, the neurological mechanisms underlying the use of sensory information during experimental conditions may differ from those operating in normal conversational speech.

6. Information concerning oral sensory function has not been shown to have clinical applicability.

7. It is important to distinguish between the effects of sensory deprivation in individuals who have already developed good speech skills and the effects in individuals with SSDs.

8. The effects of long-term oral sensory deprivation have yet to be explored.

MOTOR ABILITIES

Because speech is a motor act, researchers have explored the relationship between speech sound production and motor skills, investigating performance on gross motor as well as oral and facial motor tasks.

General Motor Skills

Studies focusing on the relationship between general or gross motor skills and articulatory abilities have yielded inconsistent and inconclusive results. It may be concluded, however, that individuals with speech sound problems do not have significant delays in general motor development unless the individual also has known neurological deficits affecting gross motor skills. As a result, the discussion that follows will focus on motor skills specific to the oral musculature.

Oral–Facial Motor Skills

Speech is a dynamic process during which fine muscle movements of the lips, tongue, palate, and jaw constantly alter the dimensions of the oral cavity. The control of these movements has been studied from at least three different perspectives, by examining rate, strength, and coordination. Relative to rate, a common approach is the use of tests of diadochokinetic (DDK) rate, which involve rapid repetition of syllables. In addition to being part of research investigations, DDK measures are also typically a part of a speech mechanism examination. These tests are intended to evaluate oral motor skills independent of phonological skills (i.e., independent of the language system). This separation is made by using nonsense syllables to prevent the speaker from accessing their long-term word storage. These tasks also typically involve early developing sounds (stops and neutral vowels) that are assumed to be the simplest in terms of motor demands. The syllables most frequently used are /pʌ/, /tʌ/, and /kʌ/ in isolation, and sequences such as /pʌtʌ/, /tʌkʌ/, /pʌkʌ/, /pʌtʌkʌ/. These tasks are typically done at maximum rates (i.e., speakers are told to produce them "as fast as possible").

DDK rate is determined either with a *count by time* procedure in which the examiner counts the number of syllables spoken in a given interval of time or a *time by count* measurement in which the examiner notes the time required to produce a designated number of syllables. The advantage of the time by count measurement is that fewer operations are required because the examiner only needs to turn off the timing device when the requisite number of syllables has been produced. Performance is then sometimes compared to normative data. Fletcher (1972) reported improvements in DDK rate with age as children increased the number of syllables produced in a given unit of time at each successive age from 7 to 13 years. Data reported by Canning and Rose (1974) indicated that adult values for maximum repetition rates were reached by 9- to 10-year-olds, whereas Fletcher's data show a convergence after age 15.

McNutt (1977) and Dworkin (1978) examined DDK rates of children with specific misarticulations (errors on /r/ and /s/) compared to their normal-speaking peers. Both investigators reported that the mean rate of utterances of the syllables tested was significantly lower in the participants with speech sound errors.

The usefulness of rapid syllable repetition tasks such as DDK to evaluate articulation skills and plan remediation has been questioned. First, such tasks involve the simple alternating contraction of opposing muscles. McDonald (1964a) noted that typical speech is different from DDK tasks because it involves the more complex simultaneous contraction of different groups of muscles, resulting in overlapping movements. The second reason to question these tasks is that they are carried out at faster than normal rate. Findings from at least two studies of speech kinematics or movement patterns (Adams et al., 1993; A. Smith et al., 1995) also suggest a different organization of the movements at fast rates compared to normal rate. Thus, DDK tasks appear to be qualitatively different from normal speech.

Winitz (1969) also pointed out that because normal speakers have a history of success with speech sounds, they may have an advantage over speakers with misarticulations on DDK tasks. Tiffany (1980) pointed out that little is known about the significance of scores obtained on DDK tasks; thus, "such measures appear to lack a substantial theoretical base" (p. 895). The one exception to this generality relates to children that might be considered to evidence childhood apraxia of speech (to be discussed in Chapters 5 and 12). Poor performance on some DDK tasks may reflect syllable sequencing problems that may be at the core of the difficulty for this population. Another exception would be clients with a history of unusual or delayed oral–motor development, which may be evidenced in sucking, feeding, and swallowing difficulties in addition to delayed speech sound development. These children may evidence problems with muscle tone and movement of the oral structures, including independent movement of the tongue and/or lips from the jaw. It is possible that slow or weak oral–motor development could be identified with DDK and may be a contributing factor to the presence of an SSD.

Owing to concerns about DDK, an alternative view on rate has been to evaluate it using real speech produced at habitual rate (the pace that speakers use most of the time). Flipsen (2002a) reviewed the available literature on the development of habituation rate in typical speakers. Although absolute values differed across studies, articulation rate (measured in either syllables or phones/sounds per second) increased significantly across the developmental period. Flipsen also presented longitudinal data from children with SSDs, which suggested that (when measured in phones per second, but not in syllables per second) articulation rate in the preschool years may be slower for these children than their typically developing peers. By adolescence, however, their rates appeared to be similar to their typically developing peers. This finding suggests that there may be at least a delay in the development of speech motor skills in children with SSDs.

The second perspective on oral–facial motor skill in SSDs has been to examine strength. Although difficult to measure in most clinical settings, tongue strength in particular has been studied by several investigators. Potter and Short (2009) reported increases in tongue strength with age in a group of 150 children aged 3–16 years. Similar findings were reported in expansion of that study by Potter and colleagues (2019), who included a total of 228 typically developing children; findings indicated rapid increases in strength from age 3–6.5 years, and then slower but steady increases up until age 17 years.

Relative to children with SSDs, differences in tongue strength compared to typically developing children have not been consistently found. Dworkin and Culatta (1985) found no significant difference in the maximum amount of tongue force that could be exerted by children with SSDs compared to children without any speech difficulties. Potter and colleagues (2019) reported no difference in tongue strength between their 228 typically developing children and 16 children with speech delay.

It has been suggested that tongue strength may be an issue in certain types of SSDs. Dworkin (1978) reported differences specific to children who were producing /s/ errors when compared to children with typical /s/ productions. Several investigators have reported reduced tongue strength in children diagnosed with childhood apraxia of speech (CAS) (Bradford et al., 1997; Murdoch et al., 1995; Potter et al., 2019). Bradford and colleagues made the comparison to those with inconsistent phonological disorder and normal-speaking children. Potter and colleagues made their comparison between children with speech delay and typically developing children. However, Robin and associates (1991) failed to find such a difference for the children with CAS in their study. The differences among the findings of these studies, however, might be accounted for by differences in criteria for diagnosing CAS (see Chapter 5).

Aside from the difficulty with routine measurement of tongue strength, the clinical value of measuring maximum tongue strength has been questioned. It has been suggested that people likely use only about 20% of their tongue strength capability during speech (Forrest, 2002). Typical measures of maximum tongue strength have not been shown to be consistently related to indices of speech production such as intelligibility measures (Bunton, 2008; Weismer, 2006). Reinforcing this lack of clinical value of tongue strength are results from Neel and Palmer (2012), who failed to find significant associations between tongue strength and either DDK rates or articulation rates.

Another perspective on tongue strength is that of Speirs and Maktabi (1990), who measured the ability to maintain a low level of target pressure for short periods. The children with SSDs in that study showed significantly less stability (i.e., poorer fine control) than children without speech errors. This is consistent with findings from Robin and colleagues (1991), who reported that children with CAS were significantly poorer at maintaining tongue pressure at 50% of maximum compared to normal-speaking children.

The third perspective on motor skill for speech production is based on the interaction of the articulators during speech. Gibbon (1999) and others (e.g., Fletcher, 1992) have pointed out that speech production normally involves the complex coordination of the movements of both clearly different articulators (e.g., lips and tongue), as well as quasi-independent regions within the tongue. Recent findings using electropalatography (EPG; to be discussed in Chapter 12) have allowed us to document the fine-grained sequencing of these speech production movements. Production of /k/, for example, requires the simultaneous bracing of the lateral parts of the tongue against the backmost upper teeth and the raising of the tongue body against the soft palate. Production of /t/, on the other hand, requires lateral bracing along all of the upper teeth and raising the tongue tip/blade to the alveolar ridge (slight variations in contact patterns related to vowel context also occur). In a /kt/ sequence, as in the word *doctor*, there are moments when both the tongue tip and the tongue body are raised simultaneously in a so-called *double articulation*. The ability to accurately and reliably coordinate such sequences in the context of rapidly produced connected speech may not reach adult skill level until the early teen years (Fletcher, 1989).

First suggested by Hardcastle and colleagues (1987), Gibbon (1999) reviewed a number of EPG studies and suggested that the motor problem may lie above the level of specific muscles or articulators. It may be that at least some children with SSDs have difficulty with precisely controlling and coordinating the movement of the various regions of the tongue; this is expressed in a poorly refined pattern of tongue to palate contact, which Gibbon referred to as an *undifferentiated lingual gesture*. A study by Lee and colleagues (2014) appeared to confirm such atypical movement patterns. During production of five different vowels, contact was observed between the tongue and the entire palate 24% of the time for 10 children with SSDs. This compared to no such contact by eight typically developing children producing the same vowels. Further study is warranted to determine how broadly this might apply to the overall population of children with SSDs.

Summary

Individuals with speech sound problems have not been shown to exhibit significantly depressed motor coordination on tasks of general motor performance. The relationship between oral–motor skills (i.e., those involving nonspeech movements) and articulation skills in SSDs of unknown origin remains uncertain. Although such individuals have been found to perform more poorly on DDK tasks than their normal-speaking peers, these results cannot be fully interpreted until the relationship between DDK tasks and the ability to articulate sounds in context is clarified. These tasks do remain a regular part of most speech mechanism examinations and may ultimately prove useful for particular subgroups of children with SSDs. For example, they may be of particular value for evaluation of children with other motor deficits (e.g., children with milder forms of cerebral palsy).

Findings of tongue strength studies suggest that although overall strength may not be a problem for children with SSDs, a more important issue may be fine tongue control or stability. It is not clear whether such findings represent children with SSDs in general, or are limited only to subgroups of this population, such as those with CAS.

Findings on articulation rate and gestural control also suggest problems with motor skills in children with SSDs. Such problems may reflect difficulty with higher-level organization of the complex movements for speech. Data supporting such a position remain limited and, however, the routine clinical application of rate and gesture measurements must await additional study.

Oral Myofunctional Disorders/Tongue Thrust

SLPs sometimes see clients who have oral myofunctional disorders (OMDs), which include such phenomena as tongue thrusting, abnormal tongue-resting postures, unusual oral movements, finger sucking, lip insufficiencies, and dental and oral structure deficiencies. The concern of SLPs relates to speech differences and disorders that may be related to such oral variations. Because tongue thrusting is the oral myofunctional disorder most commonly encountered by SLPs, this section focuses on this phenomenon.

Tongue thrust has been defined as frontal or lateral movement of the tongue during swallowing (Mason, 2011). The term itself implies that the tongue is thrust forward forcefully when in reality, such individuals do not seem to use more tongue force against the teeth than nonthrusters (Proffit, 1986). Rather, the term *tongue-thrust swallow* is more appropriately seen as a problem of directionality of tongue activity while swallowing. Hanson (1988a) suggested that a better description for these tongue position and movement behaviors would be *oral muscle pattern disorders*. Other terms sometimes used to describe these behaviors include *reverse swallow, deviant swallow*, and *infantile swallow*. The latter terms should be avoided because of their inherent faulty implications (Mason, 1988).

According to Mason and Proffit (1974):

> ... tongue thrusting is one or a combination of three conditions: (1) during the initiation phase of the swallow a forward gesture of the tongue between the anterior teeth so that the tongue tip contacts the lower lip; (2) during speech activities, fronting of the tongue between or against the anterior teeth with the mandible hinged open (in phonetic contexts not intended for such placements); and (3) at rest, the tongue is carried forward in the oral cavity with the mandible hinged slightly open and the tongue tip against or between the anterior teeth. (p. 116)

At birth, all infants are tongue thrusters because the tongue fills the oral cavity, making tongue thrust obligatory. Sometime later, the anterior tongue-gums/teeth seal during swallowing is replaced with a superior tongue-palate seal. There is some debate about when most children make this change. Hanson (1988b) suggested that this happens by age 5 years. A review of published studies by Lebrun (1985), however, concluded that "tongue thrust swallowing is the rule rather than the exception in children under 10 years of age" (p. 307). This is supported by Bertolini and Paschoal (2001), who examined a random sample of 100 Brazilian children aged 7–9 years and reported that only 24% of them presented with a normal adultlike swallow.

Tongue thrust during swallow and/or tongue fronting at rest can usually be identified by visual inspection. Mason (1988, 2011) has pointed out that two types of tongue thrusting should be differentiated. The first is described as a habit and is seen in the absence of any abnormal oral structures. The second is obligatory and may involve factors such as airway obstruction or enlarged tonsils, with tongue thrusting being a necessary adaptation to maintain the size of the airway to pass food during swallowing.

Wadsworth and associates (1998) observed a tongue-thrust swallow pattern in 50.5% of 200 children in Grades K–6 who were receiving speech-language services. In addition, a tongue-thrust swallow frequently co-occurred with resting forward tongue posture (63%), open bite (86%), overjet (57%), abnormal palatal contour (60%), and open mouth posture (39%).

Tongue Thrust and Presence of Speech Sound Errors

Investigators have reported that speech sound errors, primarily sibilant distortions, occur more frequently in children who evidence tongue thrust than in those who do not. Fletcher and colleagues (1961) studied 1,615 schoolchildren aged 6–18 years and found that children who demonstrated a tongue-thrust swallow pattern were more likely to have associated sibilant distortions than children who did not. They also reported that participants with normal swallow patterns demonstrated a significant decrease in sibilant distortion with age, whereas tongue thrusters did not. A similar relationship between tongue-thrust patterns and sibilant distortions was reported by Palmer (1962), Jann and colleagues (1964), and Wadsworth and colleagues (1998). Palmer also reported errors on /t/, /d/, and /n/, and Jann and colleagues noted additional problems with /l/.

Subtelny and colleagues (1964) used radiographic techniques to examine the relationship between normal and abnormal oral morphology and /s/ production. Their participants, 81 adolescents and adults, were divided into three groups: 1) normal speakers with normal occlusion, 2) normal speakers with severe malocclusion, and 3) abnormal speakers with severe malocclusion. In contrast to earlier investigators, these authors found that the incidence of tongue thrusting and malocclusion in normal speakers was comparable to that in abnormal speakers. This finding is consistent with the reported developmental decrease in the reverse swallow pattern. By contrast, Khinda and Grewal (1999) examined the relationship among tongue thrusting, anterior open bite, and SSDs. In a group of children with tongue thrust and normal occlusion, 30% demonstrated SSDs; by comparison, 95% of children with tongue thrusting combined with an anterior open bite were reported to have SSDs. Thus, significantly more SSDs were associated with the combination of tongue thrust and anterior open bite than with tongue thrust and normal occlusion.

Impact of Tongue Thrust on Dentition

It is generally believed that the resting posture of the tongue affects the position of the teeth and jaws more than tongue thrust or speaking does (Mason, 1988, 2011; Proffit, 1986). Tongue thrusting may, however, play a role in maintaining or influencing an abnormal dental pattern when an anterior resting tongue position is present. If the position of the tongue is forward (forward resting position) and between the anterior teeth at rest, this condition can impede normal teeth eruption and may result in an anterior open bite and/or a Class II malocclusion. However, in the absence of an anterior tongue-resting position, tongue-thrusting patients are not thought to develop malocclusions. As noted by Mason (2011), "A tongue thrust swallow represents a very brief, transient force application of the tongue against the anterior dentition. The amount of pressure exerted against the anterior dentition . . . is well within the normal range" (p. 28).

Treatment Issues

Oromyofunctional therapy (OMT) is not usually included in SLP educational programs, but some clinicians seek out this training on their own. They may then provide treatment for nonspeech oromyofunctional problems and/or incorporate such therapy into their work on speech. Training questions aside, a general concern is whether this treatment has been shown to be effective. In a review of 15 studies that examined the effectiveness of tongue-thrust therapy, Hanson (1994) reported that 14 of the investigators indicated that swallowing and resting patterns were altered successfully. Most studies reviewed patients at least a year following the completion of treatment. Only one of the studies (Subtelny, 1970) found therapy to be ineffective in correcting the disorders. Mantie-Kozlowski and Pitt (2014) documented the effectiveness of OMT for nonspeech orofacial myofunctional disorders using EPG to monitor movement patterns in three patients (two were adults).

Of most interest to SLPs would be the potential effect of OMT on SSDs. Overstake (1976) studied children aged 7–12 years with both tongue-thrust swallow and interdental /s/ production. One group ($n = 28$) received OMT only, and the second ($n = 20$) received both OMT and speech therapy. Similar percentages of the children (86% and 85%, respectively) had a normal swallow at the end of the treatment period. Similar percentages (85% and 75%, respectively) were judged to have normal /s/ production patterns. Normal in this case was based on visual appearance rather than the acoustic output. Christensen and Hanson (1981) studied 10 6-year-old children with both tongue thrust and speech sound errors. All received equal amounts of total therapy time, with half receiving a combination of OMT and speech sound therapy, and the other half receiving speech sound therapy only. The groups made equal progress on speech, but only the group receiving OMT improved tongue thrusting. Together, these findings suggest that treating a tongue thrust that is accompanied by deviant speech sound production may have a positive impact on speech production. It also suggests that, at least for some children, deviant speech production may be related to a tongue-thrust swallow.

Summary

In 1991, ASHA issued a position statement on oral myofunctional disorders. Although that statement itself has not been updated, ASHA does continue to provide basic updates on this topic in its practice portal (ASHA, n.d.-c). Currently, the following can be said about oral myofunctional disorders:

1. Existing data support the idea that abnormal labial-lingual posturing function can be identified, including abnormal tongue-resting position or thrusting of the tongue during swallowing.

2. A forward tongue-resting posture has the potential, with or without a tongue-thrust swallow, to be associated with malocclusions.

3. There is some evidence that an anterior tongue-resting posture or a tongue-thrust swallow and speech production errors coexist in some persons.

4. OMT can be effective in modifying disorders of tongue and lip posture and movement, and may help improve speech production.

5. Assessment and treatment of oral myofunctional disorders that may include some nonspeech remediation are within the purview of SLPs. SLPs wishing to provide treatment for these disorders will usually need to seek out additional training. As well, they should be prepared to engage in interdisciplinary collaboration with orthodontists, pediatric dentists, or other dentists, and with medical specialists such as otolaryngologists, pediatricians, or allergists, as needed.

6. More research is needed on the nature and evaluation of oral myofunctional disorders and the treatment of such disorders.

Pacifier Use

A topic that follows somewhat logically from oromyofunctional disorders is also one frequently raised by parents and others. Nagoda (2013) reviewed several studies and noted that between 55% and 80% of infants are reported to use pacifiers (also called dummies in Australia and the United Kingdom) at least some of the time. These devices are commonly used to soothe fussy infants, may improve sucking skills in premature infants (Kaya & Aytekin, 2017), and there has been some suggestion that their use might reduce the risk of sudden infant death syndrome (SIDS). However, a recent review (Psaila et al., 2017) indicated that no randomized trials have been conducted on the pacifier–SIDS connection. That review also noted that current thinking appears to be based primarily on a few small studies. However, out of what appears to have been an abundance of caution, the American Academy of Pediatrics (AAP, 2005) issued a policy statement on SIDS that included the recommendation that pacifiers be offered to infants under age 1 year at bedtime as a possible prevention for SIDS.

From a speech perspective, it has been suggested that the presence of a pacifier or anything else being placed in the mouth, including fingers or thumbs, might have a negative impact on speech acquisition and potentially lead to SSDs. Several possible reasons for such a connection might be proposed. First, the presence of a pacifier might alter tongue-resting posture. Second, the pacifier might affect tooth emergence and/or alignment (see Moimaz et al., 2014, but compare to Schmid et al., 2018). Third, using a pacifier has been shown to increase the risk of otitis media (Niemi et al., 2002; Rovers et al., 2008), which may then lead to an SSD. Fourth, having a pacifier in the mouth might reduce the amount of time the infant spends practicing speech. Finally, the presence of the pacifier might make parents and others less likely to interact with the infant and thereby reduce opportunities for the child to both practice speech and receive feedback from others.

The literature in this area presents a mixed picture. Baker (2002) discussed the potential pros and cons of pacifier use and suggested that there was little direct evidence of their influence on speech development. Fox and colleagues (2002) compared 65 German-speaking children aged 2;7 to 7;2 with SSDs against 48 age-matched typically developing children. They reported that children with SSDs were significantly more likely to have used a bottle as a pacifier (i.e., not just for feeding). The groups did not differ on use of pacifiers alone. A study in Chile by Barbosa and colleagues (2009) evaluated questionnaire data collected from parents of 128 children aged 3–5 years. The authors concluded that for the 42% of the children who used pacifiers, there was a threefold increase in the odds of developing an SSD. A similar study was conducted by Baker and associates (2018) of oral nonnutritive sucking in 199 Australian children (aged 46–66 months) with and without SSDs. Findings revealed no significant association with either the presence or the severity of an SSD. Nagoda (2013) looked at duration of pacifier use in 20 preschool children (15 typically developing and 5 with SSDs). Parents were asked to report the age when pacifier use started and stopped, and to estimate the average hours per day of use (while the child was awake). A total of 13 (65%) of the participants used pacifiers, but there was no difference in either the proportion of users or duration of use between the children with and without SSDs. However, when looking at the seven typically developing children who used pacifiers while awake, there was a clear trend (albeit not statistically significant) for scores on an articulation test to be negatively associated with total accumulated hours of daytime pacifier use. This suggested the possibility that the more an infant used a pacifier, the higher the risk that speech production skills might be affected.

Although further study is clearly indicated, based on the available research, the use of pacifiers likely does not interfere with acquisition of speech sounds in most children.

COGNITIVE-LINGUISTIC FACTORS

A second major category of variables that have been studied relative to a possible relationship to SSDs is cognitive-linguistic factors. Historically, the field of communication sciences and disorders has been interested in the relationship between intelligence and the presence of SSDs. In more recent years, investigators have sought to describe the relationship between disordered phonology and other aspects of cognitive-linguistic functioning. Understanding this connection is not only useful in determining the type of instructional/intervention program that may be most efficacious for the child's overall language development, but also helps to provide a better understanding of interrelationships of various components of language behavior.

Intelligence

The relationship between intelligence (as measured by IQ tests) and SSDs has been a subject of many years of investigation. Early studies (Reid, 1947a, 1947b; Winitz, 1959a, 1959b) reported low positive correlations between scores obtained on intelligence tests and scores on articulation tests. More recently, Johnson and colleagues (2010) reported findings from a 20-year follow-up study. Findings indicated no significant difference in IQ scores between those who had been diagnosed as speech impaired as preschoolers and those who had typical speech (all scored within the normal range on IQ). Thus, one did not appear to be a good predictor of the other.

A second perspective may be gleaned from studies of the phonological status of individuals with developmental delays. Prior to 1970, a number of studies explored the prevalence of SSDs in this population. In a study of 777 children aged 6–16 years with cognitive impairments (what used to be call mental retardation), Wilson (1966) concluded that "there is a high incidence of articulatory deviation in an educable mentally retarded population, and the incidence and degree of severity is closely related to mental-age levels" (p. 432). Wilson's findings also indicated that articulatory skills, which continue to improve until approximately age 9 years in the normal population, continue to show improvement well beyond that age in individuals with cognitive impairments. Schlanger (1953) and Schlanger and Gottsleben (1957) reported similar findings. Schlanger and Gottsleben also noted that individuals with Down syndrome (DS), or those whose etiologies were based on central nervous system impairment, demonstrated the most pronounced speech delay.

There is some variance in research findings for speech sound development in persons with cognitive impairments. Several studies report patterns generally similar to that of younger typically developing children (Bleile, 1982; B. L. Smith & Stoel-Gammon, 1983; Sommers et al., 1988) suggesting a straightforward delay. However, specific to children with DS, Kumin and colleagues (1994) reported a great deal of variability in the age at which sounds emerge. They also stated that these children do "not appear to follow the same order as the norms for acquisition for typically developing children" (p. 300) in addition to exhibiting a delay in emergence of some sounds as much as 5 years later than expected for typically developing children.

As a group who represents a genetically controlled subset of individuals with cognitive impairment, particular attention has been paid to individuals with DS. Sommers and colleagues (1988) presented error data on a group with DS, aged 13–22 years. Some errors were those frequently seen in error of 5- and 6-year-olds of normal intelligence (i.e., /r/, /r/ clusters, /s/, /s/ clusters, /z/, /θ/, and /v/). However, they also reported the occurrence of atypical errors such as deletion of alveolar stops and nasals.

As part of a study of overall communication profiles, Rosin and colleagues (1988) studied a group of 10 male participants with DS (chronological age [CA] = 14;7). Their performance was contrasted with a control group of individuals with other forms of cognitive impairment and two control groups of individuals with normal intelligence representing two age levels (CA = 6;1 and 15;5). They reported that as mental age (MA) increased across participants, intelligibility on a language sample increased. The

DS group was significantly different from the group of individuals with other forms of cognitive impairment and the younger-age normal group (the older group was not compared) in terms of the percentage of consonants correctly articulated on the Goldman-Fristoe Test of Articulation.

Rosin and colleagues (1988) also reported that the DS group had difficulty with production on measures that placed greater demands for sequencing (e.g., consonant-vowel repetitions, longer words). They needed significantly more cueing in order to articulate the target /pataka/ and had more variable intraoral pressure when producing /papapapa/. The mean length of utterance of the DS group was also significantly shorter than the other three groups. The authors indicated that these findings are in accord with observations of others and suggested that sequencing challenges underlie both speech motor control and language problems evidenced in participants with DS.

Shriberg and Widder (1990) summarized findings from nearly four decades of speech research in cognitive impairment as follows:

1. Persons with cognitive impairments are likely to have speech sound errors.

2. The most frequent type of error is likely to be deletions of consonants.

3. Errors are likely to be inconsistent.

4. The pattern of errors is likely to be similar to that of very young children or children with SSDs of unknown origin.

Summary

Investigators concur that there is a low positive correlation between intelligence and speech sound production skill within the range of normal intelligence. Thus, it can be inferred that intellectual functioning is of limited importance as a contributing factor to articulatory skill and can be viewed as a poor predictor of articulation in individuals within the range of normal intellectual functioning. On the other hand, a much higher correlation has been found between intelligence and articulation in individuals with cognitive impairments. The articulatory skills in a subgroup of individuals with cognitive impairment (including those with DS) were delayed and generally had error patterns similar to those seen in young normally developing children; however, they also evidenced errors that are considered different or unusual when compared to normal developing children.

Phonological Memory

It has been suggested that cognitive processing deficits may underlie some SSDs (Dodd et al., 1989; Torrington Eaton & Bernstein Ratner, 2016). One specific deficit that has been suggested is difficulty with memory (Lewis et al., 2006a; Shriberg, Lohmeier et al., 2009). Recently, both phonological short-term memory (pSTM) and phonological working memory (pWM) abilities have been specifically investigated. pSTM is the ability to briefly hold on to information and is usually measured by simple recall tasks (e.g., digit span where a series of numbers are presented and must be repeated immediately). pWM involves temporarily storing and then mentally manipulating information. It is usually measured using more complex tasks such as reverse span tasks (e.g., repeating a series of numbers backwards). The presumption is that for many children with SSDs, the individual speech sounds are not clearly represented in their long-term memory storage (what linguists call the underlying representation). A second presumption is that both pSTM and pWM are necessary in order to create those long-term representations.

Investigations in this area have yielded somewhat consistent findings. Torrington Eadie and Bernstein Ratner (2016) reported significant differences between 9 children with SSD and 42 children with typical speech (overall mean age 5;0) on a pSTM (digit span) task but not on a pWM (reverse digit span) task. Waring and associates (2017) investigated both pSTM and pWM by comparing performance from 14 children with phonological delay (PD; a subgroup of children with SSDs defined by Dodd [see Chapter 5], exhibiting errors similar to younger typically developing children) against 14 age-matched typically speaking children. Mean age for both groups was 4;4. The PD group scored significantly lower on both kinds of tasks. In addition, Waring computed difference scores between the pSTM and pWM tasks to create a manipulating score. The two groups did not differ significantly on the manipulating score, suggesting that the problem was one of holding onto the information rather than manipulation of it. The study was repeated by the same investigators in 2018 with a group of 16 children with phonological disorders (defined by Dodd as producing at least some errors not usually produced by younger typically developing children) and an age-matched group of 15 typically speaking children with a mean age of 4;1. In this case, there was no difference on the pSTM tasks, though there was a trend for the phonological disorder group to perform less well. However, there was a significant difference on the pWM tasks. This suggested that for this particular subgroup of children with SSD, the ability to mentally manipulate speech sounds in memory may be a critical issue related to SSD.

In summary, it would appear that difficulty with holding onto words in short-term memory may underlie the deficits seen in at least some children with SSDs. Depending on the speech sound error pattern, the ability to mentally manipulate those sounds within memory may also be an issue. It might lead to inaccurate or incomplete long-term representations for some speech sounds, resulting in production difficulties. It might also account for why so many children with SSDs are at risk for reading problems (to be discussed in Chapter 13). Reading requires making associations between speech sounds and written symbols, which requires the ability to hold words in memory, break them down into individual sounds, associate them with written symbols, and then reassemble them.

Phonological Encoding

Developing fully adultlike long-term representations for speech sounds is also thought to involve the ability to "... transform auditory input into phonemic, sublexical, and lexical representations ..." (Shriberg, Lohmeier et al., 2012, p. 447). In other words, aside from holding the input in working or short-term memory, that input must eventually be converted into some form that allows it to be retained in the brain. This conversion process has been termed *encoding*. The ability to encode new words into long-term representations has frequently been examined in children with language impairments using nonsense word tasks in order to get around differences in previous exposure to the words (Campbell et al., 1997). A significant challenge with using such tasks with children with SSDs is that production errors by these children are difficult to interpret. Was the error a problem of encoding or simply difficulty producing the sounds? To help get around this problem, a Syllable Repetition Task (SRT) was developed by Shriberg and colleagues in 2009, which included only four early developing consonants and a single early vowel.

At least two studies have used the SRT to examine the possibility of difficulty with encoding in children with SSDs. As part of a 2012 study of 3- to 5-year-old children, Shriberg and colleagues (2009) included 53 participants with speech delay and typical language and 43 participants with speech delay combined with delayed language. Those without language impairment were not significantly different on encoding than the 52 typically speaking participants. Those with a comorbid language impairment were, however, significantly poorer at encoding than the typically speaking participants. Roepke and colleagues (2020) conducted a similar study using 13 children aged 4–6 years in each group. In this case, the two groups with speech delay were both significantly poorer at encoding than the typical speakers. The somewhat conflicting findings between the two studies suggest the need for further investigation. It remains possible that children with SSD have problems with encoding.

Language Development

Given that the speech sound system (phonology) is part of the language system, we might expect an interaction between phonology and other aspects of language (Chapter 5 explores comorbidity or co-occurrence of SSDs and language disorders more directly). Investigators have attempted to explain the possible interaction as a way to understand the role of language development in SSDs.

The nature of the language problems experienced by children with SSDs appears to be similar to that of children whose only difficulty is with other aspects of language (i.e., those with specific language impairment [SLI]). This includes particular problems with syntax and/or morphology (e.g., Rvachew et al., 2005; Tyler & Watterson, 1991). Mortimer and Rvachew (2010) studied children with SSDs at the start of kindergarten and again at the end of first grade. All of the children (particularly those who retained low mean length of utterance values across the study period) had difficulty with finite verb morphology, which has been flagged as a potential clinical marker of SLI (Rice & Wexler, 1996). Thus, both populations (children with SSDs and those with SLI) may share a common problem with language development and impairment.

The appearance of first words is typically seen as the first real indicator of the presence of language capacity. Thus, a link between language development and SSDs might first be evident through an association between SSDs and age of onset of first words. However, both an Australian study of 1,494 children aged 4 years (Eadie et al., 2015) and an Italian study of 373 children aged 4–5 years (Salvago et al., 2019) failed to find such an association.

The role of syntax in SSDs has received particular attention. A common perception is that language is organized from the top down. In other words, a speaker organizes their output from pragmatic intent, to semantic coding, to syntactic structure, to speech sound productions. Thus, higher-level linguistic formulation may ultimately be reflected in a child's speech sound output. If this theory is accurate, it might be expected that the more complex the syntax, the more likely a child is to produce speech sound errors. Schmauch and associates (1978) studied 5-year-old children with both speech sound and language problems and reported a 17% increase in speech sound errors as the syntactic demands increased. Later developing consonants were those most influenced by syntactical complexity; while the errors tended to become more frequent, the nature of the errors changed little.

In a follow-up study by Panagos and associates (1979), 5-year-old children produced 15 target consonants in noun phrases, declarative sentences, and passive sentences, with the consonants appearing in the initial and final word positions of one- and two-syllable words. Syntax was again found to significantly influence speech sound accuracy, as did number of syllables in target words, but word position did not. The authors reported that two sources of complexity—phonologic (including difficulty with later developing consonants as well as specific contexts) and syntactic—combined additively to increase the number of speech sound errors. From the easiest context (final word position of one-syllable words in noun phrases) to the hardest (final word position of two-syllable words in passive sentences), there was a 36% increase in speech sound errors.

A second perspective on the language–phonology relationship (from the bottom up) suggests that language expression is regulated by feedback (internal and external) from speech output. The feedback is needed to maintain syntactic processing and accuracy, especially when errors occur and must be corrected. From this perspective, syntactic errors would increase as word or sound complexity increased.

Panagos and Prelock (1982) provided findings on the role of increased syllable complexity. They required 10 children with language disorders to produce sentences containing words with syllable complexity ranging from *simple* (CV) to *complex* (CVCCVC). When participants repeated sentences containing words of varying syllable complexity, they made 27% more syntactic errors on those with more syllable complexity. In addition, sentence complexity was varied from unembedded ("The girl washed the doll in the tub") to right embedded ("The cook washed the pot the boy dropped") to center embedded ("The lady the uncle liked sewed the coat"). Syntactic complexity further compounded production difficulties. From the unembedded to the center embedded, there was a 57% increase in speech sound errors.

Together, all of these studies suggest that a simultaneous top-down and bottom-up relationship exists between language and phonology. Syntactic complexity influences phonology and phonological complexity influence syntax. Another way of expressing this is to consider that children with disordered language and phonology have a limited encoding capacity; the more this capacity is strained at one level or another, the higher the probability of delay in other components of language.

One challenge to this conclusion is that these investigators have typically employed elicited imitation tasks to control the complexity of utterances. It could be argued that with this type of performance task, structural simplifications are the expected outcomes. Elicited imitation tasks do not reflect typical conversations. The complex demands of conversational speech may actually tax a child's capacity even more so than imitation tasks and may yield an even higher frequency of speech sound errors as a result.

Morphology is another aspect of language that has been investigated relative to children with SSDs. Particular attention has been paid in some studies to finite verb morphology, which may be a clinical marker for language impairment (Rice & Wexler, 1996). Using single word production data, a 2007 study by Haskill and Tyler revealed that a group of 40 children (aged 4–5 years) with both language and phonological impairments produced finite morphemes less accurately than a matched group of 23 children with language impairment only. Howland and colleagues (2019) reported similar difficulties. Rvachew and colleagues (2005) used a story retell task to study a group of 23 4- to 5-year-old children with SSDs. They specifically attended to the accuracy of /s/ and /z/ and the use of those phonemes as plural, possessive, and regular third person singular morphemes. The majority (20/23) of the children omitted these morphemes more often than expected for their age. Perhaps more importantly, the two phonemes were omitted more often in contexts where they served as a separate morpheme than when they did not, suggesting that the errors were driven by problems with morphology more than problems with phonology.

The simultaneous top-down–bottom-up relationship between phonology and other aspects of language is reflected in a synergistic view of language (Schwartz, Leonard, Folger et al., 1980; Shriner et al., 1969). This perspective assumes a complex interaction and interdependency of various aspects of linguistic behaviors, including language and phonology. Paul and Shriberg (1984), for example, suggested that children may "do things other than phonologic simplification in an attempt to control complexity in spontaneous speech" (p. 319). They noted that some children with speech delays may allocate their limited linguistic resources to realize phonologic targets consistent with their linguistic knowledge in the context of free speech, even though at other times they may use avoidance strategies or other means of reducing the encoding load.

Studies of whether intervention focused on one linguistic domain (e.g., morphosyntax) might facilitate gains in an untreated domain (e.g., phonology) may also be informative. Matheny and Panagos (1978) looked at the effects of syntactic instruction on phonologic improvement and the effects of phonologic instruction on syntactic improvement in school-age children. Each group made the greatest gains in the treated domain as compared to a control group, but also made improvements in the untreated domain. Wilcox and Morris (1995) reported similar findings. They noted that, based on comparison to a control group, children with both speech sound and language impairments who participated in a preschool language-focused program made gains not only in language but also in phonology. In a study based on two siblings from a set of triplets, Hoffman and associates (1990) also found that a narrative intervention program facilitated gains in both language and phonology for one brother, while gains only in phonology were achieved by the brother who received only phonologic instruction.

Tyler and colleagues (2002) reported one of the more comprehensive studies of cross-domain improvement between language (morphosyntax) and phonology. They compared treatment outcomes for three groups of children, all of whom had comorbid (coexisting) speech sound and morphosyntactic disorders: 1) group 1 received morphosyntactic instruction for a 12-week block followed by 12 weeks in phonology, 2) group 2 reversed the order of the 12-week blocks, and 3) group 3 served as the control group. These investigators reported that in comparison to the control group, both interventions were effective; however, only morphosyntactic instruction led to cross-domain improvement (i.e., language therapy improved phonology, but not the reverse). These findings have not been supported in other studies. Tyler and Watterson (1991) reported that participants with a severe overall language and phonological disorders made improvements in language when presented with language therapy; however, gains were not made in phonology (they actually reported a tendency for performance to become slightly worse). On the other hand, participants with mild-moderate but unequal impairments in phonology and language improved in both areas when presented with phonologic therapy. The authors suggested that a language-based intervention program may not result in improvement in phonologic as well as other language skills for children whose disorders are severe and comparable in each domain. However, children with less severe problems in one or both domains may benefit from therapy with either a language or phonology focus.

Fey and colleagues (1994) conducted an experimental treatment program with 26 participants, aged 44–70 months, with impairments in both grammar and phonology. Eighteen children received language intervention (grammar facilitation), and eight children served as controls. Results indicated that despite a strong effect of intervention on the children's grammatical output, there were no direct effects on the participants' speech sound productions. The authors indicated that trying to improve intelligibility by focusing on grammar is not defensible for children in the age and severity range of their participants. They further indicated that for most children who have impairments in both speech and language, intervention should focus on both areas. Tyler and colleagues (2002) have indicated that differences in findings between their study and that of the Fey and colleagues study may be due to differences in goal selection, intervention techniques, or measures used to determine changes in phonology.

Further clinical studies are needed to clarify the synergistic relationship between language and phonology, including cross-domain improvements. The influence of age, nature and severity of both language and SSDs, treatment approaches employed, and measures used to ascertain progress all need further study. Each of these variables should be carefully considered when SLPs launch an intervention program for children who evidence communication disorders that reflect both language delay and SSDs.

Summary

Language and phonology may be related in what has been termed a *synergistic relationship*. Investigators face the challenge of further defining the intricacies of the relationship between phonology and other linguistic behaviors in terms of both development and clinical management of disorders. It appears that for children with language impairment and moderate to severe SSDs, direct phonologic intervention may be required to impact phonology in most children. Further research in cross-domain generalization is needed to guide clinical practice in this area.

Academic Performance

The relationship between SSDs and academic performance is of interest to clinicians working with school-age children because oral language skills are fundamental to the development of many literacy-related academic skills such as reading and spelling. Because the use of sounds in symbolic lexical units is a task common to learning to speak, read, and write, researchers for many years have studied the co-occurrence of reading and SSDs, and have discussed possible common factors underlying the acquisition of literacy and other language-related skills.

A number of investigators have found that a significant portion of children with SSDs have difficulty with reading readiness (Fitzsimons, 1958; Weaver et al., 1960) and/or end up with reading and spelling difficulties (Hall,1938; Weaver et al., 1960). Such problems are not always transitory and may persist into adulthood. Lewis and Freebairn-Farr (1991), for example, examined the performance of individuals with a history of a preschool SSD on measures of phonology, reading, and spelling. Participant groups included at least 17 individuals from each of the following categories: preschool, school age, adolescence, and adulthood. Typical developing comparison groups at each age level were also tested. Significant differences between the disordered and typical groups were reported on the reading and spelling measures for the school-age group and on the reading measure for the adult group. Although the reading and spelling measures for the adolescent group and the spelling measure for the adult group did not reach significance, the trend was for the individuals with histories of SSD to perform more poorly than the typically developing individuals. Similar findings have been reported elsewhere (Felsenfeld et al., 1995; Overby et al., 2012). Given that reading plays such an important role in academic success, it is not surprising that these children are also more likely to have other academic difficulties (Templin & Glaman, 1976).

To appreciate the specific connection between SSDs and reading, recall that written language is based on spoken language. With an alphabetic language like English, the written symbols represent the sounds of the language (albeit imperfectly, because the Latin alphabet was not originally intended for English). To both decode (read) and encode (spell) words, the reader/speller must 1) appreciate that words are composed of smaller units and 2) learn the relationships between the written symbols (letters) and the spoken symbols (phonemes) they represent. Put another way, the successful reader must have *phonological awareness* and understand the *letter–sound correspondences* (these will be discussed in more detail in Chapter 13). Children with SSDs overall have been shown to have difficulty in both of these areas (Bird et al., 1995; Sutherland & Gillon, 2005). Recall also the earlier discussion in this chapter on phonological memory.

There is also evidence that the specific nature of a child's speech difficulties may be especially crucial to determining whether a reading problem will emerge (Bishop & Adams, 1990; Catts, 1993). Children whose difficulty is more with how speech sounds are used to contrast meaning in the language (i.e., whose problem is phonological) are more likely to have reading problems than children whose difficulty is with how to produce the sounds (i.e., whose problem is articulatory). Children who produce atypical errors (in addition to typical errors) may also be especially at risk (Dodd et al., 1989; Waring et al., 2017, 2018). A spoken language basis for reading and spelling difficulties is also supported by follow-up studies. Children with SSDs who end up with difficulty reading have been shown to have spelling errors that bear a striking resemblance to the kinds of errors they might have made in their earlier speech (Clarke-Klein & Hodson, 1995; Hoffman & Norris, 1989). Finally, a phonological disorder implies some difficulty with language learning. We should not, then, be surprised and would expect that children with SSDs who have additional language impairments are also more likely to exhibit reading difficulties (Lewis & Freebairn-Farr, 1991; Raitano et al., 2004).

Summary

Young children with SSDs appear to be at greater risk for academic difficulties because of potential challenges with reading and spelling. This seems to be particularly true for those whose difficulty is phonological rather than articulatory. It may also be the case that severity of involvement is a factor (i.e., the more speech sound errors a child has, the more likely it is that they will have difficulty with reading and spelling). Finally, children with SSDs who have co-occurring language disorders may be particularly susceptible to academic problems.

PSYCHOSOCIAL FACTORS

Psychosocial factors represent the third cluster of variables that have long fascinated clinicians in terms of their potential relationship to SSD. Age, gender, family history, and SES have been studied in an effort to better understand factors that may precipitate or otherwise be associated with phonologic impairment.

Age

As discussed in Chapter 3, investigations have revealed that children's articulatory and phonologic skills continue to improve until approximately 9 years of age, by which time the typically developing child has acquired most aspects of the adult sound system. Fine tuning of these skills appears to continue until at least puberty and likely well into adolescence (Flipsen, 2002a; Kent, 1976).

Several large studies were conducted prior to the widespread availability of speech and language services which offer some insight into the role of maturation on speech sound skills acquisition. Roe and Milisen (1942) sampled 1,989 children in Grades 1 through 6 who had never received any formal speech therapy. They found that the mean number of articulation errors decreased significantly each year between Grades 1 and 4. In contrast, the difference in the mean number of errors between Grades 4 and 5 and Grades 5 and 6 was not significant. The authors concluded that maturation was responsible for improvement in articulation performance between Grades 1 and 4 but was not an appreciable factor in articulation improvement in grades 5 and 6. A subsequent study by Sayler (1949) assessed articulation in 1,998 students in Grades 7 through 12 as they read sentences orally. He observed a slight decrease in the mean number of speech sound errors at each subsequent grade level, but because the improvement was so small, he concluded that maturation does not appear to be an appreciable factor in improvement in the middle school and secondary grades.

At least two large studies had a specific focus on SSDs. The National Speech and Hearing Survey (NSHS) (Hull et al., 1976) sampled more than 38,000 school-age children in the United States just prior to widespread availability of speech-language services. They reported a gradual decline in the occurrence of SSDs from kindergarten through twelfth grade. Finally, McKinnon and colleagues (2007) conducted a survey of teachers serving more than 10,000 Australian schoolchildren in kindergarten through Grade 6. Their findings indicated a decreasing proportion of SSDs across grade levels. The authors reported that, unlike in the United States where speech-language pathology services are mandated in the public schools, in Australia "once these children go to school, their access to speech-language pathology services often is limited" (p. 13).

Summary

A positive correlation between improvement in speech sound production and age in typically developing children has been reported. Findings from at least two large population studies suggest that maturation generally may be a factor in speech sound acquisition, and improvement in articulation skills may continue after age 9 years in typically developing children. However, after about age 9, the amount of improvement in speech sound acquisition, absent of intervention, is limited in typically developing children. Interestingly, however, findings from both the NSHS and McKinnon and colleagues (2007) suggest that for some children with SSDs, their difficulty resolves without intervention. This highlights the need to carefully document the progress that clients make in order to ensure that the changes observed are actually the result of interventions and not just maturation. Chapter 8 revisits this issue.

Gender

Child development specialists have long been interested in contrasts between males and females in speech sound acquisition, and SLPs have investigated the relationship between gender and speech sound production. Research in this area has focused on a comparison of 1) phoneme acquisition in males and females and 2) the incidence of SSDs in males and females.

Dawson (1929) examined the articulatory skills of 200 children from Grades 1 through 12 and reported that until approximately age 12, girls produced slightly higher scores than boys. Templin (1963) reported similar findings: "In articulation development, girls consistently are found to be slightly accelerated . . . in all instances the differences are relatively small and often are not statistically significant" (p. 13).

Smit and colleagues (1990) conducted a large-scale normative study of speech sound development in children aged 3 through 9 years from Iowa and Nebraska. They reported that the girls in this study appeared to acquire sounds at somewhat earlier ages than boys through age 6 years. The differences reached statistical significance only at age 6 and younger, but not in every preschool age group. Kenney and Prather (1986), who elicited multiple productions of frequent error sounds, reported significant differences favoring girls aged 3 through 5 years.

Additional information can be gleaned from a review of the normative data from a range of single-word tests of speech sound productions of children. Flipsen and Ogiela (2015) reported that 8 of the 10 tests they examined considered the question of gender differences when constructing their comparison groups for scoring the tests. Separate norms for males and females were provided whenever differences were found. Such a separation was provided for children up to age 6 years for one test, up to age 7 years for one test, and up to age 9 years or older for three tests. Developers of three tests did not find any gender differences at any age.

Relative to gender and the incidence of SSDs, surveys conducted by Hall (1938), Mills and Streit (1942), Morley (1952), Everhart (1960), and Hull and associates (1971) all indicated that the incidence of SSDs was higher in males than females regardless of the age group studied. Smit and colleagues (1990) stated that "it is a well-known fact that boys are at much greater risk than girls for delayed speech, and this propensity continues to be reported" (p. 790).

Gender differences have been reported by Shriberg (2010) for specific subgroups of children within his Speech Disorders Classification System (SDCS), which will be discussed in more detail in Chapter 5. For example, in older children with persisting speech errors, /r/ errors appear to be more common in males, and /s/ errors appear to be more common in females.

Summary

The sex of a child appears to have some impact on speech sound acquisition. At very young ages, females tend to be slightly ahead of males, but the differences disappear as the children get older. As a consequence, many current tests of speech sound acquisition include separate normative data for males and females. Gender differences are reflected by the identification of significantly more male than female children as having SSDs.

Family Background

Researchers have been interested in the influence of family background, both environmental and biological, and how it may affect a child's speech and language development. The following paragraphs review literature related to family background and phonology organized around three topics: 1) SES, 2) family tendencies, and 3) sibling influences.

Socioeconomic Status

The SES of a child's family, as measured by parents' educational background, occupation, income, and/or location of family residence, is a significant part of the child's environment. Because some behavioral deficiencies occur more frequently in lower socioeconomic environments, SES has been of interest to speech-language clinicians as a possible factor in speech and language development.

Early studies of this question (Everhart, 1953, 1956; Prins, 1962a; Templin, 1957; Weaver et al., 1960) relied on parental occupation as the sole measure of SES and yielded conflicting findings. The studies by Everhart and that of Prins reported no significant association, but the studies by Templin and by Weaver and colleagues indicated that the poorest articulation skills were exhibited by those from the lowest SES households.

Smit and colleagues (1990) in the Iowa-Nebraska normative study used parental education level and reported no significant relationship to speech sound performance. A similar conclusion was reached by Keating and associates (2001) with data from the Australian Health Survey, which used a combination of household income and parental occupation and education as a measure of SES. Based on the study of more than 12,000 children aged birth to 14 years, the authors also reported no significant association between SES and child speech disorders (which included both SSDs and stuttering). Another Australian study (McLeod et al., 2015) measured SES using geographical location (i.e., postal address) in a study of the speech of 803 children aged 4 and 5 years. Using a rating scale measure of how understandable the children's speech was to a variety of listeners, McLeod and colleagues reported no differences based on SES. In a related study, Johnson and colleagues (2010) examined whether having an SSD affects SES in the long term. They found that as adults individuals with a history of preschool SSDs did not end up with any lower rated SES (based on their own occupations) than those with normal speech histories.

These findings overall suggest that SSDs are not strongly associated with low SES (i.e., growing up in a low SES household does not appear to increase the risk of having an SSD). However, it is still possible that low SES may interact with other factors, such as medical attention, preschool stimulation, and opportunities for spoken interaction, to influence speech sound production.

Familial Tendencies

It is not uncommon for SLPs to observe a family history of speech and language disorders in their clients, and this has been confirmed by several studies. Neils and

Aram (1986) obtained reports from the parents of 74 preschool language-disordered children and indicated that 46% reported that other family members had histories of speech and language disorders. Of this group, 55% were reported to have SSDs, the most prevalent familial disorder reported. Shriberg and Kwiatkowski (1994) reported data from 62 children aged 3–6 years with developmental phonologic disorders. They found that 39% of the children had one member of the family with a similar speech problem, whereas an additional 17% (total = 56%) had more than one family member with a similar speech problem. A study in Jordan (Alaraifi et al., 2014) found that 21 of 45 (46.7%) patients with SSDs had reported a family history of articulation disorder.

Two studies of twins have been reported that contribute to our understanding of familial influences, including genetic factors that may relate to SSDs. Matheny and Bruggeman (1973) studied 101 same-sex twin sets, 22 opposite-sex twin sets, and 94 siblings between the ages of 3 and 8 years. With regard to speech sound performance scores, monozygotic twins correlated more closely with each other than did dizygotic twins. The authors concluded that there is a strong hereditary influence on articulation status. In addition, sex differences were found to favor females. Locke and Mather (1987) examined speech sound productions in 13 monozygotic and 13 dizygotic twin sets. They reported that the identical twins were more similar in their error patterns than the fraternal twins.

Familial tendencies are also supported by sibling data. Lewis and colleagues (1989) reported that siblings of children with severe SSDs performed more poorly than siblings of a control group on phonology and reading measures. Participants with SSD had phonologic skills which correlated positively with those of their siblings, whereas scores of controls did not. Families of children with SSD reported significantly more members with speech and language disorders and dyslexia than did families of controls. Sex differences were reflected in the incidence but not in the severity or type of disorder present. The authors concluded that their findings suggested a familial basis for at least some forms of severe SSDs.

Felsenfeld and colleagues (1995) also provided data that supported familial tendencies. In comparison to the control group, children of the 24 adult participants that had a documented history of a phonological-language disorder performed significantly more poorly on all tests of articulation and expressive language functioning. These children were also significantly more likely to have received treatment for SSDs than were the children of the 28 control participants.

A 2007 study by Lewis and colleagues compared parents of children with SSDs who themselves had histories of SSDs with parents of similar children without such histories. The parents with histories of SSDs themselves performed significantly more poorly on standardized tests of spoken language and spelling.

It may be inferred from these studies that genetic or biological inheritance factors may precipitate some SSDs; yet it is often difficult to separate environmental from genetic/biological influences. Parlour and Broen (1991) examined environmental influences on SSDs. Their research was predicated on the possibility that individuals who themselves experienced significant speech and language disorders as children are likely to provide a less than optimal cultural or linguistic milieu for their own families. Using the same data set as Felsenfeld and colleagues (1995), Parlour and Broen employed two environmental measures, the Preschool HOME Scale and the Modified Templin Child-Rearing Questionnaire. These measures allowed them to ascertain qualitative aspects of a child's environment, including physical, emotional, and cognitive support available to preschool children, and child-rearing practices based on direct observation of the examiner, parental reports, and parental responses to a written questionnaire.

The two groups performed in a comparable manner for all of the environmental domains sampled with one exception, acceptance, which assessed disciplinary practices. Parlour and Broen (1991) reported that families with a history of SSDs relied more on physical punishment than did control families. In terms of future research efforts, the authors suggested that although differences were generally not significant between the groups, the disordered group received lower mean scores than controls on each of the HOME subscales, suggesting that some subtle differences may have been present, particularly for domains involving the use of punishment, learning, and language stimulation.

Recent advances in molecular genetics are allowing us to look more directly for genetic differences in individuals with SSDs. Lewis (2009) reminded us of the complexity of the search because genes don't directly lead to the disorder, but rather, direct the production of proteins that then influence various aspects of development. She also points out that speech and language behaviors are likely related to a variety of neurological and biochemical processes, each of which may be active to differing degrees at different points in the developmental period. Those processes may also be involved with various speech and language behaviors (see our discussion of comorbidity in Chapter 5). It is likely, therefore, that multiple genes are involved. Despite the complexity of the task, Lewis notes that candidate gene regions on several different chromosomes (e.g., 1, 3, 6, 7, 15) have been implicated as possible sources of speech sound production disorders by different investigator groups. A discussion of the fine details of these findings is beyond the scope of the current text, but will be revisited again in Chapter 5.

Sibling Influences

Another factor of interest to investigators of SSDs has been sibling number and birth order. Because the amount of time that parents can spend with each child decreases with each child added to a family, some clinicians have asked whether sibling order is related to articulatory development. Koch (1956) studied the relationships between certain speech and voice characteristics in young children and siblings in two-child families. In this study, 384 children between 5 and 6 years of age were divided into 24 subgroups matched individual by individual on the basis of age, socioeconomic class, and residence. Data on speech and voice characteristics consisted of teachers' ratings. Koch reported that firstborn children had better articulation than those born second, and the wider the age difference between a child and their sibling, the better the child's articulation. Likewise, Davis (1937) reported that children without siblings demonstrated superior articulatory performance to children with siblings and to twins. On the other hand, Wellman and colleagues (1931) did not find a significant relationship between the number of siblings and level of articulation skill for 3-year-olds.

Twins have been reported to present unique patterns of speech sound acquisition (Perkins, 1977; Powers, 1957/1971; Winitz, 1969). From birth, twins receive speech stimulation not only from others within their environment but also from each other. Powers indicated that the "emotional ties of twins, too, are likely to be closer than

those of singled siblings, which further augments their interdependence in speech"
(p. 868). It is not uncommon for twins to reflect unique phonologic patterns and use
similar phonologic patterns. Schwartz and colleagues (1980) reported, however, that
in the very early stages of phonologic acquisition (the first 50 words), similarities in
phonemes used, including phonologic patterns and lexical items, were not present.
Unique patterns of speech are occasionally found in twins 2 years and older who have
little resemblance to adult models and have meaning only to the twins; these speech
patterns are termed *idioglossia*.

Summary

Little relationship exists between SES and SSDs based on available reports. Although
a higher number of misarticulating children tend to be found in lower socioeconomic
groups (especially children under 4 years) than in middle or upper SES, SES by itself
does not appear to contribute significantly to the presence of an SSD.

Studies of phonologic development in twins as well as in families with a history
of phonologic impairment suggest familial propensity toward the presence of such a
disorder. Investigations examining phonologic status and sibling relationships are
limited and the data are dated, but findings have been fairly consistent. Firstborn and
only children exhibit somewhat better articulation performance than children who
have older siblings or twins during the preschool years. The age span between siblings
also appears to affect phonologic proficiency, with better articulation associated with
wider age differences. One can speculate that firstborn and only children receive better speech models and more stimulation than children who have older siblings. The
possibility also exists that older siblings produce normal developmental phonologic
errors and, thus, at points in time present imperfect speech models to younger siblings. Unique patterns of sound productions have been reported in twins; reasons for
these patterns are speculative and tend to focus on the stimulation each twin receives
from the other. Unique speech patterns have, however, been reported, even in very
young twins (i.e., around age 2–3 years).

Genetic studies offer a tantalizing promise for tracking down the ultimate cause
of at least some SSDs. Preliminary work in this area suggests we may not be far from
identifying specific genes involved. Although the genetics question remains, there is
evidence that familial influence is a likely factor in the presence of an SSD in some
children.

The preceding discussion suggests a tension between the influence of the family
environment (siblings, birth order, parenting style, SES) and genetic endowment on
SSDs. Neither likely tells the whole story. As with most aspects of human behavior, it
is probable that speech sound development and disorders reflect a complex interaction
among many of these factors.

Personality

The relationship between personality characteristics and phonologic behavior has
been investigated to determine whether particular personality patterns are likely to
be associated with SSDs. Researchers have examined not only the child's personality
traits but also those of the child's parents, using various assessment tools.

Bloch and Goodstein (1971) concluded, in a review of the literature, that investigations of personality traits and emotional adjustment of individuals with SSDs

have shown contradictory findings and attributed this to two major problems with the investigations: 1) the criteria for defining articulatory impairment has varied from one study to the next and 2) the validity and reliability of tools or instruments used to assess personality and adjustment have varied.

In a causal correlates profile based on 178 children with SSDs, Shriberg and Kwiatkowski (1994) presented data on psychosocial inputs (parental behaviors) and psychosocial behaviors (child characteristics) that were descriptive of this population. Of the parents, 27% were judged to be either somewhat or considerably ineffective in terms of behavioral management, and 17% were either somewhat or overly concerned about their child's problem. An even smaller percentage of parents indicated that it was their perception that their child had difficulty with initial acceptance by peers. Over half of the children (51%) were described as somewhat too sensitive (easily hurt feelings), and an additional 14% were described as overly sensitive (very easily hurt feelings). Shriberg and Kwiatkowski (1994) reported that their descriptive data indicated that "a significant number of children with developmental phonologic disorders experience psychosocial difficulties" (p. 115). They indicated, however, that one cannot be completely certain that sampling biases did not inflate the magnitudes of the findings or whether the participants' data would differ significantly from data in a group without speech delay.

Summary

Although certain personality characteristics have been linked to some children with SSDs, no clear picture of personality variance from typically developing children has emerged in this population. Likewise, certain parental/home variables have been associated with this population, but the strength of that association is weak. Additional studies involving typical–disordered child comparisons are necessary before a definitive statement regarding this association can be made.

CONCLUSION

A great deal has been discovered about factors related to SSDs in children that can assist the SLP in assessing phonologic status, planning remediation programs, and counseling clients and their parents. Yet, many questions remain unanswered. One truth that emerges from the literature, however, is the absence of any one-to-one correspondence between the presence of a particular factor and the precise nature of most individuals' phonologic status. Prediction of cause–effect relationships represents a scientific ideal, but determination of such relationships in the realm of human behavior, including communication disorders, is often difficult. The likelihood of multiple factors being involved in cases of SSDs complicates the search for such relationships. At this point in time, the most that can be said is that certain of the factors discussed here may, either individually or in combination, be associated with SSDs.

QUESTIONS FOR CHAPTER 4

1. What is the relationship of speech sound perception and speech sound errors?
2. What is the relationship between phonological disorders and morphosyntactic language impairments?

3. How is each of the following factors related to clinical phonology and speech production?

   a. Otitis media

   b. Tongue thrusting

   c. Missing teeth

   d. Tonsils

   e. Cognitive impairment

   f. Phonological memory

   g. Lower SES

   h. Family history of phonological difficulties

   i. Removal of part of the tongue

4. What is the relationship between intelligence and SSDs?

5. How might the presence of a co-existing language impairment impact the expression of an SSD and vice versa?

6. Discuss how having an SSD might impact academic performance.

7. Does a child's gender matter in terms of whether they have an SSD? In what way?

8. Describe possible family tendencies within SSDs.

5

Classification and Comorbidity in Speech Sound Disorders

PETER FLIPSEN JR., JOHN E. BERNTHAL, AND NICHOLAS W. BANKSON

LEARNING OBJECTIVES

This chapter discusses how speech sound disorders (SSDs) are classified and examines associated conditions that may co-occur with them. By the end of this chapter, the reader should be able to:

- Describe the broad difference between organically based and idiopathic SSDs.
- Discuss the potential impact of several major deviations in the structure of the speech mechanism on SSDs.
- Briefly delineate what is known about some of the more common genetic conditions that include SSDs.
- Discuss the impact of hearing loss on speech sound development.
- List some common and uncommon speech errors produced by individuals with hearing loss.
- Distinguish between dysarthria and apraxia of speech (AOS).
- Discuss the controversy surrounding the category childhood apraxia of speech (CAS).
- Delineate the three broad causes and the core problem associated with CAS.
- Identify and briefly describe diagnostic markers for CAS.
- Explain the relationship between factors underlying idiopathic SSDs and the search for subgroups.
- Distinguish among three perspectives for the classification of SSDs.
- Discuss the three broad categories and nine subgroups of the Speech Disorders Classification System (SDCS).
- Distinguish among Dodd's five symptomological subgroups of SSDs.
- Discuss why different communication disorders might coexist in the same individual.
- List and describe how some common disorders might coexist with SSDs.

Chapter 1 described in a broad sense what we identify as SSDs. In recognition of the many variations of SSDs that are seen in children, speech-language pathologists (SLPs) have sought to classify or group SSDs into various subgroups. Although the field's knowledge in this area remains limited, progress has been made on this issue, and in this chapter we attempt to outline the research on this topic. Following that, we also explore the question of comorbid, or coexisting, disorders.

For many years, SLPs have divided the population of children with SSDs into two relatively large groups. The first group of children who have what is often referred to as *organically based disorders* includes those children whose difficulty with speech sounds can be readily linked to an obvious organic etiology or cause. This group includes subgroups based on specific causes. The second large group is those for whom there is no obvious cause. This latter group has been much more elusive and more difficult to identify and classify. This second group of SSDs have had many labels over the years, including functional articulation disorders, developmental phonological disorders, and speech delay of unknown origin. Most recently these have been called *idiopathic SSDs*.

ORGANICALLY BASED SPEECH SOUND DISORDERS

The following discussion is not meant to be all inclusive; it is meant only to survey a representative sample of organically based SSDs. The information is also not intended as an exhaustive coverage of any of the particular groups that are identified. Entire textbooks have been devoted to discussions of the assessment and treatment of the speech sound problems experienced by some of these populations (e.g., Kummer, 2020; Tye-Murray, 2020).

Major Structural Variations of the Speech Mechanism

It is not surprising that significant anomalies of the oral structures are frequently associated with specific speech problems. Oral structural anomalies may be congenital (present from birth) or acquired. Cleft lip and/or palate is perhaps the most common congenital anomaly of the orofacial complex. Acquired structural deficits may result from trauma to the orofacial complex or surgical removal of oral structures secondary to oral cancers. For individuals with orofacial anomalies, the course of habilitation or rehabilitation often includes surgical and/or prosthetic management, and therefore the speech clinician must work closely with a team comprised of various medical and dental specialists.

Lips

Surgical repair of clefts of the lip can result in a relatively short and/or immobile upper lip. Although this might be expected to adversely affect articulation skills, this is not generally the case. A retrospective study by Vallino and colleagues (2008) reported that only 12/90 (13%) of children with an isolated cleft lip were identified as having an SSD. Note the similarity of that percentage with the 11%–16% of preschool children who have SSDs, as highlighted in Chapter 1. The fact that the numbers are so similar suggests that having an isolated cleft lip may not increase the chances of having an SSD. Earlier studies (e.g., Laitinen et al., 1998; Riski & DeLong, 1984) have reported similar percentages and, thus, support this conclusion.

Tongue

The tongue is a muscular structure capable of considerable changes in length and width. Because the tongue is such an adaptable organ, speakers are frequently able to compensate for having both less and more of it (i.e., loss or removal of extensive amounts of the tongue or having a tongue that is larger or smaller than normal).

Surgical removal (or accidental loss) of some or all of the tongue is called a *glossectomy;* it is typically motivated by the presence of oral cancer or traumatic injury to the tongue. Clinical investigators have repeatedly reported intelligible speech production following partial glossectomies. For many patients, however, speech production is affected to varying degrees. Furia and colleagues (2001) reported pretreatment and post-treatment intelligibility scores for 27 adult glossectomy patients. The group included 6 with total removal, 9 with removal of all but the tongue base (subtotal), and 12 with partial removal. As one would expect, those individuals in the partial group demonstrated the best speech intelligibility post-surgery. A study by Skelly and colleagues (1971) noted a similar outcome pattern.

Leonard (1994) reported a study in which listeners were asked to evaluate consonants produced by 50 speakers with various types of glossectomy. She indicated that fricatives and plosives were most frequently judged to be inaccurate, whereas nasals and semivowels were less affected. A case study by Kaipa and colleagues (2012) of a single female who underwent total glossectomy revealed similar mixed outcomes. Acoustic analysis of the vowel area suggested improvements over a 3-month period following surgery, but listener judgments of consonant accuracy suggested a deterioration over the same period.

For patients with partial glossectomy, the specific surgical procedure used and/or the particular muscles removed may impact speech outcomes (Bressmann et al., 2004; Sun et al., 2007).

Individuals have been shown to be able to compensate for changes in the tongue to some extent. Skelly and colleagues (1971) noted that the compensatory articulatory patterns differed depending on the extent of the surgery. Partial glossectomy patients utilized the residual tongue stump to modify articulation; total glossectomy patients made mandibular, labial, buccal, and palatal adjustments. Skelly and colleagues also noted that unilateral tongue excision (removal of one half of the tongue only) required fewer speech adaptations than excisions involving the entire tongue tip.

In a 2014 study, Bressmann and colleagues recorded 15 patients with tumors on their tongue who were scheduled for partial glossectomy as they produced a set of tongue twisters (e.g., "Kate takes cakes to Tate"). Before surgery, the tongue twisters were produced more slowly, but just as accurately, compared to a group of age-matched control speakers. Thus, presurgical patients seemed to be able to compensate for a tongue that was enlarged due to the presence of a tumor. Six to nine weeks after surgery, their rate of speech had not changed, but the number of errors increased. In addition, pauses between repetitions of the tongue twisters were longer after surgery, suggesting that the individuals were attempting (albeit less successfully) to compensate by taking more time to plan their speech.

Some post-surgical (medical) interventions have led to improvements in speech production skill. For example, the use of a *palatal augmentation prosthesis (PAP)* in which "the palatal vault is re-established at a lower level than normal, requiring less bulk and mobility of the tongue for appropriate palatolingual contacts during speech" (Marunick & Tselios, 2004, p. 67). Another approach has been the use of artificial grafts, where the reduced tongue mass is surgically supplemented with collagen covered in a silicone layer. After several days, the silicone cover is removed. A study by Terai and Shimahara (2004) of nine adult patients who underwent this procedure revealed significantly more intelligible speech after 6 months and a small amount of additional improvement 6 months later.

An important question for SLPs is whether speech treatment will be effective for these patients. There are no definitive answers (Blyth et al., 2014), but some evidence for therapy effectiveness is emerging. A very early case study (Backus, 1940) recorded the speech pattern of a 10-year-old boy after excision of the tongue tip and the left half of the tongue. Initially, numerous consonant substitutions were observed, but after a period of treatment, he was able to produce all consonants with little identifiable deviation. The Furia and colleagues (2001) study described previously included 3–6 months of therapy following surgery, but only the total and subtotal groups made significant intelligibility improvements (no gains were made by the partial glossectomy group). A 2016 report by Blyth and colleagues from two patients following partial glossectomy suggested that therapy using feedback from ultrasound (to be discussed in Chapter 12) might be effective for this population. Both patients improved their consonant accuracy scores, but neither showed improvements in intelligibility at the sentence level.

In contrast to glossectomy, a tongue that is abnormally large is called *macroglossia*. A distinction must be made here between *true macroglossia*, in which the tongue is larger than expected, and *relative macroglossia*, in which a normal-size tongue occurs with an oral cavity that is too small (Vogel et al., 1986). True macroglossia is thought to reflect an active growth process, such as a tumor or a vascular malformation, or it may reflect certain genetic conditions, such as Beckwith-Wiedemann syndrome (BWS) (Van Lierde et al., 2010). A well-known example of relative macroglossia is seen in individuals with Down syndrome (DS). In either type of macroglossia, speech may be affected because the tongue essentially has less room within which to move. A survey by Van Borsel and associates (1999), for example, indicated articulation difficulties in 29/40 (73%) of individuals with macroglossia associated with BWS. Reduced intelligibility is a common issue in individuals with DS (Kumin, 1994), and their relative macroglossia has been assumed to be a major factor.

In cases of true macroglossia, a glossectomy procedure may be performed and can lead to improved speech skills (Heggie et al., 2013; Shipster et al., 2006; Van Lierde et al., 2010). Glossectomy is not usually performed in cases of relative macroglossia. This is likely because studies of glossectomy outcomes in individuals with DS have generally revealed poor outcomes (Klaiman et al., 1988 Margar-Bacal et al., 1987; Parsons et al., 1987). If the surgery is not performed, individuals with macroglossia must learn or be taught to compensate (Mekonnen, 2012; Stephens, 2011; Van Borsel et al., 2000).

Another tongue anomaly that is occasionally encountered is a bifid or split tongue. This may be an isolated phenomenon (e.g., Bressmann, 2006; Surej et al., 2010), or it may be a feature of certain genetic syndromes such as Smith-Lemli-Opitz syndrome (Rojare et al., 2019) and Goldenhar syndrome (Bogusiak et al., 2017). Although there has been limited study of this condition, Bressmann (2006) suggested that one speech consequence would be mild distortions of /s, z/.

Finally, it has also been suggested in some case studies (e.g., Dunn & Reeves, 2004) that additions to the tongue, such as tongue piercing, may negatively affect speech. However, it appears likely that most speakers are able to adapt quickly, resulting in normal or near-normal speech (Van Borsel & Cornelis, 2009). A study by Heinen and colleagues (2017) compared 20 adults with pierced tongues to a matched control group. The groups did not differ significantly on the clarity, rate, fluency, rhythm, or prosody of both spontaneous and read speech. As well, removal of the pierced ornament did not result in a significant change on any of those same speech dimensions.

Hard Palate

The removal of any part of the maxilla, which includes the hard palate (e.g., as necessitated by oral cancer) creates a serious problem for the speaker if it is not restored surgically or prosthetically. Many patients can achieve palatal closure after being fitted with a prosthetic (dental) appliance, sometimes called an obturator. Sullivan and colleagues (2002) reported results from 32 patients who had palatal defects because of surgical removal of a portion of the palate as a result of cancer of the maxillary sinus and alveolar ridge. One month after obturation mean speech intelligibility improved from 61% to 94%, speaking rate improved from 138 to 164 words per minute, and nasality (on a 0- to 7-point scale, where 7 is hypernasal and 0 is hyponasal) improved from 5.8 to 1.6. The patients rated themselves as having a communication effectiveness of 75% of what it was prior to the cancer. The authors concluded that "obturation is an effective intervention for defects of the maxillary sinus and alveolar ridge on speech performance. Variations in effectiveness were noted based on site of defect and patient satisfaction with the intervention" (p. 530). A similar study of 12 patients by Rieger and colleagues (2002) reported positive results. Speech intelligibility with the obturator was not significantly different from speech intelligibility before surgery.

For children born with clefts of the hard palate, the palate is typically repaired within the first 12–14 months of life. Scarring associated with the surgery has not been found to interfere with articulatory production in most cases. Obturators may also be used to create temporary closure in cases where surgery is delayed for medical reasons or if an initial palatal repair is unsuccessful.

Soft Palate

The relationship of the soft palate (velum) to speech sound production has been a topic of considerable research, much of it focusing on the velopharyngeal port and the effect of velopharyngeal competence on articulation. *Velopharyngeal competence* refers to the valving or sphincteral closure that takes place to separate the nasal cavity from the oral cavity during production of nonnasal speech sounds. As mentioned in Chapter 4, in most cases referral for assessment and management of problems with velopharyngeal functioning are made to cleft palate or craniofacial teams.

Velopharyngeal incompetence or insufficiency is often associated with individuals with clefts of the soft palate. Some speakers without clefting also demonstrate velopharyngeal incompetence; for example, individuals with dysarthria related to neurogenic paresis or paralysis of the velopharyngeal muscles (Johns et al., 2003). Management in such cases is almost always surgical or prosthetic in nature. The exception is for cases of phoneme-specific nasal emission. This is a learned behavior that may be responsive to therapy (see discussion on the soft palate in Chapter 4).

When the oral cavity communicates with (is open to) the nasal cavity, for example, through palatal fistulae (openings in the palate) or following ablative surgery (removal of part of the soft palate) or velopharyngeal incompetence, varying degrees of hypernasality will usually result. On the other hand, hyponasality (denasality) may result when the nasopharynx or nasal cavity is obstructed during speech production. Inflammation of the mucous membranes of the nasal cavity, enlarged tonsils or adenoids, or a deviated septum may also cause hyponasality.

Inadequate velopharyngeal closure is also frequently associated with changes to specific speech sound types. These include: 1) hypernasal (excessive nasal) resonance of vowels, glides, and liquids; 2) reduced or diminished intraoral pressure during production of pressure consonants (i.e., obstruents, which include fricatives, stops, and affricates); 3) nasal air emission accompanying production of pressure consonants; or 4) unusual substitutions, such as the use of glottal stops for stop consonants and pharyngeal fricatives for sibilants. These latter substitutions are sometimes referred to as *compensatory articulations*. In such cases, speakers unable to close off the air stream in the oral cavity may attempt to create closure at a location where it is possible for them to do so (i.e., below the level of the velum and other velopharyngeal muscles).

In addition to immediate problems associated with speech production, children born with clefts of the soft palate also experience a higher frequency of middle ear infections (otitis media) than children without clefts (Sheahan et al., 2003). As discussed in Chapter 4, a higher incidence of otitis media may be important for speech because it may be associated with mild-moderate or moderate hearing loss (albeit temporary), which may potentially impact speech sound acquisition. The frequency of otitis media in children born with clefts appears to be the result of problems with either the structure or function of the eustachian tube mechanism, which develops at about the same time in the embryo as the palate. Kemaloglou and colleagues (1999) reported shorter and more horizontal eustachian tubes in children with clefts of the palate compared to children without clefts. Matsune and associates (1991) reported that the tensor veli palatini muscle (which is responsible for opening the eustachian tube) is often abnormally inserted into the cartilage of the tube in cases of cleft palate. This may make it more difficult for the tube to be opened.

Nasopharynx

The nasopharyngeal tonsils (adenoids) are located at the upper, or superior, pharyngeal area. Hypertrophied (enlarged) adenoids may compensate for a short or partially immobile velum by assisting in velopharyngeal closure, thus, their removal may result in hypernasality (Haapanen et al., 1994; Maryn et al., 2004; Wachtel et al., 2000; Witzel et al., 1986). The adenoids may, however, become sufficiently enlarged that they constitute a major obstruction of the nasopharynx, resulting in hyponasal speech. Enlarged adenoids may also interfere with eustachian tube function in some individuals. When adenoids constitute an obstruction of the eustachian tube, they may be removed for medical reasons.

Summary

Although individuals with major oral structural deviations frequently experience articulation problems, the relationship between structural deficits and articulation skills is not highly predictable. The literature cites many instances of individuals with structural anomalies who have developed compensatory gestures to produce acoustically acceptable speech, whereas others with similar structural anomalies do not. It is not known why some individuals are able to compensate for relatively gross abnormalities and others are unable to compensate for lesser deficits. A speech-language clinician who evaluates or treats individuals with oral structural anomalies must work collaboratively with various medical and dental specialists during speech habilitation or rehabilitation.

Genetic Disorders

We have long known that genetic endowment combines with various environmental influences to yield individual physical and behavioral characteristics. As discussed in Chapter 4, gene regions on several different human chromosomes have been implicated as possibly underlying sources for at least some SSDs. And recently, the possibility of the interaction of multiple genes during early embryonic development has been explored (Eising et al., 2019). The idea of multiple genetic influences on SSDs is reinforced by findings such as those emerging from the Cleveland Family Speech and Reading Study (ongoing since 1988). These data suggest a great deal of genetic variation within the population of individuals with SSDs (Lewis & Iyengar, 2018).

In general, the role of our genes in SSDs is highlighted by: 1) gender differences in the occurrence of specific SSDs, 2) the tendency of certain disorders to run in families, and 3) the association of speech and language impairments with known genetic disorders and syndromes. An excellent source of more detailed information about specific genetic syndromes is Shprintzen (1997). We highlight a few here.

A classic example of a genetic condition with implications for speech sound production is *Down syndrome (DS)*, which is thought to occur once in about every 700 live births. In most cases, DS results from an extra copy of chromosome 21 (hence, it is often called trisomy 21). Several features associated with this syndrome likely contribute to difficulties with speech in this population. First, DS usually includes varying degrees of cognitive impairment that may lead to an overall delay in speech sound acquisition. Second, as mentioned previously, individuals with DS have relative macroglossia, or a normal-size tongue in a relatively small oral cavity, which results in less space for the tongue to maneuver during connected speech production. This likely explains why reduced intelligibility in conversation is such a significant concern in this population (Kumin, 1994). Individuals with DS have also been shown to have reduced muscle tone or hypotonia specific to the articulatory system (Bunton & Leddy, 2011), as well as smaller brains, including a cerebellum that is disproportionately small (Pinter et al., 2001). They have also been shown to have a high frequency of otitis media associated with eustachian tube problems (Laws & Hall, 2014; Marder & Cholmain, 2006). Some controversy remains about whether the overall pattern of speech sound acquisition in DS is similar to that of typically developing children (but simply delayed) or if it actually follows a different course. A review by Kent and Vorperian (2013) suggested that error patterns representing both normal and disordered development are likely to occur in this population.

Another genetic disorder that has been shown to include difficulty with speech sounds (without clefting) is *fragile X syndrome (FXS)*. Somewhat less common than DS, FXS is thought to occur once in about every 4,000 live births. In this case, a mutation turns off a particular section of the X chromosome, resulting in failure to produce a particular protein. Males have only a single X chromosome and so are much more likely to be affected by FXS than females (for whom the mutation might be present on only one of their two X chromosomes). FXS shares two broad features with DS, including varying degrees of cognitive impairment that may delay speech sound acquisition, and speech that is frequently difficult to understand. Studies of boys with FXS by both Roberts and colleagues (2005) and Barnes and colleagues (2009) reported that the error patterns of boys with FXS more closely resembled those of younger typically developing children (i.e., their speech was delayed and not necessarily different).

Recall also the previous discussion of true macroglossia and BWS. In addition to speech concerns related to macroglossia, this genetic disorder may also include hemihyperplasia, in which one side of the body (or just one side of some structures) is overdeveloped. This sometimes co-occurs with clefts of the palate. Both of these issues (macroglossia, hemihyperplasia) may contribute to the difficulty these individuals have with anterior speech sounds, although macroglossia is likely the major factor (Stephens, 2011; Van Borsel et al., 2000).

Another example of a genetic disorder that has been associated with SSDs is *galactosemia*. This disorder occurs once in about every 53,000 live births. It manifests primarily as an enzyme deficiency that prevents the complete metabolism of the milk sugar lactose. Toxic by-products of incomplete metabolism accumulate and can lead to severe liver and neurological damage, and potentially death (Hoffmann et al., 2011). Lactose-free diets reportedly halt any ongoing damage, but cognitive and speech deficits may remain. Hoffman and colleagues studied 32 children and adults with this condition (age range 9–37 years). These authors reported that only 9/32 (28%) had full-scale IQ scores above 85 and only 5/32 (16%) produced no errors on a test of German speech production. Shriberg, Potter, and associates (2011) reported that 8/33 (24%) of children with galactosemia presented speech characteristics that were consistent with a diagnosis of CAS (a condition to be discussed later in this chapter and in Chapter 12).

Data are emerging on specific speech deficits and error patterns in several other genetic syndromes. These include 22q deletion syndrome, which is also called velocardiofacial syndrome and DiGeorge syndrome (Baylis & Shriberg, 2019), cri du chat syndrome (Kristoffersen et al., 2014), Williams syndrome (Huffman et al., 2019), and 5p deletion syndrome (Garmann et al., 2018).

Clinical Vignette 5.1

It Runs in the Family

Author Peter Flipsen Jr. recalls working with a 5-year-old boy, Aaron (a pseudonym), who was having difficulty with production of /r/. Although, based on developmental norms, many clinicians might not have targeted this phoneme at this age, his parents specifically asked for services. Family history appeared to justify doing so. It turns out that Aaron had four older brothers, and all of them had previously been seen for speech services. Interestingly, all had worked on correcting errors with /r/.

Was this a clear-cut case of genetics being the cause? Perhaps, but two facts complicate such an interpretation. First, Aaron's younger sister had speech skills within normal limits, and it was not expected that she would need therapy. And second, neither parent had received any speech or language services as a child and not been identified as needing services.

Hearing Loss

A third subgroup of organically based SSDs includes individuals with significant hearing loss. One of the most important elements underlying the production and comprehension of speech, as well as the monitoring of one's own speech, is an auditory system that is sensitive in the frequency range where most speech sounds occur (500–4,000 Hz). Individuals with more severe hearing loss will have difficulty decoding the incoming sound signal and will perceive words differently than individuals with normal hearing mechanisms.

The child who is hard of hearing or deaf faces the challenging task of learning how to produce speech without adequate auditory input. Learning to discriminate and produce speech must then be accomplished by watching how sounds look on the face, how they feel through vibrations, and what can be perceived from a distorted auditory signal. A certain level of hearing is required to learn and maintain normal speech production. Ling (1989) summarized this relationship by noting that the more normal a person's hearing, the more natural their speech is likely to be.

Several aspects of hearing loss have been shown to affect speech perception and production; these include the level of hearing sensitivity, speech recognition ability, and configuration of the hearing loss. Individual hearing losses can range from mild to severe or profound (more than 70 dB HL). Labels such as hard of hearing and deaf are frequently applied to persons with varying degrees of hearing impairment.

Hearing sensitivity typically varies somewhat from one frequency to another, with speech and language differentially influenced by the frequency configuration and severity of the hearing loss. Although information recorded on an audiogram is a useful prognostic indicator of speech reception ability, children with similar audiograms may not perceive and process speech sounds in the same way. A pure-tone audiogram cannot measure a person's ability to distinguish one frequency from another or to track formant transitions (a skill critical to speech perception). Variables related to intervention, such as age of fitting and full-time use of amplification or the quality of early intervention programs, may also impact speech perception and the intelligibility of the speech these individuals produce.

A second hearing-related factor important to speech sound acquisition is the age of onset and the age of detection of the hearing loss. If a severe loss has been present since birth, normal acquisition of language—including phonology, syntax, and semantics—is difficult, and specialized instruction and other interventions are necessary to develop speech and language. Such instruction may rely on visual, tactile, and kinesthetic cues and signing, as well as whatever residual auditory sensation the person possesses or has been afforded via technology. For a discussion of the influence of hearing loss on infants' and toddlers' phonologic development, see Stoel-Gammon and Kehoe (1994). Children and adults who suffer a serious loss of hearing after language has been acquired usually retain their speech sound production patterns for a time, but frequently, their articulatory skills deteriorate. Even those who are assisted with amplification may find it difficult to maintain their previous level of articulatory performance, particularly for sounds with high-frequency components (e.g., sibilant sounds).

The speech of individuals with significant hearing loss is often very difficult to understand. Gold (1980) stated that, for most listeners, it may be possible to understand only 20% of what speakers with congenitally severe or profound hearing loss are attempting to say. The difficulty with understanding the speech of these individuals appears to be problems at both the segmental and suprasegmental levels. At the segmental level, errors on both consonants and vowels are observed (Levitt & Stromberg, 1983; Paterson, 1994). At the suprasegmental level, persons who are deaf or hard of hearing generally speak at a slower rate than normal-hearing speakers; this is manifest as a longer duration during the production of consonants and vowels. They also use more frequent pauses and slower articulatory transitions. Stress patterns may also differ from those of normal-hearing speakers because many persons who are deaf or hearing impaired do not distinguish duration or pitch associated with stressed and unstressed syllables. Persons who are deaf or hearing impaired sometimes use too high or too low a pitch and nonstandard inflectional patterns. Harsh or breathy voice quality and hypo- or hypernasal speech are also commonly reported (Dunn & Newton, 1986).

As noted previously, even in cases of severe and profound hearing impairment, the specific types of perception problems and speech production errors are difficult to predict. There is a great deal of individual variability. It is more difficult to predict outcomes for individuals with mild to moderate hearing losses than for those with more severe losses. What is known is that, in general, the earlier intervention is provided the better the outcomes.

Calvert (1982) reported that errors of articulation common to children who are deaf are not confined to productions of individual phonemes; errors also occur because of the phonetic context in which the phones are embedded. Calvert documented specific examples of omission, substitution, distortion, and addition errors relative to particular target phonemes, classes of phonemes, and phonetic contexts. These are highlighted in Table 5.1.

The preceding discussion is most relevant for describing only those individuals with hearing loss who use hearing aids. Both the introduction of universal newborn hearing screening and the development of multi-channel cochlear implants have significantly altered the speech production outlook for the hearing-impaired population. The net result has been far fewer delays in identifying children with congenital hearing loss (i.e., most are now identified at birth) and much earlier intervention. For those with severe/profound hearing losses, these developments have together meant that their speech, language, and academic outcomes (including reading) are generally much better than for those who rely on hearing aids. A review by Flipsen (2008) revealed that the conversational speech produced by children with cochlear implants can be highly intelligible (up to 90% in some cases). However, other studies have shown types of errors and error patterns (albeit occurring less frequently) similar to those found in individuals who are hearing impaired and use hearing aids (Chin & Pisoni, 2000; Flipsen & Parker, 2008; Grogan et al., 1995). It should be noted that all of this assumes that there are no other impairments present and that

Table 5.1. Common speech errors seen in deaf speech

1. Errors of omission	a. Omission of final consonants
	b. Omission of /s/ in all contexts
	c. Omission of initial consonants
2. Errors of substitution	a. Voiced for voiceless consonants
	b. Nasal for oral consonants
	c. Low feedback substitutions (substitution of sounds with easily perceived tactile and kinesthetic feedback for those with less (e.g., /w/ for /r/ substitution)
	d. Substitution of one vowel for another
3. Errors of distortion	a. Degree of force (stop and fricative consonants are frequently made with either too much or too little force)
	b. Hypernasality associated with vowel productions
	c. Imprecision and indefiniteness in vowel articulation
	d. Duration of vowels (speakers who are deaf tend to produce vowels with undifferentiated duration, usually in the direction of excess duration)
	e. Temporal values in diphthongs (speakers who are deaf may not produce the first or the second vowel in a diphthong for the appropriate duration of time)
4. Errors of addition	a. Insertion of a superfluous vowel between consonants (e.g., /sʌnoʊ/ for /snoʊ/)
	b. Unnecessary release of final stop consonants (e.g., [stopʰ])
	c. Diphthongization of vowels (e.g., *mit* → [mɪʌt])
	d. Superfluous breath before vowels

Source: Calvert (1982).

instruction/therapy is provided along with the implant. See Table 5.2 for a list of error patterns that have been observed in both children with hearing aids and those who use cochlear implants.

In addition to errors on specific speech sounds or sound combinations, the suprasegmental aspects of speech may continue to be of concern for even the most successful cochlear implant recipients. Abnormal resonance and difficulty with the use of syllable and word-level stress may continue to be a problem for some of these children (Anderson, 2011; Lenden & Flipsen, 2007).

It should be noted, of course, that, as with children fitted with hearing aids, outcomes for children fitted with cochlear implants (although generally much closer to typical) can be quite variable (Geers, 2006). Age at implantation continues to be a crucial variable, with children receiving their implants at younger ages clearly evidencing better outcomes. Current criteria for implantation set by the U.S. Food and Drug Administration permit implantation in children as young as age 12 months, but there is ongoing debate about implantation at even younger ages. In some European countries, children are receiving implants as young as 4 months of age. Amplification by itself is not generally considered sufficient for fully successful outcomes, and the early provision of speech and language services remains crucial (Geers, 2002).

Regardless of the age limits for implants, not all children with hearing impairments are identified as early as they should be. Newborn infant hearing screening is not infallible and some children are missed, whereas a small percentage of others may not have had access to a screening program.

Likewise, implantation may be delayed for many reasons, including health issues, parental concerns about surgical risks, or insurance issues. On a positive note, many aspects of eligibility for implantation are also changing. For example, more children with some degree of residual hearing in at least one ear are receiving implants. Preliminary data suggest that outcomes in such cases are better than for children with no residual hearing. Such children may especially benefit if a hearing aid is provided for their nonimplanted ear. This arrangement (cochlear implant in one ear and hearing aid in the other) is referred to as *bimodal hearing*. In addition,

Table 5.2. Speech sound error patterns observed in both children who use hearing aids and children who use cochlear implants

Developmental patterns[a]	Nondevelopmental patterns[b]
Assimilation errors	Initial consonant deletion
Consonant cluster reduction	Glottal stop substitution
Final consonant deletion	Backing
Liquid simplification	Vowel substitution
Palatal fronting	Diphthong simplification
Stopping	
Unstressed (weak) syllable deletion	
Velar fronting	

[a] Error patterns seen in younger typically developing (normal hearing) children.
[b] Error patterns not usually seen in younger typically developing (normal hearing) children.
Source: Parker (2005).

many child implant candidates now receive cochlear implants in both ears (*bilateral implantation*). Some recent studies have shown that bimodal hearing (Ching et al., 2006; Madell et al., 2004) and bilateral implantation (Biever & Kelsall, 2007; Galvin et al., 2007) both result in significant improvements in speech perception outcomes over a single implant alone. Data still appear to be lacking, however, on long-range speech production outcomes for these groups. Finally, cochlear implants are also being provided to children with other impairments, with findings indicating that such children are also able to benefit significantly (Ahn & Lee, 2013; Corrales & Oghalai, 2013; Hans et al., 2010).

Neuromotor Disorders

A fourth group of children with organically based SSDs are those with identifiable impairments of speech movement control (i.e., those with neuromotor impairments). Speech production at the motor level requires muscle strength, speed of movement, appropriate range of excursion, accuracy of movement, coordination of multiple movements, motor steadiness, and muscle tone (Darley et al., 1975; Duffy, 2020). Damage that impairs one or more of these neuromuscular functions may affect motor speech production, including phonation, respiration, or velopharyngeal function. Neuromotor speech disorders occur more typically in adults than children because they are often associated with strokes or other forms of brain injury. When these disorders are present at birth or shortly thereafter, they are often described as being one of various forms of cerebral palsy.

Neurologists and SLPs have long sought to understand the possible relationship between the clinical (behavioral) responses associated with neurologically impaired individuals and the site and extent of the neurological lesions (brain damage). The reason for such inquiry is to identify potential commonalities across patients between the nature and site of lesion and the concomitant cognitive, speech, and/or language impairment.

Although, as noted earlier, entire books are devoted to motor speech disorders (e.g., Duffy, 2020), the following text offers a brief introduction to this topic.

Dysarthrias

The *dysarthrias* are neurologic motor speech impairments characterized by slow, weak, imprecise, and/or uncoordinated movements of the speech musculature. Yorkston and colleagues (2010) stated that "dysarthrias form a group of disorders marked by impaired execution of the movements of speech production" (p. 4). Because dysarthrias are caused by different types of lesions, trauma, or disease that cause central or peripheral nervous system damage, they cannot be described by a single set of specific characteristics.

Dysarthrias are generally characterized by a paralysis, weakness, or incoordination of the speech musculature, which may result from localized injuries to the nervous system, various inflammatory processes, toxic metabolic disorders, vascular lesions or trauma of the brain, and lesion, disease, or trauma to the nervous system. The most significant characteristic of dysarthric speech is reduced intelligibility. Dysarthric speech may reflect specific disturbances in respiration, phonation, articulation, resonance, and prosody, or combinations thereof. Phonemes misarticulated in spontaneous speech are also likely to be misarticulated in other situations, such as in reading and imitation tasks.

Apraxia of Speech

Apraxia is a motor speech disorder also caused by brain damage, but it is differentiated from the dysarthrias as a separate clinical entity. *Apraxia of speech (AOS)* is characterized by an impairment of motor speech programming with little or no weakness, paralysis, or incoordination of the speech musculature. Whereas dysarthrias frequently affect all motor speech processes—respiration, phonation, articulation, resonance, and prosody—apraxia primarily affects articulatory abilities with secondary prosodic alterations. Duffy (2005) described some of the clinical characteristics of apraxia:

> Deviant speech characteristics associated with AOS [apraxia of speech] include a number of abnormalities of articulation, rate, prosody, and fluency. The characteristics that best distinguish it from other motor speech disorders (the dysarthrias) are distorted sound substitutions and additions, decreased phonemic accuracy with increased rate, attempts to correct articulatory errors that cross phonemic boundaries, groping for articulatory postures, greater difficulty on volitional than automatic speech tasks, and greater difficulty on SMR [sequential motion rate] and multisyllabic word tasks than AMR [alternate motion rate] and single syllable tasks. . . . Articulatory distortions, reduced rate, and various prosodic abnormalities help distinguish AOS from aphasic phonologic errors. (p. 330)

Some clients who demonstrate AOS (or verbal apraxia) also demonstrate similar difficulty in volitional oral nonspeech tasks, a behavior described as oral apraxia (Duffy, 2005). For example, an individual may protrude their tongue during eating but may be unable to perform this act voluntarily. Although oral apraxia often coexists with verbal apraxia, this is not always the case.

Duffy (2005) notes the following differences between AOS and dysarthria: 1) muscle strength, tone, range, and steadiness of movement are clearly affected in dysarthria but do not account for the deficits seen in AOS; 2) respiration, phonation, articulation, resonance, and prosody may all be affected in dysarthria, whereas AOS is limited to problems with articulation and prosody; 3) language difficulties (called *aphasia* in adults) are rarely seen in dysarthria but often co-occur with AOS; 4) speech errors are typically quite consistent in dysarthria, whereas inconsistency is more typical of AOS; 5) distortions and substitution of simpler sounds are most common in dysarthria, but AOS may also include omissions, substitutions of more complex sounds, repetitions, or prolongations; and 6) trial and error groping and self-corrections are common in AOS but uncommon in dysarthria. These two disorders (AOS and dysarthria) may also co-occur (Lapointe & Wertz, 1974).

CHILDHOOD APRAXIA OF SPEECH

One of the least understood SSD categories is *childhood apraxia of speech (CAS)*. This condition has also been known by several other names, including developmental AOS and developmental verbal dyspraxia. Two reasons appear to have spawned the difficulty with this diagnosis. First, there have been disagreements about the specific distinguishing characteristics of this condition, or, in the past, even whether such characteristics exist. Several attempts have been made to summarize this work over the years (e.g., Davis et al., 1998; Velleman & Strand, 1994). These reviews have highlighted the fact that many of the characteristics suggested as indicating CAS are not necessarily unique to it. Investigators who have tried to identify such unique characteristics do not always agree with one another. For example, Yoss and Darley (1974) reported that 16 children with delayed speech who also met their definition of CAS performed significantly poorer on non-speech praxis abilities compared to 14 children with delayed speech who did not meet their definition of CAS. On the other hand, Aram and Horwitz (1983) reported no such difference.

Some have argued that such conflicts may simply reflect coexisting oral apraxia in some children with CAS. As noted previously, this is also an issue in adult AOS. The failure to identify the unique features of CAS led some in the past to suggest that this disorder may not exist as a unique diagnostic entity. Those taking this position argued that it simply represented the most severe form of speech delay of unknown origin (to be discussed later). However, others argue that CAS is a unique diagnostic category and can be manifest along the entire continuum from mild to severe.

The second reason for the previous controversy surrounding CAS stems from concerns about applying the label apraxia because, unlike the adult form of apraxia, it is usually not possible to document specific neurological damage that might have led to the problem. This latter question is another reason that CAS is often included with SSDs of unknown origin. However, in some cases, a potential causal agent can be identified. Thus, because CAS may not clearly fit into either the organic or idiopathic (unknown origin) group, we discuss it separately here.

Defining the Disorder

Historically, overriding the discussion of CAS has been the lack of a clear definition of what constitutes this condition. This lack of consensus probably accounts for the conflicting findings noted previously because, frequently, different investigators have used different participant selection criteria.

In 2002, in an effort to resolve the issue, the American Speech-Language-Hearing Association (ASHA) established an ad hoc committee on CAS. The committee reviewed the extensive and somewhat confusing literature in this area and presented its findings in 2007. After considerable feedback, ASHA's legislative council adopted a position statement and the committee's technical report (ASHA, 2007a, 2007b). Refer to the ASHA website, where both documents can be obtained for more detailed study.

The ASHA position statement makes clear that CAS exists as a unique diagnostic category (i.e., it is not just a severe form of delayed speech). This designation is now generally accepted within the profession as a defined subpopulation of those with SSDs of unknown etiology. The position statement specifically defines CAS as follows:

> Childhood apraxia of speech (CAS) is a neurological childhood (pediatric) speech sound disorder in which the precision and consistency of movements underlying speech are impaired in the absence of neuromuscular deficits (e.g., abnormal reflexes, abnormal tone). CAS may occur as a result of known neurological impairment, in association with complex neurobehavioral disorders of known or unknown origin, or as an idiopathic neurogenic SSD. The core impairment in planning and/or programming spatiotemporal parameters of movement sequences results in errors in speech sound production and prosody. (2007a, pp. 1–2)

Note that the definition limits CAS to problems with speech. The possible coexisting but separate difficulties that children with CAS may demonstrate with nonspeech oral movements are thought to indicate the comorbidity of either an oral apraxia or an underlying neuromuscular problem (i.e., dysarthria).

Causes

The ASHA definition also emphasizes that although CAS may be a neurological problem, it may arise in one of at least three general ways. First, it may be a reflection of a known neurological condition, such as cerebral palsy. Second, it may also be comorbid with known neurobehavioral disorders, such as fragile X syndrome, galactosemia, or Rett syndrome. Note that at one point, autism was included in the list of neurobehavioral disorders, but some recent analyses suggest that the speech errors seen in that population are qualitatively and quantitatively different from those seen in CAS (Shriberg et al., 2011). Finally, the third and most common origin of CAS is that the cause is unknown.

The Core Deficit

As the definition indicates, the primary deficit in CAS appears to be one of planning and/or programming the movements necessary for speech. Such planning and programming, or what Shriberg and colleagues (2012) have called transcoding, is part of how many clinicians and researchers would describe the process of generating speech, which may be outlined as follows:

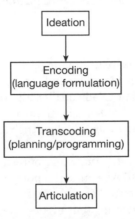

Using this outline, the speaker starts by deciding what idea or ideas they want to express (*ideation*). This is conceptual, and the linguistic details are undefined. Then the speaker selects the sentence structure and specific words to use (*encoding* or *language formulation*). Note that encoding here is the inverse of the process of phonological encoding discussed in Chapter 4, whereby language input is converted to a long-term representation in the brain. For speech production, this includes determining the particular phonemes and allophones to express the words. The next step of *transcoding* (planning/programming) involves translating the linguistic message into the details of which particular muscles are to be moved, including their sequence and timing, in order to express the message. This is what is meant in the preceding CAS definition by "the spatiotemporal parameters of movement sequences." For many in the field, transcoding is referred to as *motor planning*. Once the plan is created, it is sent via the nerves to the speech musculature, and the physical movements (i.e., *articulation*) are carried out. Relative to ASHA's definition, the core deficit in CAS is in the motor planning or transcoding step. The speaker has difficulty either creating the motor plan or accessing an already existing plan. Many current psycholinguistic models (e.g., Stackhouse & Wells' [1997] model, to be discussed later) assume that mature language users store motor plans along with word meanings and phonological details in the underlying representation for words in their brains. This allows for rapid generation of speech as the need arises (sometimes called automatized speech).

Although the preceding outline is helpful, as we know from the adult (acquired) form of apraxia, the problem of CAS may not always be limited to motor planning. It has long been acknowledged that adult apraxia may be accompanied by difficulty with language formulation (called aphasia in adults) and/or dysarthria. This may also be true in CAS. And if that weren't complicated enough, during both language formulation and motor planning, the speaker must have sufficient working memory to hold on to the linguistic message while generating the motor plan (recall our discussion in Chapter 4 about phonological memory).

Shriberg and colleagues (2012) tried to determine whether children with CAS also had problems with either their representations or memory. They used a nonword syllable repetition task (SRT) to compare 40 children with CAS against 119 typically developing children, and 210 children with non-CAS speech delay (70 of whom also had coexisting language impairments). They concluded that, in addition to problems with transcoding (motor planning), the children with CAS also had deficits in their underlying representations and problems with memory.

Diagnostic Markers

Although there seems to be consensus among professionals in the field on the underlying problem, there is not yet a specific list of diagnostic features that are unique to CAS. As early as 1981, Guyette and Diedrich identified a circularity problem. The challenge is that we want to know what features make this group distinct, but we need to know what those features are in order to select the right group of children to look for those features.

In an attempt to identify the unique characteristics of this population, the ad-hoc committee drafting the ASHA technical report on CAS (2007b) used the existing literature to identify three potential speech production features that may be unique to CAS. The first of these is inconsistent errors on vowels and consonants; in this case, the term *inconsistent* refers to multiple attempts at the same word that result in different productions. Thus, a child with CAS who attempts the word *cup* several times might produce /t ʌ p/, /t ʌ d/, and /ʌ p/. Some investigators (e.g., Murray, McCabe, Heard, et al., 2015) have questioned the diagnostic utility of this feature of inconsistency. Findings from a Brazilian study by de Castro and Wertzner (2011) would initially support this. Results indicated that inconsistency differentiated the speech of 51 children with idiopathic SSDs (what they called phonological disorder, not CAS) from that of 50 typically speaking children. Iuzzini-Seigel and associates (2017) noted that context may be crucial. They reported that inconsistency differentiated children with CAS from those with other forms of speech delay and from those with language impairment, but only when using monosyllabic words. Inconsistency on production of multisyllabic words or short phrases did not completely differentiate the groups. Interestingly, an examination of the stimuli used in the de Castro and Wertzner study revealed that 14 of the 25 words they used had three or more syllables (only three were monosyllabic). Multisyllabic words may simply be more difficult for all children with SSDs.

A second feature of CAS is difficulty with prosody, particularly as it relates to the use of phrasal or lexical stress. Shriberg and colleagues (1997b), for example, noted a tendency toward excessive and equal stress in two-syllable words. For example, production of the word *music* by a child with CAS may be perceived as MUSIC instead of the normal MUsic (equal stress on both syllables rather than just the first). One study suggested that the difference between the syllables may be present, but it may not always be perceptible to listeners (Munson et al., 2003).

The third emerging feature of CAS cited in the position statement (which may be difficult to see in most clinical situations) is lengthened and disrupted transitions between syllables and sounds. A study by Maassen and colleagues (2001), for example, compared children with CAS to typically speaking children. The children with CAS tended to pause longer before consonant clusters and pause more often between elements of a cluster.

The combination of these three characteristics (inconsistency, prosodic issues, problems with transitions) was supported by a factor analysis of the speech of 57 children independently diagnosed with CAS conducted by Chenausky and colleagues (2020). This constellation of characteristics reinforces the idea that CAS may be more than a purely motor speech disorder (also supported by the previously discussed findings from Shriberg et al., 2012). Marquardt and associates (2004) noted that the inconsistency observed in CAS may just as easily be a product of an imprecise underlying phonological representation rather than a pure speech motor programming problem. Problems with the prosody of speech feature (i.e., excessive and equal stress) may indicate some problem in the underlying representation about the hierarchical organization of speech. Reports that children with CAS exhibit difficulty with reading and spelling (Gillon & Moriarty, 2007; McNeill et al., 2009) also suggest some difficulty with underlying representations for speech. Together, this suggests that CAS is the result of a combination of both representational and motor speech difficulties (McNeill, 2007).

Some recent studies (e.g., Ballard et al., 2010; Maas et al., 2012; Preston, Leece, et al., 2016; Preston, Maas et al., 2016; Thomas et al., 2018) have used these three features to define the presence of CAS. Other investigators have included some or all of these features in combination with other feature lists compiled by experienced clinicians (e.g., Shriberg et al., 2012). Murray, McCabe, Heard, and colleagues (2015) used the three features in the ASIIA technical report along with those from Shriberg and colleagues (2012) in their study of 47 Australian children aged 4–12 years who were suspected of having CAS. Findings indicated that 32 children presented with all three features from the ASHA technical report and also had at least five of the features specified in Shriberg and colleagues. Two complete examples of recently used feature lists are shown in Table 5.3.

Additional possible features have received some recent attention. The ability of children with CAS to make use of available feedback was examined by Iuzzini-Seigel and associates (2015) with participants defined by the criteria from Shriberg and colleagues (2012). These investigators studied 30 children aged 6–17 years and measured variability in some acoustic parameters of speech during exposure to masking noise (i.e., that which would limit their ability to hear their own speech). The nine children with CAS were much more variable in their output than the 10 children with non-CAS speech delay or the 11 typically speaking children. The authors interpreted these results to suggest that the children with CAS were relying more on their own auditory feedback than on feedback from their articulators. This might, at least in part, account for findings that older children with CAS appear to benefit from supplemental visual feedback such as that provided by ultrasound (Preston, Brick, et al., 2013).

Table 5.3. Examples of possible diagnostic feature lists for childhood apraxia of speech

Grigos et al. (2015)	Shriberg et al. (2017b)[d]
Inconsistent errors on repeated productions[a, b]	Vowel distortions
Difficulty with transitions[a, b]	Voicing errors
Prosodic errors[a, b]	Distorted substitutions
Metathesis (correct phonemes present but out of order)[c]	Difficulty achieving initial articulatory configurations or transitionary movement gestures
Vowel errors[c]	Groping
Timing errors (expressed as problems with voicing)[c]	Intrusive schwa
Phoneme distortions[c]	Increased difficulty with multisyllabic words
Articulatory groping[c]	Syllable segregation
Impaired volitional oral movements[c]	Slow speech rate or slow DDK rates
Reduced phonetic inventory[c]	Equal stress or lexical stress errors
Poorer expressive language compared to receptive language[c]	

[a] Originally proposed in ASHA (2007b) technical report.

[b] Required for childhood apraxia of speech diagnosis.

[c] Additional features; at least 4/8 needed for childhood apraxia of speech diagnosis.

[d] At least 4/10 features needed for childhood apraxia of speech diagnosis.

As part of his work to refine his Speech Disorders Classification System (to be discussed in detail later), Shriberg, Strand, and colleagues (2017a, b) identified a single feature that appears to be unique to CAS. In this case, they proposed a *pause marker,* which is the presence of inappropriate between-word pauses in at least 5% of opportunities in a continuous speech sample. Such pauses might include those that occur at linguistically inappropriate positions or that are preceded or followed by a significant change in amplitude (loudness), frequency (pitch), or rate (six other types of these pauses were identified). Identification of such pauses would require the use of acoustic analysis procedures. In their study of this marker, Shriberg and colleagues included 60 children with suspected CAS (aged 4–25 years) and compared them to 205 children with non-CAS delayed speech (aged 3–9 years). Comparing the pause marker criterion and the criteria in the right-hand column of Table 5.3, the two procedures agreed on a CAS diagnosis in the suspected CAS group 87% of the time; they also excluded a CAS diagnosis for the non-CAS group 98% of the time. This suggests that this single feature holds significant diagnostic promise.

In spite of the lack of agreement about the specific features of CAS, research into this population continues. Using their list of features shown in Table 5.3 to identify 11 children aged 3–7 years with CAS, Grigos and colleagues (2015) used a motion capture system to examine movements of the jaw and lips during a naming task. They reported a greater amount of movement variability in the children with CAS compared to 11 children with non-CAS speech delay and 11 typically speaking children.

Prevalence

Given the widespread use of the CAS label, it should be noted that an accurate prevalence estimate for this subcategory of SSD has not been established. Unfortunately, there have been no systematic population studies (ASHA, 2007b). A recent estimate, based on data from 415 children representing six U.S. cities, who were referred for idiopathic speech delay, revealed 2.4% diagnosed as having CAS. This was interpreted to suggest an overall population prevalence of approximately one case per 1,000 children (Shriberg, Kwiatkowski, et al., 2019). As such, valid diagnoses of CAS are likely to be somewhat rare in most clinicians' caseloads.

Given that CAS is sometimes associated with complex neurodevelopmental disorders, prevalence may also vary depending on the specific disorder. Shriberg, Strand, and colleagues (2019) reported findings from a sample of 346 children with CAS values ranging from 0% in autism, to 3.6% in fragile X syndrome, to 6.5% in galactosemia, and 11.1% in DS. This will be discussed further under the section entitled Comorbidity.

Chapter 12 presents suggestions for assessment and treatment of CAS.

IDIOPATHIC SPEECH SOUND DISORDERS

The second, and by far, the largest group of children with SSDs is one that has puzzled investigators for many years—it includes those for whom there is no obvious cause. This has long raised the question: If we do not know how the problem arose in the first place, how do we help these children? Lacking clear answers, SLPs have for many years tended to do two things. First, we have often assumed that this is a single group, and second, we have tended to treat them all the same way. Until about the 1970s, most SLPs referred to these children as having *functional articulation disorders* (a term still used by some today). The word *functional* implies that these children have some sort of learning difficulty. And in this context, the word *articulation* implies that the problem is with learning to physically produce individual speech sounds. For many years, these children all received what is now called *traditional articulation therapy* (sometimes also called *phonetic therapy*), which is a motor skill and perception-oriented approach to therapy. This approach will be described in Chapter 10.

In the 1970s, the field of speech-language pathology began to be influenced by developments in the field of linguistics, particularly those brought forth by the publication of *The Sound Pattern of English* (Chomsky & Hallé, 1968), *Phonological Disability in Children* (Ingram, 1976), and *A Dissertation on Natural Phonology* (Stampe, 1979). These publications, combined with a growing interest in disorders of language (independent of difficulties with speech), forced SLPs to consider that in addition to learning how to physically produce speech sounds, children also have to learn how the sounds of their language are organized and relate to each other (i.e., they have to learn the phonology of the language).

These publications and the subsequent research they spawned also made SLPs realize that there were patterns among what had always seemed like unrelated collections of individual sound errors. For example, if a child said [wɪt] for *with,* [pæn] for *fan,* and [tu] for *Sue,* most clinicians at the time would likely have inferred that such a child had not learned to physically produce the /θ/, /f/, and /s/ sounds. Therapy would then focus on teaching the child to perceive and produce each of those sounds one by one. However, the insights gained from linguistics made SLPs consider that these three errors might be related in some way. All of the intended sounds represent fricative targets being replaced by stop consonants. In this case, the child may be having troubling learning the continuant feature, which all fricatives share.

Stampe took a different perspective and suggested that the child might have an immature speech production or perception system and thus was temporarily unable to either perceive or produce fricatives, or had a rule in their head that stops are used for fricatives. To get around this temporary limitation, Stampe suggested that the child was simplifying all fricatives to stops (a pattern known as *stopping*). As the child's perception or production systems matured, they would no longer find it necessary to simplify and would suppress the pattern (i.e., the child would, in this case, stop stopping). Ingram's book was one of the first to attempt to translate these developments in linguistic theory for the practicing clinician by speaking of explicitly principled therapy. The net result was that the field suddenly began referring to these children with SSDs as having developmental phonological disorders or simply phonological disorders. The emphasis had changed from articulation (motor-based problems) to phonology (cognitive-linguistic problems).

This change in labels was accompanied by changes in our approach to assessment and treatment. Many clinicians began to switch from teaching about the physical aspects of production to teaching children how using contrasting sounds results in changes in meaning. This focus on the phonology led to looking for patterns in the errors of children with SSDs. Instruction (therapy) focused on patterns that might generalize from instruction on one sound to a number of speech sound errors related to the same sound error pattern. This approach (described in Chapter 11) is called variously contrast therapy, phonological therapy, or phonemic therapy.

Whatever the terminology, many SLPs began to report that children who were given contrast therapy were progressing through therapy more quickly than before with a sound-by-sound approach. Researchers began to validate this observation empirically. Klein (1996), for example, retrospectively compared 19 children who had received traditional articulation therapy with 17 children who had received phonological therapy. The two groups had been treated at different times by different clinicians, but within each group, the therapy had been relatively controlled within a single university clinic. Klein reported that the children in the phonological therapy group spent significantly fewer months in therapy (13.5 vs. 22.3 months), were significantly less severely involved at their last treatment session, and were significantly more likely to have been dismissed from therapy with normal speech (17/17 vs. 2/19).

Although the overall results of this change in approach have been quite encouraging, it unfortunately has not proven to be universally successful. Not all of these children seem to benefit equally. Some actually respond better to traditional articulation therapy, and some do not respond well to either approach. It is still not completely clear how to determine which child will respond best to which form of intervention.

It may be helpful at this point to recall our discussions in Chapter 4. Much of the research on factors associated with SSDs was aimed at identifying a single factor or perhaps a few factors observed in selected children that might differentiate these children from those who were developing speech normally or from those with organically based problems. As was stated earlier, no single factor or set of factors has emerged. As quickly as one study reports some unique difference, another study asks the same question and reveals contradictory results. For example, Dworkin (1978) reported that children with functional articulation disorders had lower tongue strength and slower diadochokinetic rates than typically speaking children. However, a follow-up study by Dworkin and Culatta (1985) revealed no such differences. This has led many to conclude that we may be looking at a population with several distinct subgroups. Several teams of investigators have tried to sort out what those subgroups might be.

One suggestion has been to subdivide the group based on severity. Perhaps children with milder problems will respond better to particular treatments, and those with more severe problems will respond better to other treatments. There are at least three problems with such an approach. First, although it is certainly true that children with SSDs can be found anywhere along the continuum of severity (e.g., mild, moderate, severe), there are no gold standards for determining severity of involvement in this population (Flipsen et al., 2005). Drawing the lines between the groups is therefore problematic. Second, if subgroups actually exist based on some other dimension(s), creating subgroups based on severity would result in only somewhat smaller but still heterogeneous groups. Third, and perhaps most important, "there seems to be no evidence that severity measures discriminate between subgroups of children with speech disorder in terms of the type of intervention indicated, or outcome" (Dodd, 2005, p. 5). This is also supported by our earlier discussion of the difficulty in separating CAS from other severe forms of SSD.

At least three other perspectives (etiological, psycholinguistic, symptomological) have begun to show potential for defining subgroups of children with SSDs of unknown origin (Waring & Knight, 2013). The following sections describe these perspectives. It is important to note that despite considerable effort, there is still no strong consensus about the best way to subdivide this population.

Classification by Possible Etiology

For each of the organically based subgroups the cause was obvious. Shriberg (1982) argued that in the case of SSDs of unknown origin, the cause may simply be much more difficult to identify. Despite the added difficulty, however, isolating the specific causes offers the possibility of both better understanding the nature of the problem and finding a better match between the child's problem and the most appropriate treatment approach.

The causes of SSDs of unknown origin are frequently not obvious and are complicated because, in many cases, what originally caused the problem (a distal cause) may have led to other problems (a proximal cause) that may now be maintaining the disorder (the distal cause may or may not still be operating). To illustrate, consider the child born with a significant hearing loss. The hearing loss results in an inability to hear all of the fine details of speech. This distal cause may lead to poorly developed or distorted underlying representation of speech sounds in the brain. This may contribute to inaccurate production, because it would be difficult to accurately produce something if you do not have an accurate sense or perception of what the target is supposed to sound like. The hearing loss led to the problem originally and thus is the *distal cause* of the problem, but the poorly developed or distorted underlying representations (perception) may be the maintaining or *proximal cause* of the problem.

Shriberg and his team began the search for etiological subgroups by looking for *causal correlates,* or factors that appeared very often in the case histories of these children (Shriberg & Kwiatkowski, 1994). This yielded several candidates for possible subgroups. However, one major challenge is that detailed case history information is not always available. Parents, who are often the primary source of case history information, may not have very reliable memories about their children's histories (Majnemer & Rosenblatt, 1994). Complicating matters even further, many children present with more than one of the causal correlates. This led Shriberg and his team to also search for *diagnostic markers,* or speech characteristics unique to each of the possible subgroups. Such markers may also offer insight into the perceptual, cognitive, or speech-processing mechanisms involved. These processing mechanisms then serve as confirmatory evidence for the subgroups by suggesting theoretical pathways from a distal cause to a particular subgroup. The diagnostic markers may also be useful clinically. They may, for example, serve as potential treatment targets or at least help identify such targets. An understanding of both the diagnostic markers and the processing mechanisms leading to those markers might also help identify the best approach to treating those particular targets (Flipsen, 2002b).

Shriberg, Kwiatkowski, and associates (2019) presented the finalized version of what is called the *Speech Disorders Classification System (SDCS)*, which includes three categories containing a total of nine subgroups. These are summarized in Table 5.4. A schematic of the SDCS can be found at the Phonology Project website (https://phonology .waisman.wisc.edu/). The SDCS assumes that all children have some combination of genetic and environmental factors that operate to increase the risk of an SSD and/or provide some protection from such disorders. For children with SSDs, this combination of genetic and environmental factors leads to deficits or limitations in processing of speech. These deficits could be manifest in one of three broad ways: 1) at the level of representation (or storage) of auditory or somatosensory information about sounds and words, 2) as difficulty with planning and programming (transcoding) of the motor

Table 5.4. Shriberg's nine subtypes of idiopathic speech sound disorders

Category	Subgroup	Abbreviation	Prevalence[a] (%)	Sex	Diagnostic markers
Speech delay	Genetic	SD–GEN	56[b]	M > F	?[c]
	Otitis media with effusion	SD–OME[d]	?[b]	M = F	?[c]
	Developmental psychosocial involvement	SD–DPI[d]	?[b]	M > F	?[c]
Speech errors	Speech errors–sibilants	SE–/s/	1.5-2	M < F	> first spectral moment for /s/
	Speech errors–rhotics	SE–/r/	1.5-2	M > F	< F3–F2 for /r/
Motor speech disorder	Speech motor delay	SMD	12	M > F	Precision-stability index
	Childhood dysarthria	CD	3.4	M > F	Dysarthria index/ dysarthria subtype indices
	Childhood apraxia of speech	CAS	2.4	M >> F	Pause marker
	Childhood dysarthria + CAS	CD and CAS	0[e]	?	Precision-stability index and pause marker

[a] Within the population of children with ideopathic SSDs.

[b] Combined prevalence of SD–GEN, SD–OME, and SD–DPI may include up to 82.7% (see Shriberg, Kwiatkowski, et al., 2019)

[c] Diagnostic marker(s) not yet sufficiently validated (see text).

[d] Category not yet fully validated (currently considered a risk factor only).

[e] Not yet identified within idiopathic SSDs but estimated at 4.9% within complex neurodevelopmental disorders (see Shriberg, Strand, et al., 2019).

movements for speech, or 3) as an inability to accurately and precisely carry out those particular motor movements (execution). Prevalence estimates shown in Table 5.4 were largely derived from findings from 415 children specifically recruited for idiopathic SSD research from six different U.S. cities.

The first three of the nine subgroups in the SDCS are classed as forms of *speech delay.* In such cases, children present speech productions that are significantly behind developmental expectations during the preschool years. The speech of these children is quite likely to normalize with treatment. The next two subgroups represent variations of *speech errors,* in which no early concern is raised about speech, but the child simply fails to fully master one or two speech sounds during the developmental period (i.e., by age 9 years). As such, children in these two groups typically don't qualify for therapy until they are near the end of the developmental period (about age 9), if at all. The last four subgroups represent forms of childhood *motor speech disorder,* which may be less likely to normalize even with treatment, but these children typically qualify for and receive services.

Looking at the specific subgroups, the largest, speech delay–genetic (SD–GEN) includes up to approximately 56% of children who have one or more family members who have or have had speech or language problems. As shown in Table 5.4, this subgroup includes more males than females. Support for this category has already been discussed, but definitive diagnostic markers have yet to be validated. One proposal has been that these children produce a particularly high proportion of omission errors, occurring especially on later developing consonants (Shriberg et al., 2005). This suggests that the children may be having difficulty identifying the phonemic details of the language (a cognitive-linguistic problem). Lewis and colleagues (2007) reported findings that support a unique cognitive-linguistic proximal cause for this subgroup. In that study, parents of children with SSDs who themselves had a history of therapy for SSDs performed significantly less well compared to parents without such histories on standardized measures of spoken language and spelling. Research conducted by Felsenfeld and colleagues (1995) offers similar evidence. Using long-term follow-up data from the offspring of individuals who had originally been tested between 1960 and 1972 (reported in Templin & Glaman, 1976), the children of those individuals earlier identified as disordered performed significantly more poorly on tests of articulation than did the children of those who had earlier been classified as normal.

The next two subgroups (SD–OME, SD–DPI) are currently not fully confirmed. As such, the underlying mechanisms for these groups should only be considered as risk factors for speech delay at this time. Precise prevalence estimates for SD–OME and SD–DPI are also unconfirmed, though available data suggest that the combination of SD–GEN, SD–OME, and SD–DPI subgroups would include up to 82.7% of children with idiopathic SSDs (Shriberg, Kwiatkowski, et al., 2019).

Despite not being fully confirmed, we do know something of these two groups. The second subgroup, speech delay–otitis media with effusion (SD–OME), may include the up to 30% of these children who have histories of early and frequent episodes of OME. The proportion of males and females appears to be roughly equal in this subgroup (Shriberg, Kwiatkowski. et al., 2019). SD–OME definitive diagnostic markers have yet to be fully validated, although at least two have been proposed. Shriberg, Flipsen, and colleagues (2003) identified the *intelligibility-speech gap.* The conversational speech of these children was consistently less understandable than the speech of children without such histories. However, looking only at the portions of the child's speech that could be understood, the accuracy of their consonant productions was better than that seen in some of the other subgroups. In other words, their conversational speech was less well understood than would be expected given the accuracy of their consonant production. Shriberg, Kent, and colleagues (2003) proposed a second diagnostic marker for this subgroup involving a higher frequency of backing errors (a very atypical pattern of using posterior sounds, such as velar or palatal sounds, in place of more anterior sounds, such as alveolars). Like the SD–GEN subgroup, these two markers suggest difficulty extracting relevant phonemic details from the input language. In the case of SD–OME, the mechanism is thought to be their history of intermittent hearing loss (Shriberg, Friel-Patti, et al., 2000).

A third (and also not yet fully confirmed) subgroup is speech delay–psychosocial involvement (SD–DPI). Despite no clear prevalence data, it appears that males outnumber females in this subgroup. As with SD–OME, specific diagnostic markers have also yet to be identified. A proposed mechanism underlying this subgroup, which would be considered at least a risk factor for speech delay, appears to reflect how these children interact with others (hence the label psychosocial). Hauner and associates (2005) suggested that these children present with either 1) approach-related negative affect (i.e., described as aggressive, angry, or manipulative/control seeking) or 2) withdrawal-related negative affect (socially withdrawn, shy/fearful, or extremely taciturn). Thus, these children may have temperaments that make it more difficult for them to obtain the feedback they need to develop and/or normalize their speech skills. These children may also be easily frustrated by their inability to communicate effectively and/or be less likely to persist in their communication attempts.

The next two subgroups in the SDCS (speech errors–sibilants [SE-/s/] and speech errors–rhotics [SE-/r/]) are similar to SD–DPI in that their interactions with individuals around them may lead to their difficulty. In this case, however, they may have a "disposition to respond to the environmental press for mastery of speech sounds in the ambient language" (Shriberg et al., 2005, p. 838). In other words, they may be so motivated to communicate that they attempt to master some aspects of speech before being fully ready to do so. These children may adopt a production pattern that is less than optimal but which they retain into the school years. Available data suggest that these two subgroups combined include 3.4% of children with idiopathic SSDs (Shriberg, Kwiatkowski, et al., 2019). The two separate subgroups reflect the very different nature of the speech sounds that cause difficulty. This also accounts for the very distinct acoustic features of their diagnostic markers. It is, perhaps, noteworthy that problems with sibilants appear to be more common in females, but problems with rhotics appear to be more common in males.

It should be noted that in the SDCS, the two speech errors subgroups just described reflect only one type of production problem that might be observed beyond the normal developmental period (Flipsen, 2015). The other includes those children who present with production errors that are a remnant of an earlier history of any of the other seven subgroups. SLP services may have been previously provided, but not all errors were fully resolved. These remnant (residual) errors may include all possible error types (omissions, substitutions, and/or distortions), though distortions are the most likely. This contrasts with SE-/s/ and SE-/r/ errors, which are typically manifest as distortions only (see Shriberg, 1993). Within the SDCS, errors that are manifest after age 9 years, which often qualify for school-based services, are labeled as either persistent speech errors or persistent speech delay, depending on their origin.

To be clear, residual errors represent errors that are left over from early delayed speech where intervention likely occurred, whereas persistent errors were distortions present at an early age that did not call attention to themselves. Interestingly, although listeners cannot usually distinguish between the distortions from the two origins, significant acoustic differences have been documented with the use of instrumentation (Karlsson et al., 2002; Shriberg et al., 2001). Such distinctions may eventually allow us to both look backwards and speculate on origins where case history information is missing and/or consider different types of treatments for these errors. Additional research is needed in this area of study.

The last four subgroups in the SDCS include those categorized as *motor speech disorder* (Shriberg, Kwiatkowski, et al., 2019). The first of these is termed *speech motor delay (SMD)* (see also Shriberg, Strand, et al., 2019). This mildest form manifests itself as a delay in the overall development of precision and stability of speech motor skills. The diagnostic marker for this group is termed the precision-stability index (PSI); it reflects a combination of 32 different speech, prosody, and voice measures obtained using both perceptual and acoustic analyses from conversational speech samples. Approximately 12% of children with idiopathic SSDs qualify as SMD, and males are more likely to be affected than females. Children who meet the criteria for the three other subgroups of motor speech disorder may also qualify as SMD; in such cases they would be classified into the more severe category (CD, CAS, or CD + CAS) (Shriberg, 2017).

The second of the motor speech disorder subgroups is *childhood dysarthria (CD)*. As previously discussed, dysarthrias are a group of neurologic motor speech impairments characterized by slow, weak, imprecise, and/or uncoordinated movements of the speech musculature. They represent a range of problems with executing the movements necessary for speech. In this case, these are more subtle forms of the disorders without the usually expected obvious neurological damage (hence their inclusion with idiopathic SSDs). To distinguish CD from other motor speech disorders, Shriberg, Kwiatkowski et al. (2019) created a dysarthria index that includes 34 different speech, prosody, and voice measures that serves as a diagnostic marker. They also developed several smaller indices that allow for potential isolation of specific dysarthria subtypes (e.g., flaccid, spastic, hypokinetic, mixed), though these have not yet each been fully validated. Shriberg, Kwiatkowski, and colleagues (2019) reported 3.4% of idiopathic cases qualifying as CD, with males outnumbering females.

The third subgroup of motor speech disorder is the previously discussed CAS. In this case, only the idiopathic origin of CAS is included. This group includes 2.4% of idiopathic SSDs, with males greatly outnumbering females (Shriberg, Kwiatkowski et al., 2019). For purposes of the SDCS, the previously discussed pause marker constitutes the appropriate diagnostic marker for this subgroup (Shriberg et al., 2017a).

The final subgroup of motor speech disorder includes children who would have a combination of both CD and CAS. Such a combination has long been observed in adults with acquired motor speech disorders (Duffy, 2020). It would not, therefore, be unreasonable to expect that they might also do so in children. In the prevalence study by Shriberg, Kwiatkowski, and associates (2019) none of the 415 children met the combined criteria for this category. However, in a parallel study of 346 children with neurodevelopmental disorders, 4.9% qualified for this combined subgroup.

Shriberg's Phonology Project website (https://phonology.waisman.wisc.edu/) contains a wealth of information related to etiological classification. It includes a series of tools for collecting and analyzing conversational speech samples and the latest version of the PEPPER (Programs to Examine Phonetic and Phonologic Evaluation Records; Shriberg, 2019) software suite. With appropriate datasets, PEPPER can classify speakers using the SDCS.

Classification by Psycholinguistic Deficit

A second perspective on subdividing children with idiopathic SSDs into subgroups is to focus on the current underlying difficulty these children might be having with processing speech in the brain. Stackhouse and Wells (1997) argue that an etiological (what they term a medical) approach to identifying the problem for a particular child is limited both because reasons are often not apparent and because existing etiological schemes do not always point directly to specific treatment options. Medical history would not, however, be ignored in this approach (see Pascoe & Stackhouse, 2021); available information may be incorporated into a management plan where appropriate. From a diagnostic perspective, Stackhouse and Wells also argue that a focus on error patterns (what they term a linguistic approach) provides a description only of the output behavior and fails to explain why certain speech behaviors are occurring (i.e., it fails to account for even what we have here called the proximal cause). The better solution, according to Stackhouse and Wells, is to apply a psycholinguistic model. Psycholinguistic models (discussed briefly in Chapter 3) have been used for many years in the field of speech-language pathology (see Baker et al., 2001, for a review). Stackhouse and Wells provide a specific model for examining psycholinguistic processing in children with SSDs (see Figure 5.1).

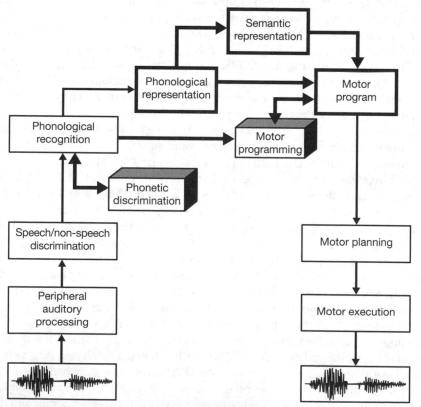

Figure 5.1.   Speech-processing model by Stackhouse and Wells (1997). Note: The broad arrows and shaded boxes represent processes hypothesized to occur off-line. From *Children's Speech and Literacy Difficulties: A Psycholinguistic Framework* (p. 350) by J. Stackhouse and B. Wells, 1997. Copyright John Wiley & Sons Limited. Reproduced with permission.

Note the term *phonological* used in Figure 5.1. In this model, Stackhouse and Wells (1997) separate a *phonological problem*—a term used to describe children's speech output difficulties in a linguistic sense—from a *phonological processing problem*—a psycholinguistic term used to refer to the specific underlying cognitive deficits that may give rise to speech and/or literacy difficulties" (p. 8). Research is ongoing for application of this model. For example, Pascoe and colleagues (2005) presented a detailed case study. Katy (a pseudonym) had difficulties with discriminating both real words and nonwords, which was interpreted as a problem with *phonological recognition*. In addition, she performed poorly on both real-word picture naming and nonword repetition, suggesting that she was having problems with her already stored *motor programs,* as well as difficulty creating new motor programs (i.e., motor programming).

Stackhouse and Wells (1997) did not initially develop their model with the specific intention of identifying subgroups. However, Vance and associates (2005) suggested that using profiles based on a particular pattern of problems might provide additional insights into the nature of a child's problem. Such insight might then be used to direct intervention. Using the model to identify subgroups seems at least plausible. One might, for example, evaluate large groups of children with SSDs of unknown origin to determine whether certain profiles are more common than others. Stackhouse (2000) used this approach in a longitudinal study to suggest how different profiles might help differentiate children with SSDs who have later literacy problems from those who learn to read normally.

Classification by Symptomatology

The third perspective on subgroups is that of Barbara Dodd and her colleagues (2005), who classify idiopathic SSDs in a different manner. Dodd and colleagues note that "there is as yet no theoretically adequate or clinically relevant explanation of disordered speech . . . current models of the speech-processing chain . . . fail to disentangle causal, comorbid, and consequent difficulties" (p. 44). Dodd and colleagues argue that surface error patterns (i.e., symptoms) provide the best perspective on classification, and that such patterns do, in fact, explain the nature of the disorder. Dodd (2014) also offers specific treatment recommendations for most of the five subgroups she proposes. The Diagnostic Evaluation of Articulation and Phonology (DEAP) (Dodd, Hua, et al., 2006) was a test specifically developed to identify subgroups of children with SSDs.

The first subgroup proposed by Dodd is *articulation disorder,* in which the child produces consistent substitution or distortion errors on a limited number of phonemes (often /s/ or /r/). Errors do not change whether the production is spontaneous or imitated. In a cohort study of 320 children with SSDs, Broomfield and Dodd (2004) classified 40 (12.5%) children into this subgroup. According to Dodd (2014), traditional motor-based therapy (see Chapter 10) may be the most appropriate treatment approach for this subgroup.

The second and largest of Dodd's subgroups, *phonological delay,* includes children whose errors can be described using phonological process (pattern) labels that are also seen in much younger typically developing children (i.e., developmental patterns). Broomfield and Dodd (2004) classified 184/320 (57.5%) children into this subgroup. Dodd (2014) suggested that this subgroup might respond best to what we have here termed linguistically based approaches (see Chapter 11).

Dodd's third subgroup, *consistent atypical phonological disorder,* includes children who produce typical error patterns, along with one or more nondevelopmental patterns (i.e., those not usually produced by typically developing children). In this case, the errors are produced consistently. Broomfield and Dodd (2004) classified 66/320 (20.6%) children into this subgroup. A specific type of linguistically based approach called *contrast therapy* may be best suited for these children, according to Dodd (2014).

Dodd's fourth subgroup, *inconsistent phonological disorder,* includes children who produce (again along with typical errors) nondevelopmental error patterns, but do so inconsistently. In this case, inconsistency refers to variations in output of repeated productions of the same words (the same description of inconsistency mentioned previously in our discussion of CAS). In this case, however, none of the other signs of CAS would be present (see Table 5.3). Broomfield and Dodd (2004) classified 30/320 (9.4%) children into this subgroup. Dodd (2014) recommended a core vocabulary approach (discussed in Chapter 12) for this subgroup.

Dodd's final subgroup is CAS. In her 2014 paper, Dodd's definition is very reminiscent of (although not identical to) our earlier discussion of CAS. She says that this subgroup demonstrates:

> Speech characterised by inconsistency, oromotor signs (e.g., groping, difficulty sequencing articulatory movements), slow speech rate, disturbed prosody, short utterance length, poorer performance in imitation than spontaneous production. CAS is rare, and reliable identification is clinically challenging. It may involve multiple deficits affecting phonological and phonetic planning as well as motor program implementation. (p. 193)

Dodd and colleagues have attempted to validate her set of categories empirically. For example, Dodd (2011) compared 23 children classified as delayed against an age-matched group of 23 children classified as disordered (producing five or more instances of at least one atypical error pattern). The delayed group made significantly fewer consonant errors overall, as well as fewer types of errors. Although the groups did not differ on general measures of language ability, the disordered group performed significantly less well on a nonlinguistic rule-learning task and showed less cognitive flexibility on two tests of executive function. Dodd interpreted the findings to mean that the disordered group was less able to sort out the sound system of the language.

Validation of Dodd's categories has also been sought by looking at differential responses to different treatment approaches, as mentioned previously. For example, Dodd and Bradford (2000) presented case study data on three children: One child with a consistent phonological disorder received the most benefit from a phonological contrast (contrast therapy) approach, whereas two children with inconsistent phonological disorders initially responded most quickly to a core vocabulary approach. Once these latter children's errors became more consistent, one of them responded more quickly to phonological contrast therapy. These same associations between subgroup membership and response to therapy were also observed in a follow-up group study that included a total of 18 children (Crosbie et al., 2005).

Summary of Classification

As comprehensive as the preceding discussion is, it represents only some current proposals as to how to classify children with SSDs. Clearly, considerable work remains. For organically based disorders, clinicians know a great deal about how to assess and treat these children. As mentioned previously, specialized texts are available that provide detailed discussions regarding various organic categories. Considerable progress has also been made in understanding the nature of the problem when the origin is currently unknown, but the field does not yet have a clear consensus about the exact nature of this group. Lacking such a consensus, SLPs are currently left to choose from a number of available options for assessing and intervening with these children. These options are outlined in subsequent chapters.

COMORBIDITY

The attempts at classification described previously assume that the child's only communication problem is difficulty with speech sounds. However, as practicing clinicians will tell you, such is frequently not the case. It is common for someone to have other communication difficulties in addition to an SSD. For example, they may also have a language disorder, a voice disorder, or a problem with fluency. Two (or occasionally more than two) disorders may coexist in the same individual. Put another way, we can say that the individual is *comorbid* for disorder X and disorder Y. The term *morbidity* arises from medicine and is just another term for illness. Physicians often talk about *morbidity rates* or rates of illness (as opposed to *mortality rates* or rates of death).

Understanding comorbidity of SSDs with other disorders has important implications for clinical practice. First, it may be important to identifying the nature of the problem. For example, if a child leaves off plural –*s* endings, we would want to know whether this is because they cannot say /s/ (a speech sound problem) or do not understand the need for the plural marker (a morphological problem). Second, it may be important to understanding the relationship between the two disorders (i.e., which came first?). For example, if a child has unintelligible speech and a rough voice quality, is the roughness of the voice making it too hard for listeners to understand them? On the other hand, perhaps the SSD came first. The child may be quite unintelligible, which makes them work harder to be understood; this may lead to excess strain on the vocal mechanism, which then leads to the voice problem. Third, there is reason to suppose that children with multiple coexisting disorders may have more serious underlying issues, which may then predict or put a child at risk for later problems. Tyler and Theodore (2015) suggested, for example, that children with comorbid SSD and language impairments may be the most at risk for literacy problems. A final reason for wanting to understand comorbidity is that it may have implications for intervention. If two problems are present, do we treat them in a particular order (perhaps treating one first will cause the other problem to take care of itself?), or do we treat them simultaneously?

But why might two disorders coexist in the same individual? Several reasons are possible, and we have already alluded to one. Certain disorders may, by their very nature, lead to other disorders. Being unintelligible because of an SSD may lead to a voice disorder. It might also lead to a language delay or disorder. When a child who is quite unintelligible attempts to communicate, others may not understand them. As a result, their conversations may end quickly because limited or no communication is occurring. During such short conversations, children may miss out on opportunities to practice formulating and producing speech as well as language. They may also miss out on the valuable listener feedback that they normally would receive. Thus, being unintelligible may indirectly lead to delayed development of language skills.

A second possible explanation for comorbid disorders stems from the fact that communication is complex and involves a number of components, all put into use at the same time. We do not normally produce speech sounds by themselves without some context. We are usually simultaneously producing morphemes (morphology), words (expressive vocabulary), and phrases and sentences (syntax). We are also modifying what we say based on our emotional state (prosody), the communicative situation (receptive language), and our conversational partner or partners at that moment and the setting (pragmatics). Two disorders of communication might therefore coexist because the SSD results from some other disorder or problem (e.g., some genetic difference) that also affects other aspects of communication.

A third possible reason for comorbid conditions may be that different aspects of language interact. Recall our earlier example of the child who leaves off the plural /s/ markers. Like many languages, English has *morphophonemic rules* in which a particular morpheme (e.g., plural markers) has several different phonetic forms (e.g., /s/, /z/, /ɪz/). The particular form used depends on the characteristics of the adjacent speech sound (i.e., is it voiceless, is it voiced, or is it another sibilant?). Producing these markers may be difficult for some children because both the sound system and the morphology must be considered at the same time. Children need to learn all aspects of communication and how they work together in order to learn the sound system and other aspects of oral communication. While attempting to master one, other aspects may lag behind, at least temporarily. Finally, we cannot dismiss the possibility that comorbid disorders may be purely accidental and, at least for some individuals, may have nothing to do with each other.

How often do we see children with more than one disorder in the overall population? Findings reported by St. Louis and colleagues (1992), who reviewed records from the 1968–1969 National Speech and Hearing Survey (NSHS), provide useful data about comorbidity. That original survey included testing of more than 38,000 school-age children (grades 1–12) from all over the United States. St. Louis and colleagues reported individual prevalence values of 9.0% for articulation disorders, 10.2% for voice disorders, and 0.8% for stuttering. The NSHS also identified that hearing impairments occurred in 2.6% of the sample. It should be noted that language was not a category included in this survey because, at the time, language disorders in children were just beginning to be recognized by our profession as a type of communication disorder that should be treated by speech pathologists. It was after this recognition that we began to refer to ourselves as speech-language pathologists.

In their review, St. Louis and colleagues (1992) reported that comorbidity appeared to be quite common. For example, only 41% of those children in the NSHS with articulation disorders had no other communication problem. "Nearly 57 percent had co-existing voice deviations... Less than 1 percent of the articulation deviant group had associated stuttering..." (p. 8). Interestingly, of those with voice disorders, only 38% had articulation disorders. Of those who exhibited stuttering, 22% also had articulation disorders. These latter numbers highlight an important issue. The percentage values for comorbidity differ depending on which group you start with (sometimes called the *index disorder*). The reasons that the index disorder makes a difference probably reflect a combination of things. First, each disorder occurs at a different overall rate in the population. Second, some disorders (e.g., SSDs) may be more likely to completely resolve than others (e.g., fluency disorders). St. Louis and colleagues reported that the percentage of children with articulation disorders declined steadily across grade levels, whereas the percentage who stuttered remained relatively consistent across grades. Third, the underlying nature of one disorder may differ from that of the other disorder, and thus each disorder may affect other aspects of communication differently.

A good illustration of this is the finding that 41% of those with articulation disorders had no other problems. The same report said, however, that this was true for only 15% of those who stuttered.

Relying on the findings of the NSHS is not sufficient, of course. First, even in 1992, St. Louis and colleagues were concerned about the age of the data in that survey (collected in 1967 and 1968). Second, definitions of disorder have changed since 1968, as have the demographics of the population. Finally, as indicated previously, the NSHS failed to examine language disorders that have since become a significant part of speech-language pathology practice.

We now turn our attention to specific comorbidities with SSDs.

Speech Sound Disorders and Language Disorders

The speech sound system (i.e., the phonology) is one component of a child's developing linguistic system along with language development. As such, phonology is frequently cited as a common link to language and is generally thought to account for comorbidity between SSDs and (spoken) language disorders. Chapter 4 also discussed this connection as a synergistic one. There has also been considerable interest in the extent to which SSDs coexist with problems not only with spoken language but also with written language (i.e., difficulties with literacy). This connection is explored in Chapter 13.

The extent of the comorbidity between SSDs and disorders of spoken language has been the subject of considerable study. One of the more extensive reviews of this literature was conducted by Shriberg and Austin (1998). Their findings for studies with speech as the index disorder (our main focus here) are summarized in Table 5.5. Using findings from those studies and some of their own data, Shriberg and Austin concluded that up to approximately 60% of preschool children with SSDs also have some type of language disorder. They also concluded that if discussion is limited to

Table 5.5. Estimates of the comorbidity of language disorders in children with speech sound disorders

Study	n	Mean age[a]	Comorbidity estimate (%)
Connell et al. (1991)	37	3	43
Shriberg et al. (1986)	33	4	60
Shriberg & Kwiatkowski (1994)	64	4	66
Shriberg et al. (1986)	38	5	50
Paul & Shriberg (1982)	30	6	66
Shriberg & Kwiatkowski (1982c)	43	6	66
Schery (1985)	718	7	75[b]
St. Louis et al. (1994)	20	7	45[c]
Ruscello, St. Louis, et al. (1991)	24	12.5	54[d]
Ruscello, St. Louis, et al. (1991)	24	12.5	21[e]

[a] Ages in years; rounded to nearest year.
[b] No index disorder in this survey.
[c] Estimated.
[d] Classified as having delayed articulation.
[e] Classified as having residual (persistent) errors.
Source: Shriberg & Austin (1998).

coexisting *receptive language disorders* (i.e., problems understanding language spoken by others), the corresponding figure drops to 20%. Consistent with Tyler and Theodore (2015), as discussed previously, Shriberg and Austin also suggested that there is some support for the idea that children who have more severe SSDs may be more likely to have comorbid expressive language disorders. Although the comorbidity estimates in Table 5.5 vary from 21% to 75%, both are noticeably higher than the 7% prevalence figure commonly cited for language disorders alone seen in the preschool population (Tomblin et al., 1997). Thus, having an SSD seems to increase the likelihood of having a language disorder, supporting a link between the two.

Murray and colleagues (2019) reported data from a study conducted in Australia from 1,494 children at age 4 years. They reported that 3.4% of the children had an SSD. Of these, 40.8% had a receptive and/or expressive language impairment (20% receptive; 36.7% expressive). In addition, 20.8% had poor preliteracy skills (assessed by examining letter knowledge). Males were twice as likely as females to have both an SSD and some type of language impairment (Eadie et al., 2015). Specific to the subgroup CAS, Murray and colleagues (2019) reported that of 26 such children, 19% and 50% met criteria for comorbid receptive and expressive language impairments, respectively.

As noted previously, the links among disorders may help inform us about the nature of the underlying problem. A study by Macrae and Tyler (2014) is a case in point. These investigators looked at the speech abilities of 28 children aged 3–5 years (13 had SSDs alone, and 15 had SSDs and comorbid language disorders). The two groups did not differ on overall speech sound accuracy. However, the children with the comorbid language impairments produced significantly more omission errors and significantly fewer distortion errors than the children without language impairments (the groups did not differ on substitution errors). The higher proportion of omission errors was interpreted to reflect a more compromised language system where more of the underlying representations for the target sounds were missing in those with comorbid language impairments.

Relative to treatment, a common clinical concern is whether there is any advantage to treating either disorder (SSD or language disorder) first, or whether they should be treated simultaneously. This question has received limited direct investigation. A study by Tyler, Lewis, Haskill, and Tolbert (2003) addressed it with 40 3- to 5-year-old children with SSD and comorbid deficits in morphosyntax. One group received 12 weeks of speech sound intervention followed by 12 weeks of morphosyntax intervention, and a second group received those interventions in the reverse order. A third group received treatment that alternated between the two on a weekly basis (i.e., 1 week of speech sound treatment, then 1 week of morphosyntax treatment). The three groups did not differ on their gains on speech sounds, but the alternating treatment group made significantly greater gains on morphosyntax. These results suggest some advantage to the alternating approach.

Speech Sound Disorders and Stuttering

Another area of comorbidity that has received considerable attention is the comorbidity of SSDs and stuttering. Several connections are possible. Van Borsel and Tetnowski (2007), for example, reported that stuttering (as noted earlier for SSDs) is more common in certain genetic disorders, such as DS and fragile X syndrome, when compared to the general population. Genetic links are also suggested by the fact that both SSDs and stuttering are more common in males than females. McKinnon and colleagues (2007) collected data on 10,425 Australian elementary school children and reported male to female ratios of 2.85 to 1 for SSDs and 7.5 to 1 for stuttering. More direct evidence for a link through genetics also comes from heritability studies. Van Beijsterveldt and colleagues (2010) looked at data from more than 10,000 pairs of 5-year-old Dutch twins and concluded that stuttering is highly heritable (i.e., genetics play a large role).

Although genetics may or may not be the distal (ultimate) connection, others have considered more proximal (immediate) connections between SSDs and stuttering. The first of these is that both are motor-based problems (i.e., problems of speech production). Perhaps a common underlying motor problem accounts for both. The higher incidence of stuttering in DS (10%–45%, according to a review by Kent & Vorperian, 2013) also supports this notion, as the speech sound problems in DS are at least partially thought of as a motor problem. An alternative perspective is that there may be a proximal connection through language (i.e., the phonology). Although we do not usually think of stuttering as a language problem, Bloodstein (2002) argued that stuttering is primarily a language problem. He notes that stuttering is most often evident at the beginning of syntactic units, is largely absent in single-word speech, and is not usually elicited by single-word tasks. Whether one considers the two disorders to be language- or motor-based, both possibilities suggest that the comorbidity between SSDs and stuttering may arise because of the child's limited capacity to manage several aspects of communication at the same time.

Relative to numbers, the bulk of the work in this area has used stuttering as the index disorder. This likely stems from the small number of individuals identified when SSDs is the index. Recall the earlier discussion of the NSHS (St. Louis et al., 1992) in which fewer than 1% of the children in that survey who had articulation problems also exhibited stuttering. On the other hand, the same survey reported that more than 20% of those who stuttered also had articulation problems. Blood and Seider (1981), who surveyed elementary school clinicians on this question, reported a similar value of 16%. Nippold (2002) cites more recent studies suggesting values in the 30%–40% range as more common. This is consistent with Arndt and Healy (2001), who reported a figure of 32%. More recently, Unicomb and colleagues (2020) reported that 6.9% of 1,607 children aged 4 years presented with both stuttering and an SSD at the same time. They noted that their lower value likely reflected their community-based sample compared to the clinical samples used for most other studies. Whichever figures one accepts, all are higher than the 3.8% of 6-year-old children with SSDs in the general population reported by Shriberg and colleagues (1999). A child who stutters appears to be at higher risk for an SSD than a child in the general population. Yaruss and Conture (1996) reached the same conclusion.

The question of treatment relative to comorbid SSDs and stuttering is a notable concern among clinicians. As previously noted, there may be some value in knowing whether to treat one or the other first or to treat them simultaneously. In the case of stuttering, however, a different issue has arisen. There has been a long-standing concern that working on speech sound production in an individual who also stutters will make the stuttering problem worse. The idea is that the stuttering may become worse in the short term because of the child's limited output capacity. Moreover, there is a greater fear that the stuttering may become worse because of the child's own negative reactions to being less fluent. Advocates of such a position would encourage an indirect approach to intervention for children who have both disorders. Nippold

(2002) reviewed a series of studies related to this question and concluded that such a position may be unfounded. She found that: 1) a higher frequency of stuttering is not associated with a higher number of speech sound errors, 2) stuttering severity has not been shown to be different in children with and without SSDs, 3) type and frequency of speech sound errors do not appear to differentiate children who stutter from those who do not, 4) stuttering is no more common on complex versus simple words, and 5) speech sound errors do not seem to be any more common on stuttered versus nonstuttered utterances. Nippold suggests, therefore, that there is little reason to expect a negative treatment interaction between stuttering and SSDs when they are treated in the same individual.

At least one more recent study offers some direct support for Nippold's conclusion. Unicomb and associates (2017) presented a series of five case studies where both an SSD and a fluency disorder were treated simultaneously in the same child. Treatment for the SSD involved either traditional articulation therapy (see Chapter 10) or minimal pairs therapy (see Chapter 11). Treatment for the fluency disorder involved the Lidcomb Program (see Onslow & O'Brian, 2013). Both fluency and speech sound accuracy improved for all five participants, suggesting that a focus on speech did not make the fluency worse.

Speech Sound Disorders and Voice Disorders

Less commonly discussed comorbidities are SSDs and voice disorders. As with stuttering, several different connections may account for the comorbidity of SSDs and voice disorders. Two have already been mentioned: 1) reduced intelligibility may lead to excess effort, resulting in some type of damage to the laryngeal mechanism and 2) poor-quality sound associated with an underlying voice disorder may reduce intelligibility and lead to reduced practice and feedback. A third possible connection could be some common underlying problem that leads to both disorders. This is suggested by studies showing the coexistence of SSDs and voice disorders (or at least voice quality differences) in three populations we have already discussed.

Individuals with significant hearing loss lack the ability to adequately monitor their output. This is believed to explain the common reports of abnormal pitch, resonance, and poor control over speech sound accuracy (e.g., Leder & Spitzer, 1990). Another population is individuals with clefts of the palate with their inability to maintain adequate intraoral pressure. This is thought to lead to both speech sound errors and excess vocal effort, which may damage the vocal folds (e.g., Leder & Lerman, 1985). The previously mentioned review by Kent and Vorperian (2013) also noted frequent reports of voice quality problems in individuals with DS. They suggested that this may reflect an extra level of effort needed to produce the voice because of either a relatively small larynx or overall low muscle tone. This " . . . may signal inefficiencies in voice production . . . " (p. 181). The increased likelihood of an SSD may then reflect the combination of inefficient voice production by an individual who is already dealing with both relative macroglossia and cognitive impairment.

Several sources for comorbidity values for SSDs and voice disorders are available. As previously mentioned, investigations based on the NSHS data suggest that almost 57% of school-age children with SSDs may also have voice disorders. Another source is Shriberg and colleagues (1992), who reported on 137 children aged 3–19 years who had speech delay of unknown origin. Their data showed that 47 (34.3%) of the children failed the laryngeal quality portion of the Prosody-Voice Screening Profile (PVSP)

(Shriberg, Kwiatkowski, & Rasmussen, 1990). Failure on this measure means that fewer than 80% of their utterances in conversation were rated as having appropriate laryngeal (i.e., voice) quality. Values from both of these reports are again in stark contrast to the 10.2% of schoolchildren overall with voice disorders reported in the NSHS and 3.9% of the 2,445 preschool-age children studied by Duff and colleagues (2004). In summary, although findings are somewhat variable, having an SSD appears to increase the risk of also having a voice disorder.

There does not appear to be much empirical investigation of treatment for comorbid SSDs and voice disorders. When there is an indication of a voice disorder most clinicians are likely to take a simultaneous approach. Given that voice disorders may involve underlying organic issues with the larynx, consultation with an otolaryngologist is indicated to either rule out those issues or provide medical or surgical intervention. Where such issues are ruled out, simultaneous counseling by the SLP to teach better vocal hygiene would appear appropriate. This would limit and hopefully prevent any vocal abuse both during therapy and in other contexts.

Speech Sound Disorders and Emotional/Psychiatric Disorders

Another area of comorbidity that has received somewhat less attention is SSD and emotional/psychiatric disorders. SLPs' caseloads often include children with other disorders such as attention-deficit disorder (ADD), attention-deficit hyperactivity disorder (ADHD), or an anxiety disorder. Although not specific to SSDs, Cantwell and Baker (1987) reported on 202 children referred for speech and/or language services. Overall, 46% also received some type of what they referred to as psychiatric diagnosis (note: The word psychiatric here encompasses a spectrum of medically diagnosed disorders that includes ADD, ADHD, and emotional problems); specifically, Cantwell and Baker reported that 17% of their participants had been diagnosed with ADD, 8% with conduct disorder, and 6% with anxiety disorder. A study by Pinborough-Zimmerman and colleagues (2007) reviewed children's records and identified 1,667 children aged 8 years in Utah with communication impairment (again, not limited to SSDs). Of these, 6.1% also had been diagnosed with ADD and 2.2% with anxiety disorder. A 2008 ASHA survey suggested that at least 60% of school clinicians provided some type of speech or language services to individuals with ADHD.

Might there be a connection between SSDs and emotional or psychiatric problems? We can once again imagine a variety of possible accounts. As noted before, children with SSDs may have considerable difficulty making themselves understood. This may lead to frustration and possibly anxiety about communicating. Conversely, the child who is by nature anxious may not be the most desirable communication partner and may become somewhat ostracized. They may then miss out on opportunities to improve their speech sound accuracy. With ADHD, the child's difficulty staying on topic may also discourage conversational partners and limit practice time with speech. The connection may be in the other direction as well. The shortened conversations that many unintelligible children often have could limit their opportunities to maintain their attention on a single topic for any length of time. Although specific evidence is not available, one might also imagine a common underlying genetic problem leading to both disorders.

Our previous discussion of Shriberg's SD–DPI category is worth recalling at this point. A prevalence of 12% with SD–DPI was suggested by Shriberg (2010). Although Shriberg does not indicate that these children would necessarily qualify for a specific psychiatric diagnosis, his description of their problem implies it might be appropriate for at least some of them. Additional comorbidity data, particularly with speech as the index disorder, are somewhat limited. Keating and associates (2001) used data from the 1995 Australian National Health Survey that included more than 12,300 children aged 0–14 years. Results showed that about 8% of children with speech disorders were reported to also have emotional problems. This contrasts with about 1% percent of children without speech disorders. That same study reported values of 5%–7% percent and 1%–2% percent, respectively, for other mental disorders.

In summary, we can conclude that an SSD presents an increased risk for psychiatric or emotional disorders, although most individuals with an SSD do not have psychiatric or serious emotional disorders. Where such problems co-occur, consultation with appropriate mental health professionals both before and during treatment for the SSD is indicated.

Speech Sound Disorders and Complex Neurodevelopmental Disorders

Work by Shriberg and others has focused attention on speech production by individuals with a variety of disorders that manifest themselves in the developmental period and appear to be at least partly neurologic in nature. That work has highlighted that these individuals may also have SSDs. As the name implies, these are complex disorders, and SLPs may already be serving these children because of other issues, such as cognitive impairments, language impairments, or behavioral issues. The possibility of also having to work on an SSD only further complicates the delivery of effective intervention to such clients.

Recall the earlier discussion of CAS and the possibility that one proposed origin of that disorder is association with disorders such as these. Recall also that the current ASHA definition of CAS includes associations with several such disorders as one possible origin. This connection led Shriberg, Strand, and colleagues (2019) to look at these disorders for signs of other motor speech disorders as well. Using a sample of 346 children, they derived a set of prevalence estimates, which are shown in Table 5.6. As can be seen, when present, the most common motor speech disorder is speech motor delay. On the other hand, for several of these populations (16p11.2, severe traumatic brain injury, autism spectrum disorder) well over half presented no motor speech disorder.

Other types of SSDs may also be possible in these populations and some data are available. Earlier in this chapter the speech delays associated with DS, fragile X syndrome, and other cognitive impairments were discussed. Relative to galactosemia, a study by Yuzyuk and colleagues (2018) reviewed clinical outcomes for 34 individuals with this condition. They found that in 13 patients over age 3 years who were most severely affected by the enzyme inactivity that is central to this condition, all had been reported to have speech deficits (details not specified). A high percentage of children with 22q11.2 deletion (also known as velocardiofacial syndrome) also present with related speech difficulties; for example, they frequently exhibit abnormal resonance, which often reduces overall speech intelligibility.

The genetic condition 16p11.2 represents a specific genetic variant linked to increased risk of autism spectrum disorder. It is characterized as either a deletion or a duplication of genetic material in that area of the person's genome. A file review by Rosenfeld and colleagues (2010) found 17 of 18 patients (94%) with the deletion had reports in their files of "... speech delays greater than other delays, poor articulation,

Table 5.6. Prevalence estimates for motor speech disorders[a] in several complex neurodevelopmental disorders

Disorder	No motor speech disorder	Speech motor delay (SMD)	Childhood dysarthria (CD)	Childhood apraxia of speech (CAS)	CD and CAS
Down syndrome (n = 45)	2.2%	26.7%	37.8%	11.1%	22.2%
Fragile X syndrome (n = 28)	35.7%	28.6%	32.1%	3.6%	0
Idiopathic intellectual disability (n = 23)	26.1%	47.8%	17.4%	8.7%	0
Galactosemia (n = 31)	41.9%	22.6%	16.1%	6.5%	12.9%
22q11.2 deletion (n = 17)	17.6%	29.4%	29.4%	11.8%	11.8%
16p11.2 (n = 108)	68.5%	27.8%	1.9%	1.9%	0
Severe traumatic brain injury (n = 52)	73.1%	15.4%	7.7%	1.9%	1.9%
Autism spectrum disorder (n = 42)	85.7%	14.3%	0	0	0

[a] Defined by using Shriberg's Speech Disorders Classification System categories (see earlier discussion on Classification).

Source: Figure 6 in Shriberg, Strand et al. (2019).

lower verbal intelligence and difficulty in reading skills" (p. 27). Relative to children with traumatic brain injury, a study of 56 children injured before age 11 years suggested that 1) children injured after age 5 years were more likely to achieve normal consonant accuracy than those injured at earlier ages and 2) age of injury was moderately correlated (0.40) with consonant accuracy 1 year following the injury (Campbell et al., 2013). Put another way, the earlier the injury the poorer the consonant accuracy outcome. Finally, for the last group listed in Table 5.6, children with autism spectrum disorder, over 85% demonstrated no motor speech impairments. Using SDCS categories (see earlier discussion under Classification), Shriberg, Paul, and colleagues (2011) tested 46 children with autism under age 9 years and estimated that 15.2% would qualify as having speech delay, while 31.8% would qualify as having speech errors (the two other broad SDCS categories).

As the name implies, these are complicated disorders and SLPs may be called on to serve children who have other conditions besides SSDs and perhaps other communication disorders, which may include motor, cognitive, and/or behavior issues. Treatment for SSDs in individuals with these disorders typically involves the SLP working on a team with other relevant professionals to balance the many needs of the client. The makeup of such teams would vary with the disorder.

CONCLUSION

For some children with SSDs, the cause of the disorder is known and specific approaches to assessment and intervention have been and continue to be developed. In other cases, however, the origin of the disorder is not known. This latter group of children does not consistently respond to the same intervention approaches, suggesting that there may be subgroups. Although many children in this population have historically been successfully provided intervention services, typically motor or linguistically oriented, several research teams continue efforts to unravel possible subgroups that may need different treatment strategies.

Children with SSDs appear to be at increased risk for other kinds of difficulties or disorders, including language impairments, stuttering, voice disorders, and psychological or emotional difficulties. Understanding the nature of these comorbidities may help us better understand the nature of the problems and how to treat them.

QUESTIONS FOR CHAPTER 5

1. What is meant by an organically based speech sound disorder? Cite some examples.

2. Briefly outline the three ways investigators have tried to identify subgroups of SSDs of unknown origin.

3. Cite specific examples wherein knowledge of etiology is highly important, if not essential, to developing an effective and efficient intervention program.

4. What is *comorbidity*, and why is it important?

5. What are some possible ways to account for comorbid conditions in the same individual?

6. How common is it for an individual who stutters to also have an SSD?

6

Assessment: Data Collection

NICHOLAS W. BANKSON, PETER FLIPSEN JR., AND JOHN E. BERNTHAL

LEARNING OBJECTIVES

This chapter discusses the first stage or initial steps in the assessment of individuals suspected of having a speech sound disorder (SSD), namely the collection of relevant data. By the end of this chapter, the reader should be able to:

- Differentiate speech sound screening from a comprehensive evaluation/ assessment.
- Discuss options for both formal and informal screening procedures.
- Identify a menu of sampling procedures that can be employed in speech sound testing.
- List the advantages and disadvantages of using single-word speech sound assessments.
- Differentiate among different elicitation formats for speech sampling.
- Explain the advantages and disadvantages of conversational speech sampling.
- Summarize considerations that are relevant for assessing speech intelligibility.
- Describe at least three different methods for assessing speech intelligibility.
- Explain what is known about the relationship between stimulability and spontaneous speech skill.
- Describe the basic procedure for stimulability testing.
- Outline the value of contextual testing.
- List some of the uses of error pattern analysis.
- Describe different options for transcribing and scoring speech samples.
- Discuss challenges faced and approaches used in testing speech sound skill in very young children.
- List and discuss several different related assessment procedures used in speech sound assessment.

ASSESSMENT PLANNING

Referrals (i.e., requests for evaluations) that are received by a speech-language pathologist (SLP) can come from a variety of sources and vary widely. They can include a family medical practitioner asking the SLP to assess speech and language development or a classroom teacher who writes, "Tom can't say /r/ correctly," or a parent who calls and says "We as a family can understand everything he says, but no one else seems to be able to." The SLP may also receive information from a colleague in the form of detailed informal observations. The referral source is asking us to make judgments about what they perceive as a problem and then offer recommendations for possible intervention. Based on this information, we proceed to develop a plan for how to collect and analyze the necessary and sufficient data in order to do this.

Typically, we begin with what some have called a *diagnostic hypothesis,* which is an initial best guess (based on whatever information we have) about what the problem might be. This allows us to select the assessment procedures we intend to use. Setting some limits on what we plan to do is important, because SLPs have a relatively broad scope of practice and typically don't have time to test everything in depth. On the other hand, the referral information is not a license to ignore other issues that we might notice. Most people are not fully aware of the extent of the SLP scope of practice; likewise, our referral source may only be focused on one aspect of communication and may not have noticed other issues. As such, we usually conduct a more comprehensive communication evaluation where, in addition to speech sound productions, we also give some attention to voice quality, resonance, fluency, syntax, semantics, pragmatics, discourse, and prosodic aspects of language. Additional related measures, such as a hearing exam and an oral mechanism examination, are also usually included.

With that context in mind, the main focus in this chapter will be on those elements of data collection most relevant to speech sound disorders (SSDs). The chapter discusses various sampling and testing procedures, as well as factors and issues to be considered when analyzing speech sound samples. Chapter 7 discusses the interpretation of speech sound sampling data and concludes with a case history of a child to whom procedures discussed in both of these chapters are applied.

SPEECH SOUND SAMPLING

One of the unique contributions of the field of speech-language pathology to the assessment of verbal behavior is the development of speech sound assessment instruments. For several decades, the use of these tools, also referred to as *phonological* or *articulation assessments,* has remained almost the exclusive domain of SLPs, although linguists, child development specialists, psychologists, pediatricians, and special and regular educators also use such tools.

Evaluation of an individual's speech sound status typically involves describing their productions and comparing them to the adult standard of the speaker's linguistic community. This type of analysis is called a *relational analysis,* a procedure that is designed to determine which sounds are produced correctly when compared to the adult standard. For young children or speakers with limited phonological repertoires, the speech sound system is sometimes described independently of the adult standard, in which case the examiner simply wants to know what speech sounds are produced, regardless of whether they are used correctly. This is called an *independent analysis.*

Although some clinicians have differentiated between delays (children whose speech sound errors are similar to those found in younger normally developing children) and disorders (children whose speech sound errors differ from normal developing children), we do not make this distinction here. In reality, most children who are having difficulty with multiple sound productions will have errors that fall into both categories.

The goals of speech sound assessment typically include one or more of the following:

1. Determining whether the speech sound system is sufficiently different from normal development to warrant intervention

2. Identifying factors that might be related to the presence or maintenance of a phonological disability/delay

3. Determining treatment direction, including selecting target behaviors and strategies to be used in intervention

4. Making prognostic statements relative to change with or without intervention/therapy

5. Monitoring change in performance across time to evaluate whether therapy is being effective and/or to make discharge decisions

In addition, the SLP might be called on to identify and describe whether any differences observed reflect dialectal variations of General American English. In most situations, such variations would not warrant remediation because they represent a valid difference rather than a disorder. In such cases, the SLP must be able to differentiate dialect differences from an SSD. However, in some cases, the need to describe such differences follows a request or inquiry related to speakers who voluntarily wish to change a regional or cultural dialect. SLPs may also receive questions about accent reduction from individuals for whom English is a second language. Issues related to dialect differences and second language learning will be discussed further in Chapter 14. Aspects of accent modification are addressed in Chapter 15.

The two most common purposes of a speech sound assessment are to determine whether an individual 1) needs instruction related to correct production and use of speech sounds and, if so, 2) the direction of treatment. To make these determinations, the clinician engages in a multistep process that involves sampling the client's speech through a variety of procedures, analyzing the data gathered, interpreting the data that have been analyzed, and then making clinical recommendations.

SCREENING FOR SPEECH SOUND DISORDERS

A complete or comprehensive speech sound assessment, including analysis and interpretation of results, is not something that can be done quickly. Because of the time required for a complete speech sound assessment, clinicians often do a screening to determine whether a more comprehensive assessment is warranted. Screening procedures are not designed to determine the need or direction of therapy, but to identify individuals who merit further evaluation as distinct from those for whom further assessment is not indicated. Screening might be used for 1) children at a Head Start program, preschool, or kindergarten to determine whether they have age-appropriate speech sound production skills; 2) older children, where maturation should have resolved most developmental errors; 3) individuals preparing for occupations such as broadcast journalism or classroom teaching that require specific speech performance standards; and 4) clients referred for other speech and language impairments (e.g., voice, language, fluency) to confirm their speech sound status.

Instruments used for screening consist of a limited sample of speech sound productions, which can often be administered in 5 minutes or less. Screening measures can be categorized as informal or formal. *Informal measures* are often used when people wish to develop their own screening tools to meet their particular needs. *Formal measures* are often employed when a clinician desires established norms for comparison purposes or testing methodologies that are more uniform.

Informal Screening Measures

The examiner usually devises informal screening measures that are tailored to the population being screened. Although informal procedures can be easily and economically devised, they do not include standardized administration procedures or normative data, which are characteristics of formal screening measures. For example, in an informal screening procedure that could be used with a group of kindergarten children, the examiner asks each child to respond to the following:

1. Tell me your name. Where do you live?

2. Can you count to 10? Tell me the days of the week.

3. What do you like to watch on TV?

4. Tell me about your favorite video game.

The focus of these questions is to engage each child in conversation so that one can obtain a sample of their typical speech sound productions.

If the screening is for adults, the examiner might ask them to do one or all of the following:

1. Read sentences designed to elicit several productions of frequently misarticulated sounds, such as /s/, /r/, /l/, and /θ/. For example, "I saw Sally at her seaside house;" "Rob ran around the orange car."

2. Read a passage with a representative sample of English speech sounds, such as the following:

   - *Grandfather Passage.* You wish to know all about my grandfather. Well, he is nearly 93 years old, yet he still thinks as swiftly as ever. He dresses himself in an old black frock coat, usually missing several buttons. A long beard clings to his chin, giving those who observe him a pronounced feeling of the utmost respect. When he speaks, his voice is just a bit cracked and quivers a bit. Twice each day, he plays skillfully and with zest upon a small organ. Except in winter when the snow or ice prevents, he slowly takes a short walk in the open air each day. We have often urged him to walk more and smoke less, but he always answers, "Banana oil." Grandfather likes to be modern in his language.

   - *Rainbow Passage.* When the sunlight strikes raindrops in the air, they act as a prism and form a rainbow. The rainbow is a division of white light into many beautiful colors. These take the shape of a long round arch, with its path high above, and its two ends apparently beyond the horizon. There is, according to legend, a boiling pot of gold at one end. People look, but no one ever finds it. When a man looks for something beyond his reach, his friends say he is looking for the pot of gold at the end of the rainbow.

3. Engage in an informal conversation about topics of interest, such as a recent trip, a television show, a recent sporting event, or another current event.

The examiner determines the criteria for the failure of an informal screening. An often-used rule of thumb is, "If in doubt, refer for further testing." In other words, if an examiner is uncertain whether the client's speech sound system is appropriate for their age and/or linguistic community, a referral should be made for a more complete assessment. The examiner can also choose to predetermine or establish ahead of time some performance standards on the screening instrument to help identify those to refer for further testing. Those individuals with the greatest need for additional testing and probable intervention are often obvious to the examiner from even a small sample of their speech and language.

Clinical Vignette 6.1

Kindergarten Screening

Faced with a community in far northern Canada that had never had speech pathology services before, author Peter Flipsen Jr. needed a way to consistently identify children in need of services. His employer was the local school board. He decided to institute a program of kindergarten screening where he would do quick evaluations of the approximately 100 children who entered kindergarten each year.

The local public health nurse screened the hearing of all children entering kindergarten each fall, so that was taken care of. But he still needed to be able to look for problems related to speech sounds, voice quality, fluency, and expressive and receptive language. He settled on the following screening procedures, which took about 15 minutes per child:

1. Administer a test of receptive vocabulary.

2. Give the child a wordless (picture) storybook. Ask them to look at the pictures and tell the story. This was recorded for later transcription.

3. Make observations during the story production about voice quality, speech sound errors, or fluency.

Step 1 provided information on receptive language and Step 2 took care of the rest. Screening took place in January of each year and took about 3 weeks to complete the procedure for 100 children. Performing the screening in January allowed the kindergarten teachers sufficient time to get to know the children. Initial findings were then discussed with each teacher to see if the screening observations were consistent with any observations the teacher had made. For any child where both the SLP and the teacher had concerns, the parents were contacted, and arrangements were made for a more comprehensive evaluation. Each year 15–20 children underwent those more comprehensive evaluations and several were enrolled in therapy.

Formal Screening Measures

Formal screening measures include published elicitation procedures for which normative data and/or cutoff scores are usually available. These formal measures are typically one of two types 1) tests that are related to or are part of a more comprehensive speech sound assessment and 2) tests that screen for speech sounds as well as other aspects of speech and language. Tests designed explicitly for the screening of speech sounds are often used for formal screening. Those instruments that combine speech sound screening with other aspects of language screening are most commonly used for more general communication disorders screening in which information on phonology is just one part of the communication assessment.

Available formal measures typically require production of 10–25 words intended to elicit production of common error sounds. These procedures typically take 2–5 minutes to administer. Some involve spontaneous naming of pictures or objects, whereas others require immediate imitation of examiner productions.

The following are examples of formal screening measures that are part of a more comprehensive assessment of phonology.

- *Diagnostic Screen* (Dodd, Hua et al., 2006)

  The Diagnostic Screen is related to the Diagnostic Evaluation of Articulation and Phonology (DEAP) instrument. The screening portion includes 22 pictures that are imitated following examiner production (model), requires 5 minutes to administer, and provides an indication of whether further assessment could be appropriate. The authors indicate that the screening test is especially useful with children who are shy, immature, or have a short attention span.

- *Preschool/Multisyllabic Screens* (Hodson, 2004)

  The Preschool Phonological Screen (PPS) and the Multisyllabic Word Screen (MWS) are both related to the Hodson Assessment of Phonological Patterns (HAPP-3) instrument. For the PPS the child is required to name 12 objects. Similarly, in the MWS (intended for children aged 8 years and older) the child names 12 pictures. Each require 2–3 minutes to administer and include cutoff criteria that indicate when a problem may be present and whether more extensive evaluation (such as giving the full HAPP-3) should be conducted.

The following tests include screening of phonology as part of an overall speech and language screening.

- *Fluharty Preschool Speech and Language Screening Test* (2nd ed.) (Fluharty, 2001)

  This test was designed for children aged 3 through 6 years. The speech sound assessment portion of the test includes 15 pictured objects designed to elicit 30 target speech sounds. Some stimulus items assess two speech sounds. Standard scores and percentiles for the articulation (speech sound) subtest are included.

- *Speech-Ease Screening Inventory* (K–1) (Pigott et al., 1985)

  This test was designed for kindergartners and first-graders. The overall test takes 7–10 minutes to administer, with the articulation section comprising 12 items. Through sentence completion items, 14 phonemes and 3 blends are assessed. Cutoff scores, which suggest the need for further testing, are provided.

- *Preschool Language Scale* (5th ed.) (Zimmerman et al., 2012)

  This test includes a supplemental articulation screener used to assess speech sounds for children aged 2;6 to 7;11. The child is required to name 14 pictures. Age-expected performance levels are provided, which signal whether further testing is needed.

- *Test of Language Development, Primary* (5th ed.) (Newcomer & Hammill, 2019)

  This test looks at several aspects of language. It includes a supplemental word articulation subtest that requires production of 25 words. Percentile ranks and scaled scores can be derived on the subtest.

Summary

Screening procedures are not designed to determine the need for or direction of treatment. Rather, their purpose is to identify individuals who merit further testing. The criteria for failure on informal screening tests are often left up to the examiner. When available for formal screening tests, standard scores, percentile ranks, and cutoff scores can aid the examiner in establishing such criteria. It is common for scores of one standard deviation or more below the mean to be used as a cutoff for further testing. For some formal instruments, cutoff scores or age expectation scores are also provided.

COMPREHENSIVE SPEECH SOUND ASSESSMENT: THE ASSESSMENT BATTERY

Sampling procedures involved in comprehensive speech sound assessments are more in-depth and detailed than those described for screening. When doing such an assessment and analysis, the clinician usually employs several testing instruments and sampling procedures because no one sampling procedure or test provides all a clinician needs to know when making case selection decisions and/or determining the direction that an intervention program should take. The evaluation typically involves speech sound productions in speech samples of varying lengths and complexities (e.g., syllables, words, phrases), phonetic contexts, and responses to various elicitation procedures (e.g., picture naming, imitation, conversation). This collection of samples is often referred to as an *assessment battery*.

The use of an assessment battery provides insight into how different types of cognitive, linguistic, and speech-motor demands affect the client's performance. For example, telling a narrative involves much more cognitive focus, linguistic formulation skill, and motor output planning than naming single pictures. One might expect fewer errors on the latter task than the former. A study of children with SSDs by Klein and Liu-Shea (2009) supported this; these investigators reported more and different types of errors in continuous productions than in single-word productions.

The influence of different speaking demands may also manifest itself through the use of different formats to obtain speech samples (see Box 6.1). For example, studies comparing responses elicited via imitation with those elicited through spontaneous picture naming have produced inconsistent results. Investigators studying children between the ages of 5 and 8 years have reported that responses elicited via imitation tasks yield more correct responses than those elicited via spontaneous picture naming (Carter & Buck, 1958; Siegel et al., 1963; M. W. Smith & Ainsworth, 1967; Snow & Milisen, 1954). Other investigators who studied children ranging in age from 2 to 6 years reported no significant differences in results from elicitation via picture naming and imitation (Paynter & Bumpas, 1977; Templin, 1947). However, it is best simply to assume that children, especially of school age, do better on imitation as compared to spontaneous picture-naming tasks.

The intersection of the demands of different tasks and different formats was studied by Dubois and Bernthal (1978), who compared productions of the same word stimuli elicited through a picture-naming task, a delayed imitation task, and a spontaneous storytelling task. They reported that the highest number of errors was found on the storytelling task and the smallest number on the picture-naming task. Although the differences between the methods were statistically significant, the authors

---

BOX 6.1   Elicitation Formats

Samples of speech production can be elicited in a variety of formats, including:

Spontaneous—speaker responds to a question, picture, or object by providing the required target without having heard the examiner produce it. For example, the clinician shows the child a picture of a house and asks, "What's this?" The child responds, "House."

Delayed Imitation—the examiner produces the target, adds some additional verbiage, and then asks the speaker to produce the target. For example: "This is a picture of a house. People can live in a house. What's in this picture?"

Direct Imitation—the examiner asks the speaker to produce the target (e.g., "Say house").

Co-Production—also called choral speech. Examiner and client produce words, phrases, or sentences at the same time. Occasionally used in therapy for fluency disorders or in integral stimulation therapy (a form of speech sound intervention for children with severely delayed speech and/or childhood apraxia of speech [CAS]). Not typically used in assessment.

   Ideally, all speech samples would be produced spontaneously, as this represents what most speakers do most of the time. It is also the most complex format, as it requires the speaker to think of the word, plan its production, and then produce it. Sometimes a child may not be familiar with a particular word or may simply not remember it at that moment. In such cases, clinicians typically try to elicit the target by delayed imitation. If that doesn't work, then direct imitation is used. Clinicians typically will note whether imitation or delayed imitation is required for more than a few items. This may reflect a reduced level of vocabulary development or difficulty with verbal recall.

---

interpreted the differences as clinically nonsignificant. They did, however, report that some individuals varied from group trends in their production of certain sounds depending on the task; for example, some children made significantly more errors on the delayed imitation task than on the picture-naming task.

   Recall that the two major purposes of a speech sound assessment are to determine the need for and direction of treatment. It is for these purposes that most of the writing, research, and testing materials on SSDs have been developed. The following pages present components of a comprehensive battery with an emphasis on procedures for obtaining speech sound samples. Following this, analysis of data collected through sampling procedures is discussed.

Speech Sound Samples Included in the Assessment Battery

Connected/Conversational Speech Sampling Rationale

Rationale. All speech sound evaluations should include a sample of connected speech. Because the ultimate objective of treatment is the correct production of sounds in spontaneous conversation, it is important that the examiner observe speech sound productions in as natural a speaking context as possible. Such samples allow one to transcribe phoneme productions in a variety of phonetic contexts, observe error patterns, and judge the severity of the problem and the intelligibility of the speaker in continuous discourse. Sounds produced in connected speech can also be studied in relation to other factors such as speech rate, intonation, stress, and syllable structure. In addition, connected speech samples allow for multiple productions of sounds across different lexical/vocabulary items.

Because spontaneous connected speech samples are the most valid and representative sample of phonological performance, some clinicians suggest that speech sound assessment should be exclusively based on this type of sample (Morrison & Shriberg, 1992; Shriberg & Kwiatkowski, 1980; Stoel-Gammon & Dunn, 1985). Connected speech samples have the advantage of allowing the examiner to transcribe sound productions within the context of the child's own vocabulary and in running speech, which includes their natural prosodic patterns. In addition, these samples can be used for other purposes, such as examining fluency, voice quality, and/or other aspects of language production. However, the following is a listing of practical problems associated with relying solely on such samples: 1) Many individuals with severe communication problems may be unintelligible, and it can be impossible or very difficult to reliably determine and/or transcribe what they are attempting to say; 2) some children can be reluctant to engage in conversational dialogue with an adult they do not know; 3) it can also be very difficult to obtain a spontaneous speech corpus that contains a representative sample of English phonemes; and 4) as Ingram (1989a) has pointed out, sounds missing from a conversational sample can reflect a selective avoidance by the child. The child may choose not to produce them. In summary, although connected speech samples are an essential part of an assessment battery, most clinicians do not rely on this type of sample exclusively.

Elicitation Procedures.   The customary and preferred method for obtaining a sample of connected speech is to engage a client in spontaneous conversation. Similar to what was suggested earlier for informal screening procedures, the clinician can talk with the client about such things as their family, television shows, favorite activities and games, or places the client has visited. The samples should be recorded so that the clinician can play them back as often as required to accurately transcribe the client's utterances. To facilitate later transcription, clinicians should also make notes about topics covered and errors observed.

Some clinicians have the client read a passage orally as an alternative method for obtaining a connected sample of speech. Although this procedure provides a sample of connected speech, it has been demonstrated that fewer errors usually occur in a reading sample than in a corpus of conversational speech (Wright et al., 1969). Moreover, clinicians frequently test children who have not yet learned to read, in which case this procedure is obviously not a viable option.

To encourage the production of specific target words (and thus specific target sounds) in a connected speech context, some clinicians use stories. In this case, the clinician tells a short story and then asks the child to tell the story back to them. Often the story is told while jointly looking at a set of related pictures. During the retell stage these pictures help remind the child of the storyline and specific target items within the story. This is a form of delayed imitation.

Some speech sound tests specify procedures for obtaining a sample of connected speech. For example, in the Glaspey Dynamic Assessment of Phonology (GDAP; Glaspey, 2019), it is recommended that the child be given a wordless storybook and asked to (spontaneously) tell the story that goes with the pictures. In some tests, a more structured format is provided. For example, in the Sounds-in-Sentences subtest of the Goldman-Fristoe Test of Articulation (3rd ed.) (GFTA-3; Goldman & Fristoe, 2015), the client listens to a story while viewing accompanying pictures. The clinician then tells the story a second time but asks the child to repeat each sentence in the story (one at a time) immediately after it is produced (a form of direct imitation). One advantage to this more structured approach is that often (as is the case with the GFTA-3) standardized scores can be generated for making case selection eligibility decisions.

Summary.   A connected speech sample is a crucial part of any speech sound assessment battery because it allows 1) assessment of overall intelligibility and severity, 2) determination of speech sound usage in its natural form, and 3) a database from which to judge the accuracy of individual sounds, patterns of errors, and consistency of misarticulations/speech sound errors. The preferred method for obtaining connected speech samples is to engage the client in spontaneous conversation. If, for some reason, this cannot be accomplished, alternate procedures that can be used include 1) eliciting conversational responses via picture stimuli or toys, 2) utilizing a reading passage, or 3) retelling a story following the clinician's model (delayed imitation).

Assessing Intelligibility

Rationale.   The primary objective of all communication interactions is to achieve some goal. The intent may be to convey information, acquire information, seek assistance with some task, or simply continue a social interaction. Whatever the goal, it is usually imperative that listeners understand what was intended. *Intelligibility* is a measure of the listener's ability to understand the intended message. Given its importance, intelligibility measurement should be included in all comprehensive speech sound assessments.

The measurement of speech intelligibility involves listeners making a perceptual judgment of the acoustic signal being transmitted. The extent to which this actually happens will depend broadly on 1) the listener's ability to hear and understand the language being spoken, 2) the listening conditions, and 3) a variety of factors related to the speaker and the message they are trying to convey. Typically, we control the first two of these by having intelligibility judgments made by listeners with normal hearing who understand the language, and by making the judgments in quiet conditions without any interruptions. What remains to affect our results are only factors related to the speaker and the message being conveyed.

Speaker factors that influence speech intelligibility include the number and types of speech sound errors, consistency of the errors, frequency of occurrence of the impacted sounds in the language, and phonological patterns used. As to number of errors, in general, the more of a speaker's productions that differ from the adult standard, the more intelligibility is reduced. However, a simple tally of the number of sounds in error is not an adequate index of intelligibility. As Shriberg and Kwiatkowski (1982a) reported, there is often a low correlation (they reported $r = .42$) between the percentage of consonants correct and the intelligibility ratings of a speech sample. Similarly, Namasivayam and colleagues (2013) reported correlations of .377 and .241 (both not statistically significant) between GFTA-2 scores and intelligibility measured in single words and sentences respectively.

Relative to the nature of the client's errors, deleting a sound usually affects intelligibility more than a distortion or substitution for the sound. The types of error patterns being used may also be crucial. We will discuss error patterns in more detail next but, in general, the more common the error pattern, the more predictable the intended words may be and the less the impact on intelligibility. For example, final consonant deletion (e.g., saying *key* instead of *keep*) is a common error made by young children. Conversely, less common or unusual error patterns (e.g., initial consonant deletion where a child might say *eat* instead of *feet*) may be more distracting for the listener and may make it more difficult to follow the intended message.

Even among the more common error patterns, specific patterns may have different effects on intelligibility depending on how often they occur. Klein and Flint (2006) found that when the opportunities for error patterns to occur were equalized, velar fronting had less impact on intelligibility than either stopping or final consonant deletion at low or moderate levels of occurrence (i.e., less than 30% of opportunities). At high levels of occurrence (i.e., at least 50% of opportunities), however, all three patterns affected intelligibility equally. Intelligibility is also affected by consistency; if errors are very consistent, intelligibility may be less affected, as the listener may quickly learn to predict what was intended. Likewise, the more frequently the target sounds that are in error occur in the language, the more likely the listener is to have difficulty understanding the message.

Factors other than the individual's speech output may also influence intelligibility judgments. These include the level of communication (single words, conversation), topic under discussion, as well as prosodic factors including speaker's rate, inflection, stress patterns, pauses, voice quality, loudness, and fluency. Familiarity with the speaker's pattern of errors may be particularly important. Parents are often better judges of what their children intend than unfamiliar adults (Flipsen, 1995). Likewise, SLPs have an advantage over non-SLPs, even during an initial encounter. And as we work with our clients in therapy over extended periods, we may become even more familiar. To avoid potential bias in making both initial and follow-up intelligibility measures, unfamiliar listeners are strongly recommended.

When one takes all of these factors together, it is clear that making oneself understood is a complex process involving many factors. Despite a temptation to rely heavily on single-word speech sound measures (to be discussed in a later section), such measures are not sufficient. Put another way, asking, "How well did he say those individual speech sounds?" is not the same as asking, "What do you believe he meant to say?" Both questions are important. Both can be asked using single words, but intelligibility should be measured directly.

Norm-referenced procedures for measuring intelligibility have yet to be developed. This is largely because it is unclear how to control all of the factors involved. Two general principles can, however, guide our decisions: 1) the poorer the intelligibility, the more likely the need for intervention and 2) the degree of intelligibility needs to be judged relative to age expectations. In addition to the discussion of intelligibility in Chapter 3, the following guideline from Bowen (personal communication, 2002) appears appropriate. Expectations for intelligibility (percentage of words understood in conversation with an unfamiliar adult) are: 1 year, 25% intelligible; 2 years, 50% intelligible; 3 years, 75% intelligible; and 4 years, 100% intelligible. Bowen arrived at this percentage by dividing a child's age in years by 4.

Elicitation Procedures.   There is no single standard procedure for quantifying the intelligibility of young children's speech. Gordon-Brannan (1994) identified three general approaches: 1) *open-set word identification,* in which the examiner transcribes a speech sample and determines the percentage of words identifiable; 2) *closed-set word identification* (also called multiple-choice procedures), in which a listener identifies words produced using prescribed word lists as a reference; and 3) *rating scale* procedures, which may take the form of either an interval scaling procedure, in which a listener assigns a rating (number along a continuum of 5–9 points) or a direct magnitude scale from which a judgment of a speech sample is made relative to a standard stimulus. Although rating scales are often used because of their simplicity and efficiency, Schiavetti (1992) has pointed out that listeners have difficulty dividing interval scales evenly, and often it is difficult to establish reliability of listeners, particularly in the middle part of a scale.

Open-set word identification tasks include calculating the actual percentage of words understood in a speech sample, and this may be the most reliable way to determine intelligibility. One notable concern with such an approach is not knowing the words the speaker intended to say. Gordon-Brannon (1994) suggested that the procedure could be enhanced by including orthographic transcription by a caregiver as a reliability check. However, even parents may not know all of the words the child intended. Thus, whether or not parents are involved, it is very difficult to count the number of intended words in longer stretches of unintelligible speech. Shriberg and Kwiatkowski (1980) suggested that transcribers can reliably count and record the number of syllables produced. This is possible because each syllable contains only a single vowel, and vowels are louder than consonants; each syllable thus stands out as a peak of loudness. The syllables identified are then grouped into words using a 3:1 a rule. Every five unintelligible syllables would be assumed to include three single-syllable words and one two-syllable word. Shriberg and Kwiatkowski labeled their procedure an *intelligibility index (II).* A study by Flipsen (2006b) compared Shriberg and Kwiatkowski's syllable identification and grouping procedures with several other methods. Flipsen reported that the differences among the methods were small enough to reflect measurement error and, for clinical use, the original approach (counting intelligible words) had higher practical efficiency. Flipsen concluded that intelligibility of conversational speech of children can be reliably quantified.

An example of a closed-set word identification procedure for estimating speech sound intelligibility is the Children's Speech Intelligibility Measure (CSIM) that was developed by Wilcox and Morris (1999). This is a commercially published measure that involves a client imitating a list of single words after the examiner's model, with responses tape recorded. Words are drawn from a pool of 600 that are grouped into 50 sets of 12 phonetically similar words. One word from each of the 50 sets is randomly chosen as a target item for each CSIM administration. Because of this large pool of items, intelligibility estimates may be repeated with a new set of similar words each time it is administered. Following the recording, two or three independent judges listen to the tape and score the 50 words, selecting a response for each word from a list of 12 words that contain 11 phonetically similar foils. Although this test produces a quantitative index of intelligibility, it is based on single-word productions and, thus, may not be fully representative of conversational speech.

Another formal closed-set measure of intelligibility that can be used with young children is the Beginner's Intelligibility Test (BIT; Osberger et al., 1994). It was originally designed for children with hearing impairment, but could be used with any preschool child. The test consists of four sets of short sentences (see Box 6.2). The child is asked to repeat after the clinician saying each of the 10 sentences in one of the sets. The productions are recorded (without the clinician's productions on the recording), then two or three adult listeners with normal hearing are asked to listen to the sentences and write down what they think the child said. The average of the percentage of words correctly identified can be calculated and converted to percentage understood. The initial score provides a baseline. If the child is enrolled in therapy, the test can be readministered at regular intervals (using a different list each time) to monitor progress.

As noted earlier, rating scales are commonly used to measure intelligibility. They can however be problematic. In particular, most have not been validated in any formal way. As a consequence, individual ratings are often quite variable across clinicians. One recent example of a rating scale procedure that has shown better validity is the

---

BOX 6.2 Sentence Lists for Beginner's Intelligibility Test

List 1

1. The baby falls.
2. Mommy walks.
3. The duck swims.
4. The boy sits.
5. Grandma sleeps.
6. That is a little bird.
7. The boy walked to the table.
8. My car is blue.
9. He is brushing his teeth.
10. She is taking a bath.

List 2

1. Daddy runs.
2. The baby cries.
3. The dog eats.
4. The girl drinks.
5. The clown falls.
6. That is a big bed.
7. The boy walked to the chair.
8. My van is green.
9. They are playing the drums.
10. She is talking on the phone.

List 3

1. Daddy walks.
2. The bunny drinks.
3. The dog sleeps.
4. The girl jumps.
5. Mommy reads.
6. That is a brown chair.
7. The boy is on the table.
8. My airplane is big.
9. He is tying his shoe.
10. She is brushing her hair.

List 4

1. The bear sleeps.
2. Mommy sits.
3. The rabbit hops.
4. The cowboy jumps.
5. Grandma falls.
6. That is a black hat.
7. The boy is under the table.
8. My airplane is small.
9. He is painting the chair.
10. She is cooking dinner.

From Osberger, M. J., Robbins, A. M., Todd, S. L., & Riley, A. I. (1994). Speech intelligibility of children with cochlear implants. Used with permission.

Intelligibility in Context Scale (ICS) (McLeod, 2015, 2020; McLeod et al., 2012), which involves asking parents to rate their child's speech in response to seven questions:

1. Do you understand your child?

2. Do immediate members of your family understand your child?

3. Do extended members of your family understand your child?

4. Do your child's friends understand your child?

5. Do other acquaintances understand your child?

6. Do your child's teachers understand your child?

7. Do strangers understand your child?

For each question, possible responses are 1) never, 2) rarely, 3) sometimes, 4) usually, and 5) always. A validation study (McLeod et al., 2015) with 803 Australian children found mean scores ranging from 4.7 (out of 5) for Question 1 to 4.0 for Question 7. This finding suggested that the scale is broadly sensitive to listener familiarity. For children whose parents were concerned about their speech, overall mean scores were significantly lower (3.9) than for children whose parents were not concerned about their speech (4.6). There were no differences among children of different socioeconomic status or between monolingual children and those who were learning more than one language.

Clinical Vignette 6.2

Informal Estimates of Intelligibility

Clinicians have long recognized that intelligibility values are important to the assessment process and for measuring progress in therapy. A common approach to doing so occurs while clinicians are writing their assessment reports (author Peter Flipsen Jr. admits to having done this regularly in his work as a clinician). They try to recall how the entire interaction went and they come up with an informal estimate of how much of the client's speech they could understand (e.g., "Billy was 40% intelligible overall").

At a recent workshop given by author Peter Flipsen Jr., he wanted to see how reliable such estimates were. In a theatre-style lecture hall with about 100 clinicians with varying levels of clinical experience, he played a 5-minute excerpt from a conversation between a 4-year-old child with an SSD and an SLP. He then asked attendees to estimate what percentage of the child's speech they had understood. The following is a sample of what they reported:

25%, 65%, 15%, 80%, 35%, 50%, 70%, 60%, 40%, 30%, 75%, 20%, 65%, 30%, 35%, 60%, 20%, 70%, 40%, 50%

Who was right? This is not unimportant! Depending on which of these clinicians had been doing the assessment, very different clinical decisions might have been made. The point here is that these informal estimates are not at all valid. Intelligibility measures need to be based on a more specific and more controlled basis.

Regardless of the method used for estimating intelligibility, it should be kept in mind that individual listeners can vary widely in their intelligibility judgements (Hustad et al., 2015). It is strongly recommended, therefore, that more than one listener be used and scores averaged.

Single Word/Citation Form Sampling

Rationale. From the standpoint of widespread usage, analyzing phoneme productions in a corpus of single-word productions (usually elicited by having an examinee name pictures) has been the most common method for assessing speech sounds. This is sometimes referred to as a *speech sound inventory.* Single words provide a discrete, identifiable unit of production that examiners can usually readily transcribe. Because transcribers often are interested in observing the production of only one or perhaps two segments (sounds) per word, they are able to transcribe and analyze single-word samples more quickly than multiple- or connected-word samples. Even though a test can prescribe the scoring of only one or two sounds in a word, we recommend, particularly with children exhibiting multiple errors, that the tester consider transcribing the entire word, including the vowels. The efficiency of analyzing sound productions from single-word productions has resulted in widespread use of word stimuli. As suggested earlier, this type of sampling provides data that are supplemental to information obtained from the connected speech sample.

When sampling single words, most tests typically target only one or two consonants to be scored in each word. Sounds typically are assessed in the *initial* position (sound at the beginning of a word; e.g., /b/ in /bot/), *final* position (sound at the end of a word; e.g., /t/ in /ræbɪt/), and sometimes in the *medial* position (sounds between the initial and final sounds; e.g., /ɔ/, /k/, and /ɪ/ in /wɔkɪŋ/). However, the terms initial, medial, and final have been criticized as being somewhat problematic. For example, is the /l/ in /plet/ in initial or medial position? It could be argued that it is in initial position because it is part of an initial consonant cluster; on the other hand, it is not the initial sound in the word.

Alternative labels have been used to describe sounds' positions in words. In some instances, consonants are described relative to their location within syllables. *Prevocalic* position refers to consonants that precede a vowel (CV) and, therefore, initiate the syllable (e.g., *soap, cat*). *Postvocalic* position refers to consonants that follow the vowel (VC) and, therefore, terminate the syllable (e.g., soa*p*, ca*t*). *Intervocalic* position involves a consonant that is embedded (VCV) between two vowels (e.g., ca*m*el, ea*g*er). A singleton consonant in the initial position of a word is prevocalic. Likewise, a singleton sound in word-final position is postvocalic. A consonant in the intervocalic position often serves the dual function of ending the preceding syllable and initiating the following syllable. A medial consonant can stand next to another consonant and serve to initiate (release) or terminate (arrest) a syllable and, therefore, is not necessarily intervocalic. More recently, the terms *onset* (elements of a syllable before a vowel) and *coda* (elements of a syllable after a vowel) have been used, particularly when sounds are studied as part of literacy development. Thus, references to initial, medial, and final positions refer to location of consonants in a word, whereas the terms prevocalic, intervocalic, postvocalic, onset, and coda refer to consonant position relative to syllables.

As mentioned earlier, speech sound performance may vary across different tasks owing to differing production demands. It should be noted, however, when considering such variations, that research findings have shown a positive correlation between responses obtained from naming pictures and speech sound productions in spontaneous speaking situations. In spite of this finding, clinicians need to be aware that sound productions in single words may or may not accurately reflect the same sounds produced in a spontaneous speech context. Morrison and Shriberg (1992) reviewed 40 years of studies that were designed to compare citation-form testing (single-word testing) with continuous-speech sampling. They reported that, in general, more errors occur in spontaneous connected speech as compared to production of single words, although there were instances and reports in which speech sound errors were more frequent in single words. However, in their own research, they reported that children produced sounds more accurately in connected speech when those sounds were well established but more accurately in citation-form testing when those sounds were just emerging.

The nature of the stimuli being used in these tests may affect the results obtained. Harrington and associates (1984) reported that children produced fewer errors when items were elicited via photographs as compared to line drawings. The structure of the words used in single-word tests may also be a factor. James and colleagues (2016) suggested that such tests consist largely of single-syllable words, which may not be sufficiently demanding to reveal a child's typical errors. James and colleagues reported that in a sample of 283 children aged 3;0 to 7;11 a significantly greater number of errors were produced on polysyllabic words than on single-syllable words. Work by Masso, McLeod, and colleagues (2016, 2017) supports a need to pay much more attention to performance on polysyllabic stimuli. Despite reservations about making inferences concerning conversational speech based on single-word samples, most clinicians value and include single-word productions in the assessment battery. Commercially available tests that are commonly used in the United States are highlighted in Table 6.1. A comprehensive review and comparison of these tests is beyond the scope of the current text, but many of them were reviewed by Flipsen and Ogiela (2015).

What seems appropriate to mention here is that there is considerable variation across the tests in Table 6.1. Most cover a range of ages, some allow for testing children as young as 18 months, and some can be used with adults. The number of test items varies from as few as 30 to as many as 80. These tests also vary in other ways. For example, one test can present items in the developmental sequence of sound mastery, whereas another can organize the analysis according to place and manner of articulation. Many employ colored drawings that are especially attractive to young children; however, others elicit responses with photographs or line drawings. Some tests elicit responses through imitation tasks rather than naming pictures, photographs, line drawings, or toys.

For clinicians, single-word tests offer several distinct advantages over conversational speech sampling. They include most, if not all, of the consonants in a language and do so in a relatively short time period. In addition, for unintelligible clients, the examiner has the advantage of knowing the words the client has attempted to say. Another advantage is that for purposes of determining eligibility for services, particularly in the public schools, clinicians can generate standardized scores. These are available because the test developers have administered the test to a large sample of the general population as a basis for comparison. It should be noted that, as shown in Table 6.1, the term *large* has been defined differently by different test developers, as the size of the normative samples ranges from 650 to more than 3,000.

In addition to concerns about whether they represent typical production, single-word tests also have other limitations. Such measures do not allow children to use their own words but involve production of a set of predetermined syllable and word shapes. Clinicians should recognize that syllable shape and stress patterns of stimulus words can affect speech sound productions. As well, citation tests primarily consist of nouns because they can be pictured; thus, they do not reflect all the parts of speech used in connected conversational speech.

Table 6.1. Single word citation tests

Test name	Age range[a]	Size of normative sample	Number of test words	Word positions tested
Arizona Articulation and Phonology Scale (4th ed.; AAPS-4; Fudala & Stegall [2017])	1;6 to 21;11	3,192	53	I, F
Bankson-Bernthal Test of Phonology (2nd ed.; BBTOP-2; Bankson & Bernthal [2020])	3;0 to 9;11	770	80	I, F
Clinical Assessment of Articulation and Phonology (2nd ed.; CAAP-2; Secord & Donahue [2014])	2;6 to 11;11	1,486	44	I, F
Diagnostic Evaluation of Articulation and Phonology (American edition; DEAP; Dodd, Hua, et al. [2006])	3;0 to 8;11	650	30	I, F
Glaspey Dynamic Assessment of Phonology (GDAP; Glaspey [2019])[c]	3;0 to 10;11	880	49	I, F
Goldman-Fristoe Test of Articulation (3rd ed.; GFTA-3; Goldman & Fristoe [2015])	2;0 to 21;11	1,500	60	I, M, F
Hodson Assessment of Phonological Patterns (3rd ed.; HAPP-3; Hodson [2004])	3;0 to 7;11	886	50	n/a[b]
LinguiSystems Articulation Test (LAT; Hardison et al. [2010])	3;0 to 21;11	3,030	52	I, M, F
Photo Articulation Test (3rd ed.; PAT-3; Lippke et al. [1997])	3;0 to 8;11	800	72	I, M, F
Structured Photographic Articulation Test featuring Dudsbury (3rd ed.; SPAT-D-3; Tattersall & Dawson [2016])	3;0 to 9;11	2,473	51	I, M, F
Woodcock-Camarata Articulation Battery (WCAB; Woodcock et al. [2019])[c]	2;0 to 90;0	1,096	varies	I, M, F

[a] Expressed in years; months.

[b] Assesses errors based on phonological patterns only (not standard word positions).

[c] Uses nontraditional approach to scoring (see text).

Source: Flipsen & Ogiela (2015). *Key:* I, initial; M, medial; F, final.

Another difficulty with single-word tests designed to elicit a sample via picture naming is that they often elicit only a single production of a given sound in each of either two or three word positions. During phonological development, inconsistency in production is common, even in the same stimulus word. Because the production of a sound can fluctuate, the client's customary articulatory patterns can be difficult to determine with only one to three samples of a sound. The clinician can increase the number of sound samples obtained through a single-word test by transcribing all the sounds in each stimulus (lexical) item instead of focusing only on one or two sounds in each stimulus item. They can also add words that include particular phonemes in order to provide additional opportunities to produce sounds of interest.

On balance, single-word tests remain a valuable and widely used tool. Largely because of concerns with obtaining speech samples that more closely represent what speakers typically do, we strongly recommend that both types of samples (single words and conversational speech) be included in the assessment battery.

Elicitation Procedures.   Single-word citation tests involve having a client name single words in response to picture stimuli. These tests employ very common words that most children likely know. However, when testing very young children (or those with comorbid language delays), the previous discussion about spontaneous versus imitated productions should be kept in mind. In order to compare a child's score to developmental norms for the test it is necessary for the client to produce all of the words on the test. For children who don't know the words, clinicians may need to rely heavily on imitated productions. To avoid this issue or to supplement it when it arises, single-word samples can also be obtained by having a child name toys or objects, or by asking questions that might lead to spontaneous productions. The clinician may also simply wish to transcribe single-word productions the child produces spontaneously during conversational or play interactions.

Scoring Procedures.   Typically, all of the items on a citation test are presented to the client and any errors present are noted. For most tests, errors are noted for each individual phoneme and classified by traditional articulatory error type (e.g., substitution of /p/ for /f/) and/or by phonological pattern type (e.g., final consonant deletion). The total number of errors is then compared to the developmental norms provided with the test to yield one or more types of norm-referenced scores.

Two recently published tests listed in Table 6.1 are scored somewhat differently. For the GDAP (Glaspey, 2019), the initial attempt at each word is first examined for errors. Any error is then probed using a series of supportive prompts to determine if correct production can be elicited. This is a form of stimulability testing (to be discussed next) and performance is scored from 1 to 15 based on the amount of support needed to elicit a correct response (if at all possible). Those stimulability scores are then totaled and compared against the developmental norms for the test.

With the Woodcock-Camarata Articulation Battery (WCAB; Woodcock et al., 2019), scoring is computer-based and initially each word production is only scored for total correctness. For any words where errors are observed, syllable and phoneme judgments can be made, but transcription is not required. Camarata and colleagues (2019) noted that the reasoning behind using word-level accuracy judgments is that they are much more reliable than phoneme-based scoring. The software uses decision-tree logic to generate norm-referenced scores as well as a *relative mastery index (RMI)*. RMI represents the percentage of error-free productions relative to age-mates. Complete phoneme-level analysis is also possible for generating treatment goals.

Assessment of Vowels

As stated previously, one concern with published single-word tests is their heavy focus on consonants; they have traditionally placed little emphasis on the assessment of vowels. Our assessment tools are not completely lacking, however. Some published single-word articulation tests do allow for more detailed vowel analysis. For example, the GFTA-3 (Goldman & Fristoe, 2015) includes a vowel screener. As well, vowel analysis is possible using the DEAP (Dodd, Hua, et al., 2006), the Arizona Articulation and Phonology Scale (AAPS-4; Fudala & Stegall, 2017), and the Kaufman Speech

Praxis Test for Children (Kaufman, 1995). Another assessment instrument that targets the assessment of vowels in addition to consonants is the Toddler Phonology Test (McIntosh & Dodd, 2013). This is intended for assessment of 2-year-old children and allows for evaluation of both consonants and vowels. It does not have normative data for American English but does allow for a systematic examination of early vowel productions.

The lack of attention to vowels is undoubtedly a reflection of the fact that most preschool and school-age children with SSDs have problems primarily with consonants and that vowels are typically mastered at a relatively early age. However, SLPs are increasingly involved in early intervention programs for children at risk for communication impairments. As well, at least three other populations wherein vowels are more of a concern have been receiving more of our attention. These include 1) second-language learners (see Chapter 14), 2) individuals with significant hearing impairment (Ertmer et al., 1996; Levitt & Stromberg, 1983), and 3) individuals with CAS (Jacks et al., 2013). As such, vowel productions have been increasingly scrutinized (see Ball & Gibbon, 2002, 2013, for a discussion).

As recommended earlier, it is suggested that when using commonly used speech sound instruments, clinicians should transcribe the entire response to the stimuli word rather than just the sound focused on by the test developers. This is especially important with children who reflect multiple misarticulations. The transcription for the entire word will capture some of the client's vowel performance. To conduct a comprehensive review of vowels and diphthongs, it may be necessary to supplement existing stimuli with additional vowels, diphthongs, and contexts not included in standard tests. Pollock (1991) has suggested the following approach:

1. Clients should be provided multiple opportunities to produce each vowel.

2. Vowels should be assessed in a variety of different contexts, including a) monosyllabic and multisyllabic words, b) stressed and unstressed syllables, and c) a variety of adjacent preceding and especially following consonants.

3. Limits for the range of responses considered correct or acceptable should be established because cultural or dialect influences can affect what is considered correct. This will be discussed again in Chapter 14.

Informal analysis of vowel accuracy is also possible. For example, it can be calculated from conversational speech samples using metrics such as percentage vowels correct (PVC; Shriberg, Austin, et al., 1997). Identification of problems with specific vowels would require a more comprehensive analysis. A set of single-word productions that samples all of the vowels and diphthongs could be elicited for this purpose. One such sample that could potentially be appropriate for young children (adapted from Penney et al., 1994) is shown in Table 6.2 (note that some words are repeated as they sample more than one vowel). These words may be elicited using a combination of picture stimuli and imitation.

Summary.   Single-word samples, usually obtained via speech sound tests, provide an efficient and relatively easy method for obtaining a sample of speech sound productions. Although they can be a valuable part of the speech sound assessment battery, they should not constitute the only sampling procedure. Among their limitations are the small number of phonetic contexts sampled, the failure to reflect the effects

Table 6.2. Single-word stimuli for sampling American English vowels in young children

Vowel	Monosyllabic words			Polysyllabic words	
	V-initial	Open syllables	Closed syllables	Stressed	Unstressed
/i/	eat	key	wheel	Easter	movie
		bee	seal	zebra	bunny
/ɪ/	in		fish	pillow	sandwich
			pig	sister	
/e/	eight	day	cake	crayon	Sunday
			rain	table	
/ɛ/	'F'		red	feather	hello
/æ/	ant		cat	apple	snowman
	and		mask	candle	
/u/		shoe	boot	Snoopy	bathroom
				balloon	
/ʊ/			book	cookie	
			foot	woolly	
/o/	old	no	soap	bowling	pillow
			boat	snowman	radio
/ɑ/	on	saw	dog	pocket	peacock
				water	
/ʌ/	up		duck	bubble	
			sun	bunny	
/ə/					zebra
					wagon
/aɪ/	ice	pie	knife	tiger	bye-bye
	eyes	tie	five	lion	
/aʊ/	out	cow	clown	tower	bow-wow
			down	cowboy	
/ɔɪ/	oink	toy	noise	noisy	cowboy
				poison	
/ɝ/		fur	bird	turtle	
				Ernie	
/ɚ/					feather
					sister

of conversational context, the questionable representativeness of single-word naming responses, limited attention to vowels, and factors associated with variations of syllable shape, prosody, word familiarity, and parts of speech (e.g., nouns, verbs). Additional informal analysis is also suggested.

Stimulability Testing

Rationale.   Another sample of speech sound productions frequently included in a test battery is obtained through stimulability testing; that is, sampling the client's ability to imitate the correct form (adult standard) of error sounds when provided with stimulation. Traditionally, this testing has examined how well an individual imitates, in one or more phonetic contexts (i.e., isolation, syllables, words, phrases), sounds that were produced in error during testing.

Stimulability testing has been used 1) to determine whether a sound is likely to be acquired without intervention, 2) to determine the level and/or type of production at which instruction might begin, and 3) to predict the occurrence and nature of generalization. In other words, these data are often used when making decisions regarding case selection and determining which speech sounds to target in treatment.

Investigators have reported that the ability of a child to imitate syllables or words is related to normal speech sound acquisition, as well as to the probability of a child spontaneously correcting their misarticulations (Miccio et al., 1999). Pretest and post-test comparisons with kindergarten and first-grade children have indicated that untreated children with high stimulability skills tended to perform better than children with low stimulability scores. For participants who were not stimulable, direct instruction on speech sounds was found to be necessary because most did not self-correct their errors.

It has also been reported that good stimulability also suggests more rapid progress in treatment (Carter & Buck, 1958; Farquhar, 1961; Irwin et al., 1966; Sommers et al., 1967). Carter and Buck reported, in a study of first-grade children, that stimulability testing can be used for such prognostic purposes. They reported that first-grade children who correctly imitated error sounds in nonsense syllables were more likely to correct those sounds without instruction than children who were not able to imitate their error sounds. Kisatsky (1967) compared the pre- to post-test gains in articulation accuracy over a 6-month period in two groups of kindergarten children, one identified as a high stimulability group and the other as a low stimulability group. Although neither group received articulation instruction, results indicated that significantly more speech sounds were self-corrected by the high stimulability group in the 6-month post-test when compared to the low stimulability group.

It could be inferred from these studies that individuals with poor stimulability skills should be seen for treatment because it is unlikely that such children will self-correct their speech sound errors. Children with good stimulability skills tend to show more self-correction of their speech sound errors; however, this finding is not true for all children. As a result, stimulability is only one factor to be used in making decisions about treatment and target selection (see also Clinical Vignette 6.3).

Stimulability has also been found to be an important factor in generalization. Elbert and McReynolds (1978) noted that generalization of correct /s/ production to a variety of contexts occurred as soon as the children learned to imitate the sound. In addition, Powell and colleagues (1991) reported that stimulability was the most decisive variable they examined in explaining generalization patterns and could be used to explain and predict generalization patterns. They concluded that clinicians should target nonstimulable sounds first because nonstimulable sounds are unlikely to change, whereas children may self-correct many stimulable sounds during treatment even without direct instruction on those stimulable sounds. Note once again, however, that this does not apply to all children with SSDs. This may be because (as discussed in Chapter 4) being stimulable may not be a sufficient marker for target selection.

   The concept of stimulability has been used in various ways. Glaspey (2012) noted that early use of the term referred to a global score of overall ability, but more current use is relative to performance for individual phonemes. Clinicians seek to determine whether the child either is stimulable or not stimulable for a particular sound. In addition, clinicians often specify the level to which the child is stimulable (e.g., X was stimulable for word initial /k/ at the syllable and word levels but not the phrase level). Glaspey went on to suggest the need for a broader application of the concept that involves ". . . continual assessment throughout the treatment process to determine changes in a child's abilities as a result of participation in treatment" (p. 12). In other words, it can be used as both a measure of potential for change as well as an index of change itself. Such use would be based on the systematic application of additional stimulation support, such as placement instruction and visual/tactile imagery to determine the level of support the child needed to correctly produce the sound. Now published as the GDAP (Glaspey, 2019; see also Table 6.1), the child's performance for a particular sound is assigned a score from 1 to 15 based on a matrix of the amount of support needed and the highest level of linguistic complexity at which the sound is correctly produced. As the child progresses through therapy, the procedure is readministered at regular intervals. The utility of this measure is the subject of ongoing investigation.

Clinical Vignette 6.3

Stimulability and Readiness?

Author Nicholas Bankson recalls the situation of his preschool daughter who consistently produced a /θ/ for /s/ substitution. He administered a sound in isolation and nonsense syllable assessment when she was aged 4 years, and she could produce /s/ correctly in all contexts. As an SLP, Dr. Bankson was curious to see whether his daughter would self-correct the /s/ sound.

   By the time his daughter reached kindergarten, no change in production had occurred. Because her consistent lisping was bothering his SLP sensibilities, Dr. Bankson decided she would be a good client at the university clinic for a practicum student. However, once his daughter was told she was going to be getting some help for her /s/ problem (and without any instruction from her dad) she began to self-correct and the error very quickly disappeared.

   Who knows what the dynamics were that fostered this change, but at a basic level, her stimulability appeared to allow her to change her speech and forgo an intervention program. It should perhaps be added that the university clinic director was sorry to lose what appeared to be an ideal candidate for a clinician's initial clinical experience.

   Beyond the GDAP, few standardized procedures for conducting stimulability testing are available. Some tests, such as the Goldman-Fristoe Test of Articulation (GFTA-3; Goldman & Fristoe, 2015) and the Bankson-Bernthal Test of Phonology (BBTOP-2; Bankson & Bernthal, 2020), include stimulability subtests. As an alternative, Adele Miccio (personal communication, 2002) suggested an informal but systematic measurement probe that would assess a child's stimulability for consonant errors by reviewing whether a client can imitate an error sound in isolation and then in the initial, medial, and final positions when juxtaposed to the vowels /i/, /ɑ/, and /u/. For example, if /s/ is the target error sound, the client would be asked to imitate the sound in isolation and then in the following syllable contexts: /si, isi, is, sɑ, ɑsɑ, ɑs, su, usu, us/. Thus, the child would be imitating the target sound in 10 productions, for which a percentage of correct productions for each sound would then be obtained. This stimulability probe is similar to that originally suggested by Carter and Buck (1958). The 2019 edition of the BBTOP-2 includes a very similar subtest to that proposed by Miccio.

Elicitation Procedures.   In the typical approach (similar to that of both Miccio and Carter & Buck [1958]), the instruction prior to production is, "Look at me, listen, and say what I say." The examiner typically does not point out where teeth, tongue, or lips are positioned during production or provide any other cues or instruction. If the client is unsuccessful at imitating the sound, some examiners engage in cueing or trial instruction, providing directions for how to make sounds. The GDAP described previously represents a highly structured approach to such trial instruction. Information obtained through such trials may also be used in selecting targets and determining the direction of treatment.

The focus of stimulability testing usually includes only imitative testing of those sounds produced in error in single-word and/or conversational samples. Clinicians usually want to assess imitation in isolation, nonsense syllables (usually in prevocalic, intervocalic, and postvocalic positions), and words (again, across-word positions). Cooperation of the child, number of sounds produced in error, and success with imitation are factors the clinician should consider when deciding how extensive the stimulability assessment should be.

As an example, in the case of a client with a /θ/ for /s/ error or [θʌn] for [sʌn], the client could be asked to initiate /s/ as follows:

1. Isolation: /s/ 6 trials

2. Nonsense syllables:

    /si/   /isi/   /is/

    /sɑ/   /ɑsɑ/   /ɑs/

    /su/   /usu/   /us/

3. Words:

    sail   bicycle   ice

    sun   baseball   horse

    seal   missile   bus

Summary.   Stimulability testing is generally considered useful in identifying those individuals most likely to need phonological intervention (those with poor stimulability performance) and for determining stimulus items for initiation of instruction. Stimulability performance has been found to have some prognostic value for identifying those speech sound errors a child will likely self-correct and/or that will generalize most quickly in therapy. However, other factors may be involved. For example, as discussed in Chapter 4, stimulability and speech perception skills likely interact somewhat in determining whether performance will improve on its own.

Contextual Testing

Rationale.   As indicated earlier, speech sound errors, especially in children, can be variable and inconsistent. Some of this inconsistency may reflect the fact that sounds are often easier to produce in some contexts as opposed to others. It should not be surprising, therefore, that identifying those contexts that are more or less difficult for an individual client (i.e., contextual testing) can be used when making treatment decisions, such as choosing sounds or sound patterns to work on in therapy or identifying a particular phonetic context that facilitates accurate sound production.

Contextual influences are based on the concept that sound productions influence each other in the ongoing stream of speech. McDonald (1964a) and others have suggested that valuable clinical information can be gained by systematically examining a sound as it is produced in varying contexts. McDonald coined the term *deep test* to refer to the practice of testing a sound in a wide variety of phonetic contexts. Coarticulatory effects consist of mechanical constraints associated with adjacent sounds and simultaneous preprogramming adjustments for segments later in the speech stream. This overlapping of movements (preprogramming) can extend as far as six phonetic segments away from a given sound (Kent & Minifie, 1977). Although the primary influence would appear to be sounds immediately preceding or following a target sound (Zehel et al., 1972), we know that as a result of coarticulatory effects, segments can be produced correctly in one context but not in another. Such information is of value to the clinician who seeks to establish a particular sound segment in a client's repertoire and can be useful to determine a starting point in therapy.

Elicitation Procedures.   Several procedures are available to assess consistency-contextual influences. These include the Secord Contextual Articulation Tests (S-CAT) (Secord & Shine, 1997a) and the Contextual Test of Articulation (Aase et al., 2000). The S-CAT consists of three components: 1) Contextual Probes of Articulation Competence (CPAC), 2) Storytelling Probes of Articulation Competence (SPAC), and 3) Target Words for Contextual Training (TWAC; Secord & Shine, 1997b). The CPAC and SPAC are designed to assess 23 consonants and vocalic /ɚ/ in various phonetic contexts through word and connected speech samples and can be used with clients from preschool through adult. The Contextual Test of Articulation tests 5 consonant sounds and 15 consonant clusters through sentence completion items in several vowel contexts.

In addition to published contextual tests, an informal contextual analysis can be performed by reviewing a connected speech sample for contexts in which a target sound is produced correctly. Occasionally, facilitating contexts can be found in conversations that are not observed in single words or word pairs. For example, the /s/ sound might be incorrect in production of /sʌn/ but be produced correctly when the /s/ sound is juxtaposed with /t/, as in /bæts/ or /stɔp/. Phonemes can also be examined in various morphophonemic alterations to determine the effect of morpheme structure on phonological productions. Such alterations can be examined by having the client produce a sound in differing morphophonemic structures. For example, to determine whether word-final obstruent /g/ has been deleted in /dɔg/ (i.e., [dɔ]), the examiner might assess whether /g/ is produced in the diminutive /dɔgi/. Likewise, when the child misarticulates /z/ in the word /roz/, the examiner might also want to observe /z/ production in the morphophonemic context of /rozəz/ to determine whether the error is a sound production problem or a problem with marking plurality (a language-related difficulty).

Consonants can also be examined for correct phoneme productions in the context of consonant clusters. Although it is true that, in most instances, a consonant is more likely to be produced correctly as a singleton rather than in consonant clusters, it is not unusual for sounds to be produced correctly in the context of a cluster, even when misarticulated in a singleton context. For example, a child might produce a correct /s/ in *stick* but not in *sick,* or a correct /r/ in *grain* but not in *rain.*

Summary. Contextual testing is conducted to determine phonetic contexts in which a sound error may be produced correctly. These contexts can then be used to identify a starting point for remediation. Contextual testing is also used as a measure of consistency of misarticulation. It should be pointed out that although contextual testing can be very helpful to a clinician, this type of assessment is not a routine part of a speech sound assessment, largely because of the amount of time required in testing and analysis. Thus, it is often identified as a supplemental aspect of a testing battery, formally employed when it would appear to be particularly useful with a given client who likely is a candidate for treatment services.

Error Pattern Identification

For children with multiple errors, the assessment battery usually includes a measure designed to identify sound error patterns or commonalities that occur across error productions.

Rationale. In an effort to obtain an understanding of speech sound errors in a client with multiple errors, clinicians need to identify error patterns that encompass several individual speech sound targets. A phonological pattern (the preferred term rather than process, which is also a term that continues to be used) is typically defined as "a systematic sound change or simplification that affects a class of sounds, a particular sequence of sounds, or the syllable structure of words." The identification of phonological patterns assumes that children's speech sound errors are not random but represent systematic variations from the adult standard.

One of the reasons pattern analysis procedures have appeal is that they provide a more complete description of the child's overall phonological system. For example, if a child leaves the phonemes /p, b, k, g, t, s, z/ off the end of words, the pattern can be described as final consonant deletion. Khan (1985) furnished another illustration of a phonological process/pattern. A child who substitutes /wawa/ for *water* might be described in a traditional substitution analysis as substituting [w] for /t/ and substituting [a] for final /ɚ/. On the basis of what we know about speech sound acquisition, the [wawa] for *water* substitution is more accurately described as syllable reduplication, a common pattern seen in young children. The child in this instance is probably repeating the first syllable of the word *water,* /wa/, rather than using individual sound substitutions for target sounds in the second syllable. In this example, the child is also demonstrating knowledge of syllable structure because *water* contains two syllables, as does the production /wawa/. Consistent with the theory of natural phonology (discussed in Chapter 3), the child appears to understand at some level what the target is supposed to be but is temporarily limited in their ability to fully express and produce it.

A second reason for doing a pattern analysis is the potential for facilitating treatment efficiency. When a pattern reflecting several sound errors is targeted for treatment, the potential exists for enhancing generalization across sounds related to that pattern by working on one or more sounds that reflect that pattern and looking for generalization to other sounds reflected in the same error pattern.

Systems of pattern analysis, whether based on the relatively simple place-manner-voicing analysis or the more commonly employed phonological pattern procedures, are most appropriate for the client who has multiple errors. The intent of the analysis is to determine whether there are patterns (commonalities) or relationships among speech sound errors. In contrast, for a child who makes only a few speech sound errors, a phonological pattern analysis would provide minimal additional insight into the child's phonological system. For example, if a client is misarticulating only two consonants, /s/ and /r/, the clinician would likely develop a remediation plan that targets both consonants for direct instruction.

Phonological patterns identified in the child's speech can also aid in treatment target selection. For example, if a child has eight speech sound substitutions reflecting three error patterns (e.g., stopping of fricatives, gliding of liquids, fronting), remediation would likely focus on the reduction of one or more of these phonological patterns. The modification of one or more speech sounds (exemplars) reflecting a particular error pattern frequently results in generalization to other speech sounds reflecting the same error pattern. For example, establishment of /p/ and /f/ in word-final position for a child who deletes final consonants may generalize to other stops and fricatives deleted in word-final position.

Another example of a pattern-oriented remediation strategy for instruction would be to target all speech sounds that appear to be simplified in a similar manner, such as fricatives being replaced with stops (i.e., stopping). In this instance, the clinician might focus on the contrast between stops and fricatives. By focusing on sounds that reflect a similar error pattern, treatment should be more efficient than if it were to focus on individual sounds without regard to phonological patterns. To borrow an old expression, the clinician may be killing two (or more) birds with one stone.

Elicitation Procedures.   Several analysis procedures that are based on identifying phonological patterns have been published. These include several of the single-word tests listed in Table 6.1 (e.g., AAPS-4, BBTOP-2, Clinical Assessment of Articulation and Phonology [CAAP-2, Secord & Donahue, 2014], DEAP, HAPP-3, Structured Photographic Articulation Test [SPAT-D-3; Tattersall & Dawson, 2016]). Pattern analysis can also be carried out on data from the GFTA-3 using the Khan-Lewis Phonological Analysis (3rd ed.) (KLPA-3; Khan & Lewis, 2015). In addition to these published analysis procedures, productions recorded during connected speech sampling and/or single-word testing can be analyzed manually for the presence of error patterns (pattern definitions are provided in Chapter 7). It should also be pointed out that several computer-based programs can assist the clinician in analyzing error patterns (discussed in Chapter 7). As well, some test publishers are beginning to create online platforms where transcriptions can be entered and then are scored automatically (e.g., KLPA-3).

Summary.   Phonological pattern analysis facilitates identification of commonalities among error productions. This analysis offers the potential to make target selection, treatment structure, and generalization more efficient.

Criteria for Selecting Phonological Assessment Instruments

Clinicians have a number of formal published test instruments to consider for use. Reviews of both single-word tests (Flipsen & Ogiela, 2015) and tests that provide procedures for the analysis of phonological patterns (Kirk & Vigeland, 2014, 2015) can be consulted for additional details of their content. Selection is, however, up to each clinician and should be appropriate to the individual being tested. The clinician should carefully consider the sample the instrument is designed to obtain, the nature of the stimulus materials (e.g., how easily recognized are the target pictures or objects?), the scoring system, and the type of analysis facilitated by the instrument. Practical considerations in test selection include the amount of time required to administer the instrument and analyze the sample obtained, as well as the cost of purchasing the test and any test forms. The following is a discussion of some of these variables in more detail.

Sample Obtained

Test instruments vary in the representativeness of the speech sample obtained. Variables to evaluate include the specific consonants, consonant clusters, vowels, and diphthongs tested, as well as the units in which sounds are to be produced (i.e., syllables, words, sentences). In addition, stimulus presentation and type of sample elicited (e.g., picture naming, sentence completion, imitation, delayed imitation, conversation) should also be considered when selecting instruments.

Material Presentation

Another practical factor that should be considered when selecting commercially available tests is the attractiveness, compactness, and manipulability of materials. Size, familiarity, and color of stimulus pictures and appropriateness to the age of the client can influence the ease with which the clinician obtains responses to test stimuli. In addition, the organization and format of the scoring sheet are important for information retrieval. Tests with familiar and attractive stimulus items and score sheets that facilitate analysis are desirable.

Scoring and Analysis

Because the scoring and analysis procedures that accompany a test determine the type of information obtained from the instrument, they are important considerations in test selection. Currently available assessment instruments are designed to facilitate one or more of the following types of analysis: 1) analysis of consonant and vowel sounds of the language; 2) sound productions in a variety of word or syllable positions and phonetic contexts; 3) place, manner, voice analysis; 4) phonological pattern/process analysis; 5) age appropriateness; 6) speech sound stimulability assessment; and 7) contextual assessment. Some tests provide guidance relative to how to score productions from speakers of nonstandard dialects or second language learners, which may also be a consideration. A practical consideration relates to how much time is required to complete an analysis versus the value of information obtained. A careful study of the test manual is usually a good first step in making a determination of which assessment instrument to use for a given exam.

Transcription and Scoring Procedures

Methods for Recording Responses

The recording systems used by clinicians vary according to the purposes of testing, the transcription skills of the examiner, and personal preferences. The type of response recording the examiner employs will, however, determine the type of analysis the clinician is able to perform with the sample obtained. In turn, the type of analysis conducted can significantly influence instructional decisions, which frequently include a recommended treatment approach.

In the least sophisticated scoring procedure, speech sound productions are simply scored as correct or incorrect based on the examiner's perception of whether the sound produced is within the acceptable adult phoneme boundary. This type of scoring is sometimes used to assess day-to-day progress, but is not recommended when doing a speech sound assessment designed to determine eligibility for or the direction of treatment because more detailed description is required for this purpose.

The most common transcription system for recording sound errors is the International Phonetic Alphabet (IPA), which includes a different symbol for each phoneme. As indicated in Chapter 2, more than 40 such symbols are utilized to identify the phonemes of the English language. This broad transcription system, supplemented with a set of *diacritics* (narrow markers), usually provides sufficient detail for speech-language clinicians to adequately describe speech sound productions. For example, in a broad transcription of the word *key,* one would transcribe the initial segment with the symbol /k/. A more precise transcription of the initial /k/ would include the diacritic for aspiration [ʰ] following word initial [kʰ] because aspiration occurs in production of /k/ in word-initial contexts. The aspiration modifier [ʰ] in this transcription represents one example of a diacritic. Use of diacritics, sometimes called a *close* or *narrow transcription,* allows for recording of specific topographical dimensions of individual segments and is recommended when broad transcription does not adequately describe an error. For example, if /s/ in the word /sʌn/ is lateralized (air emitted sideways rather than forward), the diacritic for lateralization is placed under the /s/, thus [s̪ʌn]. See Table 6.3 for a list of common symbols and diacritics for clinical use.

Table 6.3.   Symbols and diacritics

[x]	Voiceless velar fricative, as in *Bach*
[ɸ]	Voiceless bilabial fricative
[β]	Voiced bilabial fricative
[ʔ]	Gottal stop, as in [mʌʔi]
[ɹ̪]	r with [w] like *quality*
Stop release diacritics	
[ʰ]	Aspirated, as in [tʰæp]
[˭]	Unaspirated, as in [p˭un]
Diacritics for nasality	
[˜]	Nasalized, as in [fæ̃n]
[x̃]	Denasalized
[˷]	Produced with nasal emission
Diacritics for length	
[ː]	Lengthened
Diacritics for voicing	
[̥]	Partially devoiced, as in [spuṇ]
Diacritics for tongue position or shape	
[̪]	Dentalized, as in [tɛṉθ]
[̺]	Lateralized, as in [s̺op]

Diacritic markers are especially useful when describing the speech of individuals whose speech sound productions cannot be adequately described by broad phonetic symbols. For example, in assessing the speech sound status of an individual with a cleft condition who is unable to achieve velopharyngeal closure for certain speech sounds, diacritics indicating nasal emission on consonants (šneɪl) or nasalization of vowels (bæn) can be useful in the description of the client's production of such segments. Similarly, when assessing the articulation of an individual with impaired hearing, symbols to indicate appropriate vowel duration (e.g., [siː] for lengthened), devoicing (e.g., [b̥]), and denasalization (e.g., ræ̃n) are recommended if these characteristics are present in productions. Likewise, with developmental articulation errors characterized by lateralization (e.g., frequently observed with [s̞]), dentalization (e.g., [s̪]), and devoicing (e.g., [n̥]), diacritics should also be utilized. As suggested previously, the frequency with which diacritic markers are utilized is highly dependent on the nature of the types of clients seen by a clinician, as well as the types of speech sound errors that are observed.

Accuracy of Transcriptions

One of the major concerns regarding transcription of responses relates to accuracy. Clinicians must be concerned with whether their transcriptions are a valid representation of a client's productions. Beginning clinicians in particular often worry about the consistency of their transcriptions. Findings from a study by Munson and colleagues (2012) suggested, however, that they need not despair, as their abilities are likely to improve as they gain more clinical experience.

For most aspects of clinical phonology, auditory perceptual judgments by the examiner remain the primary basis of judgments and intervention decisions. Because of the dependence on perceptual judgments, it is important for clinicians to establish the reliability and validity of their perceptual judgments.

Interjudge Reliability.   Traditionally, clinicians have used agreement between two independent transcribers as a means of establishing reliability of judgments. *Interjudge agreement,* or *reliability,* is determined by the comparison of one examiner's transcriptions with those of another and is essential for reporting the results of speech sound research. In addition, for students beginning to make judgments about accuracy of speech sound productions, establishing interjudge reliability with a more experienced person can assist in the development of accurate judgments. A commonly used method called *point-to-point agreement* compares the clinicians' judgments on each test item. The number of items judged the same is divided by the total number of items being judged to determine a percentage of agreement between judges. As an example, if two judges were to agree on 17 of 20 items and disagree on 3, they would divide 17 by 20 and get 0.85, which would then be multiplied by 100 to obtain an interjudge reliability index of 85% agreement.

Intrajudge Reliability.   Along with knowing that their judgments agree with those of another examiner, the clinician also wants to know that their standards for judgments are consistent over time. Comparison of judgments made when scoring the same data on two separate occasions is referred to as *intrajudge reliability.* Recordings of responses are used to determine this type of reliability because two judgments of the same responses are made.

In a study of point-to-point reliability of judgments of broad and narrow phonetic transcription, Shriberg and Lof (1991) reported that for interjudge and intrajudge reliability, average agreement for broad transcriptions exceeded 90%, and for narrow transcriptions was 65% (interjudge) and 75% (intrajudge). As noted in the literature, formal assessment of the reliability of judgments is essential when doing speech sound research, but also important when one developmentally establishes the reliability of their perceptual judgments of speech sound productions.

Auditory perceptual judgments are occasionally supplemented with physiological measures (such as aerodynamic measures) and acoustical measures (such as that obtained from spectrographic analysis). The emergence of free acoustical analysis software such as PRAAT, developed by Boersma and Weenink (2021), has made the use of acoustic analysis by clinicians a much simpler proposition.

It should be remembered that data from these three types of measures might not always be consistent with each other. For example, a glottal substitution for a stop in word-final position could be identified via a spectrographic analysis, yet a listener might not hear the glottal production and, thus, will transcribe it as a deletion (omission). It must be recognized, however, that even the more objective measures of speech segments (i.e., acoustical and physiological recordings) are not devoid of human interpretation and no one-to-one correspondence exists among a phoneme production, perception, and/or acoustical and physiological measurements.

ASSESSMENT IN VERY YOUNG CHILDREN

Phonologic evaluation of young children (infants and toddlers) presents a series of clinical challenges. Anyone who has spent much time with this population will attest to the difficulty in keeping them focused on any one thing for more than a few minutes. Their small size and high-pitched voices means their voices don't carry far and, thus, clinicians may have difficulty hearing young children and knowing what they are saying. As well, much of their speech may be unintelligible and make judgments of productions difficult. Perhaps most importantly, such assessments must be accomplished within the broader context of evaluating overall communicative behavior. Because speech sound development is integrally related to development of cognition, language, and motor skills, those other aspects of a child's development generally need to be considered. However, for purposes of this text, it is useful to isolate phonologic considerations from the overall communication process.

As discussed in Chapter 3, much variability exists among young children in terms of the age at which specific speech sounds are acquired. Such variability makes it difficult to formulate strict developmental expectations and guidelines for the assessment of speech sound productions in infants and toddlers. Some guidelines can, however, be offered and are useful in the assessment of very young children. One of the first assessments of phonologic development involves determining whether the infant is progressing normally through the stages of infant vocalization. Speech sound productions emerge within the context of infant vocalizations at the prelinguistic level. Information presented in Chapter 3 regarding the characteristics of these stages is helpful in knowing about sound productions that typically occur during this developmental period, including the gradual shift from prelinguistic to linguistic behavior that typically occurs during the first year.

The point in time and/or development of young children when clinicians frequently become involved in assessing phonology occurs after 18–24 months. By this age, children typically have acquired approximately 50 words and are stringing two words together. With enough meaningful language production to examine, clinicians are usually interested in determining how the child is doing in comparison to age expectations (i.e., they do a relational analysis). In principle, this can be accomplished using some of the commonly used single-word tests listed in Table 6.1 (AAPS-4, GFTA-3, CAAP-2), which have children under age 3 years included in their test norms. As noted earlier, however, keeping these children focused long enough to complete these formal assessments can be a challenge. Two additional tests, the Toddler Phonology Test (TPT; McIntosh & Dodd, 2013) and the Profiles of Early Expressive Phonology (PEEPS; Stoel-Gammon & Williams, 2013) were both specifically developed with this very young population in mind.

For children younger than 18 months, or those older than this with limited vocal repertoires, the clinician seeks to describe the sounds the child uses for communication regardless of correct usage (i.e., an independent analysis). In typically developing children, first words typically occur at about 12 months of age, the transition stage occurs between 12 and 18 months, and two or three words are put together in sequence (strings) around 24 months. In children with speech delay, obviously these stages can occur at a later chronological age. Procedures for eliciting vocalizations from young children depend on the level of the child's development and can include a range of activities. These include such things as stimulating vocalizations during caregiving and feeding activities; informal play with a caregiver, sibling, or clinician; structured play; interactive storytelling; sentence repetition; retelling of a story told by the clinician (delayed imitation); narrative generation (about a favorite book); and spontaneous conversation.

Stoel-Gammon (1994) reported that at age 24 months, children can be categorized into three groups: 1) those who are typical in terms of linguistic development, 2) those who are slow developing (late talkers) but evidence no major deviations from patterns of normal acquisition, and 3) those whose developmental patterns deviate substantially from the broadest interpretation of norms in terms of order of acquisition or achievement of certain milestones. Stoel-Gammon indicated that the first group includes 85% of children, with the remaining 15% split between the second and third groups. Those in the second group would likely have a vocabulary of fewer than 50 words, a phonetic inventory with only four to five consonants, and a limited variety of vowels. They would otherwise be following the normal order of phoneme acquisition and not have unusual error types. These children should be monitored every 3–6 months to be certain that they catch up with the typical group. Children in the third group are those who should be considered for an early intervention program.

An independent analysis of phonology is typically based on some type of continuous speech sample and is designed to describe a child's productions without reference to adult usage. It would typically include the following (Stoel-Gammon & Dunn, 1985):

1. An inventory of sounds (consonants and vowels) classified by word position and articulatory features (e.g., place, manner, voicing).

2. An inventory of syllables and word shapes produced (e.g., CVC, CV, VC, CCV). For example, a toddler who says /tu/ for *soup* would be given credit for a CV utterance. Likewise, a production of /wɑwɑ/ for *water* would count as a CVCV production.

3. Sequential constraints on particular sound sequences (e.g., /ɛfʌnt/ for /ɛləfʌnt/).

One concern with using the spontaneous output of such young children is test–retest reliability of the sample being obtained. Morris (2009) examined this based on independent analyses of speech sound productions from 20-minute toddler play sessions. She examined speech sound inventories in initial and final position, word shapes, syllable structure level, and an index of phonetic complexity. She reported the highest degree of test–retest reliability for syllable structure level and phonetic complexity. Reliability values for the other measures were not statistically significant. She interpreted her findings to suggest that analysis of phonetic and word-shape inventories would likely require longer samples to yield reliable data.

Summary

Phonological evaluations with infants and toddlers are usually done within the context of an overall communication assessment because phonological development is integrally related to other aspects of development, such as cognition, motor development, and other aspects of linguistic development. Informal assessment involving independent analyses is typically done with very young children and for those with limited verbal repertoires. Usually, an independent analysis includes an inventory of sounds, syllables, and word shapes produced and phonological contrasts employed. Once a child has a vocabulary of approximately 50 words, relational analysis typically is employed as part of the assessment battery.

RELATED ASSESSMENT PROCEDURES

The assessment of a child with an SSD almost always includes testing and data-gathering procedures supplemental to those focusing directly on speech sound behavior. Information is gathered to provide a more comprehensive picture of an individual client and thereby contribute to a better understanding of their phonological status. It can also influence treatment recommendations that are made regarding a given client.

   These additional assessment procedures often include a case history; an oral cavity examination; and hearing, language, fluency, and voice screenings. These procedures can aid the clinician in identifying factors that may contribute to or be related to the delay or impairment of speech sound development. They may also help identify comorbid conditions or lead to referral to other specialists. As such, they may have a significant influence on treatment decisions. If, for example, a child has an issue with closure of the velopharyngeal port, referral to a cleft palate team might result in pharyngeal flap surgery or the fitting of an intraoral appliance, such as a palatal lift, prior to speech intervention.

   Appropriate related personnel (e.g., audiological, medical) must corroborate the presence of suspected sensory, structural, or neurological deficiencies, and their recommendations must be considered part of the assessment. Any of these factors can be important in making decisions regarding the need for therapy, the point at which therapy should begin, and the treatment to be prescribed. Although language, fluency, and voice screening are part of overall communication evaluations, they are not reviewed here.

Case History

To facilitate an efficient and effective assessment, a case history is usually obtained from the client or a parent/primary caregiver prior to collecting data directly from the child. This allows the clinician to identify 1) possible etiological factors; 2) the family's or client's perception of the problem; 3) the academic, work, home, and social environment of the client; and 4) medical, developmental, and social information about the client. It may also assist the clinician with establishing the initial diagnostic hypothesis or best guess as to what the core deficit might be. This may help with selecting specific test instruments for the direct assessment of the child.

Case history information is usually obtained in a written form completed by the client or parents. It is frequently supplemented by an oral interview. Specific questions on the phonological status of a young child might include the following:

1. Did your child babble as an infant? If so, can you describe it?

2. When did your child say their first words? What were they? When did they start putting words together?

3. Describe your child's communication problem and your concerns about it.

4. How easy is your child to understand by the family and by strangers?

5. What sounds and words does your child say?

6. What do you think caused your child's speech difficulty?

7. Is there any family history of speech difficulties and, if so, how would you describe them?

8. Have there been any issues with your child's ears and/or hearing?

For many clinicians, Items 3 through 8 may be of primary usefulness in the case history.

Although case histories obtained from the client and/or the client's family are products of memory and perception and, therefore, might not reflect total accuracy (Majnemer & Rosenblatt, 1994), parents and clients in general are fairly reliable informants. Thus, the case history provides the clinician with important background information that frequently influences assessment decisions and subsequent management recommendations.

Oral Cavity Examination

Oral cavity (oral mechanism) examinations are administered to describe the structure and function of the oral mechanism for speech purposes. In particular, dentition is observed for bite and missing teeth, and hard and soft palates are examined for clefts, submucous clefts, fistulas, and fissures. Size, symmetry, and movement of the lips; size and movement of the tongue; and symmetry, movement, and functional length of the soft palate are assessed.

To examine the intraoral structures, it is recommended that the client be seated immediately in front of the examiner with their head in a natural upright position and at a level that allows easy viewing. The examiner should wear surgical gloves. If the client is a young child, the examiner might have the child sit on a table, or the examiner can kneel on the floor. Although it might seem that the oral cavity would be viewed best when the client extends their head backward, such a position can distort normal relationships of the head and neck. The client's mouth usually should be at the examiner's eye level. A flashlight or other light source together with a tongue depressor aids in the examination. Observations should start at the front of the oral cavity and progress to the back. Because the oral cavity examination is important in identifying possible structural abnormalities, a description of how an examination is conducted follows.

For a more complete presentation of procedures for conducting an oral mechanism examination, see St. Louis and Ruscello (2000).

Dentition

For the examiner to evaluate the occlusal relationship (i.e., alignment of upper and lower jaws), the client should have the first molars in contact with each other because the occlusal relationship of the upper and lower dental arch is made with reference to these molar contacts (recall the discussion from Chapter 4). The upper dental arch is typically longer and wider than the lower dental arch; therefore, the upper teeth normally extend horizontally around the lower dental arch and the maxillary (upper) incisors protrude about one-quarter inch in front of the lower teeth and cover about one-third of the crown of the mandibular incisors. Such dental overjet is the normal relationship of the dental arches in occlusion.

The teeth are said to be in open bite when the upper teeth do not cover part of the lower teeth at any given point along the dental arch. Mason and Wickwire (1978) recommended that when evaluating occlusal relationships, the clinician should instruct the client to bite on the back teeth and to separate the lips. They further stated that while in occlusion the client should be asked to produce several speech sounds in isolation, especially /s/, /z/, /f/, and /v/. Although these sounds may not normally be produced by the client with teeth in occlusion, the standardization of air space dimensions and increases in pressure in the oral cavity can unmask a variety of functional relationships. For example, the child who usually exhibits an interdental lisp may be able to articulate /s/ surprisingly well with teeth together. This occluded position can also unmask and/or counteract habit patterns related to the protrusion of tongue and mandible on selected sounds.

Mason and Wickwire (1978) also suggested that when an individual with excessive overjet has difficulty with /s/, they should be instructed to rotate the mandible forward as a means of adaptation to the excessive overjet. As pointed out in Chapter 4, however, dental abnormality and speech problems are frequently unrelated; thus, a cause–effect relationship between occlusion deviation and articulation problems should not be assumed.

Hard Palate

The hard palate (i.e., the bony portion of the oral cavity roof) is best viewed when the client extends their head backward slightly. Normal midline coloration is pink and white. When a blue tint on the midline is observed, further investigation of the integrity of the bony framework is indicated. Such discoloration can be caused by a blood supply close to the surface of the palate and is sometimes associated with a submucous cleft (an opening in the bony palatal shelf). But a blue tint seen lateral to the midline of the hard palate usually suggests only an extra bony growth, which occurs in approximately 20% of the population.

When a submucous cleft of the hard palate is suspected, palpation (rubbing) of the mucous membrane at the midline of the most posterior portion of the hard palate (nasal spine) is recommended. Normally, at the back edge of the hard palate the posterior nasal spine points toward the back of the pharynx. A submucous cleft is indicated by the combination of 1) a missing posterior nasal spine, 2) a zona pellucida or translucent area in the midline of the soft palate, and 3) a bifid or divided uvula (Calnan, 1954; Reiter et al., 2011). Although many SLPs note the height of the hard palatal vault, most individuals with high palatal vaults use compensatory movements that allow for adequate speech sound production.

Soft Palate or Velum

The soft palate should be evaluated with the head in a natural upright position. When it is not in that position, changes in the structural relationships in the oral cavity area can prevent the viewing of velar function as it occurs during speech.

Mason and Wickwire (1978) cautioned that the assessment of velar function, especially velar elevation, should not be done with the tongue protruded or with the mandible positioned for maximum mouth opening. They recommended a mouth opening of about three-quarters of the maximum opening because velar elevation might be less than maximum when the mouth is open maximally.

The coloration of the soft palate, like that of the hard palate, should be pink and white. The critical factor in velar function is the effective or functional length of the velum, not the velar length per se. Effective velar length is the portion of tissue that fills the space between the posterior border of the hard palate and the posterior wall of the pharynx. Effective velar length is only one factor in adequate velopharyngeal sphincter function and provides little or no information concerning the function of the sphincter's pharyngeal component (see the following description), another critical factor for adequate velopharyngeal valving.

The final velar observation typically made is velar symmetry and elevation. When asked to sustain a vowel such as "ahhh," the client's velum should rise vertically and not deviate to either side. When the velum does not elevate, an inadequately functioning velopharyngeal sphincter should definitely be suspected. If it does elevate, it indicates normal movement, but seeing movement alone is not sufficient. Velopharyngeal closure also involves movement of the posterior and lateral pharyngeal walls, which cannot be viewed from the mouth. Confirming that velopharyngeal closure is normal requires specialized procedures 1) by an otolaryngologist viewing closure from the top with a nasendoscope inserted through the nose, 2) by a radiologist using a lateral fluoroscopic x-ray, or 3) by a speech pathologist using specialized equipment to study airflow and pressure through the mouth and nose (speech aerodynamics). However, if a child has normal resonance (nasality), one can assume that the velopharyngeal sphincter is working normally for speech purposes.

The posterior-most appendage or extension of the velum is the uvula, which has little or no role in speech production in English. However, a bifid uvula should alert the clinician to other possible anatomical deviations. A bifid uvula appears as two appendages rather than one and, as noted previously, is occasionally seen in the presence of submucous clefts and other abnormal anatomical findings. By itself and in the absence of excess nasality in speech, a bifid uvula is of limited diagnostic value.

Fauces

The next area to observe in the oral cavity is the faucial pillars and the tonsillar masses. Only in rare instances are these structures a factor in speech production (but recall Clinical Vignette 4.2). The presence or absence of tonsillar masses is noted and, if present, their size and coloration are observed. Redness or inflammation could be evidence of tonsillitis, and large tonsillar masses could displace the faucial pillars and reduce the isthmus (or space between the pillars).

Pharynx

The oropharyngeal area is difficult to view in an intraoral examination. The pharyngeal contribution to velopharyngeal closure cannot be assessed through intraoral viewing because pharyngeal valving occurs at the level of the nasopharynx, a level superior to that which can be observed through the oral cavity. In some individuals, movement of tissue to form a prominence or ridge (Passavant's pad) can be seen on the posterior wall of the pharynx. Passavant's pad is not visible at rest but (if present) can usually be seen during sustained phonation. Passavant's pad is present in approximately one-third of individuals with cleft palates but is otherwise rare. Because its presence may reflect a compensatory mechanism, the examiner should be alert to possible velopharyngeal valving problems. The presence of Passavant's pad could suggest that adenoidal tissue is needed for velopharyngeal closure, and this factor is usually considered in surgical decisions regarding adenoidectomies.

Considerable research has been conducted in the development of instrumental measures that can help in the assessment of velopharyngeal adequacy and function. Such measures are used to supplement clinical perceptions related to the adequacy of velopharyngeal function. Inadequate velopharyngeal function frequently is associated with hypernasal resonance, weak production of pressured consonants (i.e., stops, fricatives, and affricates), and nasal emission of air. A number of direct and indirect instrumental procedures can help to assess velopharyngeal function; for example, nasometer, videofluoroscopy, nasopharyngoscopy, and airflow (aerodynamic) measures. For more information about such techniques, see chapters in Kummer (2020).

Tongue

As pointed out in Chapter 4, the tongue is a primary articulator, and individuals are able to modify tongue movements to compensate for many structural variations in the oral cavity. In terms of tongue size, two problematic conditions are occasionally found. The first, termed *macroglossia,* is an abnormally large tongue. Although the incidence of this condition is relatively low, historically some have associated it with Down syndrome. Research data, however, indicate normal tongue size in this population, but low muscle tone in the tongue and an undersized oral cavity may be present (the combination of a normal-size tongue in a small oral cavity is what we previously termed *relative macroglossia*). The condition in which the tongue is abnormally small in relation to the oral cavity is termed *microglossia,* but this condition rarely, if ever, causes a speech problem.

It has been pointed out that tongue movements for speech activities show little relationship to tongue movements for nonspeech activities. Unless motor problems are suspected, little is gained by having the client perform a series of nonspeech tongue movements. Protrusion of the tongue or moving the tongue laterally from one corner of the mouth to the other can provide information about possible motor limitations or problems with control of the tongue.

The rapid speech movements observed in diadochokinetic tasks (syllabic repetition; e.g., /pʌ pʌ pʌ, pʌ tʌ kʌ/) provide some information with respect to speech function. The absolute number of syllables that an individual can produce in a given unit of time usually bears little relationship to articulatory proficiency, except when gross motor problems are present. For a discussion of the relationship between diadochokinetic testing and articulation, see Chapter 4. Mason and Wickwire (1978) suggested that the clinician focus on the pattern of tongue movement and the consistency of contacts during diadochokinetic tasks.

A short lingual frenum can restrict movement of the tongue tip. As discussed in Chapter 4, most individuals, however, acquire normal speech in spite of a short lingual frenum. If the client can touch the alveolar ridge with the tongue tip, the length of the frenum is probably adequate for speech purposes. In the rare instance in which this is not possible, surgical intervention may be necessary.

Summary

In an oral cavity examination, the clinician assesses the adequacy of structure and/or function that might contribute to speech sound errors. When concerns arise, several options are available: 1) refer the client to other professionals (e.g., otolaryngologist, orthodontist, cleft palate team) for assessment and possible intervention, 2) engage in additional observation and testing to verify the earlier observation and note its impact on speaking skills, and 3) provide instruction related to compensatory or remedial behaviors.

Audiological Screening

The primary purpose of audiological screening is to determine whether a client exhibits a hearing loss or reduction of auditory function, which could be an etiological factor associated with an SSD. Audiological screening is usually conducted with pure tones and/or impedance audiometry prior to or as part of the phonological assessment. Most audiological screening by SLPs is done with pure tone testing.

Pure tone screening typically involves the presentation of pure tone stimuli at 500, 1,000, 2,000, and 4,000 Hz at a predetermined intensity level in each ear. Usually, 20 dB HL is used for screening, but this level can be altered to compensate for ambient noise in the room. The pure tone frequencies used in screening are those considered most important for perceiving speech. The loudness of the pure tone stimuli reflects threshold levels needed to function adequately in the classroom and in the general environment.

Impedance screening measures eardrum compliance (movement of the eardrum) and middle-ear pressure as air pressure is altered in the external auditory canal. This screening test also yields basic information about the functioning of the tympanic membrane by eliciting the acoustic reflex. The acoustic reflex can be measured by presenting a relatively loud signal to the ear and observing the presence or absence of a change in the compliance of the eardrum. Screening of the acoustic reflex usually involves the presentation of a 1,000 Hz signal at 70 dB above a person's threshold. The acoustic reflex is a contraction of the stapedial muscle when the ear is stimulated by a loud sound and serves as a protective device for the inner ear. The client who fails a pure tone or impedance screening should be referred to an audiologist for a complete audiological assessment.

Summary

As indicated in Chapter 4 in the discussion of hearing as it relates to an individual's speech sound productions, it is critical to know the status of a client's hearing. There is some indication that recurrent middle ear problems can contribute to SSDs. In the case of more severe auditory impairments, a relatively high positive correlation between extent of hearing loss and level of speech and language development occurs frequently. Given this relationship, audiological screening must be a routine part of speech sound assessment procedures.

Speech Sound Perception/Discrimination Testing

A review of the literature concerning the relationship between speech sound perception and articulation is presented in Chapter 4. The information presented there provides a background for the assessment of speech sound perception, which follows.

In the earlier years of the SLP profession (1920–1950), clinicians assumed that most children with speech sound errors were unable to perceive the difference between the standard adult production and their own error production, and then inferred that many phonological problems were the result of faulty perception. As a result of this assumption, speech sound discrimination testing that covered a wide variety of sound contrasts became a standard procedure in the assessment battery. These general discrimination tests did not examine contrasts relevant to a particular child's error productions (e.g., target sound vs. error sound—*rabbit* vs. *wabbit*) but sampled a wide variety of contrasts. An example of a general test of discrimination is the Goldman-Fristoe-Woodcock Test of Auditory Discrimination (Goldman et al., 1970).

Investigators have reported research findings that have cast doubt on the relationship between general speech sound discrimination and SSDs (Schwartz & Goldman, 1974; Sherman & Geith, 1967). The result has been that today, general speech sound discrimination tests are almost never used in clinical assessment. However, speech sound discrimination testing is recommended for those few clients suspected of having a generalized perceptual problem (e.g., inability to differentiate a wide variety of minimal pair sound contrasts). The type of testing recommended for more routine clinical use is a task based on testing discrimination of the child's particular production error(s). Two approaches can be taken to such assessment: judgment tasks and contrast testing.

Judgment Tasks

At least two different judgment tasks could be used to assess discrimination skills. The first of these is the Speech Production Perception Task (SP-PT) (Locke, 1980b). Words are verbally presented one at a time by the clinician, and the client must decide (i.e., make a judgment) about whether the word was produced correctly. The SP-PT is focused on a child's perception of their articulatory errors. It involves no preselected stimuli; rather, the stimuli are based on the child's error productions. See Table 6.4 for the format for this task and Box 6.3 for instructions on how to administer the procedure.

Preliminary to the presentation of the SP-PT, the child's speech sound errors must be identified. The child's error productions and the corresponding adult standard (correct) forms are then used to construct the perception task. In this procedure, the adult norm is identified as the stimulus phoneme (SP), the child's substitution or deletion as the response phoneme (RP), and a perceptually similar control phoneme is identified as CP. The control phoneme is one that the child produces correctly and is as similar as possible to both the target and the child's error. For example, if the client substitutes [wek] for /rek/, the SP would be *rake* /r/, the RP would be *wake* /w/, and an appropriate CP could be *lake* /l/ because /l/ is a liquid, as is /r/.

To administer the task, the examiner presents a picture or an object to the child and names it either correctly, using the target phoneme, using the client's incorrect response (error) phoneme, or using the control phoneme. For each presentation, the child has to judge whether the word was produced correctly. The number of correct responses to the three types of stimulus items (target, error, control) are tabulated. A similar 18-item test is constructed for each sound substitution in which perception is to be examined in depth.

A similar measure to the SP-PT called the Speech Assessment and Interactive Learning System (SAILS; Rvachew & Herbay, 2017) has been developed as a tablet-based application. As with the SP-PT, the software focuses on perception of individual phonemes rather than overall perceptual skills. But rather than relying on the clinician

Table 6.4. Speech production perception task

Speaker's name _____ Sex _____ Date of birth_____			
Test date:		Test date:	
Usual error pattern / / [a] → / / [b]		Usual error pattern / / [a] → / / [b]	
Target sound / / Error / / Control / / [c]		Target sound / / Error / / Control / / [c]	
Stimulus – Category	Response[d]	Stimulus – Category	Response[d]
1. / / - Error	yes NO	1. / / - Target	YES no
2. / / - Control	yes NO	2. / / - Control	yes NO
3. / / - Target	YES no	3. / / - Target	YES no
4. / / - Target	YES no	4. / / - Error	yes NO
5. / / - Error	yes NO	5. / / - Control	yes NO
6. / / - Control	yes NO	6. / / - Error	yes NO
7. / / - Target	YES no	7. / / - Target	YES no
8. / / - Control	yes NO	8. / / - Error	yes NO
9. / / - Error	yes NO	9. / / - Target	YES no
10. / / - Target	YES no	10. / / - Control	yes NO
11. / / - Error	yes NO	11. / / - Control	yes NO
12. / / - Control	yes NO	12. / / - Error	yes NO
13. / / - Error	yes NO	13. / / - Target	YES no
14. / / - Target	YES no	14. / / - Control	yes NO
15. / / - Error	yes NO	15. / / - Error	yes NO
16. / / - Control	yes NO	16. / / - Target	YES no
17. / / - Target	YES no	17. / / - Control	yes NO
18. / / - Control	yes NO	18. / / - Error	yes NO
Mistakes: Error ____ Control ____ Target____		Mistakes: Error ____ Control ____ Target____	

Misperception, 3+ mistakes on "Error."

[a] Phonetic transcription of target word for this task.

[b] Phonetic transcription of what the speaker usually says in place of the target word.

[c] Control sound should be similar to both target sound and usual error but produced correctly.

[d] Correct responses shown in UPPERCASE.

Source: Locke (1980b).

to present live-voice examples, the child is presented with recorded productions from a range of speakers producing both correct productions and a variety of incorrect productions. The child then makes a judgment about what they heard by selecting the picture that corresponds to the target word (if they believe the production was correct) or a large X (if they believe it was incorrect). The software can track judgment accuracy, and thus can be used for both assessment of initial perceptual skills and to monitor progress in therapy. The judgment task itself also works as a therapy activity. Several studies using an earlier CD-ROM based version of this approach (now available as a tablet-based application) have shown it to be effective as a therapy tool and will

BOX 6.3 Instructions for the Speech Production Perception Task

Note that each form can accommodate testing for two different speech errors.

1. Identify the target sound and the child's usual error for that target. Also identify a control sound that is similar to both the target and the child's error but that the child produces correctly. For example, if the child says *fumb* for *thumb*, /θ/ would be the target sound, /f/ would be the child's error, and /s/ might serve as the control (assuming the child usually says /s/ correctly).

2. Under Production Task, list the target word and the substitution. For example, if they said *fumb* for *thumb*:

thumb → fumb

3. Indicate the target sound in the space marked Target (θ in the previous example), the substituted sound in the space marked Error (*f* in the previous example), and a related sound as a control in the space marked Control (it should be similar to both the target and the error but one that the child produces correctly; *s* might be a good one for the previous example).

4. In each of the 18 spots under Stimulus–Class, fill in the appropriate sounds from Step 2, depending on the item that is listed. For example, if the item says Target, write θ; if it says Error, write *f*; and if it says Control, write *s*. This creates the stimuli for the test.

5. Using the target picture or an object as the visual cue, ask the speaker to judge whether you said the right word. For example:

   a. Is this some?

   b. Is this fumb?

   c. Is this thumb?

   d. Is this thumb?

   e. Is this fumb? etc.

   If the speaker answers "yes," circle *yes* next to the item. If the speaker answers "no," circle *no*.

6. If the word *yes* or *no* appears in uppercase letters, that indicates the correct response. If it is in lowercase letters, that indicates it would be a mistake in perception.

7. Count the mistakes (the number of lowercase responses) in each category (Target, Error, Control).

8. The speaker is said to have a problem with perception if three or more mistakes in perception are noted in response to the error stimuli. Because there are six possible error stimuli, the child has then produced at least 50% incorrect responses and thus appears to be having trouble distinguishing what they usually say from what they should be saying.

9. If the child makes three or more mistakes on the control sound, this suggests the child may not fully understand the task. Results of testing should be discarded and the test attempted at a later date.

be discussed further in Chapter 10 (e.g., Rvachew, 1994; Rvachew & Brosseau- Lapré, 2012, 2015; Rvachew et al., 2004).

Contrast Testing

An alternative to perceptual tasks outlined previously is the use of sound contrast testing. Once again, words are presented one at a time. In this case, the client is shown two pictures and must select the picture that corresponds to the word(s) that were just spoken. The names for the pictures reflect a contrast between the client's production error and some other sound (perhaps the client's usual error). For example, for a child who substitutes /w/ for /r/, the two pictures might represent *ride* and *wide*. The contrast could also be with some similar sound, so the pictures might represent *lake* and *rake*. In-depth perceptual testing of an error sound requires numerous phonemic pairings, all focusing on contrasts of the error sound with the target or similar sound.

Contrast testing is particularly useful with individuals learning English as a second language. Frequently, it is difficult for such people to hear sound differences that involve sounds not used in their native language. For example, native Japanese have trouble differentiating /r/ and /l/, and Spanish speakers sometimes have trouble differentiating /ɪ/ and /i/.

Assessment of a child's awareness of phonological contrasts provides the clinician with data relative to the child's phonemic system at a perceptual level. Most clinicians improvise assessment tasks requiring the child to indicate awareness that certain contrasts are in their perceptual repertoire. For example, a child with sound substitutions of /t/ for /s/ could be shown pictures of the following pairs of words that contrast s/t, s/ʃ, and s/θ and be asked to pick up one picture from each pair as it is named:

| sea | sea | some |
| tea | she | thumb |

A child who cannot readily perceive these contrasts might be a candidate for perceptual training (to be discussed in Chapter 10).

Summary

If it is suspected that a child's speech sound errors are related to faulty perception, perceptual testing or contrast testing is appropriate. The primary concern relates to the child's ability to differentiate between the adult standard and their error productions. Perceptional testing should be based on the child's specific errors with assessment items based on phonemic contrasts the individual does not produce in their speech sound productions. Although our understanding of the relationship between phonological productions and perception is incomplete, it appears that improving perceptual skills may be useful in helping some children improve their speech sound productions. For individuals who are second language learners, perception testing is a very useful component to the assessment battery.

CONCLUSION

Speech sound assessment may consist of screening and/or a comprehensive assessment. The former provides a quick evaluation to determine whether a problem may be present and whether more complete assessment is needed. A comprehensive assessment battery includes connected speech and single-word sampling, as well as stimulability and contextual testing. The battery also often includes supplemental procedures, such as the collection of a case history, an oral cavity examination, audiological screening, and perceptual testing. All of these data are then compiled and interpreted. Such interpretation is the subject of Chapter 7.

QUESTIONS FOR CHAPTER 6

1. What is the purpose of a speech sound screening, and what are some examples of when this would occur?

2. Describe the elements of a speech sound assessment battery and how each is accomplished.

3. What related assessments need to accompany the speech sound assessment battery?

4. What are the strengths and limitations of citation testing and spontaneous speech assessment?

5. What is meant by a pattern analysis, how is it done, and how may the results impact intervention decisions?

6. What is the purpose of the case history? What elements of the history are likely to be of prime importance to the clinician?

7. Distinguish among target phonemes, error phonemes, and control phonemes used for speech perception testing. When is perception assessment recommended?

8. What is a diacritic marker and when is it used?

9. How is the accuracy of one's scoring of responses assessed? Why is this important?

10. What is included in an oral cavity examination, and what variations may be most likely to occur? What should a clinician do if there is an item of concern in this examination?

7

Assessment: Decision Making

JOHN E. BERNTHAL, NICHOLAS W. BANKSON, AND PETER FLIPSEN JR.

LEARNING OBJECTIVES

This chapter discusses various aspects of interpreting the data collected during assessment of a possible speech sound disorder (SSD). By the end of this chapter, the reader should be able to:

- Describe different criteria for making case selection eligibility decisions.

- Discuss how intelligibility data may be related to case selection decisions.

- Differentiate between intelligibility and severity of involvement as they relate to SSDs.

- Illustrate how to calculate percentage of consonants correct (PCC) and use the value obtained to assess severity of involvement.

- Identify and contrast three categories of speech sound patterns.

- Discuss the rationale for taking a pragmatic approach to determining the nature of a speech sound problem and how this relates to one's approach to therapy.

- Contrast a developmental approach with a complexity approach to target selection.

- Describe how intelligibility, stimulability, frequency of occurrence, and contextual analysis might be used to select treatment targets.

- Briefly explain how dialect or second language learning may impact treatment decisions.

- Discuss how treatment decisions might be affected by varying social-vocational expectations.

- List the advantages and disadvantages of computer-assisted analysis of SSDs.

After the various types of speech samples are collected, the clinician reviews responses to the speech sound assessment tasks and interprets the data to make appropriate and efficacious decisions. Specifically, the data gathered during the assessment are analyzed and interpreted to determine such things as 1) whether there is a problem that justifies intervention, 2) how severe the problem is, 3) the nature of the problem, and 4) what to target in intervention.

CASE SELECTION

Addressing the previous issues is not always straightforward. For example, determining whether there is a problem requires more than simply looking at test scores to see whether they meet some predetermined cutoff value (this is, however, an important step in the process). It includes examining the client's ability to make themselves understood (intelligibility), determining severity of involvement, looking for broader patterns in the client's errors, assessing stimulability, and examining case history and file data to identify possible causal factors. Interpreting the data also includes deciding whether referrals to other professionals for assistance is necessary.

Eligibility

To determine whether children in the public schools should receive therapy for speech sounds, several factors are considered. First, scores on standardized tests, such as the single-word tests (described in Chapter 6), are often examined. Typically, each jurisdiction (e.g., school district) establishes a minimum cutoff score (e.g., 1.5 standard deviations below the mean or below the 10th percentile) that a child must meet to qualify for services. Although a heavy emphasis is often placed on such scores, they should not be the sole basis for eligibility decisions. Children can usually qualify for services if their speech and language disorders interfere with their educational performance.

   U.S. federal law requires that special education services be available if educational performance is negatively affected by a speech and/or language disorder. However, there has been considerable variability in how this should be interpreted (Farquharson & Boldini, 2018). In particular, clinicians differ in whether the presence of an SSD in the absence of any academic deficits is sufficient to require provision of speech-language pathologist (SLP) services. Although in this book we have made the case that SSDs put children at risk for academic difficulties, some of these children manage just fine academically. As outlined in Box 7.1, it appears clear to us that even children without academic deficiencies should be eligible for speech services. The potential negative social stigma that these children often face (Krueger, 2019; Silverman, 1989), as well as any parental concerns about social, emotional, and/or career consequences, warrant our serious consideration in making eligibility decisions.

   Overall scores on standardized tests remain the most common mechanism for qualifying children with SSDs for services in the public school. However, Storkel (2019) and others have made the argument that rather than using a single test score, eligibility for speech sound intervention services could also be based on comparison to developmental norms for individual speech sounds. Indeed, on some occasions (as described in Clinical Vignette 7.1) a child might qualify for services based on an overall test score but an initial analysis might suggest there would not be any eligible speech sound targets. Storkel argued that in such cases a more detailed analysis might be in order. By looking at either phonological pattern occurrence or the specific kinds of errors being produced, specific therapy targets might be identified.

   For example, many clinicians would not work on /s, z/ in a 6-year-old child based strictly on developmental norms. However, most children of that age who produce errors on those sounds are producing dentalized distortions (Smit, 1993a, 1993b). If the child in question were substituting stops /t, d/ for /s, z/ that would be quite atypical. Thus, the error pattern alone could justify intervention. A similar argument could be made for the 6-year-old child who lateralized /s, z, ʃ, tʃ, dʒ/; errors of this type are very rare at this age (Smit, 1993a). The idea that unusual errors might be reasonable

---

BOX 7.1   What Does "Adversely Affects Educational Performance" Mean?

As noted by Farquharson and Boldini (2018), the Individuals with Disabilities Education Act (IDEA, 2004) sets three criteria for children to be eligible for SLP services in the public schools: ". . . (a) the child is diagnosed with a qualifying disability, (b) the disability adversely affects a child's educational performance, and (c) specialized instruction and related services are necessary for the child to make progress" (pp. 1–2). However, no specific definition of "adversely affects educational performance" is provided in the law, leaving it open to some degree of interpretation (Thomas, 2016).

Some have argued that the term *educational performance* includes more than academics. In order to clarify, ASHA sought guidance from the U.S. Department of Education (USDOE). The 2007 response from the USDOE Office of Special Education and Rehabilitative Services (OSERS) appears to confirm that academic failure is not necessary:

> It remains the Department's position that the term "educational performance" as used in IDEA and its implementing regulations is *not limited to academic performance.* Whether a speech and language impairment adversely affects a child's educational performance must be determined on a case-by-case basis, depending on the unique needs of a particular child and not based only on discrepancies in age or grade performance in academic subject areas. (OSERS, 2007; p. 1, emphasis added)

---

justifications for the need for therapy is also supported by data from a longitudinal study of 1,494 children by Morgan and colleagues (2017). In that study, children with typical errors at age 4 years were far more likely to resolve those errors by age 7 years than children who had produced unusual errors at the earlier age.

Clinical Vignette 7.1

No Treatable Targets?

Following kindergarten screening, a 5-year-old boy, Jordan (a pseudonym) was referred for a comprehensive assessment. Findings indicated his conversational speech was about 75% intelligible; he also achieved a standard score of 73 (more than 1.5 standard deviations below the mean) on a single-word articulation test. By both of those measures, he met eligibility requirements for therapy. He was stimulable for most of his errors to at least the word level.

When examining his specific speech sound errors, however, and comparing them against developmental norms, none of the sounds met criteria for treatment (assuming mastery to be the age at which 90% of children were correctly producing the sound). In other words, there did not appear to be any specific speech sound targets to work on.

As it turned out, Jordan had a low shallow palate and a small overjet (his lower front teeth were noticeably behind his upper front teeth). This combination resulted in a restricted space in the front of his oral cavity. This might have accounted for his reduced intelligibility, as you may recall from your phonetics class that many speech sounds are produced around the alveolar ridge.

Medical and dental examinations suggested no immediate need for intervention. Given Jordan's age, his mandible (the slowest growing part of the human face) would likely continue to grow and the overjet might eventually resolve itself. There were no other issues of language or communication to motivate therapy. Under the circumstances, therapy was not recommended and Jordan was placed on a watch-and-see list.

One year later, Jordan's parents and his teacher reported that his speech was fully intelligible, and they were no longer noticing any speech sound errors.

Ultimately, qualifying children for speech sound intervention requires the school-based SLP to collaborate with a school-based diagnostic team to establish the need for services consistent with federal guidelines, as well as state and local eligibility criteria. Whereas these are particularly relevant for school-based therapy programs, they may also be employed when selecting clients in other clinical service venues.

Intelligibility

Perhaps the factor that most often brings young children to an SLP's attention is the intelligibility or understandability of their speech. This is also the factor most frequently cited by both SLPs and other listeners when judging the severity of a phonological problem (Shriberg & Kwiatkowski, 1982a). It should be pointed out, however, that severity of an SSD and speech intelligibility are different, though related, concepts. To put it more succinctly, intelligibility is how much of the message is understood, whereas severity is how bad/significant the problem is. Hence, we treat intelligibility and severity separately here.

As the goal of most communicative interactions is for the listener to understand the intended message, full intelligibility is frequently cited as the main long-term goal for most SSDs. This, then, mandates that SLPs document it adequately and monitor progress toward that goal. Specific formal procedures for doing so were described in Chapter 6.

If being understood is the objective, it makes sense that significantly reduced intelligibility could also be a basis for a child receiving speech services. Although, as discussed in Chapter 6, there are no norm-referenced intelligibility tests available, we could use what we know about normal development as a frame of reference. We know that the vast majority of children are fully intelligible by age 4 years (though they may not yet have mastered all of the speech sounds). This would suggest that any child over age 4 years who is not yet fully intelligible could justifiably be considered eligible for services.

Severity

Once eligibility has been determined (or sometimes as part of the process of determining eligibility), another commonly asked question relates to the severity of the SSD. *Severity* of a phonological disorder refers to the significance of an SSD and is associated with labels such as *mild, moderate,* and *severe.* Severity may also be looked at as representing the degree of impairment.

How well the message is being understood (i.e., intelligibility) is clearly a factor related to how significant an SSD might be. It is not, however, the only factor that is typically considered. A study of judgments of severity of children with SSDs by Flipsen and colleagues (2005) revealed that experienced clinicians considered intelligibility as well as such things as number, type, and consistency of errors, along with whole-word accuracy, in making such determinations.

Although severity ratings are not always required, many jurisdictions and/or insurance companies may use them to determine funding for the length or frequency of services. For example, mild cases may warrant a single weekly session for a fixed number of weeks, whereas more severe cases may be allotted treatment two to three times per week for the same number of weeks. Likewise, severity ratings may also be used by clinicians or administrators to manage busy caseloads. Mild cases may receive services in groups or as part of a classroom activity. More severe cases may be seen individually or in some combination of individual and group intervention as well as classroom activities.

Assessing Severity

There are currently no gold standards for determining severity for SSDs, nor is there a consensus on which specific factors to consider. Some states provide specific guidelines for determining severity of involvement for SSDs in school-age children. For example, the Tennessee Department of Education (2009) asks clinicians to consider sound production, stimulability, motor sequencing, and intelligibility (with specific descriptors for each rating value on each factor). An overall score is then generated and translates to a particular severity category ranging from mild to profound. A similar approach is followed by the North Dakota Department of Public Instruction (2010), although the factors to be considered are slightly different (intelligibility or PCC, speech sounds or phonological processes, stimulability, educational impact).

In most instances, however, clinicians must use their own judgment and decide on their own which factors to consider and how to weigh each of the factors (Spaulding et al., 2012). Without some guidance, however, the risk is inconsistency across clinicians in the assignment of severity. A high amount of variability in ratings was confirmed in the previously mentioned study of experienced clinicians' judgments of severity by Flipsen and colleagues (2005). This raises serious questions about the usefulness of such measures.

One attempt to develop a more objective way of determining the degree of severity is that of Shriberg and Kwiatkowski (1982a). These researchers recommended the calculation of PCC as an index to quantify severity of involvement. Their research indicated that among several variables studied in relation to listeners' perceptions of severity, the PCC correlated most closely. In other words, PCC appears to best correlate with SLPs' severity ratings of continuous speech.

The PCC requires the examiner to make correct–incorrect judgments based on a narrow phonetic transcription of a continuous speech sample. Such judgments were found to be a reasonable measure for the classification of many children's SSDs as mild, mild-moderate, moderate-severe, or severe. Procedures outlined by Shriberg and Kwiatkowski (1982a) for determining PCC are as follows:

> Tape record a continuous speech sample of a child following sampling procedures. Any means that yield continuous speech from the child are acceptable, provided that the clinician can tell the child that his exact words will be repeated onto the "tape machine" so that the clinician is sure to "get things right." (p. 267)

Sampling Rules

1. Consider only intended (target) consonants in words. Intended vowels are not considered.

   a. Addition of a consonant before a vowel, for example, *on* [hɔn], is not scored because the target sound /ɔ/ is a vowel.

   b. Postvocalic /r/ in *fair* [feɪr] is a consonant, but stressed and unstressed vocalics [ɝ] and [ɚ], as in *furrier* [fɝiɚ], are considered vowels.

2. Do not score target consonants in the second or successive repetitions of a syllable, for example, *ba-balloon,* but score only the first /b/.

3. Do not score target consonants in words that are completely or partially unintelligible or where the transcriber is uncertain of the target.

4. Do not score target consonants in the third or successive repetitions of adjacent words unless articulation changes. For example, the consonants in only the first two words of the series [kæt], [kæt], [kæt] are counted. However, the consonants in all three words are counted as if the series were [kæt], [kæk], [kæt].

Scoring Rules

1. The following six types of consonant sound changes are scored as incorrect:

   a. Deletions of a target consonant.

   b. Substitutions of another sound for a target consonant, including replacement by a glottal stop or a cognate.

   c. Partial voicing of initial target consonants.

   d. Distortions of a target sound, no matter how subtle.

   e. Addition of a sound to a correct or incorrect target consonant, for example, *cars* said as [kɑrks].

   f. Initial /h/ deletion (*he* [hi]) and final n/ŋ substitutions (*ring* [rɪŋ]) are counted as errors only when they occur in stressed syllables; in unstressed syllables, they are counted as correct, for example, *feed her* [fidɚ]; *running* [rʌnin].

2. Observe the following:

   a. The response definition for children who obviously have speech errors is "score as incorrect unless heard as correct." This response definition assigns questionable speech behaviors to an "incorrect" category.

   b. Dialectal variants should be glossed as intended in the child's dialect, for example, *picture* "piture," *ask* "aks," and so on.

   c. Fast or casual speech sound changes should be glossed as the child intended, for example, *don't know* "dono," and "*n*," and the like.

   d. Allophones should be scored as correct, for example, *water* [wɑrɚ], *tail* [teɪl̩].

Calculation of PCC:

$$PCC = \frac{\text{number of correct consonants}}{\text{number of correct + incorrect consonants}} \times 100$$

Based on research that related PCC values to listeners' perception of degree of handicap, Shriberg and Kwiatkowski (1982a) recommended the following scale of severity:

85%–100%	Mild
65%–85%	Mild/moderate
50%–65%	Moderate/severe
<50%	Severe

Shriberg, Austin, and colleagues (1997) have described extensions of this PCC metric to address concerns related to what were perceived as limitations in the original procedure. Thus, the authors have presented additional formulas (e.g., percentage of vowels correct [PVC]; percentage of phonemes correct [PPC]; PCC adjusted [PCC-A]) that address such variables as frequency of occurrence of sounds; types of errors, including omissions and substitutions; the nature of distortions; and vowel and diphthong errors. Flipsen and colleagues (2005) examined these measures along with several others as potentially more valid ways to determine severity. None of the alternatives appeared to be any better than the original PCC at capturing severity as judged by experienced clinicians.

A long-standing concern about using PCC as just described is the need for narrowly transcribing a continuous speech sample and the amount of time required to do so. As a possible alternative, Johnson and associates (2004) derived PCC scores for 21 children aged 4–6 years with speech delay from an imitative sentence task and compared them to PCC scores from the conversational task recommended by Shriberg, Austin and colleagues (1997). Findings indicated that PCC scores did not differ significantly, with results indicating clinical equivalency. They cited advantages of sentence imitation samples that included providing opportunities to observe infrequently occurring speech sounds, reducing problems with knowing what the target words might be, and providing for replicated samples in pre- and post-treatment assessment. Overall, the use of sentence imitation made more efficient use of clinician and client time than conversational sampling and analysis.

Quantitative estimates of severity, such as the PCC, provide the clinician with another means for determining the relative priority of those who may need intervention and a way to monitor progress/change.

Pattern Analysis

In addition to considering intelligibility and severity, the data obtained are also reviewed to determine whether a child is using patterns of speech errors at a level appropriate to the child's age. When conducting a pattern analysis, the clinician reviews and categorizes errors according to commonalities among them. As mentioned in Chapter 6, determination of a child's patterns may be based on any one of several formal assessment instruments. These include several of the single-word tests listed in Table 6.1 (e.g., AAPS-4, BBTOP-2, CAAP-2, DEAP, HAPP-3, SPAT-D-3). Pattern analysis can also be carried out on data from the GFTA-3 using the Khan-Lewis Phonological Analysis (3rd ed.) (KLPA-3; Khan & Lewis, 2015). As with those single-word tests discussed in Chapter 6, a comprehensive review of these pattern analysis procedures is beyond the scope of this text, but a review by Kirk and Vigeland (2014) is available.

To reinforce our earlier recommendation that connected speech samples should always be included in a comprehensive assessment, the clinician may also examine errors produced during a connected speech sample and apply a manual determination of error patterns.

Types of Pattern Analyses

Place-Manner-Voicing Analysis.   The simplest type of pattern analysis involves classifying substitution errors according to place, manner, and voicing characteristics. A *place-manner-voicing analysis* facilitates the identification of patterns, such as voiced for voiceless sound substitutions (e.g., voicing errors—/f/ → [v], /t/ → [d]), replacement of fricatives with stops (e.g., manner errors—/ð/ → [d], /s/ → [t]), or substitution of lingua-velar sounds for lingua-alveolar sounds (e.g., place errors—/k/ →[t], /d/ → [g]). Another example is a child whose speech patterns reflect correct manner and voicing but production of errors in place of articulation, such as fronting of consonants (e.g., /k/ → [t], /g/ → [d]). In this instance, the child is fronting consonants and substituting sounds that are correctly produced in the front of the oral cavity (the manner is consistent with the target sound) for those in the back or posterior of the oral cavity.

Phonological Pattern/Process Analysis.   A second and more frequently used type of pattern analysis is sometimes called a *phonological process (pattern) analysis*. As already discussed, phonological pattern analysis is a method for identifying commonalities among errors. Before discussing interpretation of such analyses, we would like to review again some of the more common patterns (presented in Chapter 3 in terms of speech acquisition and discussed in Chapter 5) observed in the speech of young children. Although there are differences in pattern terminology and listings of phonological patterns employed by various authors, most are similar to those shown next. This list is not exhaustive, but represents most of the common patterns seen in normally developing children and have been commonly used in analyzing the sound errors of phonologically delayed children.

Whole Word (and Syllable) Patterns.   Whole word and syllable structure patterns are changes that affect the syllabic structures of the target word.

1. *Final consonant deletion.* Deletion of the final consonant in a word. For example:

boot	[bu]
cap	[kæ]
fish	[fɪ]

2. *Unstressed syllable deletion (weak syllable deletion).* An unstressed syllable is deleted, often at the beginning of a word, sometimes in the middle. For example:

potato	[teto]
telephone	[tɛfon]
pajamas	[dʒæmiz]

3. *Reduplication.* A syllable or a portion of a syllable is repeated or duplicated, usually becoming CVCV. For example:

dad	[dædæ]
water	[wɑwɑ]
cat	[kækæ]

4. *Consonant cluster simplification.* A consonant cluster is simplified by a substitution for one member of the cluster. For example:

black	[bwæk]
ski	[sti]
ask	[æst]

5. *Consonant cluster reduction.* One or more elements of a consonant cluster are deleted. For example:

stop	[tɑp]
last	[læt]
string	[tɪŋ]

6. *Epenthesis.* A segment, often the unstressed vowel [ə], is inserted. For example:

black	[bəlæk]
sweet	[səwit]
sun	[sθʌn]
long	[lɔŋg]

7. *Metathesis.* There is a transposition or reversal of two segments (sounds) in a word. For example:

basket	[bæksɪt]
spaghetti	[pʌsgɛti]
elephant	[ɛfəlʌnt]

8. *Coalescence.* Characteristics of features from two adjacent sounds are combined so that one sound replaces two other sounds. For example:

swim	[fɪm] /f/ combines the fricative feature of /s/ and the labial feature of /w/
close	[toz] /t/ combines the stop feature of /k/ and the alveolar feature of /l/

Assimilatory (Harmony) Patterns.   In this type of error pattern, one sound is influenced by another nearby sound (usually within the same word) in such a manner that one sound assumes features of a second sound. Thus, the two segments become more alike or similar (hence, the term *harmony*) or even identical. Types of assimilation include:

1. *Velar assimilation.* A nonvelar sound is assimilated (changed) to a velar sound because of the influence, or dominance, of a velar. For example:

duck	[gʌk]
take	[kek]
coat	[kok]

2. *Nasal assimilation.* A nonnasal sound is assimilated and replaced by a nasal because of the influence, or dominance, of a nasal consonant. For example:

candy	[næni]
lamb	[næm]
fun	[nʌn]

3. *Labial assimilation.* A nonlabial sound is assimilated to a labial consonant because of the influence of a labial consonant. For example:

bed	[bɛb]
table	[bebu]
pit	[pɪp]

Segment Change (Substitution) Patterns.   In these patterns, one sound is substituted for another, with the replacement sound reflecting changes in place of articulation, manner of articulation, or some other change in the way a sound is produced in a standard production.

1. *Fronting.* Substitutions are produced anterior to or forward of the standard production. This category is sometimes subdivided into velar fronting (e.g., / d/ → [g]) and palatal fronting (e.g., /ʃ/ → [s]). For example:

go	[do]
monkey	[mʌnti]
she	[si]

2. *Stopping*. Fricatives or affricates are replaced by stops. For example:

> *sun*   [tʌn]
> *peach*   [pit]
> *that*   [dæt]

3. *Gliding of liquids*. Prevocalic liquids are replaced by glides. For example:

> *run*   [wʌn]
> *yellow*   [jɛwo]
> *leaf*   [wif]

4. *Affrication*. Fricatives are replaced by affricates. For example:

> *saw*   [tʃɑ]
> *shoe*   [tʃu]
> *sun*   [tʃʌn]

5. *Vocalization (or vowelization)*. Liquids or nasals are replaced by vowels. For example:

> *car*   [kʌo]
> *table*   [tebo]
> *tire*   [taɪo]

6. *Denasalization*. Nasals are replaced by homorganic stops (place of articulation is similar to target sound). For example:

> *moon*   [bud]
> *nice*   [daɪs]
> *man*   [bæn]

7. *Deaffrication*. Affricates are replaced by fricatives. For example:

> *chop*   [sɑp]
> *chip*   [ʃɪp]
> *page*   [pez]

8. *Glottal replacement*. Glottal stops replace sounds usually in either intervocalic or final position. For example:

> *cat*   [kæʔ]
> *tooth*   [tuʔ]
> *bottle*   [bɑʔl]

9. *Prevocalic voicing*. Voiceless consonants (obstruents) in the prevocalic position are voiced. For example:

> *paper*   [bepɚ]
> *Tom*   [dɑm]
> *table*   [debo]

10. *Devoicing of final consonants*. Voiced obstruents are devoiced in final position. For example:

> *dog*   [dɔk]
> *nose*   [nos]
> *bed*   [bɛt]

Multiple Pattern Occurrence

The examples of phonological patterns just presented included lexical items that reflect only a single pattern for each example. In reality, the child may produce forms that reflect more than one pattern, including some that are not reflected in the preceding definitions and descriptions. A single lexical item may have two or even more patterns operating or interacting. When such productions occur, they are more complex and difficult to unravel than words that reflect a single pattern. For example, in the production of [du] for *shoe,* Edwards (1983) pointed out that the [d] for /ʃ/ replacement reflects the phonological pattern of 1) depalatalization, which changes the place of articulation; 2) stopping, which changes the manner of articulation; and 3) prevocalic voicing, which changes a voiceless consonant target to a voiced consonant. In the substitution of [dar] for *car,* the [d] for /k/ substitution is accounted for by the patterns of both velar fronting and prevocalic voicing. The identification of the sequence of steps describing how interacting patterns occur is called a *derivation* or *pattern ordering.*

Unusual Pattern Occurrence

As indicated throughout this book, a great deal of individual variation exists in children's phonological acquisition. Although most children use common developmental phonological patterns, the patterns observed across individuals vary. This is especially true in the speech of children with SSDs. Unusual phonological patterns (e.g., use of a nasal sound for /s/ and /z/), called *idiosyncratic processes* or *patterns,* differ from the more common phonological patterns we have identified previously and are seen in children with both normal and delayed phonological development. Some examples of unusual patterns were presented in Chapter 5 (see Table 5.2).

The greatest variation in phonology occurs during the early stages of development and is probably influenced, in part, by the lexical items the child uses when acquiring their first words. Recall that unusual errors are less likely to resolve on their own compared to normal error patterns (Morgan et al., 2017). This supports a long-standing argument that the presence of unusual errors may be used to justify therapy much earlier than using developmental norms for acquisition of the target sound (Leonard, 1973; Smit, 1993a, 1993b; Stoel-Gammon & Dunn, 1985; Storkel, 2019).

Sound Preferences

Another type of sound pattern that some clinicians have reported is called *systematic sound preference.* In these situations, children seem to use a segment (sound) or two for a large number of sounds or for an entire sound class(es). Sometimes, a particular sound is substituted for several or even all phonemes in a particular sound class (e.g., /p/ for all fricatives). Other children may substitute a single consonant for a variety of segments, such as [h] for /b, d, s, ʒ, z, dʒ, tʃ, ʃ, l, k, g, r/ (Weiner, 1981a). It has been postulated that such preferences may indicate that some children are avoiding the use of certain sounds that are difficult for them to produce.

Interpreting Phonological Pattern Data

Young children during the phonological acquisition stage simplify their productions as they learn the adult phonological system. For example, a child attempting to say the word *dog* might produce [dɔ] instead. For most children such patterns are temporary. When they persist, however, SLPs should identify these patterns to aid in the description of the child's phonological system.

A variety of efforts have been made to explain why some children have a propensity to produce these patterns. One of these is based in the theory of natural phonology, which was discussed in Chapter 3. This theory assumes that young children have adultlike underlying representations for the speech sounds of the language. As a consequence of a temporary limitation during the developmental period, however, children are unable to translate those underlying sound representations into correct speech sound productions. Rather, they simplify their productions into something they are currently capable of producing. Using the previous example, it could be hypothesized that adding a final consonant onto the end of an open syllable is difficult for this child.

A second account of this same error arises from the theory of generative phonology. In the course of trying to identify the rules of the language, the child establishes a temporary language rule that assumes that all (or most) words end in open syllables. Hoffman and Schuckers (1984) suggested at least three other plausible explanations for such errors: 1) the child misperceives the adult word; for example, they perceive [dɔg] as [dɔ]; 2) the child's underlying representation for dog is [dɔ], so that is what they produce; or 3) the child has a motor production problem (i.e., they may have the appropriate perception and underlying representation but do not possess the necessary motor skill to make the articulation gesture to produce the sound).

If the only evidence we have is that the child produced [dɔg] as [dɔ], there is no way to know the actual reason for the error production. Referring to the child's error pattern as *final consonant deletion (FCD)* does not explain the reason for the error. The same might be said for the child who produces *tea* when intending to say *key*. We can refer to this production pattern as *velar fronting* (or simply fronting), but we do not know why the child made that particular error. Thus, labels attached to phonological patterns do not explain why the child has made the error. Such labels only describe what is being observed in the child's speech output.

That is not to say that labels for phonological patterns have no value. They can be useful for at least two reasons. First, we can use them to help determine whether a child is eligible for services by comparing their occurrence to developmental norms, such as those discussed in Chapter 3 (see Table 3.9). Second, if we notice that a particular pattern, such as final consonant deletion, occurs frequently and includes a variety of different final consonants, we may be able to treat multiple targets simultaneously (see Chapter 11). Thus, identifying phonological patterns can be a useful clinical tool for both assessment and treatment, even though the patterns themselves do not explain the nature or reason for the child's problem.

The first step in a phonological pattern analysis is to examine individual sound errors to identify possible pattern(s) that might be present, including how frequently the pattern(s) occur. Next, the clinician should determine whether intervention for the pattern use is warranted. If a formal test with normative data was used in the assessment, the scores on the test can be compared to local eligibility criteria. When connected speech samples are being analyzed, all errors should be examined to identify what patterns might be occurring and what percentage of opportunities included the use of the pattern (e.g., if you are focused on final consonant deletion, of all the possible final consonants, what percentage were deleted?). These values can then be compared to reference data, such as those in Grunwell (1987) and Roberts and colleagues (1990), or by consulting Table 3.9.

Stimulability

Another factor often considered in case selection is stimulability. In Chapter 6, procedures for conducting and interpreting stimulability testing were presented.

Investigators have reported that the ability of a child to imitate the correct form of an error sound in isolation, syllables, and/or words increases the probability that the child will spontaneously correct their misarticulations of that sound or make faster progress in therapy on stimulable sounds. The fact that a young child acquiring phonology can imitate error sounds suggests that the child may be in the process of acquiring those sounds. On the other hand, the use of stimulability testing for predicting spontaneous improvement or the rate of improvement in remediation has not been documented sufficiently to make definitive prognostic statements.

Stimulability testing is only a general guide for the identification of clients who may correct their phonological errors without intervention and sounds that will show relatively quick success in treatment. False positives (i.e., clients identified as needing instruction but who ultimately will outgrow their problems) and false negatives (i.e., clients identified as not needing instruction but who ultimately will require intervention) have been identified in all investigations focusing on stimulability as a prognostic indicator. These findings must be considered when results from stimulability testing are used to make predictive statements regarding general clinical outcomes or outcomes for specific sounds that are stimulable.

Relative to deciding whether treatment itself is warranted, our inability to be certain about prognosis from stimulability testing creates a dilemma. If some or all of a child's error sounds are stimulable, and that means those sounds are likely to emerge on their own, why would we intervene? Why would we use up valuable clinician time, as well as the child's learning time, for therapy? Couldn't that time be better used for other needs? However, our limited ability to predict outcomes from stimulability testing means that most clinicians prefer not to take the chance; most would not use stimulability as the sole basis for deciding if a child should receive therapy. Stimulability data are only one of several factors to consider when making judgments relative to providing services or as a prognostic tool.

Causal Correlates

Some of the information gathered during the assessment process (particularly the case history information) may offer some insight into case selection. A family history of speech or language impairments, for example, increases a child's risk for related difficulties. Thus, a child with such a history whose test scores might not otherwise justify intervention might qualify. Likewise, a child with documented nervous system impacts (e.g., an episode of meningitis or a blow to the head causing a concussion or a period of unconsciousness) or noticeable delays in gross or fine motor development, would likely warrant close monitoring of speech and language development. This same information may also prove useful in helping sort out the nature of a documented SSD (to be discussed later).

Outside Referrals

As broad as scope of practice is, SLPs cannot sort out all problems that might impact SSDs. This means we must be prepared to make referrals to other professionals. Two examples come immediately to mind. First, SLPs routinely screen hearing. A child who fails such a screening should be rescreened soon thereafter. A second screening failure warrants referral to an audiologist. The second example is where the oral mechanism examination reveals significant dental issues. In such cases, parents should be advised to seek evaluation by a dentist. Although managing the hearing or dental issues will not likely immediately resolve the SSD (see, however, Clinical

Vignette 7.2), such team management may improve the chances for success with our interventions.

Clinical Vignette 7.2

Dental Referral

An SLP conducted an assessment on a 6-year-old boy, Andrew (a pseudonym). His parents were concerned about his speech. Test results revealed correct production of all speech sounds except consistent substitution of /θ/ for /s/ and /ð/ for /z/. He was stimulable for his errors in isolation only. His hearing and language skills were within normal limits, and he was not experiencing any academic difficulties.

During his oral mechanism examination, however, a large anterior open bite was found. When Andrew closed his mouth and smiled, his back teeth came together but his upper incisor teeth sat at least one-half inch above his lower incisors. On several occasions during the assessment, he was seen sucking on two of his fingers. His mother noted that this behavior was common for him, despite frequent requests from her that he not do it. It appeared that the presence of Andrew's fingers in his mouth was altering the position of his teeth, likely causing the large open bite. This likely meant that when he spoke his tongue would slide forward to fill the open space. This, then, likely accounted for his speech errors.

Andrew's mother was advised to consult with the family dentist. She reported that the dentist had suggested the use of a dental appliance, which Andrew then wore for the next 6 months. The appliance clipped onto his upper back teeth and had two small prongs that hung down behind his upper incisors. Whenever he put his fingers in his mouth, they would be gently but firmly poked by these prongs.

No speech services were provided. At the end of 6 months, Andrew was reevaluated. His mother reported that he was no longer sucking on his fingers. His open bite had disappeared, and his speech errors did as well. His file was closed.

Case Selection Guidelines

The first question that must be answered with data from speech sound assessment is whether there is a phonological problem that warrants intervention. By reviewing formal test scores, the intelligibility of the speaker, the severity of the problem, stimulability results, and the error patterns that may be present, a decision can be made regarding whether intervention is warranted.

As a general guideline for initiating intervention, a child typically would be one standard deviation or more (some state guidelines call for 1.5–2 standard deviations) below their age norm on a standardized measure of phonology. The clinician should recognize, however, that this is only a general guideline and that the other factors mentioned, such as intelligibility, the nature of the errors and error patterns, consistency of errors, impact of the disorder on academic performance, the child or parent's perception of the problem, and other speech-language characteristics, might also be important in intervention decisions.

Children between 2.5 and 3 years old who are unintelligible are usually recommended for early intervention programs, which typically include parental education and assistance. Children aged 3 years or older who evidence pronounced intelligibility problems or who evidence idiosyncratic phonological patterns are also usually candidates for intervention. Children aged 8 years and younger whose speech sound performance is at least one standard deviation below the mean for their age are frequently candidates for intervention. Most children 9 years or older are recommended for intervention if they consistently produce speech sound errors—often called *residual* or *persistent errors*. Teenagers and adults who perceive that their phonological errors constitute a handicap should also be considered for instruction. Likewise, children of any age should be considered for evaluation when they or their parents are overly concerned about their speech sound productions.

THE NATURE OF THE PROBLEM

Once the need for intervention is established, the next logical step would be to try to determine what specific type of problem is occurring. This is sometimes called generating a diagnosis, or what Rvachew and Brosseau-Lapré (2012) have said is "...your best hypothesis about the underlying nature of the [problem] ..." (p. 505). Doing so would seem to make sense because this should help focus our intervention efforts. As discussed previously, for the organically based disorders, we usually have a clear sense of what is causing the difficulty with speech sounds and thus have developed specific interventions that appear to work for most individuals. For children born with clefts of the palate, for example, the primary problem is with the physical structures used for speech, which prevent proper speech learning. Medical or prosthetic interventions are carried out to address the physical defect, and SLPs then focus their efforts on teaching the physical aspects of speech production.

In the case of an SSD for which the cause is unknown, our ability to identify the underlying problem is limited. Recall the overall discussion of classification systems from Chapter 5; all three systems (etiology, symptomatology, processing) were intended to define subgroups of individuals with SSDs that identify the problem. The labels should, in principle, lead to particular types of treatments. In the case of Dodd's approach, research is emerging suggesting particular subgroups may benefit best from particular approaches (e.g., Dodd & Bradford, 2000). But there is still no broad consensus on the subgroups and, thus, there is no clear consensus on the specific treatments to be recommended. Even for the one subgroup that we agree on (childhood apraxia of speech [CAS]), our ability to distinguish it from other subgroups remains somewhat clouded. Understanding the core problem has, however, led to investigations of particular treatments (to be discussed in Chapter 12).

Recall also from Chapter 5 the outline presented for speech generation (reproduced here). The implication of that outline is that a problem at each step should lead to a specific label and perhaps a specific kind of treatment. Problems with ideation would reflect either cognitive or psychological issues, but treating those sorts of problems would be outside the SLP scope of practice in most cases. But the other three boxes certainly apply to our field. If we believe the problem is with sorting out how particular sounds function within the language system (e.g., does substituting one sound for another result in a change in meaning?), we would call it a *phonological disorder*. In such cases, we might be more inclined to use a linguistically based intervention (see Chapter 11). If we think the problem involves difficulty with transcoding (planning/programming), we might call it CAS and focus our intervention on that problem. And if we believe the problem is primarily a difficulty with physically producing the speech sounds, we would say it is an *articulation disorder* and be more inclined to use a motor-based intervention (see Chapter 10).

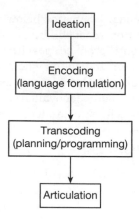

Even assuming this outline may be helpful, a major challenge is identifying the specific tasks that might help sort out the differences among problems in each of the steps in the speech generation outline. Unfortunately, there is still no consensus on what those tasks might be. If an individual has problems in more than one area (e.g., encoding and transcoding or transcoding and articulation) the task becomes even more complicated. Finally, it should be noted that this outline ignores speech perception. Although, as discussed previously, children with SSDs don't have general problems with speech perception, research suggests that as many as one-third of preschool children may have speech perception problems specific to their production errors (Eilers & Oller, 1976; Locke, 1980a; Rvachew et al., 1999).

The task is made even more complicated by the possibility that a particular child may have more than one problem at the same time. At the very least, speech acquisition involves sorting out 1) the perceptual attributes of each sound, 2) how each sound fits in the phonological system of the language, and 3) the motor movements required to produce them. Given the gradual nature of speech acquisition, it is conceivable that a child with three speech errors may have perceptual difficulty with one, a phonological issue with another, and an articulatory challenge with the third. Support for this idea of mixed disorders within individual children is found in a study by Dodd, Reilly, and colleagues (2018). These investigators reported findings for 4-year-old children who were producing non–age-appropriate errors. For purposes of that study, an articulation error required that the child be producing mostly distortion errors and not be stimulable for the error. Phonological errors consisted of mostly substitution or omission errors and were stimulable. Here are the findings:

14 children	Articulation errors only
1 child	Lateralized fricatives and phonological errors
13 children	Dentalized fricatives and phonological errors
13 children	Phonological errors only

Given the lack of consensus and difficulty pinning down the nature of the underlying problems, it should come as no surprise that, historically, clinicians have mostly ignored the question. Prior to the 1970s, all problems with speech sounds were assumed to be articulation disorders (and possibly problems with speech perception). Then there was a switch to thinking that almost all of these problems are phonological. As discussed earlier, studies such as those of Klein (1996) indicated that the switch in focus was largely positive, but not all children with SSDs were best helped with a phonological (linguistic) approach.

A Pragmatic Approach

Without specific recommendations grounded in research, how might one decide what to do? Some clinicians continue to ignore the distinctions between types of SSDs, and they treat all problems with speech sounds the same way. Although such an approach appears to lack a theoretical underpinning, it may not. By choosing a particular treatment, clinicians are actually making assumptions about the nature of the problem. For example, those who apply a motor-based therapy are effectively saying they believe that the problem is with physically producing the speech sounds (it is an articulation disorder). A recent study by Brumbaugh and Smit (2013) actually suggested that more clinicians use traditional motor-based therapy than other approaches. Likewise, those who apply a linguistically based therapy are really saying the problem is with sorting out how the sound units function to create meaning within the language (it is a phonological disorder).

Many clinicians recognize that SSDs do not all reflect the same problems. However, when lacking specific direction from the research evidence, they take a somewhat pragmatic approach. They do this by 1) assuming that speech perception problems are rare, if nonexistent (in the absence of a documented hearing loss), and largely ignore them; 2) assuming that a child with only a few errors must have an articulation disorder; 3) assuming that a child with many errors, especially where such errors can be described using phonological pattern labels, must have a phonological problem; and 4) assuming that children with the most severe problems and who progress the slowest must have CAS.

Such an approach raises several concerns. First, as discussed in Chapter 4, speech perception problems do occur in perhaps as many as one-third of preschool children. These are not general problems of perceiving speech but (where they exist) are likely specific to one or more speech sounds that the child is having difficulty producing. Thus, we recommend that speech perception skills be evaluated on all potential therapy targets using procedures such as the Speech Production Perception Task (Locke, 1980b) described in Chapter 6.

A second concern with the pragmatic approach is that the number of errors may not be an ideal indicator of the nature of the problem. As discussed earlier, just because it is possible to apply a phonological pattern label to an error or even to a group of errors does not by itself mean the underlying problem is phonological. A child may, for example, produce multiple errors because of difficulty with learning the motor movements for many sounds. That said, recall that studies such as that of Klein (1996) showed that a linguistically based treatment for children with multiple errors resulted in superior outcomes to a motor-based approach. Although such an approach is not universally successful, it may be a reasonable assumption that most children with multiple errors have a phonological disorder.

Likewise, the inverse situation needs to be considered. Farquharson (2019) presented a case of a child with a single sound in error who (based on an analysis of their spelling errors) appeared to have a poorly developed phonological representation for that sound. The problem would then appear to be at least partly phonological rather than articulatory. This led Neal (2020) to recommend examining each child's progress with reading and spelling to rule out phonological issues. Lacking such concerns, it seems reasonable to assume that a child with only a few errors likely has an articulation disorder.

The most problematic aspect of this pragmatic or atheoretical approach may be the assumption that the child who progresses slowly in treatment has CAS (see also Velleman, 2003). As was discussed in Chapter 5, given the array of treatment options (discussed in Chapters 10–12), slow progress in therapy may simply mean the best approach has yet to be applied; likewise, it may be that the child simply has difficulty learning to physically produce sounds or learning the rules of the phonology of the language. Consequently, separating CAS from a severe phonological disorder remains a challenge. Applying some of the CAS criteria discussed in Chapter 5 may be useful. One of the challenges we still face as professionals interested in SSDs is to develop more refined assessment tools so that we can make better predictions regarding the nature of a disorder and, thus, be more efficient and effective when we determine how we will approach intervention.

TARGET SELECTION

As a final aspect of the assessment process, sampling data are further reviewed to determine goals or targets for intervention. Note that while to some extent the selection of targets is specific to particular treatment approaches, the following covers some general considerations.

Developmental Appropriateness

Many clinicians follow what is sometimes called *developmental logic*. That means they assume that therapy should mimic the typical developmental sequence. In the process of speech sound acquisition, children typically produce errors. Using this approach, the goal is to determine whether particular speech sounds have not been mastered that should have been mastered at the child's current age. Any sounds that are deemed to be behind are then rank ordered from most to least behind and then treated in that order. In other words, target those sounds that are normally acquired earliest in the developmental sequence. A similar approach can be taken with phonological patterns (i.e., treat the earliest patterns that typically developing children no longer use).

Individual Speech Sounds

As discussed in Chapter 3, when deciding what is developmentally appropriate for particular sounds, one must be cautious when assigning an age to a particular sound. Investigators have attached an age expectation to specific speech sounds by listing the age levels at which a given percentage of children in a normative group have mastered each sound tested. Table 3.3 in Chapter 3 provides a detailed summary of these investigations. Sander (1972) pointed out that such normative data are group standards that reflect upper age limits (i.e., 75% or 90% of children at a particular age produce the sound) rather than average performance or customary production (50% of children at a particular age produce the sound). Sander stated that "variability among children in the ages at which they successfully produce specific sounds is so great as to discourage pinpoint statistics" (p. 58). Storkel (2019) extends this point by arguing that this variability provides clinicians with flexibility. Depending on the circumstances, a case could be made for using 50%, 75%, or 90% as the cutoffs for defining normal acquisition and for justifying when to work on particular sounds.

The studies outlined in Table 3.3 are based on large groups of children. Keep in mind that when using the data from any large group study, individual developmental data are obscured. Although the precise sequence and nature of phonological development varies from one person to another, in general, certain speech sounds are mastered earlier than others, and this information can be used in identifying appropriate speech sound targets. For example, if 6-year-old Kirsten says only the sounds usually produced by 75% of 3-year-old children but is not yet using sounds commonly associated with 4-, 5-, and 6-year-olds, her phonological productions would be considered delayed.

Although there is some variability across the normative studies of speech sound development, there is considerable agreement from one data set to another. Clinicians typically select one study (or more if they produced similar findings) as their reference point. Some have suggested that target selection might be based on the concept of relating age and sound errors to the early eight, middle eight, and late eight developing sounds (Shriberg, 1993) that were discussed in Chapter 3. Bleile's (2013) book titled *The Late Eight,* is a resource for teaching the late eight developing sounds (/ʃ, θ, s, z, ð, l, r, ʒ/). He indicated that these sounds are most likely to challenge school-age children and non-native speakers, both children and adults. This does not necessarily mean that these sounds should be the first sounds targeted. As pointed out, other variables are taken into consideration when determining sounds to be initially focused on for instruction.

Phonological Patterns

Rather than focusing on individual speech sounds, clinicians may consider the age appropriateness of certain phonological processes/patterns that may be present in a young child's speech. Several investigators have provided data that are relevant to young children's use of phonological processes (see also Table 3.9 in Chapter 3). In a cross-sectional study, Preisser and colleagues (1988) examined phonological patterns used by young children. Between ages 24 and 29 months, the most commonly observed patterns were cluster reduction, liquid deviation (which included deletions of a liquid in a consonant cluster; e.g., *black* → [bæk]), vowelization (e.g., *candle* → [kændo]), and gliding of liquids (e.g., *red* → [wɛd]). Next most common were patterns involving the strident feature.

Roberts and colleagues (1990) observed a group of children aged 2;5 to 8 years in a quasi-longitudinal study; that is, children were tested a varying number of times over the course of the study. They reported a marked decrease in the use of patterns between the ages of 2;5 and 4. They also reported that at age 2;5, the occurrence for the following patterns was less than 20% of opportunities: reduplication, assimilation, deletion of initial consonants, addition of a consonant, labialization shifts, methathesis, and backing. By age 4, only cluster reduction, liquid gliding, and deaffrication had an occurrence of 20% or more.

Stoel-Gammon and Dunn (1985) reviewed studies of pattern occurrence and identified those patterns that typically are no longer present by age 3 years and those that persist after age 3 in normally developing children. Their summary is:

Patterns Disappearing by 3 Years	Patterns Persisting After 3 Years
Unstressed syllable deletion	Cluster reduction
Final consonant deletion	Epenthesis
Consonant assimilation	Gliding
Reduplication	Vocalization (vowelization)
Velar fronting	Stopping
Prevocalic voicing	Depalatalization
	Final devoicing

Bankson and Bernthal (1990) reported data on the patterns most frequently observed in a sample of more than 1,000 children, 3–9 years of age, tested during the standardization of the Bankson-Bernthal Test of Phonology (BBTOP). The BBTOP ultimately included the 10 patterns that appeared most frequently in children's productions during standardization testing. The patterns that persisted the longest in children's speech were gliding of liquids, stopping, cluster simplification, vocalization (vowelization), and final consonant deletion. These data are almost identical to those reported by Khan and Lewis (1986), except they later (2002) found that velar fronting also persisted longer in young children's speech.

Hodson (2010a) suggested that clinicians focus on facilitating appropriate phonological patterns (rather than eliminating inappropriate ones). For highly unintelligible children, she suggested focusing on stimulable patterns so that the children can experience immediate success. As a general guide, Hodson delineates the following potential primary targets:

1. *Syllableness.* For omitted vowels, diphthongs, vocalic/syllabic consonants resulting in productions limited to monosyllables; using two-syllable compound words, such as *cowboy,* and then three-syllable word combinations, such as *cowboy hat*

2. *Singleton consonants in words.* Prevocalic /p, b, m, w/; postvocalic voiceless stops; pre- and postvocalic consonants, such as *pup, pop;* intervocalic consonants, such as *apple*

3. */s/ Clusters.* Word initial, word final

4. *Anterior/posterior contrasts.* Word-final /k/, word-initial /k/, /g/ for fronters; occasional /h/; alvolars/labials if backers

5. *Liquids.* Word-initial /l/, word-initial /r/, word-initial /kr/, /gr/—after the child readily produces singleton velars; word initial /l/ clusters—after the child readily produces prevocalic /l/

Complexity (Nondevelopmental) Approach

An alternative to using developmental logic is to take a complexity approach (i.e., treat the later developing or most complex sounds first). Research by Gierut and associates (1996) has suggested that for children with multiple errors, treatment of later as opposed to earlier developing sounds results in greater overall improvement in the client's phonological system than does targeting early developing sounds. This finding is in keeping with other research (Dinnsen et al., 1990; Tyler & Figurski, 1994) that suggests targeting sounds evidencing greater as opposed to lesser complexity is a more efficient way to proceed with speech sound intervention. These researchers reported that there was more generalization to other sounds when later or more complex sounds were targeted rather than earlier sounds (which are assumed to be easier to produce). Gierut (2001) suggested that by targeting the following, a greater impact might be made on a child's overall sound system:

1. Later developing as contrasted with early developing sounds

2. Nonstimulable as contrasted with stimulable sounds

3. Clusters as contrasted with singletons

4. Difficult to produce as contrasted with easy to produce sounds

Rvachew and Nowak (2001) reported data that do not support these assertions from a study of children with moderate or severe phonological delays. These investigators found that children who received treatment for phonemes that are early developing and associated with some degree of correct productions (productive phonological knowledge) showed greater progress toward production of the target sounds than did children who received treatment for late developing phonemes associated with little or no productive knowledge.

Tambyraja and Dunkle (2014) attempted to resolve the conflicting evidence for this approach by reviewing six available studies. They could not conclude that either a developmental or nondevelopmental approach was more effective overall. However, a nondevelopmental approach did appear to promote greater generalization to untreated sounds, particularly if the chosen treatment targets were not stimulable before the start of therapy.

Unusual Patterns/Errors

As noted earlier, unusual errors are far less likely to resolve on their own than typical errors (Morgan et al., 2017; Storkel, 2018a, 2019). As such, targeting sounds for which unusual errors are being used could easily be justified. For example, lateralization errors (which often occur with sibilant sounds) are not common at any age and are known to be difficult to remediate. When such errors are observed, ignoring developmental norms and targeting them early is recommended. Information on error frequency at various ages is available from Smit (1993a, 1993b).

Overall Intelligibility

On rare occasions (recall Clinical Vignette 7.1), a child is deemed eligible for therapy (e.g., by a normed test score), but on closer examination, none of the speech sounds or phonological patterns are judged to be developmentally delayed. In such cases, the clinician may opt for a watch-and-see approach where the child is monitored regularly to see if they are making progress. This is a less desirable approach for many parents. An alternative might be to make a more general instructional target, such as improving overall intelligibility. Although such a target is often the long-term goal for many individuals with SSDs, in this case, it becomes the central focus of intervention. One might approach such a target using the naturalistic approach (Camarata, 2021). This will be discussed in Chapter 11.

Stimulability

Another factor to be considered in selecting treatment targets is stimulability. Recall the earlier discussion of stimulability and case selection. The same considerations apply to target selection. Many clinicians have postulated that error sounds that can be produced through imitation are more rapidly corrected through intervention than sounds that cannot be imitated. McReynolds and Elbert (1978) reported that once a child could imitate a sound, generalization occurred to other contexts. Thus, imitation served as a predictor of generalization. Powell and colleagues (1991) also reported that stimulability explained many of the generalization patterns observed during treatment. They found that sounds that were stimulable were most likely to be added to the phonetic repertoire regardless of the sounds selected for treatment. Miccio and Elbert (1996) suggested that teaching stimulability may be a way to facilitate phonological acquisition and generalization by increasing the client's phonetic repertoire.

Although there seems to be general agreement that stimulability is associated with more rapid success in therapy, some clinicians assign such stimulable sounds a lower priority for remediation. The presumption is that they are more likely to improve on their own and therapy time might better be spent on treating nonstimulable sounds. Likewise, it has been reported that teaching sounds on which the child is not stimulable has the greatest potential to positively affect the child's overall phonological system, although such sounds may be more difficult to teach (Powell et al., 1991).

Recall, also, the earlier discussion of the complexity approach. In sum, there is justification for choosing both stimulable sounds as targets (e.g., faster progress in therapy) and nonstimulable sounds as targets (e.g., more overall gains in the child's system or less likely to self-correct). The evidence for either choice is not absolute and, therefore, each clinician must decide for themselves based on an individual client and the preferences of the clinician. Many take a mixed approach by choosing stimulable targets initially to promote early success in therapy, but switching to nonstimulable targets as therapy progresses. A somewhat concrete variation on the stimulable versus nonstimulable approach is that used in the Glaspey Dynamic Assessment of Phonology (Glaspey, 2019); in this case targets are rank ordered based on level of stimulability. Depending on one's choice to favor or disfavor stimulable sounds, speech sounds that are either the most or least stimulable could be targeted first.

Frequency of Occurrence

Another factor used in target sound selection is the frequency with which the sounds produced in error occur in the spoken language. Obviously, the higher the frequency of a sound in a language, the greater its potential effect on intelligibility if corrected through instruction. Thus, treatment may have its greatest impact on a client's overall intelligibility if frequently occurring segments produced in error are selected for treatment.

Shriberg and Kwiatkowski (1983) compiled data on the rank order and frequency of occurrence of the 24 most frequently used consonants in conversational American English from a variety of sources. Their compilation indicated that 11 consonants /n, t, s, r, l, d, ð, k, m, w, z/ occur very frequently in connected speech, so errors on these sounds are likely to have the most adverse effect on intelligibility. The data reported by Shriberg and Kwiatkowski also show that almost two-thirds of the consonants used in conversational speech are voiced, 29% are stops, 19% are sonorants, and 18% are nasals. Dental and alveolar consonants accounted for 61% of the productions, and labial and labiodental sounds for 21%. In other words, over four-fifths of consonant occurrences are produced at the anterior area of the mouth.

Contextual Analysis

As stated earlier, contextual testing examines the influence of surrounding sounds on error sounds. Contextual testing may identify *facilitating phonetic contexts*, which are defined as surrounding sounds that have a positive influence on production of error sounds (Kent, 1982). Thus, contextual testing provides data on phonetic contexts in which an error sound can be produced correctly, which could be a helpful beginning point for treatment. Through the identification of such contexts, the clinician might find that a specific sound doesn't have to be taught but should instead be isolated and stabilized in a specific context because it is already in the client's repertoire. Both the client and clinician may save the time and frustration that often accompany initial attempts to establish a speech sound by focusing first on contexts in which the sound is produced correctly and then gradually shifting to other contexts. For example, if a child lisps on /s/ but a correct /s/ is observed in the /sk/ cluster in [bɪskɪt] (biscuit), one could have the client say *biscuit* slowly, emphasizing the medial cluster (i.e., sk), and hopefully hear a good /s/. The client could then prolong the /s/ before saying the /k/ (i.e., [bɪs ss kɪt]) and ultimately say the /s/ independent of the word context (i.e., /sss/). This production could then be used to transfer and generalize to other contexts using the stabilized /s/ production.

In general, when contexts can be found where target sounds are produced correctly, such sound contexts can be used efficiently in remediation. The number of contexts in which a child can produce a sound correctly in a contextual test may provide some indication of the stability of the error. It seems logical that the less stable the error, the easier it might be to correct. If a client's error tends to be inconsistent across different phonetic contexts, one might assume that the chances for improvement are better than if the error tends to persist across different phonetic contexts or situations.

Contextual analysis can also be applied to phonological patterns. For example, does stopping affect only certain sounds? Is it perhaps limited to only the sibilant fricatives? Does fronting occur only in initial position of words? By determining the scope of each pattern, we are able to target our intervention efforts more specifically. Because contextual testing is somewhat time-consuming to accomplish, particularly if a formal measure is employed, it is one of the less frequently employed speech sound assessment approaches.

OTHER FACTORS TO CONSIDER IN INTERVENTION DECISIONS

Dialects and Second Language Learning

As will be discussed in detail in Chapter 14, the linguistic culture of the speaker is a factor that must be considered when deciding on the need for speech-language intervention or the targets to be addressed. This is particularly true for clients from ethnic or minority populations for whom one of the standard varieties of English might not be the norm. *Dialect,* as discussed in Chapter 14, refers to a consistent variation of a language, reflected in pronunciation, grammar, or vocabulary, that a particular subgroup of the general population uses. Although many dialects are identified with a geographical area, those of greatest interest to clinicians are often dialects related to sociocultural or ethnic identification.

The phonological patterns of a particular dialect may differ from the general cultural norm, but these variations reflect only differences, not delays or deficiencies, in comparison to the so-called standard version of the sound system, as well as broader aspects of language. To view the phonological or syntactic patterns used by members of such subcultures as delayed, deviant, or substandard is totally inappropriate. As F. Williams (1972) put it years ago, "The relatively simple yet important point here is that language variation is a logical and expected phenomenon, hence, we should not look upon nonstandard dialects as deficient versions of a language" (p. 111). This perspective has obvious clinical implications. Persons whose speech and language patterns reflect a nonstandard cultural dialect should not be considered for remediation or instruction unless their phonological patterns are outside the cultural norm for their region or ethnic group, or the individual wishes to learn a different dialect.

Phonological differences may also occur in the speech of individuals within subcultures. The speech and language patterns of African American people who live in New York City, for example, may be quite different from African Americans who live in New Orleans. One cannot use normative data based on General American English (GAE) to judge the phonological status of individuals of some subcultures, nor should one assume that members of certain subcultures have homogeneous linguistic patterns, especially when geographic or ethnic factors are considered. Again, refer to Chapter 14 for additional information on this topic. Phonological assessment and analysis procedures for 14 different languages are available at: http://phonodevelopment.sites.olt.ubc.ca/

Clinicians must take similar consideration when asked to work with individuals learning English as a second language. All such individuals will take time to master the elements of their new language. This means that the length of time a speaker has been learning the language is critical to what we should expect from them. Independent of that, it must be remembered that the individual may have underlying speech or language learning problems that are independent of the second language learning process. SLPs are not usually expected to teach English per se, but may be asked to consult in cases where the process is atypical or much slower than expected. Likewise, SLPs may be asked to work with individuals whose speech retains influences from their first language (i.e., those who have a foreign accent). This topic will be covered in more detail in Chapter 15.

Clinicians need to know about a child's linguistic and cultural background in order to make appropriate assessment-related decisions, including the need for intervention and instructional goals. Peña-Brooks and Hegde (2000) suggest that clinicians need to know:

1. The language and phonologic characteristics, properties, and rules of the linguistically diverse child's primary language

2. How the primary language affects the learning of the second language

3. How to determine whether there are language or phonologic disorders in the child's first language, second language, or both

In the event that a speaker wishes to modify their dialect or accent, the clinician may wish not only to use traditional sampling methods to describe the child's phonology, but also to employ measures specifically designed to assess the dialect and nonnative speaker's use of English phonology. Instructional decisions are then based on samples obtained and the variations that exist between standard English and the person's dialect or accent.

Social-Vocational Expectations

Another factor to consider in the analysis and interpretation of a phonological sample is the attitude of the client or the client's parents or caregivers toward the individual's speech sound status. In cases when a treatment recommendation is questionable, the attitude of a client or family may be a factor in decisions for or against intervention. This is particularly important for older children and adults. Extreme concern over an articulatory difference by the client or the client's parents may convince the clinician to enroll an individual for instruction. For example, the child who has a frontal lisp and has a name that begins with /s/ may feel very strongly that the error is a source of embarrassment, even though the lisp has minimal effect on intelligibility or academic learning. Crowe-Hall (1991) and Kleffner (1952) found that fourth- and sixth-grade children reacted unfavorably to children who had even mild articulation disorders. The literature contains many reports in which elementary children have recounted negative experiences in speaking or reading situations when they produced only a few speech sounds in error. Even minor distortions can influence how one is perceived. Silverman (1976) reported that when a female speaker simulated a lateral lisp, listeners judged her more negatively on a personality characteristics inventory than when she spoke without a lisp.

Overby and colleagues (2007) reported that second-grade teachers had different expectations of children's academic, social, and behavioral performances when making judgments of children who were moderately intelligible and those with normal intelligibility. One-third of the teachers related children's school difficulty to their SSDs and made expectations based on the speech intelligibility of the children.

The standard for acceptance of communication depends to a large extent on the speaking situation. People in public speaking situations could find that even minor distortions detract from their message. Some vocations; for example, radio and television broadcasters, may call for very precise articulation and pronunciations, and thus, some individuals may feel the need for intervention for what could be relatively minor phonetic distortions or even dialectal differences. We suggest that if an individual, regardless of age, feels hampered or vocationally limited by speech errors or speech differences, treatment/instruction should at least be considered.

DIGITAL/ONLINE PHONOLOGICAL ANALYSIS

Any discussion of phonological analysis and interpretation would be incomplete without calling attention to the fact that computer/digital programs are available to assist with the analysis of phonological samples in clients who exhibit multiple errors. Masterson and associates (1998) indicated that there are two primary reasons for using this type of analysis of a phonological sample: 1) it saves time and 2) it provides more detail of analysis than one typically produces with traditional paper and pencil (manual) analysis procedures.

In a study of time efficiency of procedures for phonological and grammatical analysis, comparing manual and computerized methods, Long (2001) reported that without exception for both phonology and language, computerized analyses were completed faster and with equal or better accuracy than were manual analyses. Phonological analyses included the evaluation of variability, homonymy, word shapes, phonetic inventory, accuracy of production, and correspondence between target and production forms. Long further indicated that the time needed for analyses, both computer and manual, was affected by the type of analysis, the type of sample, and the efficiency of individual participants.

Relative to the commercially available tests (i.e., those listed in Table 6.1), rapidly changing digital technology in the last 20 years has meant that these tools currently vary considerably in terms of the availability of digital analysis capabilities. The variations includes no digital scoring or analysis (DEAP, PAT-3, SPAT-D-3), CD-ROM-based scoring and analysis systems (HAPP-3; available separately from https://www.myphonocomp.com/), tablet-based apps (CAAP-2; LAT), and cloud-based scoring and analysis (AAPS-4; GDAP; GFTA-3). Where available, digital scoring and analysis involves inputting phonetic transcriptions from a computer or tablet keyboard and/or selecting from predetermined stimuli. Unfortunately, speech recognition technology is not yet adequately developed to allow for direct computer transcription from live or recorded speech samples. Once the transcriptions have been entered, various types of analyses (including generation of standard scores or percentile ranks and phonetic or phonemic inventories) can be conducted, displayed, and stored.

For informal assessments, including conversational speech samples, several programs have been developed over the years that provide systematic digital analysis. As with the commercially available tests, these require the clinician to transcribe the sample and enter the transcription manually. Two free programs are described next. Each program has its own strengths and limitations and, undoubtedly, future procedures will add new and helpful procedures for clinicians.

Computerized Profiling is a set of programs designed for both language and phonological analysis developed by Long and colleagues (2002). Analyses includes both relational and independent analyses of consonants and vowels, word position analysis, syllable shapes used, patterns among errors, and calculation of PCC. It can be downloaded from https://sites.google.com/view/computerizedprofiling.

The most recent version of Programs to Examine Phonetic and Phonological Evaluation Records (Shriberg, 2019) is a suite of programs that provides a variety of different analyses, including classification of the sample into a diagnostic category (as discussed in Chapter 5). This is available at https://phonology.waisman.wisc.edu/.

CASE STUDY: ASSESSMENT DATA

The anonymized case study that follows considers a young child referred to an SLP for evaluation. Introduced here, the case will be revisited in later chapters to exemplify varied perspectives on treatment and intervention.

Assessment: Phonological Samples Obtained

Client: Kirk

Age: 3;0 years

Reason for Referral: Parental referral due to Kirk's poor intelligibility even when speaking with familiar listeners, and only slightly better (but still poor) when speaking with those who know him well.

Case History/Speech and Hearing Mechanisms Status

The case history submitted by the parents and supplemented with an interview at the time of the examination revealed typical motor and language development; however, speech sound development was delayed. Hearing screening indicated that hearing was within normal limits. A speech mechanism examination indicated normal structure and function.

Language

Vocabulary, syntax, and pragmatics appeared typical based on case history, language sample obtained, and social interaction between Kirk and the examiner. Language skills, as measured by the Peabody Picture Vocabulary Test and the Preschool Language Scale, indicated language within normal limits. Poor intelligibility made it difficult to assess expressive morphosyntactic structures; however, a spontaneous speech sample obtained through storytelling evidenced four 6-word utterances, a seemingly rich vocabulary, and appropriate concepts for a 3-year-old child. Based on these data, Kirk's language skills were determined to be within normal limits. This will however, need to be confirmed later once his intelligibility improves.

Fluency and Voice

Fluency was regarded as normal. However, a hoarse voice was noted. It was determined that vocal quality should be monitored over time by the parents and clinician to determine whether a problem was developing.

Speech Sound Samples Gathered

The examiner gathered the following samples:

- Conversation connected speech sample of 180 words was obtained, with Kirk telling the story of the *Three Little Pigs*. This story was used because Kirk was familiar with it, and words in the story were known to the examiner, thus facilitating phonological analysis.

- Single-word productions were obtained through the BBTOP. All consonants and vowels produced by Kirk in the stimulus words were transcribed.

- Stimulability testing was done in isolation, syllables, and words for all target sounds produced in error.

Phonological Results and Analysis

The transcription of the connected speech sample and the single words from the BBTOP were analyzed with the Proph phonological analysis component of the Computerized Profiling (Long et al., 2002) program. Individual sound transcriptions were entered into the program and served as the basis for the analysis.

Phonological Analysis Outcomes

The PCC was determined based on the connected speech sample. The PCC value was 34%, which translates to a rating of severe for connected speech.

Segmental Analysis

Segmental analysis revealed numerous sound substitutions, particularly the use of /d/ in place of fricatives, affricates, and some clusters. In addition, there were inconsistent initial and final consonant deletions, including deletion of the initial /h/, /r/, and /l/. Other substitutions included /f/ for /s/ and some prevocalic voicing. These errors were evidenced in both single-word productions and in running speech, although higher accuracy was reflected in single-word productions. Table 7.1 reflects consonant singleton transcriptions from single-word productions. Figures in the table indicate percent accuracy of production.

Table 7.1. Consonant singleton productions in Kirk's single-word productions, including percentage accuracy of production

		Error productions		
Target	Error	Initial (%)	Error	Final (%)
p		100		100
b		100		100
m		100		100
w	Ø	0		
f	/d/	0	/s/	0
v	/d/	0		100
θ	/d/	0	/t/	0
ð	/d/	0		
t		100		100
d		100		100
s	/d/	0	/f/	50
z	/d/	0	/v/	0
n		100		100
l	Ø	0	/o/	0
ʃ	/d/	0	/f/	0
tʃ	/d/	0		100
dʒ	/d/	0		
j	Ø	0		
r	Ø	0		
k		100		100
g		100		100
h	Ø	0		

Key: Ø, omission error.

Stimulability Analysis

Imitative testing (stimulability) was conducted for all sounds produced in error. Kirk was instructed to "Look at me, listen to what I say, and then you say it." This was followed by a model of the correct sound. Responses were solicited for sounds in isolation, syllables, and the initial position of words.

Kirk was stimulable for most error sounds in isolation, syllables, and initial word position. He did not correctly imitate any of the clusters that were in error. The following sounds were not stimulable: /ʃ/, /tʃ/, /z/, /dʒ/, /r/, and /ɝ/. The /s/ was stimulable only in isolation, even though it was observed in the word-final position of some spontaneous words produced during testing.

Pattern Analysis

A phonological pattern analysis was completed through the Proph program (Long et al., 2002) to determine error patterns that were evidenced in Kirk's single-word as well as connected speech sample. This analysis revealed that the most prevalent pattern was stopping, with all fricatives and affricates impacted (85% of possible occasions in connected speech and 44% occurrence in stimulus words from the BBTOP, particularly initial position). The most prevalent example of stopping was the use of /d/, which was substituted for initial /f/, /v/, /θ/, /ð/, /s/, /z/, /ʃ/, /tʃ/, and /dʒ/, and the clusters /sl/, /sn/, and /fl/. Kirk used frication (e.g., /s/, /f/, although inappropriately) when producing some single words. A diagram of his sound collapses for /d/ is as follows:

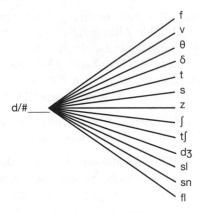

Clusters were simplified approximately 75% of the time in both isolated words and connected speech samples. Less frequently occurring patterns included context-sensitive voicing (prevocalic voicing) and initial consonant deletions. Prevocalic voicing occurred in less than 25% of possible instances and initial consonant deletions less than 12%.

Vowel Analysis

The Proph program assesses vowel accuracy and, as might be expected for his age, Kirk's vowel productions were almost entirely accurate in both running speech and single-word productions. Inconsistent misarticulations were observed on the vowels /ɛ/ and /ʊ/ in running speech.

Summary

These data reflect a 3-year-old boy with an SSD that, according to his PCC, BBTOP norms, and examiner's subjective evaluation, is severe in nature. Although intelligibility was not formally measured, understanding his verbal productions was difficult even for family members. Most of Kirk's errors were sound substitutions, with some deletions in both initial and final word positions. Substitution errors were predominately the /d/ being substituted for fricatives and affricates. The presence of initial consonant deletions is developmentally an unusual process, but it is present only for the aspirate /h/ and liquids. Final consonant deletion is a process usually no longer seen in children by age 3 years and was observed only occasionally in Kirk's speech. Inconsistencies in all types of error productions were noted.

Speech sound errors for which Kirk was not stimulable included the fricative /ʃ/, the affricates /tʃ/ and /dʒ/, the prevocalic /r/, and the vocalic /ɝ/. These error sounds will likely need to be stabilized in isolation and/or syllables and will require motor practice in single words before they are incorporated into word pairs that reflect relevant sound contrasts. For /h/ and /k/, which were easily stimulated at the word level, it is likely that Kirk needs instruction in how these sounds are used contrastively in the language, or it might be necessary only to monitor these sounds to make sure they are acquired.

Assessment: Interpretation

Case Selection

Intervention is warranted for Kirk. Factors that influenced this recommendation are as follows:

1. Normative data indicate that most normally developing 3-year-old children are approximately 75% intelligible. Although Kirk has just turned 3, we would nonetheless expect him to be more intelligible than he is. Intelligibility was not formally determined in our assessment battery, but observational data, as well as reports from his family, indicate that much of Kirk's speech is unintelligible. This factor weighed heavily in our decision regarding Kirk's need for intervention.

2. With a PCC value in running speech of less than 40%, Kirk's impairment is regarded as severe in nature. This rating relates to level of handicap reflected in his speech.

3. Phonological analysis evidences numerous substitution errors, some deletions, and several phonological patterns that one would not expect in a child of his age. Positive indicators regarding Kirk's phonological status include the fact that he uses almost all vowels and some consonants correctly in his speech and is stimulable (with effort) for many of his error segments. His relatively large vocabulary and the length of his utterances suggest that his linguistic deficits are confined to articulation and phonology, another positive indicator.

4. Intervention appears favorable because Kirk is stimulable for many of his error sounds, is highly verbal, has appropriate language skills, and is not reluctant to speak.

Target Selection

Because Kirk has numerous misarticulations and because these errors fall into patterns, target selection should begin with a review of these patterns. The error pattern that occurred most frequently was that of stopping, with several initial sounds, predominately fricatives and glides, collapsed into /d/. He also evidenced voicing of voiceless consonants in the initial position, gliding of liquids, and cluster reductions.

Although stopping is a pattern that persists in children sometimes past the age of 3, it is unusual for a child of this age not to be using more fricatives in speech. Most children are expected to use /f/ correctly by this age, and many are using /s/ as well. Because the fricative feature is diminished in Kirk's speech, reduction of stopping is the phonologic target of choice for initial therapy. The other two patterns evidenced in Kirk's speech (i.e., voicing, gliding) will be focused on later, largely because voicing does not have a great impact on intelligibility, and gliding occurred relatively infrequently and likely does not affect Kirk's intelligibility as much as stopping.

Intervention suggestions for Kirk are discussed in detail at the end of Chapters 10 and 11. In terms of target selection, we would suggest approaches that allow for focusing on several error sounds in each lesson. Kirk's good attention span and good language skills will hopefully facilitate his handling multiple treatment goals. We would suggest addressing the sound collapses reflected in the /d/ replacement for numerous fricatives, other stops, and clusters.

Because Kirk is very young, one might choose to focus on only one or two sounds in the early sessions to avoid confusion among targets. As progress is made, additional targets can be identified and added to the sessions. If one chooses to focus on one or two target sounds at a time, our suggestion for a priority focus is /f/. This is a highly visible sound and one that develops early, would address Kirk's stopping pattern, and frequently develops in final position prior to initial position. Kirk already uses the sound as a substitution for other fricatives in the final position; for example, he says /tif/ for /tiθ/ but /lis/ for /lif/. A second treatment target, likely one to work on simultaneously, is the correct use of /s/. The /s/ is in Kirk's repertoire, however, it is used inappropriately. As stated already, length of attention span, including ability to focus on multiple sounds and/or sound contrasts simultaneously, will influence the choice of treatment approach. This issue is addressed in Chapters 10 and 11.

Summary

Kirk is a child who needs phonological intervention. The intelligibility, severity, and developmental level of his phonology support this decision. On the basis of his phonological samples, teaching frication to reduce stopping, producing sounds correctly in word-initial position, and further increasing Kirk's phonological repertoire would appear to be priority goals for initiating therapy.

CONCLUSION

Assessment data are interpreted for a variety of reasons, including deciding if there is a problem, the nature of the problem, whether treatment is indicated, and what the treatment targets might be. Each decision requires the consideration of a number of different factors. The next chapter turns to a discussion of the basic considerations for treatment.

QUESTIONS FOR CHAPTER 7

1. Discuss how the following factors may be utilized in case selection:
   a. Intelligibility
   b. Stimulability
   c. Error patterns
2. Discuss how the following factors might influence target behavior selection:
   a. Stimulability
   b. Frequency of occurrence
   c. Developmental appropriateness
   d. Contextual analysis
   e. Phonological patterns
3. Differentiate between intelligibility and severity.
4. How might treatment targets differ between a preschool child and a child aged 12 years?
5. How do dialectal considerations influence intervention decisions?
6. Discuss what we know and do not know about determining the underlying nature of SSDs.

8

Using Evidence-Based Practice in Treatment

PETER FLIPSEN JR., NICHOLAS W. BANKSON, AND JOHN E. BERNTHAL

LEARNING OBJECTIVES

The focus of this chapter is the application of general principles of evidence-based practice (EBP) to treatment for speech sound disorders (SSDs). By the end of this chapter, the reader should be able to:

- Define EBP.
- Identify the three elements of EBP that must be integrated.
- Discuss how evidence levels might be used in selecting treatment approaches.
- Contrast information provided by published (peer reviewed) evidence versus clinical evidence.
- Distinguish among treatment data, generalization data, and control data and how they might be used to detect change and determine what might have caused the change.

Before discussing particular treatment approaches, this chapter and the one that follows focus on some basic underlying concepts that should be considered when developing a treatment plan. We begin with a discussion of *evidence-based practice* or *EBP*, a system that provides a scientific perspective for application of any treatment approach. ASHA (2004b, 2005) has adopted EBP principles, which include suggestions for how clinicians can objectively document treatment outcomes.

The goal of speech-language therapy is to facilitate change in clients' communication. To do so, we typically assess baseline skill in our initial assessments, apply some type of intervention, and then reassess to see if change has occurred. When change occurs in the direction for which we aimed, then everyone is usually pleased. A critical question, however, is whether we can be certain that the observed change was the result of our intervention. As will be discussed later in this chapter, other possible causes (called extraneous effects) of the change must also be considered. This is important, because in an age of accountability, those who pay for our services deserve to know whether or not any observed changes are due to the intervention that was provided. We also should be motivated to know this because if the change was actually the result of something other than our instruction, we have wasted both valuable time (ours and that of our client) and resources. That represents time and resources that could have been better spent elsewhere.

THE BASICS OF EVIDENCE-BASED PRACTICE

EBP is a framework that allows us to be accountable to our clients, to those who pay for our services, and to ourselves. At its core, it involves the integration of three elements into the decision-making process for our clients:

1. The best available published evidence

2. Clinical evidence collected using our clinical expertise

3. The preferences and values of the client

Published evidence indicates whether or not, under somewhat controlled conditions with a particular group of clients, a particular treatment is effective at remediating a particular problem. In other words, it shows us what might work. If our client shows similar characteristics to the clients reported in published evidence, there is a good chance the treatment outcomes will also be similar. It is clearly not a guarantee, however. On the other hand, if the client is not similar to those in the published evidence, we would be less certain about whether that treatment is applicable or the most efficacious, although it may still work.

EBP definitions usually list clinical expertise as the second key element. This expertise is not simply a clinician's training and experience, although that is a major part of it. From an EBP perspective, it includes the ability to initially judge whether change is happening and, secondly, whether the change is due to the intervention or something else. This means it requires designing and implementing a system of clinical data collection to generate clinical evidence.

Client preferences and values represent choices that clients make for themselves. Based on the ethical principle of autonomy, they (or their parents/caregivers) have the right to determine what happens to them. As will be discussed in subsequent chapters, clinicians usually have a range of possible therapy options from which to choose. Before beginning therapy, we are obliged to present our client with treatment options that might be provided and discuss the possible benefits and risks of each. Although it may be subject to the limitations of our workplace and caseload, the choice of which option to use is ultimately up to them (or their parents/caregivers).

THE PUBLISHED EVIDENCE

In its definition of EBP, ASHA's position statement specifies that SLPs should use ". . . current, high-quality research evidence . . ." (ASHA, 2005; p.1). The notion of high quality implies that the quality of the available research varies. How then does one judge that quality? Although a detailed discussion of such evaluation is beyond the scope of this text, one basic way is to consider the design of the study. Over the years, the efficacy of various treatment approaches for different speech and language disorders has been evaluated using an array of different formats and study designs. Each study design provides varying degrees of control over other possible causes of change (i.e., extraneous effects). Discussion of how these designs exhibit this control is typically covered in another part of your education but, in general, it is possible to rank study designs with the rankings reflecting the degree to which extraneous effects are controlled. The results of such rankings are referred to as *evidence levels*. ASHA's (2004b) technical report on EBP includes a set of such levels, arranged to show that higher-level studies (i.e., those with a lower numerical rating) provide greater degrees of control over extraneous effects than those with a higher number. The levels are:

Level Ia   Well-designed meta-analysis of more than one randomized controlled trial

Level Ib   Well-designed randomized controlled study

Level IIa   Well-designed controlled study without randomization

Level IIb   Well-designed quasi-experimental study

Level III   Well-designed nonexperimental studies (i.e., correlational and case studies)

Level IV   Expert committee report, consensus conference, clinical experience of respected authorities

It is important to point out that the lowest level (level IV) is *expert opinion,* which includes that of both academic professionals and experienced clinicians. Although it is not a particularly high level of evidence, expert opinion can be valuable because it is usually based on extensive experience and is often where we start if a new approach appears. However, despite their experience, experts and experienced clinicians may be biased (often unknowingly) for or against a particular approach. Some of this bias arises because of time spent employing particular approaches. They may know a methodology better and thus do a better job administering it than some other approach with which they are less familiar. In addition, if an approach results in desired outcomes, clinicians can be biased to continue to use such an approach even though it might not be the most efficacious. This strong possibility of bias means that more objective evidence/documentation obtained through formal and controlled research studies (when available) should take precedence over expert opinion.

Specific research into interventions for SSDs has been ongoing for many years. Baker and McLeod (2011a) conducted an extensive review of published treatment studies conducted up to that point. They used the previous evidence level scheme to assign evidence levels to each of the studies reviewed. They excluded level IV reports but identified 134 other studies published between 1979 and 2009. Of these, Baker and McLeod found that only two meta-analyses (level Ia) had been conducted. There were also 20 randomized control trials (level Ib), but 100 (74%) of the studies were either level IIb or level III. This suggests that much of the available evidence regarding treatment effectiveness related to SSDs is at lower evidence levels. Baker and McLeod did note a positive trend in the literature for more recent studies to be of higher evidence levels than in the past. They also pointed out that the majority of the studies (63.6%) reviewed involved 10 or fewer participants, which seriously limits our ability to make broad conclusions or generalize from such studies. The bottom line appears to be that, although there is a fairly large body of treatment literature concerning SSDs, much work remains to be done.

Two sets of authors have drawn general conclusions about whether treatment for SSDs works by examining the findings of two level Ia studies. Both Law and colleagues (2004) and Nelson and colleagues (2006) looked broadly at outcome research for both speech and language interventions, and reported specific findings for SSDs. In each review, the authors examined findings from studies that spanned a number of years in which participants had been randomly assigned to experimental or control groups. Both reviews concluded that, when comparing the groups receiving intervention to those receiving no treatment, the intervention groups consistently performed better than the no-treatment groups on outcome assessment measures. This positive treatment effect was seen with a variety of outcome measures. Thus, it would appear that, at least in general terms, interventions for SSDs makes a positive difference.

Relative to specific approaches, Baker and McLeod (2011a) documented 46 different approaches, with 23 approaches studied more than once. Unfortunately, only 40 of 134 (30%) studies involved direct comparisons of different approaches. Among studies of the same approach, Baker and McLeod observed that different investigators sometimes reached different conclusions. In such cases, it may be necessary to compare research designs (i.e., evidence levels) because, as noted earlier in this chapter, different designs offer different amounts of control over the influence of extraneous effects. Findings from higher level studies provide us with more confidence in the outcomes. Where conflicting studies are at the same evidence level, further review will be required. More recent evidence grouped by specific approaches is also available in A. L. Williams and colleagues (2021).

Selecting an Approach

As noted, many approaches have evidence that they can work, thus resulting in the need for clinicians and clients to make choices. Given that higher level evidence provides better control over extraneous effects, approaches with the highest levels of evidence would always be preferable. Consequently, it is also important to examine the participant descriptions in the studies to see how similar the participants are to the client we have in front of us. The more similar the participants in a study are to our client, the greater the likelihood that the treatment will be effective with our client.

CLINICAL EVIDENCE

The second element of EBP is clinical expertise. This includes the collection of clinical data to determine both if change is occurring and whether or not the treatment is responsible for the change. Doing so requires selecting the appropriate measures to use and being able to interpret what they mean.

Measuring Change

From a clinical perspective, there are at least three types of change to consider. First, there is the overall change that reflects progress toward the long-term goal. Such goals typically involve achievement of both near error-free production, as well as full message intelligibility. As discussed in Chapter 6, norm-referenced tests, such as the Goldman-Fristoe Test of Articulation, the Clinical Assessment of Articulation and Phonology, and the Bankson-Bernthal Test of Phonology, can be used to determine eligibility for therapy and are designed for that purpose.

It is tempting to simply readminister these tests on a regular basis and look for changes in test scores as a measure of progress. This is not a wise practice for several reasons. First, with such a practice, there is a statistical problem known as *regression to the mean* (to be discussed later in this chapter). Second, and from a more practical standpoint, such tests typically provide only a limited sample of the child's speech. They often include only a single word that tests performance on each sound in each word position (e.g., word-initial /s/). It is possible that when such a test is readministered the child might remember having problems with that particular word during testing and may have practiced the word. The child may then appear to have mastered the sound but is not necessarily able to produce that same sound in other words. On the other hand, the child may have become hypersensitive to that particular word because of their failure and might continue having difficulty with it, even when they are perfectly capable of producing that sound in many other words. Thus, norm-referenced tests may simply not be sensitive enough to capture change in speech sound performance. Such tests are also not consistent indices of intelligibility and may not be appropriate to assess progress toward intelligibility goals.

A more appropriate procedure for tracking overall change would be the use of recording and transcription of conversational speech samples. As suggested by Newbold and associates (2013), change could be tracked using segmental measures, such as percentage consonants correct (PCC), or word-level measures, such as proportion of whole-word proximity (PWP).

The second and more immediate type of change to be considered is the moment-to-moment performance on the specific therapy targets being practiced. This is sometimes referred to as *treatment data*. The context of these treatment data will vary widely depending on how therapy is progressing. It may, for example, reflect performance on the target sound produced in isolation, in word contexts, or embedded in a conversational interaction. Over time, as speech sound skill improves, accuracy on these targets is expected to improve. These data are typically recorded at the end of each treatment session as percentage correct.

The third type of change to be considered is the degree to which the skill being taught in therapy has generalized beyond the specific items that are being worked on in therapy. This topic will be covered in more detail in the next chapter but, broadly speaking, *generalization* is the extent to which the skills taught in therapy can be used in other communicative contexts. Without such generalization, every communication skill would need to be taught in every possible context, which would be highly impractical. For example, if the client is taught to produce /s/ in 25 different words containing /s/, we would expect that the client would come to be able to correctly produce /s/ in other words where that sound occurs, not just that particular set of 25 words. Likewise, we would expect that skill/production with /s/ might generalize to similar sounds such as /z/. We might also expect that both /s, z/ would also be produced correctly in interactions with other people besides the clinician or in other physical locations besides the therapy room.

The degree to which skills are generalizing must be measured, and this is typically done using what are known as *probes* (sometimes called *generalization probes*) for each target sound being worked on in therapy (see Elbert et al., 1967). Such probes might include several words (typically 8–15) that contain the target sound but which have not been used in therapy activities. The S-CAT probes (Secord & Shine, 1997a) discussed in Chapter 6 can be used or adapted for this purpose. Using words that are not practiced in therapy helps determine whether the child is actually learning the sound and generalizing that sound into new/novel words in their sound system. Having a sound incorporated into the child's speech sound system allows the child to correctly produce any word containing the sound, even if that word has seldom been encountered before.

Without such probes, clinicians can never be certain that the child isn't simply memorizing the set of speech movements for the particular words being practiced in therapy. Probes generally are not administered during each treatment session because clinicians do not want the child to become overly familiar with the words used in the probe. A more typical practice is to administer a probe every four or five sessions, once a month, or at the point when the child reaches some predetermined production criterion on the practice words used during instruction. Generalization probes are also occasionally administered in other physical settings and with other communication partners.

Determining What Caused the Change

Change either happens or it doesn't. Clinicians collect treatment data and administer generalization probes to determine whether the child is developing the targeted skill and incorporating the targeted sounds or patterns into their sound system. If a client is not showing improvement, the speech-language pathologist (SLP) has to decide whether to continue the intervention plan or modify it. On the other hand, an SLP who sees change has confirmation that the intervention is meeting the goal for the clients to make progress toward normal speech sound skills and produce intelligible speech. Yet, as noted earlier, seeing change and positive outcomes may not be enough. By themselves, changes observed in treatment data and generalization probe data do not always mean that the treatment was responsible for the change. It is still quite possible that something else may be responsible.

Other Factors Possibly Responsible for Clinical Change

What else might have caused the change in the individual's speech? If the clinician provided intervention and the child improved, is it not reasonable to assume that the treatment caused it? Perhaps it did, but there is a possibility that the change was unrelated to the treatment. Other influences could have been involved.

If you enter a room and flip on a light switch and a light turns on, you would likely assume that it was your action of moving the switch that caused the light to go on. That may not be the only explanation, however. Perhaps there was a motion sensor in the room that turned on the light. Your act of flipping the switch may just have been coincidental. If there's a motion sensor, it was your movement as you entered the room that actually turned on the light. On the other hand, what if the light was really turned on by sound activation? Your footsteps or the noise of turning the door handle as you entered the room would be what turned on the light. Again, your flipping the switch on would have been just coincidental. Alternatively, what if a wireless device held by a friend who was with you controlled the light, and your friend actually turned on the light using that device just as you flipped the switch? Or, finally, what if there were a timer on the light and you happened to flip on the switch exactly as the timer was turning the lights on? In either of these circumstances, your act of flipping on the switch may have been a coincidence. The light just happened to come on right after you flipped the switch.

These are far-fetched examples, but they serve to illustrate that clinicians should not be too quick to assume that observed changes resulted from their efforts. In clinical situations, a number of different things (sometimes called extraneous effects) might really have caused the change instead of, or in addition to, a clinician's intervention. Gruber and colleagues (2003) identified several such effects of which practicing clinicians need to be aware. One of the first factors to consider when working with children is normal development or maturation. It is always possible that a child's maturational development (e.g., fine-motor skills, auditory discrimination skills, grasp of a particular phonemic contrast) may have changed on its own, so that the child is now capable of producing the sound on which the clinician and child have been working. The change may have had little or nothing to do with the intervention. This is part of what Gruber and colleagues called the *natural history effect,* or the normal course of a condition over time, and can be either positive (i.e., the condition improves) or negative (such as in certain genetic or degenerative disorders). For children, the natural history effect includes factors such as normal development. For adults, the natural history effect includes things like normal recovery from neurological insult or the expected deterioration seen over time from a degenerative disorder such as Parkinson disease.

A second extraneous effect is the well-known *placebo effect,* in which improvement results from intervention of any sort being applied. Gruber and colleagues (2003) document a wide range of studies (in speech-language pathology and other disciplines) demonstrating this type of effect. Any attention being paid to the speech of young children has the potential to lead the child to focus on their speech and make changes that have nothing to do with the specific intervention that is being applied. Such changes may be temporary or even permanent. A variation on the placebo effect is the *Hawthorne effect,* in which the client improves because they become convinced that the particular treatment they are receiving is working. A fourth extraneous effect discussed by Gruber and colleagues is the *experimenter effect,* or *Pygmalion effect,* in which the client responds positively to clinician attention, signals, and/or interactions with the clinician so that change occurs. The client may have such high confidence in the skill of the clinician that they assume the treatment must be working. For all three of these effects (placebo, Hawthorne, and Pygmalion), the client may put forth extra effort or place extra focus on treatment. It may also be the case that the client or their family reports improvement to the clinician when in fact there is none. Clinicians cannot monitor clients' speech all the time, so they often rely on reports from the client or client's family to help determine therapy success and/or change in the speech of an individual.

Finally, there is also the previously mentioned *regression to the mean.* This is a statistical (but very real) phenomenon. It involves the very high probability that anyone who achieves an extremely low or extremely high score on some measurement will produce a subsequent score on that same measurement that is closer to the average (or the mean). People vary in their behavior from moment to moment, and that is certainly true of children with SSDs. When the SLP measures a child's performance on a norm-referenced test, the SLP obtains a sample of the child's behavior. If at one point the child produces a very low score, part of the reason for that low score may be because they were not necessarily performing at their best on that particular day. Indeed, the child may have been performing at their worst. Statistically speaking, when the clinician measures their performance at a later time, the probability is very high that the child will have a better day and their score will go up (i.e., be closer to the mean). The higher score may have nothing to do with a change in the child's skill resulting from therapy.

In addition to the extraneous effects discussed by Gruber and colleagues (2003), there are also potential influences from outside therapy sources. Some children, for example, may be attending private therapy in addition to receiving services from clinicians in the public schools. Alternatively, parents or teachers who are often aware of the intervention goals may be emphasizing correct articulation in their interactions with the child, such as during book-reading activities. Such additional input or instruction is certainly a potentially positive influence, but it serves to complicate the question of what caused the change.

Adding Control Data

Given that clinicians cannot assume that observed changes are always due to therapy, what can be done about it? The solution lies in collecting control data (Baker & McLeod, 2004). These are data obtained from treatment targets for which no therapy is being applied and which are different enough from the current treatment targets so that no generalization would be expected. The client ends up serving as their own control. It is very similar to a research strategy known as a *single subject design*. It is also often called a multiple baseline design. Progress on treated targets is compared against progress on untreated control targets. Change is expected to only occur on the treated targets (and on the generalization probes) but not on the control targets. Eventually, treatment would be applied to the control targets and, at that point, change would be expected on those targets. This illustrates a concept known as *experimental control*, in which change only occurs when treatment is applied and not at any other time. In other words, the client is serving as their own control, from a research design perspective.

This strategy is illustrated in Figure 8.1 with a hypothetical example of a child who has as the treatment goal to improve their production of both /s/ and /r/. On the horizontal axis of each half of the figure is the number of the session in which performance is measured. On the vertical axis of the top half is the percentage correct for /s/ and on the vertical axis of the bottom half is the percentage correct for /r/. Sessions 1 through 3 are baseline sessions in which no treatment was provided and, as shown, no improvement was noted for either target. Such baseline measurements are important to establish that the behavior you are measuring is not beginning to change on its own. During sessions 4 through 7, treatment was provided for /s/ (treatment I) but not yet for /r/, which serves as the control sound. Notice an increase in the percentage correct for /s/ but no change in the percentage correct for /r/. At that point, treatment is introduced for /r/, and an improvement is seen in the percentage correct for /r/ during sessions 8 through 11.

How does this approach account for extraneous effects? The change was seen when treatment was applied to each target, but no change was observed when treatment was not applied. And when the focus of treatment changed to a new target, change was seen on the new target. There is a direct connection between when treatment is applied and when change occurs. It appears that the treatment was responsible for the change. If any extraneous effects had been operating, improvement might have been seen on at least some (if not all) of the targets that were not receiving treatment. When this happens, the value of our intervention could be called into question. Lof (2010) described the collection of data to control for extraneous effects in this way as the generation of practice-based evidence.

To summarize, three different kinds of clinical data are required:

1. *Treatment data.* Performance on the specific targets being used in therapy sessions

2. *Generalization probes.* Performance on related or similar targets that are not currently being worked on in therapy but where generalization might be expected

3. *Control probes.* Performance on unrelated, untreated targets

Treatment data are useful to determine whether change is taking place. Generalization probes indicate whether the client is integrating (generalizing) the new target into their speech and language system. Control probes can help indicate whether

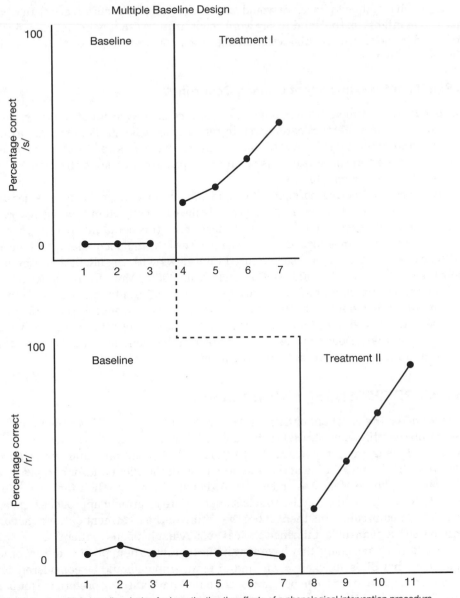

Figure 8.1. A multiple baseline design for investigating the effects of a phonological intervention procedure.

extraneous factors might be influencing the change. From the perspective of wanting to know if the treatment is causing the change, we hope for change on both the treatment data and the generalization probes, but no change on the control probes. Refer again to Figure 8.1 for an illustration of this. When treating a fricative like /s/ (treatment I), we would not expect change to occur on a liquid like /r/, because the two sounds are very different in terms of how they are produced and their acoustic characteristics. Thus, /r/ was serving as the control sound during our treatment of /s/. Seeing change on /s/ but no change on /r/ suggests that no extraneous factor is influencing the change on /s/, and the change is the result of our treatment. If change had occurred on /r/ when we were not treating it, we could not be certain as to why /s/ had improved.

During each treatment phase, we would also be checking for generalization. In treatment I, we might ask the child to say words containing /s/ that were not specifically practiced in the treatment. Likewise, during treatment II, we might do the same with untreated /r/ words.

Is Significant and Important Change Occurring?

It is one thing to demonstrate that change is occurring as a result of treatment; it is quite another to say that the degree or quality of the change is significant or important. Olswang and Bain (1994) suggested that the clinician can answer "yes" to this question only if broader generalization is occurring. The nature of generalization will be discussed in the next chapter.

Another perspective on significant and important change is to consider the degree to which the client or their caregivers believe that any change being observed is having a positive effect on their lives. Determining this could involve simply asking the client or caregiver directly about their sense of the impact of therapy (Krueger, 2019) or even conducting more structured interviews with the client and others in their life (e.g., Barr et al., 2008; McCormack et al., 2009). More formal measures of how the child is functioning socially can be completed by parents, teachers, and others in the child's life. Examples of such measures include the Strengths and Difficulties Questionnaire (Goodman, 1997) and the Pediatric Quality of Life Inventory (Varni, Seid, & Rode, 1999). Documenting change with such instruments would require that they be administered before and after treatment.

CLIENT PREFERENCES AND VALUES

The idea of asking the client or their caregivers for their opinion about the impact of therapy on their life suggests that their perspective may be as important as that of the clinician. This is, in part, why the ASHA (2004b) EBP position statement requires that, from the very beginning of the interactions with the client and/or caregiver, we also consider their preferences and values. Although clients and their families rarely have the knowledge and expertise to select appropriate treatment approaches, engaging in EBP means educating them about the nature of the treatment options that are available so they can make informed choices about what happens to them.

In addition to ensuring they have a say in the therapy to be applied, there are other aspects of what SLPs do where client and/or family input should be considered. For example, there are times when parents (or the child) have a strong preference for particular speech sound targets, which may be very important to them (e.g., names of siblings or pets). Another area where input should be sought is in the use of reinforcement for positive responses. Some clinicians like to use tangible reinforcements (e.g., tokens, prizes, food items), but some parents may object to these in general, seeing them as a form of bribery. In the case of food reinforcements in particular, many parents have strong feelings about what their children eat. Parents may also identify food allergies that were not documented in their child's file. Another aspect of therapy for which parents may want to be consulted is the choice of stimulus items. Some may have objections to the use of words related to particular topics. On the other hand, they may have suggestions for particular words that also happen to fit their child's therapy goals (e.g., particular words that begin with /s/ or that end with /k/). Regular positive dialogue with parents is strongly recommended.

CONCLUSION

In order to be effective, efficient, and accountable, interventions must be approached systematically. This involves employing what we know from the existing literature, as well as EBP principles for making informed decisions regarding every step in the process. The next chapter discusses practical considerations for the application of any therapy approach.

QUESTIONS FOR CHAPTER 8

1. Describe the three components of EBP that must be integrated.

2. What information do treatment data, generalization probes, and control probes provide?

3. What does practice-based evidence tell us that published research does not?

9

The Basics of Remediation

NICHOLAS W. BANKSON, PETER FLIPSEN JR., AND JOHN E. BERNTHAL

LEARNING OBJECTIVES

This chapter discusses the basic elements of remediation of speech sound disorders (SSDs). By the end of this chapter, the reader should be able to:

- List and discuss the various elements of a framework for organizing speech sound remediation.
- Compose basic short, intermediate, and long-term goals for speech sound remediation.
- Distinguish among different intervention styles.
- Describe the three basic components involved in effective stimulus presentation.
- Compare and contrast vertical, horizontal, and cyclical goal attack strategies.
- Discuss the various aspects involved in measuring treatment intensity.
- Distinguish between pull-out and classroom-based intervention.
- Discuss the advantages and disadvantages of individual versus group intervention.
- Differentiate among treatment data, control data, and generalization data, and describe how such data might be collected.
- Discuss various types of generalization and how they might be facilitated.
- Discuss the factors involved in deciding when to dismiss a client from therapy.
- Describe some of the challenges of working with both very young and older children.

Once a determination has been made that an individual's speech sound production is disordered or delayed and warrants intervention, the speech-language clinician is faced with the task of identifying the most appropriate treatment approach. Before discussing the specifics of particular treatment approaches in the next three chapters, this chapter focuses on some basic underlying concepts that should be considered when developing a treatment plan. Although the focus is on disordered phonology, the concepts and principles described in this chapter may also be useful in terms of instruction related to other speech/language disorders, as well as accent/dialect modification. This lays the groundwork for specific treatment approaches to be discussed in subsequent chapters.

A FRAMEWORK FOR CONDUCTING THERAPY

Hart and colleagues (2014) have suggested a useful framework for therapy that includes three main components: 1) treatment targets (i.e., those specific things that the clinician is trying to change), 2) treatment mechanisms (i.e., how the treatment is expected to work), and 3) treatment ingredients (i.e., what the clinician does to affect the change). This section reviews each of these components and discusses strategies for their application.

Treatment Targets

The choice of specific instructional targets was previously discussed in Chapter 7 as a basic element of decision making following a comprehensive assessment of an individual with an SSD. Broadly speaking, clinicians target one or more of the following: 1) production accuracy of individual speech sounds, 2) reduction in the use of phonological patterns, 3) overall message intelligibility, or 4) functional communication. As discussed in Chapter 7, the selection of individual speech sounds or patterns is typically made using either developmental appropriateness or a complexity approach. Stimulability and/or frequency of use of the sound in the language may also be considered in target selection.

Treatment Goals

Choosing a target behavior by itself is not sufficient as a treatment goal. In order to be functional, treatment goals need to also include a specific time frame to achieve the goal and a criterion for success. Time frames used may be short-term, intermediate-term, or long-term; these time frames may mean different things in different settings. In a public school setting, a short-term time frame frequently is a semester. Intermediate-term time frames may refer to an academic year or the next scheduled review of the individualized education program (IEP); these typically happen at least once every 3 years. Long-term time frames typically refer to the point at which the client is eligible to be discharged from the caseload.

The ultimate long-term goal for most speech sound therapy will be adultlike accuracy of all the speech sounds of the language, as well as 100% intelligibility of the message to all users of the language. In some cases, such as where physical disabilities limit precise speech motor control, perfect accuracy may be less important than functional communication (i.e., do most listeners understand the intended message?). Some other examples of treatment goals include:

Short term: By the end of the fall semester Rashid will produce the phonemes /f/ and /v/ with 90% accuracy when repeating 5- to 7-word sentences.

Intermediate term: By the end of the school year Aaron will reduce the use of stopping of fricatives and fronting of velars to less than 30% when naming picture stimuli.

Long term: By the time of her next scheduled IEP (in 3 years) LaToya will be at least 95% intelligible in conversational speech with unfamiliar adult listeners.

Practice Stimuli

The majority of clinicians appear to focus on either accuracy of individual speech sounds or reduction in the use of phonological patterns. With motor-based approaches (see Chapter 10) production practice typically begins with the sound in isolation and gradually moves up through syllables, words, phrases, sentences, and conversation. With linguistically based approaches (see Chapter 11) practice typically begins at the word level. In either case, at some point specific word stimuli must be selected.

Storkel (2018b) noted that for most clinicians the choice of particular practice words is not given much consideration. She points out, however, that there is considerable research available suggesting that certain word characteristics may have a positive influence on treatment success. In particular, she points to word frequency, neighborhood density, age of acquisition, and lexicality as potentially influencing speech sound outcomes.

Word frequency relates to how often a word occurs within the language. High-frequency words (e.g., road) are used more often in the language than low-frequency words (e.g., raccoon). Neighborhood density refers to how many phonologically similar words occur in the language. For example, the word *road* would be a high-density word, as it shares sounds with many words, such as node, load, code, toad, sewed, rid, raid, ride, read, red, rude, roam, rope, rose, row, and ode. Storkel (2018b) reviewed several treatment studies looking at the impact of word frequency and neighborhood density. She concluded that both high-density and high-frequency words appear to promote better speech sound generalization than low-frequency or low-density words.

Relative to age of acquisition, Storkel (2018b) reminds us that, like speech sounds, children do not all acquire words at the same age. This is a reflection of both the conceptual complexity of the words and their frequency of use in the language. Gierut and Morrisette (2012) reported that more speech sound generalization occurred when using later-acquired words than early-acquired words (regardless of how frequent the words were in the language).

Finally, Storkel (2018b) discussed lexicality, or whether or not the stimulus is a real word or a nonword (nonsense word). She notes that if young children are able to master sounds using late-acquired word stimuli (which they are likely unfamiliar with), this suggests they may not need to know the meaning of the words themselves. She then reviewed several studies and concluded that the use of nonwords may promote more rapid speech sound learning than real words. For example, Cummings and Barlow (2011) used a multiple baseline design with four children aged 3;3 to 6;9. Two children were treated with high-frequency real words and the other two were treated with nonwords. The authors concluded that nonwords resulted in more change, slightly more generalization, and less error variability than real words. One caveat, as noted in Chapter 5, is that many children with SSDs have comorbid language impairments. In such cases the use of real words offers the added advantage of being able to simultaneously work on vocabulary.

Treatment Mechanisms

The presumption underlying most treatment approaches is that the approach is directed at addressing the underlying problem. Motor-based approaches generally assume that the underlying problem is either perceptual or motor learning. As such, motor learning principles (to be discussed in Chapter 10), combined with a bottom-up skill-learning process, underlie those approaches. Linguistically based approaches (Chapter 11), on the other hand, assume that the child has failed to sort out some or all of the rules of the speech sound system. Most of these approaches assume that the child has failed to identify the particular speech sounds that are used to communicate meaning within the language.

Such assumptions lead to three characteristics common to most linguistically based approaches. First, they make use of either real words (or nonwords that have been assigned fictitious meanings). Second, they also are structured to include natural communicative consequences (i.e., feedback indicating whether the correct meaning was conveyed or not). And thirdly, they assume that the goal is to teach the child about the sound system, not individual sounds. This then means that not all possible speech sounds need to be taught. Generalization from the specific therapy target to other related targets is expected. More details on the specific mechanisms for change will be discussed where available, along with each approach in subsequent chapters.

Treatment Ingredients

Regardless of the specific approach, clinicians have considerable flexibility regarding how treatment is organized and presented to the client. Available options reflect a variety of dimensions, which will be discussed next.

Intervention Style

Therapy activities vary in their style of presentation. The key issue here is the amount of structure that may be prescribed for or tolerated by a given client. Shriberg and Kwiatkowski (1982b) described the structure of treatment activities as ranging from drill (highly structured therapy) to play (little structure to therapy). These authors described the following four modes (what we call styles) of intervention:

1. *Drill.* This type of therapy relies heavily on the clinician presenting some form of antecedent instructional events followed by client responses. The client has little control over the rate and presentation of training stimuli.

2. *Drill-play.* This type of therapy is distinguished from drill by the inclusion of an antecedent motivational event (e.g., activity involving a spinner, roll of dice, card games).

3. *Structured play.* This type of instruction is structurally similar to drill-play, however, training stimuli are presented as play activities. In this mode, the clinician moves from formal instruction to playlike activities, especially when the child becomes unresponsive to more formal instruction.

4. *Play.* The child perceives what they are doing as play; however, the clinician arranges activities so that target responses occur as a natural component of the activity. Clinicians may also use modeling, self-talk, and other techniques to elicit responses from a child.

Shriberg and Kwiatkowski (1982b) conducted several studies with young children with SSDs to compare the relative effects of these four treatment modes. They reported that drill and drill-play modes were more effective and efficient than structured play and play modes. In addition, drill-play was as effective and efficient as drill. Clinicians' evaluation of the four modes indicated that they felt drill-play was most effective and efficient for their clients, and they personally preferred it. Shriberg and Kwiatkowski urged that three factors be considered when making a choice of management mode: 1) a general knowledge of the child's personality, 2) the intended target response, and 3) the stage of therapy.

Stimulus Presentation and Feedback

Regardless of the target, intervention approach, or style, almost all therapy involves the same basic interaction sequence with three components. This sequence is outlined as follows:

Antecedent events (AE). Delineation of stimulus events designed to elicit particular responses (e.g., auditory/visual modeling or pictures presented by the clinician, followed by a request for the client to imitate the model or name a picture)

Responses (R). Production of a target behavior (e.g., often a particular sound in isolation or sound productions in a given linguistic and/or social context)

Consequent events (CE). Reinforcement or feedback that follows the response (e.g., the clinician says "good" if a response is accurate or may say "try again" if inaccurate; tokens to reinforce correct responses)

Antecedent events (AE) are the stimulus events presented during or just prior to a response. Such events typically consist of a verbal model, a picture, printed material, or verbal instructions designed to elicit particular verbal responses. For example, if a client is working on /s/ at the word level, the clinician may show the child a picture of soap and ask the child, "What do we wash with?" The child may be further asked to "say the word three times," or to "put it in a sentence." The type of antecedent events vary depending on whether the clinician is seeking to establish and/or practice a motor behavior, teach a phonological rule or contrast, or help the client use a newly learned production in a phrase or sentence.

Responses (R) are the behaviors the clinician has targeted for the client. These may range from approximations of the desired behavior (e.g., movement of the tongue backward for production of /k/) to production of the correct behavior (e.g., /k/) in connected speech. The clinician is concerned with the functional relationship between an antecedent event and a response or, in other words, the likelihood that a given stimulus will elicit the desired response. Movement to the next level of instruction is often contingent on a certain number of correct responses. It is important in the establishment of a speech sound that clients have the opportunity to produce many productions in the course of a therapy session. A high rate of production provides the opportunity for both the clinician's external monitoring and the client's automatization of the response. It is usual that responses are stabilized at one level of complexity before proceeding to the next level (e.g., sounds are often easier to produce in syllables than in words; single words are easier to produce than words in phrases or sentences).

The third aspect of the temporal sequence for instruction is *consequent events (CE)*, which occur following a particular response and usually are labeled reinforcement or punishment. Whether a response is learned (and how quickly it is learned) is closely related to what happens following the occurrence of a behavior or response. The most frequently used consequent event in clinical speech instruction is *positive reinforcement*. Tangible consequents such as tokens, points, chips, and informal reinforcers, such as a smile or verbal feedback, are typically used. Consequent events intended to reinforce should immediately follow the correct or desired behavior and should be used only when the desired or correct response is produced. Reinforcement is defined by an increase in a behavior following the presentation of consequent events. Providing a positive consequence after an incorrect production sends the wrong message to the speaker, possibly reinforcing an incorrect response, and does not facilitate

Table 9.1. Sequential series of antecedent events, responses, and consequent events

Step	Antecedent event	Response	Consequent event
1	Clinician: Put your tongue behind your teeth, have the tip of your tongue lightly touch the roof of your mouth as if you were saying /t/, and blow air. Say /s/.	/t/	Clinician: No, I heard /t/.
2	Clinician: Keep your tongue tip a little bit down from the roof of your mouth and blow air. Say /s/.	/s/	Clinician: Good! Perfect!
3	Now say /s/ three times.	/s/, /s/, /s/	Clinician: Great!
4	Now say /sɑ/.	/sɑ/	Clinician: Super!

learning of target responses. The use of punishment as a consequence is seldom if ever used in treatment.

Instructional steps are organized so that a sequential series of antecedent events, responses, and consequent events is followed as one progresses through various levels of therapy (more on these levels in Chapter 10). See Table 9.1 for an example of a sequential series.

Use of Tabletop Versus Digital Materials

Historically, the stimuli for therapy are presented as words spoken aloud by the clinician, as hard copy pictures, or as physical objects. Such presentations are usually described as tabletop materials. The advent of the microcomputer in the 1980s, followed by subsequent development of other digital devices, including laptop computers, tablets, and smartphones, has provided clinicians with a set of new options for presenting the therapy stimuli.

It has long been suggested that young children are highly motivated by information and entertainment presented on digital screens. It stands to reason, therefore, that the presentation of therapy stimuli in digital format might have a facilitating therapeutic effect. There is a growing body of literature that has examined this question. At least five studies (Jesus et al., 2019; McLeod et al., 2017; Shriberg, Kwiatkowski, & Snyder, 1989; 1990; Wren & Roulstone, 2008) have directly compared tabletop stimuli with stimuli presented via digital media. All revealed equivalent outcomes using both methods, suggesting that the use of digital media can be at least as effective as tabletop materials. All five studies noted some variability in response across individuals. Shriberg, Kwiatkowski, and Snyder (1990) also noted that digital presentations appeared to be somewhat less effective than tabletop presentations in the initial establishment of the target sound. Taken together, these findings suggest that use of the digital format is worth considering, particularly for individual clients who find digital presentation motivating.

Goal Attack Strategies

An early intervention decision relates to determining the number of treatment goals targeted in a given session. Fey (1991) described three goal attack strategies applicable to children with SSDs. The first strategy is called a *vertically structured treatment program,* in which one or two goals or targets are trained to some performance criterion before proceeding to another target. Treatment sessions of this type involve a high response rate for a single target, involving lots of repetition of that target. The traditional approach to treatment of SSDs, to be described in detail later in this book, is an example of a vertically structured program. In this approach, one or two phonemes are targeted for treatment and are worked on until they are produced in conversation, before training is initiated on other target sounds. For a client who exhibits five different phonologic patterns, the clinician may target one pattern and focus treatment on one or two sounds related to that process/pattern until some criterion level is reached before proceeding to the next target process. Elbert and Gierut (1986) termed this vertical type of strategy *training deep*. The assumptions behind the vertical strategy are that 1) mass practice on a restricted number of target sounds with a limited number of training items facilitates generalization to other nontrained items and 2) some clients are best served by focusing on one or a few targets rather than many.

A second instructional strategy is a *horizontally structured treatment program* (Fey, 1991; A. L. Williams, 2000b), or what Elbert and Gierut (1986) have called *training broad*. Using this strategy, the clinician addresses multiple goals in each session. Thus, more than one goal may be incorporated into each session, and goals may change across sessions. By working on several sounds or patterns in the same session, the client will presumably learn commonalities or relationships among sound productions, and treatment may be more efficient. In contrast to the vertical approach, the client receives less intense training on specific targets, but the training presented is focused on a broader range of components of the sound system. The concept behind training broad is that limited practice with a range of exemplars and sound contrasts is an efficient way to modify a child's phonological system. The goal is to expose the child to a wide range of target sound productions so that this broad-based training facilitates simultaneous acquisition of several treatment targets.

A third strategy (Fey, 1986), which combines aspects of the vertical and horizontal approaches, is a cycles, or *cyclically structured,* treatment program (Hodson, 2010a; Hodson & Paden, 1991). In this approach, a single target (or pattern) is addressed for a period of a week or more. After a fixed amount of therapy time (e.g., a total of 2 hours), another goal is addressed. The movement from goal to goal is essentially a horizontal approach to treatment, whereas the focus on a single sound for a fixed time period may be viewed as vertical.

Historically, the most common strategy employed in speech sound remediation was the vertical approach, but many clinicians favor the horizontal or cyclical approach. A. L. Williams (2010) has suggested a combination approach where a vertical approach is used until clients can produce a sound at the motor level with some consistency, which would then be followed by a horizontal or cyclical approach. With children who produce multiple errors, all three approaches have been shown to improve speech sound skill, but horizontal and cyclical strategies may be preferable because they offer variety within or across treatment sessions. For clients who evidence one or two errors, such as those who misarticulate /r/, /s/, /l/, or /θ/ (persistent or residual errors), a vertical approach is the usual option.

Treatment Intensity

As will be discussed in subsequent chapters, there is significant evidence that many different treatments can and do work to remediate SSDs (see Baker & McLeod, 2011a). But regardless of which approach is taken, how much of that treatment must be applied to affect the desired change? At least two comprehensive reviews of the treatment literature have examined this question (e.g., Kaipa & Peterson, 2016; Sugden et al., 2018a). Unfortunately, neither group of authors were able to conclude much beyond the fact that more treatment is better than less treatment. This may reflect the fact that researchers and clinicians vary widely on how to define what is meant by treatment intensity. Warren and colleagues (2007) suggest that a complete understanding of intensity requires specifying at least five different intensity-related variables:

- *Dose:* "... the number of properly administered teaching episodes during a single intervention session." (p. 71). This is similar to the number of trials or opportunities to attempt the target (e.g., 50 trials per 30-minute session).

- *Dose form:* "... the typical task or activity within which the teaching episodes are delivered." (p. 71). This is similar to our earlier discussion of intervention style (e.g., drill-play using single-word stimuli).

- *Dose frequency:* "... the number of times a dose of intervention is provided per day and per week." (p. 72). For example, one 30-minute session, twice per week.

- *Total intervention duration:* "... the time period over which a specified intervention is presented." (p. 72). For example, 9 months.

- *Cumulative intervention intensity:* "... the product of dose x dose frequency x total intervention duration." (p. 72). Dose form can also be specified. Using the previous examples: 50 trials x 2x per week x 40 weeks = 4,000 total single word trials using drill-play.

Although these definitions offer a useful starting point, they offer little day-to-day guidance for clinicians. As was done in Chapter 7, a pragmatic approach may again be needed. Of the previous variables, the last one, cumulative intervention intensity, is simply the product of the others. Of the remaining four, clinicians often have little control over dose frequency; it is often dictated by either caseload size and/or set by default by the work setting. This is also true for total intervention duration. In private practice settings it is typically determined by whoever is paying the bill, and in school settings it is somewhat open-ended and dictated by federal and state laws (i.e., intervention will last until the child is eligible for dismissal) and district policies.

It may be worth noting that Taps (2008) reviewed 821 files of public school children with SSDs and reported that they had received 50–100 hours of treatment prior to discharge. A similar review of 203 files by Bruce and associates (2018) found they needed an average of 82 hours of treatment before discharge. Relative to dose form (i.e., intervention style) clinicians may choose, but recall that the two most structured options, drill and drill-play, have been shown to be the most efficient (Shriberg & Kwiatkowski, 1982b). This, then, leaves dose (i.e., number of trials per session) as the one variable that clinicians have most control over to determine the efficiency of intervention in most situations.

What treatment dose might be reasonable? An examination of current practice might offer some real-world insight. Surveys in the United States suggest that a typical session length in the schools is 20–30 minutes (ASHA, 2018; Mullen & Schooling, 2010). A survey of Australian clinicians suggested 30–44 minutes (Sugden et al., 2018a). Taking the middle point, how many trials might be expected in 30 minutes? This may depend somewhat on the nature of the task the client is asked to carry out. Sugden and colleagues reported that more than 50% of clinicians used fewer than 20 trials in a session for perceptual or conceptual tasks. The next highest frequency was 21–49 trials per session used for both kinds of tasks. On the other hand, values were higher for production tasks, with 40% of clinicians reporting that they used

50–99 trials per session, while 38% used 21–49 trials per session. This would suggest most clinicians are presenting 50–60 production trials in a 30-minute session.

Rvachew and colleagues (2018) would refer to such a dose as a low-intensity session. A medium-intensity session would include up to 100 trials, whereas a high-intensity session of the same length might include up to 300 trials. How might one explain such a large range of trials in the same length of time? The difference may reflect how far along the child happens to be in the therapy process. Preston, Leece, and colleagues (2019) suggested that early on, when there was much instruction and a high frequency of feedback occurring, the number of trials might be lower. Later in therapy, when learning was becoming automatized and feedback had been reduced, the number of trials would be higher. In reviewing six studies using speech motor chaining (to be discussed in Chapter 10) they reported an average of 218 trials during 40- to 52-minute sessions over the course of an entire treatment cycle. This would suggest that clinicians should set a target over the course of therapy to average 100–125 production trials in a 30-minute treatment session (fewer trials early on, more later).

ADDITIONAL SERVICE DELIVERY CONSIDERATIONS

In addition to the choices that the clinician must make regarding the individual client, clinicians must also consider their overall caseload and the work setting. The following section discusses these considerations, which may impact aspects of treatment.

Scheduling of Instruction

Another consideration in planning for speech sound intervention relates to the scheduling of treatment sessions. Relatively little is known about the influence that scheduling of instruction has on remediation efficacy, and there are insufficient research reports to determine which scheduling arrangements are most desirable. In addition, it is often not practical to schedule treatment sessions on an ideal basis. One recent treatment study by Allen (2013) looked at 54 children randomly assigned to one of three conditions where total amount of treatment was the same for each group. One group received speech sound intervention three times per week for 8 weeks. A second group received the same intervention once a week for 24 weeks. The third group received a control (storybook) treatment that did not focus on speech sounds. The children in the first group made significantly greater gains in speech sound skill compared to the children in the other two groups. This suggested that more intense treatment over a shorter period was superior to less frequent treatment spread out over a longer period.

Treatment scheduling is usually determined by such factors as the client's age, attention span, and severity of the disorder, along with practical realities, such as financial resources available, availability of instructional services, size of the clinician's caseload, and treatment models being employed by a school system (e.g., pull-out vs. classroom-based instruction). Investigators who have studied scheduling have generally focused on the efficacy of intermittent scheduling versus block scheduling of treatment sessions. *Intermittent scheduling* usually refers to two or three sessions each week over an extended period of time (such as 8 months), whereas *block scheduling* refers to daily sessions for a shorter temporal span (such as an 8-week block).

Several older studies have compared dismissal rates associated with intermittent and block scheduling, primarily for public school students with articulation disorders (see review by Van Hattum, 1969). Based on these studies, Van Hattum reported that block scheduling was a more efficient way to achieve articulatory/phonological progress than was intermittent scheduling. Unfortunately, however, variables such as disorder severity, stimulability, and treatment methodology employed were not well enough controlled or described to make definitive clinical recommendations from these investigations.

Bowen and Cupples (1999) described a scheduling protocol in which children were seen once weekly for approximately 10-week blocks, followed by approximately 10 weeks without treatment. They reported positive results with this treatment schedule. It should be pointed out, however, that their treatment included multifaceted components, including parent education. The specific influence of the break in treatment schedule on treatment outcome is unknown.

Although there are few controlled experiments on scheduling, the following suggestions for scheduling speech sound intervention (where flexibility is available) seem appropriate:

1. Scheduling interventions four to five times per week for 8–10 weeks may result in slightly higher dismissal rates than intermittent scheduling for a longer period of time, with the greater gains being made early in the treatment process. Some children, especially preschoolers, can generalize correct productions without a lot of instruction.

2. Intensive scheduling on only a short-term basis does not appear to be as appropriate with clients who have severe articulation/phonological disorders and need ongoing services.

3. Scheduling a child for more but shorter sessions per week appears to yield better results than fewer but longer sessions.

Pull-Out Versus Classroom-Based Instruction

A consideration related to treatment is the place and format of school-based service delivery. One decision relates to whether treatment is provided through a *pull-out model* (the client is instructed in a treatment room) or *inclusion model* (the client is instructed in a classroom setting), or a combination of the two. Historically, the pull-out model was the choice for articulation/phonological treatment. In recent years, an emphasis has been placed on integrating speech and language services within the classroom. Data reported by Mullen and Schooling (2010) suggested that over 98% of K–12 services for SSDs was being provided via pull-out (in either individual or small group formats).

The opportunity to incorporate a child's instruction with the academic curriculum and events associated with a child's daily school routine is the optimal way to enhance the efficiency and effectiveness of therapy. Classroom inclusion may also capitalize on the opportunity for collaboration among regular educators, special education educators, speech-language pathologists (SLPs), and other professionals within a child's educational environment. Masterson (1993) suggested that classroom-based approaches for school-age children allow the clinician to draw on textbooks, homework, and classroom discourse to establish instructional goals, target words, and instructional procedures. For preschoolers, classroom activities such as crafts, snacks, and toileting are similarly helpful activities that can be combined with language and phonological instruction. In addition, for preschool and children in the early primary grades, classroom-based phonological awareness activities may provide clinicians the opportunity to extend services to all children in a classroom as they collaborate with teachers.

Masterson further indicated that classroom-based approaches can be most useful for treating conceptual- or linguistic-based errors, as opposed to errors that require motor-based habilitation. Instruction in the context of the classroom setting is typically less direct than that for a pull-out model and requires collaborative efforts between the clinician and the classroom teacher. The vocabulary used in the curriculum can be used by the speech clinician as the basis for target practice words. Classroom instruction is particularly appropriate when a client is in the generalization, or carryover, phase of instruction, in which academic material and other classroom activities allow for an emphasis on communication skills.

It is likely that both of these models (i.e., pull-out, classroom inclusion) are appropriate for a given client during the course of intervention depending on where they are on the treatment continuum, a concept that is discussed in the next chapter.

Individual Versus Group Instruction

Clinicians must determine whether clients are treated individually or in a small group. Treatment in the public schools is frequently conducted in small groups. Brandel and Loeb's (2011) survey of school-based clinicians indicated that 73% of children on their caseloads were being seen in small groups. When children with SSDs are grouped, such groups usually consist of three or four clients of about the same age who work on similar target behaviors.

Group instruction should be different from *individual instruction in a group* (the clinician works with each client individually while the remaining group members observe). Group instruction can and should be structured so that individuals in the group can benefit from interaction with other members and from activities that involve the entire group. For example, individuals can monitor and reinforce each other's productions and can serve both as correct models for each other and as listeners to see whether the communication intent of the message is met or whether the productions are correct.

Although some findings suggest that group intervention can be effective (e.g., Skelton & Richard, 2016), empirical comparisons of individual and group instruction remain limited. Sommers and colleagues (1964) reported that 50-minute group instruction based on the pull-out model resulted in as much articulatory change as 30-minute individual instruction when both group and individual sessions were conducted four times per week for 4 weeks. In a subsequent study (Sommers et al., 1966), similar results were obtained from group sessions held 45 minutes each week and individual instruction sessions held 30 minutes each week over a period of 8.5 months.

These investigators concluded that group and individual sessions were equally effective and that neither grade level (fourth to sixth grades vs. second grade) nor severity of the SSD influenced the results. It is important to observe that in both studies by Sommers and colleagues (1964; 1966) the group therapy sessions were longer than the individual therapy sessions. As Rvachew and Brosseau-Lapré (2012) note, group therapy is often used as a way to manage large caseloads and "... SLPs in typical practice do not increase session length when implementing group therapy ..." (p. 630). The net result would be that the amount of practice each child receives is actually reduced. It might not be reasonable, therefore, to expect the same outcome in a group session of the same length as an individual session, because each child would have less actual practice time in a group session.

It is our suggestion that a combination of group and individual sessions may be advantageous for most individuals with SSDs. Furthermore, instructional groups should usually be limited to three or four individuals whose ages do not exceed a 3-year range. As well, each child in the group should have an opportunity to practice their own goals at whatever production level is appropriate for them. Some investigators suggest that when children are learning the motor skills involved in the production of a given sound, individual instruction is perhaps the best format, if only for a limited number of sessions or parts of sessions. Once a sound is in the child's production repertoire, group and classroom activities can easily be incorporated into the instructional plan.

Summary of Service Delivery

Prior to (or perhaps along with) choosing a therapy approach, the basic structure of therapy needs to be set up, and clinicians should consider each of the following:

1. Treatment goals, including specific targets and the stimuli to be used

2. Style of intervention: drill, drill-play, structured play, play, or some combination

3. Whether tabletop or digital materials will be used

4. Goal attach strategy: vertical, horizontal, or cyclical

5. Intensity of treatment: session length, sessions per week, dose per session

6. Treatment schedule

7. Pull-out or classroom-based instruction

8. Individual or group instruction

TRACKING PROGRESS IN INTERVENTION

As discussed in Chapter 8, it is the responsibility of the clinician to collect relevant data to ensure that 1) change is occurring, 2) any change observed is due to the treatment being applied and not to some extraneous influence, and 3) relevant generalization (see the next section) is taking place. This means collecting treatment data, control data, and generalization data. The specific data to be collected should, of course, be relevant to the goals being targeted.

Before discussing the specifics of how to engage in data collection, it is important to note one thing not to do. The use of norm-referenced tests to monitor progress in therapy is not appropriate. Several different reasons for not doing so were highlighted by McCauley and Swisher (1984). First, they note that such tests ". . . will rarely be sensitive enough to behavioral change to document progress . . ." (p. 346). These tests are intended to compare the child against their peers by comparing performance on behavior patterns that are relatively stable. Such stability ensures that variations seen are a reflection of individual differences and not due to the inherent variability of the task.

The task stability of single-word articulation tests is also problematic because they assess skill on a task that is not representative of either everyday communication or the typical demands of therapy. Everyday communication involves production of connected speech rather than single words. Most therapy situations involve responding to a random presentation of many different words containing the target sound. This is contrasted with single-word articulation tests that typically evoke performance on any one phoneme using only a single word.

A second concern with using norm-referenced tests to monitor progress raised by McCauley and Swisher (1984) is the idea of regression to the mean. Poor performance on a norm-referenced test during an assessment may, in part, have been the result of the child having a very bad day (e.g., they didn't get enough sleep, they had a fight with a sibling, they forgot their lunch). Statistically, the odds of all those negative things operating again when the test is readministered are very low. Any improvement in their performance may simply reflect them having a better day.

A third reason why readministering a norm-referenced test is not a good idea is that the child may simply have learned the test items. They may remember having struggled with some of the words and may have spent some of the intervening period practicing those particular words. As well, most single-word articulation tests include common or high-frequency words, which may inadvertently have been used as therapy targets. Indeed, earlier in this chapter we argued in favor of using such high-frequency words in therapy. But rather than worrying about not teaching to the test, the better solution is simply to avoid readministering norm-referenced tests to track progress.

Treatment data are, as the name implies, performance data on the stimuli presented during the intervention session. As stimuli are presented to the child, the clinician makes a note of whether or not the child responded correctly. A simple tally on a piece of paper (e.g., ЈЖ ЈЖ ЈЖ ЈЖ) is often sufficient. At the end of the treatment session, if the child attempted to produce the target sound in 50 single words and produced 20 of them correctly, a value of 40% correct can be entered into a log (paper or digital).

Generalization data (see the next section for various types) need not be collected every session. More typically, generalization data might be collected every few weeks or perhaps once a month. For example, if 20 stimulus words containing /s/ in word-initial position are being practiced in therapy, a check for generalization to other words containing /s/ in word-initial position might be conducted. These words can be presented to the child and, again, the percentage correct can be recorded. For generalization across different settings (e.g., the classroom vs. the clinic room) the usual therapy stimuli can be brought to the other setting and the child's success rate on those stimuli can be evaluated and recorded.

Collection of control data would be similar to generalization data in many ways. It would involve presenting stimuli containing the predetermined control sound. These would be for a sound the child does not produce correctly, which is not being worked on in therapy, and where generalization is not expected. For example, when working on /k/, a very different sound like /v/ might serve as a control sound, or if the target is /s/, a sound like /r/ could be the control sound. Whatever that sound happens to be, stimuli are presented every few weeks (or once a month) and percentage correct values tabulated and recorded.

All three types of data can be recorded in table form and/or plotted visually, as was illustrated in Chapter 8 (see Figure 8.1).

FACILITATING GENERALIZATION

Regardless of the particular instructional approach, therapy is typically thought to consist of three phases: 1) establishment, which involves the client mastering the skills being taught within the structure of the treatment sessions; 2) generalization, or the extension of the skills being taught across a variety of contexts and situations; and 3) maintenance or the development of automatic or permanent skill. It should be noted that the structure of therapy should, from the very beginning, have generalization and maintenance built into it. With that being said, it is useful to discuss each of these three somewhat overlapping phases.

Establishment is at the heart of each specific treatment approach and will be discussed in various ways in subsequent chapters. Almost all forms of intervention, though, require that clinicians deal with one of the most significant challenges, which is facilitating generalization. Teaching a child how to physically produce a sound (a motor-based approach; see Chapter 10) or teaching them where to use it to facilitate a change in meaning (a linguistically based approach; see Chapter 11), or introducing an older child with a long-established error pattern to alternative forms of feedback (see Chapter 12) does not guarantee that they will use the sound appropriately in their everyday speech. It usually requires planning for it as part of treatment. Consequently, generalization is not necessarily taught, but rather, as stated previously, it is facilitated.

What follows includes an introduction to the concept of generalization, followed by a review of 1) across-position generalization, 2) across-context generalization, 3) across-linguistic unit generalization, 4) across-sound and feature generalization, and 5) across-situation generalization.

Stokes and Baer (1977) have defined *generalization* as:

> The occurrence of relevant behavior under different non-training conditions (i.e., across subjects, settings, people, behavior, and/or time) without the scheduling of the same events in those conditions as had been scheduled in the training conditions. Thus, generalization may be claimed when no extra training manipulations are needed for extra training changes. (p. 350)

In other words, generalization (sometimes called *transfer*) is the principle that learning one behavior in a particular environment often carries over to other similar behaviors, environments, or untrained contexts. For example, if one learns to drive in a Ford Fusion, there is a high probability that one can also drive a Honda Accord. Generalization of training occurs from driving the Ford to driving the Honda. In terms of speech sound remediation, if a client learns to produce /f/ in the word *fish*, [f] production will probably generalize to other words that contain /f/, such as *fun*. If generalization did not occur, it would be necessary to teach a sound in every word and context—an impossible task. The clinician must rely on a client's ability to generalize in order to affect a change in the use of speech sounds. Generalization, however, does not occur automatically, nor do all persons have the same aptitude for it. People vary in their ability to achieve generalization, but certain activities can increase the likelihood of generalization.

One type of generalization is *stimulus generalization,* which occurs when a learned response to a particular stimulus is evoked by similar stimuli. Behaviors that have been reinforced in the presence of a particular stimulus may be said to have generalized when they occur in the presence of novel but similar stimuli, even though the response was not reinforced or taught. Consider this example: A client who utilizes the process (pattern) of velar fronting (/t/ for /k/ substitution) has been taught to produce /k/ correctly at the word level in response to the auditory stimulus, "Say *key*." The client is later shown a picture of a key and asked to name it, but no model is provided. If the client says *key* with /k/ produced correctly in response to the picture (i.e., the model is no longer necessary for a correct production), stimulus generalization has occurred.

Response generalization is another type of generalization that is especially relevant to speech sound remediation. This is the process in which responses that have been taught transfer to other behaviors that are not taught. An example of response generalization is as follows: A client with /s/ and /z/ errors is taught to say [s] in response to an auditory model of [s]. She is then presented an auditory model [z] and asked to imitate it. If the client emits a correct [z], response generalization has occurred.

Such generalization is well documented. An early study by Elbert and colleagues (1967) included children with /s/, /z/, and /r/ errors who were taught to say [s] correctly. Generalization was evident by correction of the untrained /z/, which has many features in common with /s/. However, no generalization to the untrained /r/ was noted. Obviously, sounds in the same sound class and having similar features with the target sound are those for which response generalization is most likely to occur.

Several other types of generalization can also occur during speech sound remediation, including generalization from one position to another, from one context to another, to increasingly complex linguistic levels, to nontrained words, to other sounds and features, and to various speaking environments and situations. Clinicians often attempt to facilitate generalization by sequencing instructional steps from simple to more complex behaviors. By proceeding in small, progressive steps, the clinician seeks to gradually extend the behavior developed during the establishment period to other contexts and situations.

The amount of training required for the different types of generalization has not been established and seems to vary considerably across individuals. Elbert and McReynolds (1978) reported data from five children between 5 and 6 years of age indicating that between 5 and 26 sessions were required before across-word generalization occurred. They speculated that the error patterns exhibited by the children affected both the time required and the extent of transfer that occurs.

For those clients who begin remediation with an established target behavior in their repertoire, generalization may be the primary task of instruction. Following is a discussion of the various types of generalization that are expected in the articulation remediation process.

Across-Word Position/Contextual Generalization

Generalization of correct sound productions across-word positions is well documented (Elbert & McReynolds, 1975, 1978; Powell & McReynolds, 1969). The term *across-word position* refers to generalization from a word position that is taught (initial, medial, or final) to a word position that is not taught. By teaching a sound in a particular position (e.g., initial position), generalization may occur to a second position (e.g., final position). SLPs have traditionally taught target sounds first in the initial position of words, followed by either the final or medial position. One rationale for beginning with the initial position is that, for most children, many sounds are first acquired in the prevocalic position (the most notable exception is certain fricatives (e.g., /f/) that appear first in word-final position).

Ruscello (1975) studied the influence of training on generalization across-word positions. Two groups, each containing three participants, were presented with training programs that differed with respect to the number of word positions practiced in each session. Ruscello reported significantly more generalization across training sessions for those subjects who practiced a target sound in the initial, medial, and final word positions than for the group that practiced a target sound only in the word-initial position. Weaver-Spurlock and Brasseur (1988) also reported that simultaneous training of /s/ in the initial, medial, and final positions of familiar words was an effective training strategy for across-position generalization to nontrained words.

It can be inferred from the available data that generalization from initial to final position is just as likely to occur as generalization from final to initial position. A preferred word position that would maximally facilitate position generalization has not been established. Thus, the word position in which a target sound is trained does not seem to be a factor in position generalization. In terms of clinical management, unless the pattern of errors suggests a particular word position for initial training (such as final consonant deletion), it is recommended that the clinician train the word position that the client finds easiest to produce, check for generalization to other positions, and then proceed to train the other word positions if generalization has not already occurred. Except for selected fricative sounds (those that develop earliest in the final position), the easiest position to teach tends to be the initial position. However, contextual testing could result in the identification of singleton or cluster contexts that are facilitating for an individual child. In the case of /s/, frequently it is taught in /s/-cluster contexts such as /sn/, /st/, or /ts/.

Technically, position generalization may be viewed as a type of contextual generalization. The term *contextual generalization,* however, also refers to phonetic context transfer; for example, generalization from /s/ in *ask* to /s/ in *biscuit* or to /s/ in *fist.* This type of generalization, in which a production transfers to other words without direct treatment, is an example of response generalization as previously described. When preliminary testing has indicated specific contexts in which an error sound may be produced correctly, clinicians frequently attempt to stabilize such productions; that is, they see that a target sound can be consistently produced correctly in that context and then provide instruction designed to facilitate generalization of the correct sound to other contexts.

As with all types of generalization, the client must exhibit transfer to untrained contexts at some point for the remediation process to be complete. In a study of phoneme generalization, Elbert and McReynolds (1978) reported that although facilitative phonetic contexts have been posited as a factor in generalization, their data did not support the idea that certain contexts facilitate generalization across subjects. Instead, they found a great deal of variability in facilitative contexts across individuals. The authors also reported that once a child imitated or was stimulable for the sound, generalization occurred to other contexts. They concluded that the status of the sound in the client's productive repertoire had more to do with generalization than did contextual factors.

Elbert and colleagues (1991) examined the number of minimal word-pair exemplars necessary for children with SSDs to generalize to other words. They reported that for their participants (primarily preschool children), generalization occurred using a small number of word-pair exemplars (five or fewer for 80% of the children), but there was substantial variability across individuals. The occurrence of response generalization when teaching a small number of exemplars is consistent with findings from previous treatment reports (Elbert & McReynolds, 1978; Weiner, 1981b).

Across-Linguistic Unit Generalization

A second type of generalization involves shifting correct sound productions from one level of linguistic complexity to another (e.g., from syllables to words). For some clients, the first goal in this process is to transfer production of isolated sounds to syllables and words; others begin at the syllable or word level and generalize target sound productions to phrases and sentences.

Instruction typically begins at the highest level of linguistic complexity at which a client can produce a target behavior on demand. Instruction progresses from that point to the next level of complexity. When sounds are taught in isolation, the effects of coarticulation are absent and, therefore, the potential for generalization to syllables and words may be diminished. This notion received some support from a study reported by McReynolds (1972) in which the transfer of /s/ productions to words was probed after each of four sequential teaching steps: 1) /s/ in isolation, 2) /sɑ/, 3) /ɑs/, and 4) /ɑsɑ/. Although no transfer to words was observed following training on /s/ in isolation, more than 50% transfer to words was observed following training on /sɑ/. It should be recognized, however, that the training of /s/ in isolation prior to syllables might have had a learning effect and influenced the generalization observed following syllable instruction.

Van Riper and Erickson (1996) and Winitz (1975) recommended that sounds be taught in nonsense syllables or nonsense (nonce or nonwords) words before they are practiced in meaningful words, thereby reducing the interference of previously learned error productions of the target sound. This view is in contrast with the language-based perspective that phonologic contrasts should be established at the word level because meaningful contrasts are a key to acquisition. Powell and McReynolds (1969) studied generalization in four participants who misarticulated /s/. They reported that when two of the individuals were taught consonant productions in nonsense syllables, transfer of the target sound to words occurred without additional training. The other two individuals had to be provided additional instruction specifically at the word level for generalization to words to occur. Elbert and colleagues (1990) reported that when preschool children were taught target sounds within a minimal pair contrast training paradigm, generalization occurred to other single-word productions, as well as to conversational speech. Based on a 3-month post-treatment probe, they reported that participants continued to generalize to other nontrained contexts.

In summary, it appears that some clients generalize from one linguistic unit to another without specific training; others require specific instructional activities for transfer from one linguistic unit to another. The process of generalization across linguistic units varies across individuals, as do all types of generalization.

Across-Sound and Across-Feature Generalization

A third type of generalization is observed when correct production of a target sound generalizes from one sound to another. Generalization most often occurs within sound classes and/or between sounds that are phonetically similar (e.g., /k/ to /g/, /s/ to /z/, and /ʃ/ to /s/). Clinicians have long observed that training on one sound in a cognate pair frequently results in generalization to the second sound (e.g., Elbert et al., 1967).

Generalization of correct production from one sound to another is expected when remediation targets are selected for linguistically based treatment approaches (see Chapter 11) based on pattern analysis. Often, in these approaches target behaviors that reflect patterns common to several error productions are selected. It is assumed that generalization will occur from exemplars to other error sounds within the same sound class or, in some instances, across sound classes.

A client can learn a feature and transfer the feature to other sounds without necessarily correcting a sound. For example, a client who substitutes stops for fricatives may learn to produce /f/ and overgeneralize its use to several fricative sounds. Although the client no longer substitutes stops for fricatives, they now substitute /f/

for other fricatives (e.g., [sʌn] → [fʌn], [ʃoʊ] → [foʊ]). Although the same number of phonemes is in error, the fact that the client has incorporated a new sound class into their repertoire represents progress because it involves enhancement of the child's phonological system (A. L. Williams, 1993).

Frequently, the establishment of feature contrasts is part of the effort to reduce and eliminate pattern usage and *homonomy* (in which one sound is substituted for several sounds in the language). The notion of feature and sound generalization, like other types of generalization, is critical to the remediation process. During the 1990s, several studies of children with multiple speech sound errors were conducted, and data were collected regarding the impact on generalization of various types of treatment targets. Results of these studies are relevant to our discussion of across-sound and across-feature generalization.

In a study related to teaching stimulable versus nonstimulable sounds, Powell and associates (1991) reported that teaching a nonstimulable sound prompted change in the target sound and other stimulable sounds that were produced in error. However, teaching a stimulable sound did not necessarily lead to changes in untreated stimulable or nonstimulable sounds. The implication of this study is that treatment of nonstimulable sounds may lead to increased generalization and, thus, have a more widespread impact on the child's overall sound system than treating stimulable sounds.

Gierut and colleagues (1996) examined generalization associated with teaching early developing sounds versus later developing sounds. They reported that children taught later developing sounds evidenced change in the treated sound, with generalization occurring both within and across sound classes. For those taught early developing sounds, improvements were noted on the target sound within class sounds but not across sound classes.

Studies of generalization associated with teaching sounds evidencing least versus most knowledge of sounds in the sound system (Dinnsen & Elbert, 1984; Gierut et al., 1987) have indicated that treatment focused on least knowledge resulted in extensive systemwide generalization in which treatment of most knowledge contributed to less change in a child's overall sound system. Studies comparing generalization associated with teaching phonetically more complex sounds to those less phonetically complex sounds (Dinnsen et al., 1990; Tyler & Figurski, 1994) have reported that more extensive changes were obtained when treatment was focused on more complex phonetic distinctions between error sounds, as compared to simpler distinctions between sounds.

Rvachew and Nowak (2001), however, reported findings contradictory to those of Dinnsen and colleagues (1990) and Tyler and Figurski (1994). Rvachew and Nowak studied the amount of phonological generalization associated with treatment targets that reflected early developing and more phonological knowledge (i.e., correct production in a larger number of contexts) as contrasted with later developing and little or no productive phonological knowledge. Greater treatment efficiency was associated with phoneme (sound) targets that reflected early developing and more productive phonological knowledge.

Further investigation is necessary before definitive statements may be made with regard to the issue of targeting early versus later acquired sounds, and more versus less phonological knowledge. One idea suggested is that the differences reported may reflect individual differences. Powell and Elbert (1984) investigated the generalization patterns of two groups of children with misarticulations. Specifically, they wanted to see whether the group receiving instruction on earlier developing consonant clusters (stop + liquid) would exhibit generalization patterns different from those of the group receiving instruction on later developing consonant clusters (fricative + liquid). The authors reported that no clear overall pattern was observed; instead, the six participants exhibited individual generalization patterns. All participants evidenced some generalization to both the trained and untrained consonant clusters. The most interesting finding was that generalization to both cluster categories occurred on the final probe measure in five of six participants regardless of the treatment received. Powell and Elbert attributed generalization across sound and classes, in part, to the level of pretreatment stimulability.

Across-Situations Generalization

The fourth and final type of generalization to be discussed in this chapter, called *situational generalization,* involves transfer of behaviors taught in the clinical setting to other situations and locations, such as school, work, or home. This type of generalization is critical to the remediation process because it represents the terminal objective of instruction (i.e., correct productions in conversational speech in nonclinical settings). Such generalization has also been called *carryover* in the speech-language pathology literature.

Most clinicians focus on activities to facilitate situational transfer during the final stages of remediation. Some, including the authors of this chapter, have argued that clinicians should incorporate these activities into earlier stages of instruction. For example, once a client can produce single words correctly, efforts should be made to incorporate some of these words into nonclinical settings. A major advantage of providing instruction in the classroom setting (inclusion model) is the opportunity to incorporate treatment targets into a child's natural communicative environment. For example, if a child's science lesson incorporates words containing a target sound (such as /s/), the teacher or clinician can provide the opportunity for the child to utilize their new speech sound in words like sun, solar, ice, estimate, season, and summer. Although much emphasis is placed on facilitating situational generalization, little experimental data are available to provide specific guidance to the clinician.

Studies by Costello and Bosler (1976), Olswang and Bain (1985), and Bankson and Byrne (1972) have shown that situational generalization is facilitated throughout treatment, but the extent of such transfer varies greatly from one individual to another. Costello and Bosler investigated whether certain clinical situations were more likely to evidence generalization than others. They recorded the transfer that occurred from training in the home environment to probes obtained in the following four settings:

1. A mother administered the probe while sitting across from her child at a table in a treatment room of the speech clinic.

2. An experimenter (who was only vaguely familiar to the child) administered the probe while sitting across from the child at the same table in the same room as setting 1.

3. The same experimenter administered the probe while she and the child were seated at separate desks facing each other in a large classroom outside the speech clinic.

4. A second experimenter (unknown to the child prior to the study) administered a probe while she and the child were alone and seated in comfortable chairs in the informal atmosphere of the clinic waiting room.

Although generalization occurred from the therapy setting to one or more of these testing situations, there was no evidence that generalization was more likely to occur in one environment than another. It may be that generalization variables differ so much from person to person that it is impossible to predict which environments are most likely to facilitate situational generalization.

Olswang and Bain (1985) monitored situational generalization for three 4-year-old children in two different settings during speech sound remediation. They compared conversational speech samples recorded in a clinic treatment room and recorded by parents at home. They reported similar rates and amounts of generalization of target sounds for both settings.

One strategy that has been suggested to facilitate situational generalization is the use of self-monitoring. Self-monitoring techniques have included hand raising (Engel & Groth, 1976), charting (Diedrich, 1971; Koegel et al., 1986), and counting of correct productions, both within and outside the clinic (Koegel et al., 1988).

Koegel and associates (1988) examined generalization of /s/ and /z/ in seven children. They reported that when the children self-monitored their conversational productions in the clinic, no generalization of the correct target production outside the clinic occurred. However, when children were required to monitor their conversational speech outside the clinic, rapid and widespread generalization occurred across subjects, although at slightly different rates. They reported high levels of generalization for all children. In contrast, when Gray and Shelton (1992) field-tested the self-monitoring strategy of Koegel and associates, the positive generalization effect was not replicated.

In a retrospective study of the efficacy of intervention strategies, Shriberg and Kwiatkowski (1987) identified self-monitoring procedures as a potentially effective component to facilitate generalization to continuous speech. In a subsequent experimental study, Shriberg and Kwiatkowski (1990) reported that seven of eight preschool children generalized from self-monitoring to spontaneous speech. They concluded, however, that although self-monitoring facilitated generalization, it varied in terms of type, extent, and point of onset.

Despite a paucity of data on situational generalization, available evidence indicates that, as with other forms of generalization, the extent to which it occurs in different settings varies greatly among individuals. There is also the suggestion that situational generalization may be influenced by age and the level of development of the child's phonologic system (Elbert et al., 1990). Self-monitoring may also be crucial. A step-wise approach to facilitating self-monitoring might take the following form:

1. Clinician monitors and provides verbal feedback

2. Clinician monitors and provides nonverbal cueing (raises finger, head nod)

3. Client corrects themself when they hear errors

4. Client anticipates errors and self-corrects

5. Correct productions are automatic

Parental Assistance With Generalization

Clinicians have recognized that the generalization process in speech sound remediation might be facilitated if individuals from the client's environment could be drawn into the generalization phase of the treatment process. The assumption has been that persons significant to the client, including parents, teachers, and peers, could engage in activities designed to extend what the clinician was doing in the clinical setting. A survey of 235 Australian SLPs (Sugden et al., 2018b) found that over 96% made use of parents to assist with intervention, with most doing so by providing home practice activities. Such activities were provided after most or all sessions by 90% of the respondents. A survey of 156 U.S.-based SLPs by Tambyraja (2020) suggested somewhat less frequent use of homework activities, with 53% of the SLPs providing them most of the time or always.

Several intervention programs include instructional activities designed for parents to use with their children at home (Bowen & Cupples, 1999; Gray, 1974; Mowrer et al., 1968). Sommers (1962) and Sommers and colleagues (1964) studied several variables related to articulation instruction. More improvement between pre- and post-test scores was reported for children whose mothers were trained to assist with instruction than for a control group of children whose mothers had not received training. Carrier (1970) reported a study comparing a group of 10 children aged 4–7 years old who participated in an articulation training program administered by their mothers and a similar control group who received minimal assistance from their mothers. The experimental group obtained significantly higher scores on four speech sound measures than the control group. Other investigations in which parents provided directed speech sound instruction for their children (Dodd & Barker, 1990; Pamplona et al., 1996; Rvachew & Brosseau-Lapré, 2015; Shelton et al., 1972; Shelton et al., 1975; Sugden et al., 2020) reported that parents can be successfully utilized and, when properly trained, can be at least as effective as SLPs.

When considering the assignment of homework activities, the clinician must be sensitive to the role parents and other nonprofessionals can assume in the treatment process. In such instances, there are several things that should be kept in mind. For example, can the parents/caregivers 1) provide good auditory models of target words, 2) have their child(ren) practice target words that the child(ren) can produce correctly, and 3) reinforce correct productions? Other things to keep in mind when utilizing parents include the following: First, if parents are to judge the accuracy of sound productions, they must be able to discriminate the sounds accurately. Second, the clinician should demonstrate to the parents the procedures to be used in the program, then the parents should demonstrate to the clinician the same procedures to ensure that they can carry them out. Third, the clinician must recognize that parents have only a limited amount of time; consequently, programs should be designed for short periods. Fourth, written instructions of the specific tasks should be provided. Finally, clinicians should keep in mind that parents tend to function better as monitors of productions than as teachers. Parents sometimes lack the patience and objectivity necessary to teach their own children. However, if parents or other individuals in the child's environment have the desire, skill, time, and patience to work with their children, the clinician may have helpful facilitators of the generalization process and, thus, reduce the time in treatment.

Generalization Guidelines

1. For the most rapid context and situational generalization, begin instruction with target behaviors (sounds) that are stimulable or in the client's repertoire.

2. For children with multiple errors, there are data to support each of the following as ways to facilitate generalization:

   a. Nonstimulable sounds should be treated before stimulable sounds for systemwide change.

   b. Sounds evidencing least knowledge should be treated before those evidencing most knowledge for systemwide change.

3. Because word productions form the basis of generalization, productions at the word level should be incorporated into the instructional sequence as soon as possible. When teaching a sound, words and syllable shapes within the child's lexicon should be used.

4. The more features that sounds have in common, the more likely that generalization will occur from one to another. For example, teaching /ɝ/ usually results in generalization to the unstressed /ɚ/ and the consonantal /r/; teaching one member of a cognate sound-pair, such as /s/, usually results in the client's correction of the cognate /z/.

5. Teaching a feature in the context of one sound, such as frication in /f/, may result in generalization of that feature to other untreated sounds (e.g., other fricatives such as /z/ or /v/).

6. Data to support a particular order for teaching sounds in various word positions to facilitate generalization are lacking. Beginning with the word position that is easiest for the client is often used as a starting point.

7. When selecting sounds to target phonologic patterns, choose target sounds from across different sound classes in which the pattern occurs to increase the likelihood of generalization across the sound system (e.g., for final consonant deletion, one might select /d/, /f/, and /m/).

8. Nonsense syllables may facilitate production of sounds in syllable or nonword contexts during establishment of sound production because nonsense syllables pose less interference with previously learned behaviors than do words.

9. Activities to facilitate situational generalization are advised as soon as the client can say a sound in words.

10. In the case of preschool children, generalization frequently takes place without formal instruction to facilitate situational generalization.

11. Parents, teachers, and others in the child's environment can be used effectively to facilitate phonologic change in children.

DISMISSAL FROM INSTRUCTION AND MAINTENANCE

The final phase of phonologic instruction occurs when the client habituates new target behaviors and otherwise assumes responsibility for self-monitoring target productions. This phase of therapy is an extension of the generalization phase.

    During the final phase of therapy, sometimes referred to as the *maintenance phase,* clients decrease their contact with the clinician. Shelton (1978) labeled the terminal objective of articulation remediation as *automatization* and described it as the automatic usage of standard articulation patterns in spontaneous speech. The term automatization implies that phonologic productions can be viewed as motor behavior that develops into an automatic response. When errors are linguistic in nature, maintenance may be viewed as the mastery of rules or phonemic contrasts. In reality, both the motor production and phonologic rules become part of a person's everyday productive behavioral responses by this point in treatment. The maintenance phase may be considered complete once the client consistently uses target behaviors in spontaneous speech.

As mentioned in Chapter 4 and earlier in this chapter, self-monitoring appears to be important to consolidating the skills being learned. Clients should be expected to monitor their own productions during maintenance. Having the client keep track of target productions during specified periods of the day is a procedure that might facilitate self-monitoring of target productions.

Information from the learning literature offers insights into the maintenance or retention of newly acquired phonologic patterns. *Retention,* in the context of speech sound remediation, refers to the continued and persistent use of responses learned during instruction. Once an individual learns a new pattern or response, they must continue to use (retain) the response. In clinical literature, retention is sometimes discussed in terms of intersession retention and sometimes in terms of habitual retention. *Intersession retention* refers to the ability to produce recently taught responses correctly from one session to the next. Speech clinicians frequently observe between-session forgetting in many clients. In this instance, having parents monitor a child's productions of a selected group of words may be helpful. Short practice sessions between therapy appointments may improve intersession retention. *Habitual retention* is the persistent and continued use of the response after instruction has been terminated. The term *maintenance* is also used to refer to this phenomenon. Speech clinicians occasionally dismiss clients from instruction only to have them return for additional therapy some months later. Such individuals obviously did not habituate or retain their newly learned responses.

Sommers (1969) reported that articulation errors are susceptible to regression. In a follow-up study of 177 elementary school children who had been dismissed from articulation instruction during a 6-month period, he found that approximately one-third had regressed. Based on conversational samples of target sound productions, 59% of those who had worked on /s/ and /z/ had regressed, but only 6% of those who had worked on /r/ had regressed. In contrast, Elbert and colleagues (1990) reported that for preschool children, learning continued to improve on both single-word and conversational speech samples obtained 3 months post-treatment. These data support the idea that young children are actively involved in the learning process and continue to learn more about the phonologic system after treatment has terminated. It appears that speech sound errors in preschool children are less habituated than in older school-age children and are easier to correct and maintain.

Mowrer (1982) pointed out several factors that have been shown to influence the degree to which information will be retained in the child who is dismissed from therapy, but then returns for lack of long-term maintenance, or the child who has forgotten previous learning between sessions. First, the meaningfulness of the material used to teach the new responses may affect retention, although there is little empirical evidence in the articulation learning literature on this point. In general, as the meaningfulness of the material increases, the rate of forgetting tends to decrease; thus, the use of meaningful material is recommended during remediation. Consequently, names of friends, family members, pets, familiar objects, and classroom items are appropriate choices. Although meaningfulness of material could be an important aid to long-term retention, the clinician might find, as stated earlier, that nonmeaningful material (e.g., nonsense syllables) may be useful during earlier phases of instruction (i.e., establishment). Leonard (1973) reported that when /s/ had been established in meaningful words, fewer training trials were required to transfer to other words than when nonsense items were utilized.

A second factor believed to affect retention is the degree or extent to which something has been learned. In general, the higher the number of trials during the learning process, the greater the retention. Retention improves when some overlearning of verbal material takes place. To avoid unnecessary practice, it is important to determine the minimum amount of learning trials needed to provide a satisfactory level of retention. The optimum point for stopping instruction occurs when additional training does not produce sufficient change in performance to merit additional practice; however, there are few data to guide the clinician about when this point might be.

A third factor affecting retention is the frequency of instruction or the distribution of practice. Retention is superior when tasks are practiced during several short sessions (distributed practice) than during fewer longer sessions (massed practice). On the basis of this fact, frequent short practice sessions are recommended. In his review of this topic, Mowrer (1982) concluded:

> On the basis of controlled learning experiments in psychology alone, it could be recommended that clinicians could increase retention by providing frequent instruction; but bear in mind that no data are available from speech research that confirms this recommendation ... the important factor in terms of frequency of instruction is not how much instruction ... but the total number of instruction periods. (p. 259)

A fourth factor shown to affect retention is the individual's motivation. It would seem that the more motivated a person is, the greater the extent of retention of material that has been learned. Little, if any, experimental work reported in the phonologic literature has attempted to examine motivational state during speech instruction.

Baker (2010a) reviewed eight studies that reported on children whose speech was judged to be normal at the time of dismissal. She found that a wide range of sessions and hours was required for normalization of children's speech, and a wide range of dismissal criteria were reported. The dismissal criteria for speech sounds ranged from 50% accuracy of targeted sounds during conversational speech (A. L. Williams, 2000a) to 75% accuracy on a single-word probe (McKercher et al., 1995).

Dismissal of children who have achieved intelligible speech usually occurs because treatment goals have been achieved. However, not all dismissals are the result of the child's having achieved treatment goals; they can occur for other reasons. Dismissal might occur when services are restricted by policies for enrollment or caseload size. For example, Baker (2010a) points out that sometimes dismissals are the result of the need for a clinician to serve other children who are judged to have a greater need for intervention. In such instances, it may be disheartening for both the client and the clinician, and it is best to prepare both parents and children.

Dismissal Criteria

The maintenance phase provides a period for monitoring retention, and dismissal decisions are made during this period. Limited data on dismissal criteria have been reported; thus, evidence is lacking to support a single dismissal criterion. Elbert (1967) suggested dismissal might be based on two questions: 1) Has the maximum change in this individual's speech behavior been attained? and 2) Can this individual maintain this level of speech behavior and continue to improve without additional speech instruction? No matter what criteria are used for dismissal, they should be based on periodic samples of phonologic behavior over time. The maintenance phase provides the final opportunity for the clinician to monitor, reinforce, and encourage the client to assume responsibility for habituation of the new speech patterns.

Diedrich and Bangert (1976) reported data on articulatory retention and dismissal from treatment. Some of the children studied were dismissed after reaching a 75% criterion level for correct /s/ and /r/ productions as measured on a 30-item probe word test plus a 3-minute sample of conversational speech. Four months later, 19% of the children had regressed below the 75% criterion level. No higher retention was found, however, among those children who remained in treatment until achieving higher than 75% criterion level on the probe measure. Diedrich and Bangert concluded that most speech clinicians tend to retain children with /s/ and /r/ errors in articulation instruction longer than necessary.

Maintenance and Dismissal Guidelines

1. The reinforcement schedule should continue to be intermittent during maintenance, as during the latter stages of generalization.

2. During the maintenance phase, clients should assume increased responsibility for self-monitoring their productions and maintaining accurate productions.

3. Dismissal criteria may vary depending on the nature of the client's problem and the client's age. Preschool children with multiple errors generally require less stringent dismissal criteria than older children because they have been reported to continue to improve phonologic productions without instruction once they begin to incorporate a new sound(s) into their repertoire. School-age and older clients who evidence residual /r/, /s/, and /l/ errors, and whose speech patterns are established and resistant to change, might require more stringent dismissal criteria to retain the productions.

4. It has been suggested that clinicians may tend to keep many clients enrolled for remediation longer than necessary. In other words, the cost–benefit ratio for intervention may significantly decline after a certain point is reached in treatment. No specific recommendation on what that point might be is possible at this time.

TREATMENT CONSIDERATIONS FOR VERY YOUNG CHILDREN

Much of the previous discussion assumes a child who is motivated and capable of sitting and attending to the therapy process for extended periods of time. With older children, motivation may be a challenge and many may have experienced a lack of success in therapy and/or simply developed a long-standing distortion habit. For that population, those additional issues will be addressed next. At the other end of the continuum are very young children (i.e., toddlers; typically those under age 3 years) for whom attention may be an issue. Assessment issues for this group were discussed in Chapter 6. We now turn our attention to treatment considerations.

Modifications to several of the topic areas from the previous section will need to be considered. The goals of treatment for toddlers may need to be somewhat different. They may initially consist of allowing the child to acclimate to the therapy process and environment. This would mean giving them time each session to explore the therapy room, becoming familiar with the space, the available materials, and the clinician. Expecting them to sit at a table and respond to picture stimuli may be unreasonable initially, although eventually that may become possible. Therapy objects as stimuli may be preferable to pictures at first, as toddlers are often motivated by being able to tactually explore the world around them.

Early goals for toddlers should usually focus more on overall communication, rather than on the details of speech. For those with highly unintelligible speech, their experience with turn-taking may be limited, as their difficulty making themselves understood may have resulted in much shorter verbal interactions (i.e., listeners give up quickly when the message is not being conveyed). Following the child's lead and responding to all of their communicative signals (e.g., sounds, facial expression, gestures) will encourage them to continue to try to get their message across. Asking many yes/no questions may be of benefit as well, to clarify their intentions. As their intentions become clearer, providing them with lots of verbal models (e.g., naming the things they point to or are playing with) and imitating what they say with a more fully correct example should also encourage them to continue the interactions. As their attempts become closer to the target, occasional requests for clarification can be added to encourage even closer approximations.

Relative to intervention style, play is likely to be more successful than other styles early in treatment. This style can be transitioned to structured play and perhaps eventually drill-play or even drill. The length of time spent on any one activity may be limited at first, but as a child becomes used to the setting and the activities, the amount of time focused on a given activity can slowly be increased. This will mean planning for many different kinds of activities within any one session.

As for treatment intensity, shorter more frequent sessions (when possible) typically make more sense, as toddlers are unlikely to be able to sustain their attention for very long periods of time. Likewise, the number of trials/responses may be compensated for by engaging the client in an increased number and variety of shorter instructional activities. As time moves along the dose can be expanded.

Clinical Vignette 9.1

The Shy Child: Separating From the Parent

Author Peter Flipsen Jr. recalls a 3-year-old child named Kevin (a pseudonym) who had a severe speech and language delay likely due to an episode of meningitis he had experienced at age 15 months. His speech output was quite unintelligible and he was very reluctant to separate from his mother for therapy sessions. With his mother in the room, he tended to cling to her and offered few communicative attempts.

One day Dr. Flipsen asked his mother to sit in a chair just outside the door to the therapy room. Inside were a bunch of toys Kevin liked to play with, but Dr. Flipsen told his mother (with Kevin listening) that she could not enter the room. Kevin clung to her side. Dr. Flipsen went into the room and showed Kevin all the toys he was missing. Eventually he ran in, played with a few things for a few moments, but ran back to his mother's side. This happened six or seven times over the course of the session.

At the next session his mother's chair was moved away from the doorway. His mother was told to sit with her feet sticking out so Kevin could see them. Once again, Kevin did not initially enter the room, but eventually did so. As in the previous session, he ran back to her a few times to confirm she was there, but eventually all he did was look over to make sure he could see her feet.

Two sessions later his mother was positioned so her feet were no longer visible. The next session the door was closed and Kevin spent the entire session in the room with Dr. Flipsen. For all subsequent sessions Kevin had no problem doing so, and therapy became much more productive.

THE CHALLENGES OF WORKING WITH OLDER CHILDREN

Working with older children poses its own set of challenges. For current purposes, the term older will refer to children aged 7 years and older. This age cutoff was chosen for three reasons. First, based on the reanalysis of the large cross-sectional studies of speech sound acquisition by Crowe and McLeod (2020), 90% of children whose first language is English appear to have mastered all of the speech sounds by this age. Second, this is an age at which most children are able to more actively participate in decisions about their care (see the following discussion regarding treatment decision making). And third, for children with normal cognitive abilities, this is the youngest age at which most children are able to take advantage of instrumental feedback, which will be discussed in Chapter 12.

Although working with 7-year-old children may not be that different from working with younger children, for those who are much beyond this age several aspects of intervention may need adjustment. These include factors related to motivation for therapy, treatment decision making, and the mechanics of the intervention itself.

Motivation for Therapy

Providing motivation to attend and actively participate in therapy can certainly be a challenge with older children. Consulting with their parents/caregivers about possible rewards for doing so may be of some value. However, because their speech errors are likely to be well established habits by this age, they will need to be focused and work hard in therapy to break those habits. Such focus and effort is likely to require a great deal of internal motivation.

One possible source of additional motivation for older children may be the therapeutic alliance we make with our clients. Building rapport over time, respecting their choices, and allowing them to have input into the day-to-day decisions about activities and stimuli being used makes them partners in the process. We do this in a somewhat casual, informal way with younger children. With older children, this can be done more overtly by talking with them about what they want to accomplish and how they might meet those goals. Doing so may help inspire them to be more active participants in therapy.

It is also possible that the approach being used may itself be motivating. Several of the instrumental feedback approaches to be discussed in Chapter 12 provide significant motivation because they are so different from traditional therapy. Discussing with them (in terms they can understand) the science behind what is being done may pique their curiosity and inspire them to participate more. When using such approaches, it may also be of some value to ask them to invite a peer or two to attend the therapy to share why and how they are making the effort to improve their speech skills and then to show off. This may result in the peer becoming an ally to support them in social situations.

Treatment Decision Making

As children get older, it is quite natural for them to want to have more control over the decisions that affect them. In ethical terms, this is known as the right to exercise autonomy. This is why in Chapter 8, in the discussion of evidence-based practice, client preferences and values were included. Where possible, choices are presented and the client's preferences must be considered.

For young children, offering them choices about small things, such as which particular therapy activity to use, is commonplace. But parents almost always make the major therapy decisions (i.e., whether to begin therapy, choice of overall approach, dismissal from therapy, input on treatment targets). This is understandable, as young children lack the capacity to fully appreciate what is in their best interests. At some point, however, children develop that capacity and should be involved in the decision-making process. There is no hard-and-fast rule as to when that point is reached. Legally, every state sets the age at which children can make their own decisions; prior to that age the decision is ultimately up to the parents. However, at some point most parents recognize that their child should have input into decisions related to them. Thus, it makes sense to consult with the child's parents and, with their consent, include the child in the discussion of options.

At what point should clinicians consider including the child in these discussions? A common standard in research studies may be informative. When children are being asked to participate in research studies, parents ultimately give consent, but children over the age of 7 or 8 years must usually be asked to give their assent (i.e., they are asked for their permission using simple terms). This may be a reasonable standard to use.

Clinical Vignette 9.2

Dismissal From Therapy?

One clinician recalls working with a 13-year-old girl in a small town in northern Canada. She had been in therapy for about a year, when one day she commented that she did not want to come anymore. She saw no real need for it. She commented that everyone understood her speech, no one made fun of her, and she was generally happy about her life. She was a good student academically.

The girl's mother was asked to attend the next therapy session and a three-way discussion was held. Ultimately, it was agreed that therapy would be suspended. The girl was advised that she could restart therapy at any time just by asking.

The Mechanics of Intervention

Therapy sessions are often different for older as contrasted with younger children. As discussed earlier, drill-based therapy is the most efficient treatment style. Older children may be more tolerant of drill therapy because they are usually able to stay focused on a task for longer periods than younger children. On the other hand, they may also be more easily bored with it. This may be easily managed via the therapeutic alliance discussed previously. It will generally be easier to discuss the need for a lot of practice to change old habits with older children. They will also be more likely to respond in a positive manner to the logic of such discussions. A direct extension of the need for intense practice relates to treatment intensity. Older children and adults may also be willing to attend more frequent sessions (schedule permitting) to increase the amount of possible practice. Whether discussing more exercises in the session or more frequent sessions, couching it in terms of being done with therapy faster may also be helpful.

Stimuli to be used in therapy will likely need to differ for older children as well. Their vocabularies and topical awareness will generally be different with age, so more age-appropriate targets can and should be chosen. Likewise, many older children may be able to read and, therefore, stimuli need not always be limited to those that can be presented via pictures (a common limitation of stimuli for younger children). Phrase- and sentence-level stimuli can also be read rather than presented as imitation tasks.

Generalization activities for older children can often be much more overt and the client may be given more autonomy in carrying them out. Older children can be asked to fill out a log or diary for homework on their own, for example. They can also be asked to try out their speech practice activities with peers (i.e., to practice self-monitoring) or in other nontherapy situations on their own. Clearly, the clinician will need to judge how autonomous each child can be.

CONCLUSION

In order to be effective, efficient, and accountable, interventions must be approached systematically. A framework for being systematic was presented. The age of the child will need to be taken into account as well.

The chapters that follow describe a range of intervention options from which we can determine what might be most appropriate for our client.

QUESTIONS FOR CHAPTER 9

1. When in the treatment process would it be appropriate to use continuous versus intermittent reinforcement?

2. What are critical considerations in selecting consequent events?

3. Distinguish among vertical, horizontal, and cyclical goal attack strategies.

4. Describe and give examples of three types of speech sound generalization.

5. Present five expectations relative to speech sound generalization.

6. Discuss some of the challenges of treating very young children.

7. How might treating older children differ from treating very young children?

10

Motor-Based Treatment Approaches

JOHN E. BERNTHAL, PETER FLIPSEN JR., AND NICHOLAS W. BANKSON

LEARNING OBJECTIVES

This chapter discusses motor-based approaches to the remediation of speech sound disorder (SSDs), as well as assessment and treatment of childhood apraxia of speech (CAS). By the end of this chapter, the reader should be able to:

- Differentiate among the three phases of SSD treatment.

- Discuss principles of motor learning with specific regard to pre-practice goals, principles of practice, and principles of feedback.

- Describe the use of the challenge point framework for optimizing treatment progress.

- Explain different options for perceptual training.

- Distinguish among different methods for eliciting speech sounds.

- List and describe the basic steps in traditional articulation therapy.

- Discuss different forms of contextually based treatment approaches.

- List three populations where vowel remediation may be especially relevant.

APPROACHES TO INTERVENTION

Chapter 9 discussed general concepts and principles that underlie remediation of SSDs. These principles and considerations are applicable to all the treatment approaches that are discussed in this chapter, as well as those in Chapters 11 and 12. As a supplement to these chapters, we have also included some material on accent modification (a rather specialized area) in Chapter 15.

As previously discussed, speech-language pathologists (SLPs) have historically approached the correction of speech sound errors from the standpoint of teaching a motor behavior. Most clinicians viewed speech sound errors as arising from an individual's inability to produce the complex motor skills required for the articulation of speech sounds. According to a relatively recent survey (Brumbaugh & Smit, 2013), many SLPs continue to use motor-based approaches and may be making this same assumption about the underlying problem. Since the 1970s, clinicians have also viewed SSDs from a linguistic (phonological) perspective. The linguistic perspective is based on the recognition that some individuals produce speech sound errors because they have not learned to use certain phonologic rules, especially sound contrasts, in accord with the adult norm. In other words, many error productions reflect a client's difficulty in sorting out how sounds are used to contrast meaning in the language, rather than an inability to physically produce the sounds.

Before discussing specific intervention approaches, a few general comments are in order. First, although it is convenient to dichotomize approaches to intervention into *motor/articulation* (to be discussed in this chapter) and *linguistic/phonologic* (to be discussed in Chapter 11) categories, it is important to remember that normal speech sound production involves both the production of sounds at a motor level and their use in accordance with the phonological/linguistic rules of the language. Thus, the two skills are intertwined and may be described as two sides of the same coin. As mentioned in Chapter 7, it is often difficult or impossible to determine whether a client's errors reflect a lack of motor skills to produce a sound, a lack of linguistic knowledge, or deficiencies in both. It may be that, in a given client, some errors relate to one factor, some to another, and some to both. By careful observation of a client and the nature of their problem, and at times a bit of experimentation, the clinician usually is able to determine when one type of intervention should be emphasized.

A second point to be made is that even though a disorder may be perceived as relating primarily to either the motor or linguistic aspects of phonology, instructional programs typically involve elements of both. Some therapy activities undoubtedly assist the client in the development of both linguistic knowledge and appropriate motor skills. Consequently, the intervention approaches discussed in this text have been divided primarily on the basis of the degree to which they emphasize either motor or linguistic aspects of speech sound learning.

A third point to keep in mind is that several of the treatment approaches presented in this chapter were not developed from a particular theoretical perspective. Many approaches have emerged from pragmatic origins and continue to be used simply because clinicians perceive that they work. Thus, some of the approaches described in this and the following two chapters can be related to theory, some are atheoretical, and others lie somewhere between. For each approach presented, we provide a Background Statement that reflects our perception of the theoretical perspective from which the approach has emerged. An ongoing challenge is to develop, refine, and revise theories that provide rationale, support, explanations, and direction for intervention procedures.

Lastly, as discussed in Chapters 1 and 8, we are in an era of evidence-based practice. That means that regardless of whether an approach has strong theoretical underpinnings or not, clinicians must demonstrate that the treatment being applied can and is making a real difference over and above any of the extraneous effects (e.g., maturation) that were described in Chapter 8. This includes choosing approaches based on the best available published research evidence. That evidence will be highlighted under Research Support for the approaches to be presented. The evidence will be framed based on the levels of evidence that the American Speech-Language-Hearing Association (ASHA) has adopted and that were outlined in Chapter 8.

Once an approach is chosen, SLPs must collect their own clinical evidence (data) using appropriate treatment, control, and generalization measures, also described in Chapter 8 (see also Baker & McLeod, 2004, 2011b). This combination (published evidence and clinician-generated evidence) maximizes our confidence that any change that is being observed is the result of our efforts and not some outside influence. This provides some assurance that our time and that of our clients and their families is being put to good use.

TREATMENT CONTINUUM

As noted in Chapter 9, treatment has typically been viewed as a continuum of activities comprising three phases: establishment, generalization, and maintenance. This continuum, which comes from the motor learning literature, is applicable to most types of speech and language disorders. The goal of the first phase of instruction, called *establishment,* is to elicit target behaviors from the client and then stabilize such behaviors at a voluntary level. Specific procedures for establishment vary depending on the approach. For motor-based approaches, this generally involves teaching the correct production of an individual sound, whereas for linguistically based approaches, it involves ensuring correct production of a target, along with some contrasting sound, such as the child's typical error for that sound (usually at the word level or higher). If the child's problem is judged to be primarily linguistically based, the establishment phase may be shorter than for motor-based problems because the physical skill to produce the target is often present.

Motor-based establishment procedures are often based on production tasks, as in the example of a clinician teaching a child who does not produce /l/ where to place their tongue to say /l/. In addition, for a child who can say /l/ but deletes it in the final position (e.g., *bow* for *bowl*), the contrast between word pairs, such as *bow* and *bowl* or *sew* and *soul,* may also need to be taught during the establishment phase. In cases where a perceptual problem is suspected, some form of perceptual training (to be discussed later) may also be incorporated into the establishment phase.

Once the client is able to readily produce the correct form of the sound and is aware of how it is used contrastively, they are ready to move into the second or *generalization* phase of instruction (which was discussed in some detail in Chapter 9). This second phase is designed to facilitate transfer or carryover of behavior at several generalization levels: positional, contextual, linguistic unit, sound, and situational. The treatment process for this phase includes instructional activities or strategies designed to facilitate generalization or carryover of correct sound productions to sound contrasts, words, and speaking situations that have not been specifically trained. An example of a context generalization activity would be practicing /s/ in a few key words (e.g., see, sit, seek) and then determining whether /s/ is produced correctly in other words. An example of a situational generalization activity would be practicing /l/ in sentences in the treatment setting and then observing whether the child uses /l/ in words, phrases, and sentences produced in their classroom or home.

During the generalization phase, clinicians usually follow a very predictable progression from smaller to larger linguistic units (e.g., sounds to syllables to words to sentences to conversation). Moving from one level to the next occurs once the client achieves some predetermined level of success (e.g., 80% correct across three consecutive treatment sessions). An alternative to such a predictable progression can be found in the work of Skelton and colleagues (Skelton, 2004; Skelton & Funk, 2004; Skelton & Hagopian, 2014), who have suggested that progress may be faster if, during generalization, different levels of practice are randomly presented within an activity (an approach described as *concurrent treatment*). This approach will be discussed next.

The third and final phase of remediation, *maintenance,* is designed to stabilize and facilitate retention of those behaviors acquired during the establishment and generalization phases. Frequency and duration of instruction are often reduced during the maintenance phase, and the client assumes increased responsibility for maintaining and self-monitoring correct speech patterns. The client may also engage in specific activities designed to habituate or automatize particular speech patterns. A maintenance activity could consist of a client keeping track of their /s/ productions at mealtime or use of r-clusters during 5-minute phone conversations every evening for a week. It should be pointed out that although establishment, generalization, and maintenance have been identified as discrete phases of treatment, in practice there might be considerable overlap among these phases.

It should be noted that clients may enter the treatment continuum at different points, the exact point being determined by the individual's initial articulatory/pho-nological skills. Consider these two examples: Mark is able to produce a sound cor-rectly in words and is able to perceive the target contrastively. He, therefore, begins instruction at the generalization stage and would likely focus on incorporating target words into phrases. Kristy is able to produce a sound imitatively in syllables, perceives the sound contrast in word pairs, but fails to incorporate the target production of the sound into words. She also enters the treatment continuum at the generalization stage but at an earlier point than Mark. In her case, the clinician will seek to establish the target sound in a set of target words selected on the basis, perhaps, of facilitating con-text or even vocabulary items used in her classroom. For Mark, the clinician will facil-itate generalization to phrases and sometimes other contexts. For Kristy, the clinician will facilitate generalization from syllables to words, including words not specifically focused on in a therapy session. The clinician must identify not only the appropriate phase of the treatment continuum, but also the appropriate level within a phase at which to begin instruction.

MOTOR LEARNING PRINCIPLES

Motor-based approaches to treating SSDs are designed to focus primarily on the motor (or movement) skills involved in producing target sounds. They also frequently include perceptual tasks as part of the treatment procedures. Most motor-based approaches represent variations of what is often referred to as the *traditional approach* or *traditional articulation therapy*. Treatment based on an articulation/phonetic or motor perspective focuses on the placement and movement of the articulators in com-bination with some form of perceptual training (e.g., ear training and focused auditory input). This remediation approach involves the selection of a target speech sound or sounds, with instruction proceeding through the treatment continuum described pre-viously until the target sounds are used appropriately in spontaneous conversation. Thus, from the perspective of advocates of motor-based approaches, speech produc-tion is viewed as a learned motor skill with remediation requiring repetitive practice at increasingly complex motor and linguistic levels and situations until the targeted articulatory gestures become automatic.

It is somewhat surprising that despite the long-standing use of motor-based approaches, there is limited research available about how speech motor learning occurs, particularly in children. Fortunately, research in other disciplines, such as physical therapy, as well as in adults with acquired speech disorders, has revealed a series of basic principles that may be applicable to children with SSDs. Maas and colleagues (2008) summarized much of this research into three areas: pre-practice goals, principles of practice, and principles of feedback. We now discuss each of these in turn.

Pre-Practice Goals

Prior to beginning instruction, there are several important aspects of the therapy process for clinicians to consider. First, they should help ensure the child is motivated for learning by including them (and/or their parents) in establishing goals to work on and making those goals functionally relevant. For very young children and/or those with cognitive impairments, we would likely rely more heavily on parental input for establishing goals. A second aspect to be considered is that when beginning therapy, we need to ensure that the child understands the tasks being asked of them. We do this by both using simple, easy-to-understand instructions and providing good models of both the goal behavior and what would be unacceptable productions. We may need to either practice or record examples of both correct productions and errors so we can reliably present these models to the child so that they understand what is and is not a correct production. Finally, prior to remediation planning, we need to be sure of the child's perceptual abilities (i.e., hearing acuity and sound contrast perception) to avoid frustration during the learning process. This is particularly important for preschool children who are susceptible to middle ear infections that may result in intermittent hearing loss.

Principles of Practice

As Ruscello (1984) pointed out, practice is the key variable for mastery of any skilled motor behavior. Clinicians must therefore arrange therapy so that there are lots of opportunities to practice the desired behavior. In addition, Maas and colleagues (2008) also point out that:

1. Where possible, many shorter treatment sessions have generally been shown to be more productive than fewer but longer sessions.

2. Practice under a variety of conditions (e.g., different rates with different intonation patterns) is preferable to repeating the targets many times under the same conditions.

3. Random presentation of targets is better than multiple attempts at the same target.

4. Having the child focus on correct productions of a sound is preferable to having them focus on the details of the individual articulator movements.

5. Practicing the entire speech target (even if it is only the sound in isolation) is better than breaking that target down into tiny pieces and repeating those pieces multiple times. For example, practicing production of /r/ is better than repeatedly sticking the tongue in and out of the mouth without making any sound to simulate the tongue retraction gesture of /r/.

Principles of Feedback

Maas and colleagues (2008) noted that the way feedback is provided to the child may be crucial to their learning. Early on in therapy, it appears best to provide *knowledge of performance* or feedback about what specifically they are doing correctly or incorrectly (e.g., "Don't forget to keep your teeth together when you say that /s/ sound."). But once the target begins to be established, feedback should quickly change to *knowledge of results,* or a focus on whether the target was produced correctly (e.g., "Excellent. That was a very good /s/ sound." or "No, good try but not quite right. Try that one again."). Interestingly, the research Maas and colleagues cite also suggests that less feedback is better than more because it gives the child the opportunity to reflect internally on their productions. Therapy may need to begin with a lot of feedback to maximize initial learning, but it appears best to diminish the feedback so that it becomes relatively infrequent (e.g., start with feedback for every attempt and, as the child becomes more successful, switch to feedback every third attempt, progressing to only providing feedback every tenth attempt).

To aid in the transition from frequent feedback from the clinician to limited feedback, the child may occasionally be asked to express their own opinion about their attempts (i.e., to engage in explicit self-monitoring). As the frequency of feedback is reduced, it can then also become somewhat variable (i.e., not on a strict fixed ratio schedule) in terms of when it is specifically provided. Finally, when feedback is delivered, there should be a slight delay (i.e., 1–2 seconds) to give the child the opportunity to reflect on their own (auditory, tactile, kinesthetic, and proprioceptive) feedback. However, the clinician must take care that some extraneous event doesn't occur prior to the feedback, lest the event rather than the desired behavior be reinforced.

These principles are drawn largely from research on a variety of types of motor learning, largely outside the realm of speech learning and from a small number of studies of adult speech motor learning. Thus, extending them to therapy with children evidencing SSDs is still somewhat speculative. However, many of them are consistent with what clinicians report they have been doing for years and with our discussion of shaping and positive reinforcement of behaviors discussed in Chapter 9. It should be recognized that treatment studies in the area of SSDs have often reported success when incorporating these learning principles (e.g., positive reinforcement) as part of their therapy protocols.

OPTIMIZING LEARNING: THE CHALLENGE POINT FRAMEWORK

One of the challenges in teaching any new skill and including motor skills is being efficient. In particular, the goal is to optimize both the task and the feedback so that the learner can learn as quickly as possible. In this case, learning includes both generalization and maintenance. Optimization of learning can be impeded in one of two ways. First, if too much time is spent producing targets with high accuracy (i.e., if the task is too easy), little corrective feedback is provided, and little learning is taking place. On the other hand, if errors are being made on most or all attempts (i.e., if the task is too hard), so much feedback is received that it may overwhelm the ability to deal with it, and learning is also diminished. The notion of the *challenge point* or the *optimal challenge point* was proposed by Guadagnoli and Lee (2004) as that level of difficulty that allows for enough feedback to facilitate learning but not decrease the efficiency and effectiveness of therapy.

As Rvachew and colleagues (2018) expressed it, the challenge point is the right amount of information to learn. As the child improves their skill, the challenge they face needs to increase. If therapy performance falls off too quickly, however, the clinician needs to step back a bit and make the task a little easier. It seems likely that the challenge point will vary somewhat across individuals, but one example of a set of benchmarks comes from Hitchcock and McAllister Byun (2015a) in a study of feedback for correcting /r/ in an 11-year-old girl:

Performance <50% correct   Make the task easier

Performance 51%–80% correct   Keep the task the same

Performance >80% correct   Make the task harder

In the Hitchcock and McAllister Byun (2015a) study, previous therapy had established /r/ but had failed to yield any generalization beyond the word level. The challenge point framework was used across 17 once-per-week sessions. This included 3 baseline sessions, 10 treatment sessions, 3 follow-up sessions, and a follow-up session 1 month later (no feedback was provided during baseline or follow-up sessions) using the benchmarks reported previously. Performance was measured every 10 trials, and thus the difficulty of the task was being constantly adjusted based on the child's performance. The girl achieved 100% success in both word- and sentence-level probes at the follow-up session.

Making the task easier or harder can be accomplished by making changes along any one of several dimensions, according to Rvachew and colleagues (2018). These include:

1. *Practice intensity*—more or fewer trials in the session (either by faster or slower presentation of stimuli or making the session longer or shorter)

2. *Task difficulty*—embed the target in more or less complex word shapes or longer or shorter linguistic units

3. *Degree of stimulation*—move up or down the continuum from coproduction (easiest) to direct imitation to delayed imitation to spontaneous production (hardest)

4. *Nature of the feedback provided*—move from knowledge of performance (less challenging) to knowledge of results (more challenging) to no feedback (most challenging)

5. *Frequency of the feedback*—less feedback increases the challenge

TEACHING SOUNDS/ESTABLISHMENT

For clients who do not produce target behaviors on demand or who have perceptual and/or production difficulty with particular speech sounds, the first step usually involves teaching sounds, which may include perceptual training. Clients who enter the treatment continuum at this point often include those who 1) do not have a specific sound in their repertoire and are not stimulable for that sound, 2) produce a sound in their repertoire but only in a limited number of phonetic contexts and are unable to readily produce the sound on demand, 3) do not perceive the sound in minimal pairs or in a judgment task, such as Locke's (1980b) SP-PT, or 4) produce a sound on demand but do not easily incorporate the sound into syllabic or word units.

Two basic teaching strategies are used to establish sound productions. The first involves discrimination/perceptual training prior to or along with direct production training. The second involves initiating treatment with a production focus and makes the assumption that the client will learn to discriminate and perceive the sound as an indirect benefit of production training. Perceptual instruction is frequently an inherent aspect of production training. For example, when a client is asked to say *house* but says *hout,* the clinician may say, "No, not *hout* but *house.*" In this instance, although instruction is production oriented, perceptual training is inherent to the task. Some clinicians, therefore, choose not to do perceptual training as a separate step.

Winitz (1984) suggested that auditory discrimination training precede articulation production training at each stage of production (e.g., isolation, syllable, word, sentence, conversation) until the client can make the appropriate speech sound discrimination easily at each level. The idea that perceptual training should precede production training is based on the assumption that certain perceptual distinctions are prerequisites for establishing the production of a speech sound in the child's phonologic system, although this assumption is not universally accepted. As noted in Chapter 4, there is some evidence that using concurrent perceptual training with production training may improve production skill and possibly perceptual skill as well.

Perceptual Training

Assuming that perceptual training is provided as a separate step (either prior to production training or at the same time), several options are typically used.

Traditional Ear Training

The type of perceptual training that historically is most common is called *ear training* or speech sound discrimination training or sensory-perceptual training. Instructional tasks designed to teach discrimination stem from the traditional motor approach to articulation treatment and, in its simplest form, typically involve making same–different judgments about what is heard (e.g., "Tell me if these are the same or different: *rake–wake.*").

Van Riper and Emerick (1984), Winitz (1975, 1984), Powers (1971), and Weber (1970) recommended that discrimination training occur prior to production training during the establishment phase of the treatment continuum. As discussed in Chapter 4, however, routine perceptual training may be of little value. It would appear to be more appropriate to use discrimination (or perceptual) training only in cases in which perceptual difficulties have been documented and then targeted only to sounds in which both a perceptual and a production problem are present. Such an approach is supported in a study conducted by Overby (2007), who reported that a group of second-grade children with SSDs had lower overall scores on a speech perception task than typically developing children. She did not find, however, a consistent pattern or relationship of the specific speech sound errors children made and performance on the speech perception task for the specific speech sound error. In other words, not all of the production errors were linked to a problem with perception.

Traditionally, speech sound discrimination training has focused on judgments of external (clinician-produced) speech sound stimuli. Speech sound discrimination training procedures are often sequenced so that the client goes from judgments of another speaker's productions to judgments of their own sound productions.

Methodology for Traditional Ear Training.   Van Riper and Erickson (1996) outlined the following methodology for tradition ear training:

1. *Identification.* Call the client's attention to the target sound—what it sounds like, what it looks like as you observe the lips and mouth—and, as best you can, help them be aware of kinesthetic sensations or what it feels like inside the mouth. For some children, it may help to label the sound and have an appropriate picture or object to go with it (e.g., /f/ is the angry cat sound; /t/ is the ticking sound; /k/ is the throaty sound). For a larger list of such metaphors see Bleile (1995; pp. 234–235).

    After auditorily stimulating the child with repeated productions of the target sound by the clinician, then the child is asked to raise their hand, ring a bell, or otherwise indicate when they hear the target sound in isolation. The target is intermingled with other sounds. Initially, the other sounds should have several feature differences from the target in terms of voicing, manner, and place of production (e.g., /s/ and /m/). However, as instruction progresses, the number of feature contrasts between the target and the other sounds should be fewer (e.g., /s/ vs. /θ/).

2. *Isolation.* Have the client again listen for the target sound by identifying it in increasingly complex environments. Begin by having the child raise their hand, show a happy face, or otherwise indicate when they hear the sound in a word (begin with the initial position). Then progress to having the child listen for the sound in phrases and sentences. This step might also include practice identifying the presence of a sound in the middle or at the end of the word. Note that this step may be very difficult for young children before they have learned to read and is not usually included unless the child has a good grasp of the concepts beginning, middle, and end.

3. *Stimulation.* Provide the client an appropriate auditory model of the target sound in both isolation and words. This activity might include limited amplification and varying stress and duration of the target sound. Hodson (2010a) advocates this type of activity as part of the cycles approach to remediation (to be discussed in Chapter 11) and is discussed later as *amplified auditory stimulation.*

4. *Discrimination.* Ask the client to make judgments of correct and incorrect productions you produce in increasingly complex contexts (i.e., words, phrases, sentences). In this activity, the client is comparing someone else's production with their own internal image of the correct form of a sound. For example, if a child substituted /θ/ for /s/, the clinician might say: "Here is a picture of a thun. Did I say that word right? Did you see my tongue peeking out at the beginning of the word? Did you hear /θ/ instead of /s/? See if I am right when I name this picture [picture of school]: *thcool, thcool.* Did I say that correctly?"

Perceptual Training of Sound Contrasts

One way in which linguistics has impacted clinical phonology has been on the nature of perceptual training that should either precede or be a part of phonological treatment. Rather than focus on discrimination between sounds, the phonological perspective suggests that perceptual training should focus on minimal pair-contrast training with the particular minimal pairs utilized reflecting the child's error pattern.

LaRiviere and associates (1974) first proposed this training, which focuses on the client's differentiation of minimally contrasting word pairs. For example, when consonant clusters are reduced, the child would be taught to sort contrasting word pairs (e.g., *top* vs. *stop*) into categories that reflect simplification of a consonant cluster and those that reflect appropriate production of the target consonant cluster (e.g., *sick* vs. *stick*). Another example is a task for final consonant deletion in which the client picks up pictures of *tea* and *teeth* as the clinician randomly names them.

The intent of this training is to develop a perceptual awareness of differences between minimal pairs (in this case, the presence or absence of a final consonant in the word), and the training serves to establish the appropriate phonologic contrasts. Such training might also be used for single errors (i.e., those that don't necessarily reflect a wider pattern across several sounds). For example, with the child who substitutes /t/ for /k/, the focus might be on discriminating pairs, such as *net* and *neck*. Many clinicians employ perceptual training of this type, and a method for using it is presented here. The topic is further described in Chapter 11 when contrast intervention strategies are discussed.

Methodology for Perceptual Training of Sound Contrasts.   Perceptual training for sound contrasts may be delivered through the following methodology:

1. *Introduction of the minimal pair.* Present to the client a word that contains the target sound. For example, if the child is substituting /t/ for the fricative /ʃ/, the word *shoe* might be used in a perceptual training activity. The child listens as the clinician points to five identical pictures of a shoe and names each one.

   Next, present to the client a second word, also with associated pictures of the word, which contain a contrasting sound that is very different from the target sound (i.e., has several different features from the target sound). For example, *shoe* might be contrasted with *boo* (ghost picture). The phonemes /ʃ/ and /b/ differ in voicing, manner, and place of articulation. For this step, the clinician identifies the original five pictures of a shoe plus the five pictures of boo.

2. *Contrast training.* Practice differentiating the two contrasting words at a perceptual level. Line up the 10 pictures, 5 of which are of a shoe and 5 of boo. Ask the client to hand you the picture you name. Make random requests for either boo or shoe. If the child can readily do this, they have established at a perceptual level the contrast between /ʃ/ and /b/. If the child has difficulty with this task, it should be repeated, possibly with different words. Once the child can do this task, contrast training should be repeated with minimal pairs involving the target and error sound (e.g., *shoe–two; shop–top*).

   When the clinician is satisfied that the client can discriminate the target sound from other sounds and that they can perceive the target in minimal pairs involving the target sound and error sound, the client is ready for production training. It should be pointed out that, in our experience, many children readily discriminate accurately in external monitoring tasks; that is, they can discriminate the clinician's productions although they may not produce the contrast.

Perceptual Training Software

An alternative to the classic perceptual training described previously is the use of commercially developed programs such as the Speech Assessment and Interactive

Learning System (SAILS; Rvachew & Herbay, 2017). This is a software program (now available as a tablet-based application) specifically intended to improve speech perception skills in children with SSDs. The child is presented with a variety of correct and incorrect real-speech examples of the target phoneme and is asked to make judgments about whether the production was correct. The software provides visual feedback about the accuracy of the child's judgment. According to Rvachew and Brosseau-Lapré (2010), the child usually works with an adult who also provides specific feedback about the child's judgments (e.g., "Yes, that was a good /s/ sound." or "That /s/ didn't sound right, did it?"). The software also tracks the child's success rate to assist the clinician in monitoring progress. Administration of the SAILS program can be done either prior to beginning production training or concurrently (e.g., for 5–10 minutes at the beginning of each therapy session).

There is published evidence that the SAILS program can be effective. At least three randomized controlled trials (level Ib) have been conducted using it. One of these (Rvachew, 1994) was discussed in Chapter 4. More recently, Wolfe and colleagues (2003) conducted a study with nine preschool children who had SSDs. Five of the children received production training only, and four received a combination of production and SAILS training. The two groups performed equally well overall, but performance was better with the SAILS training on targets when perceptual skills were poor at pretreatment testing.

Rvachew, Nowak, & Cloutier (2004) conducted the third randomized controlled trial involving SAILS. A group of 34 preschool children with SSDs received weekly treatment sessions for a variety of targets with whatever production approach their clinician thought was appropriate. In addition, half the children underwent SAILS training sessions whereas the other half (controls) listened to computerized stories and answered questions about the stories. The children who received the SAILS training demonstrated better speech production skills at the end of 16 weeks of therapy; in addition, prior to entering first grade, 50% of those who received SAILS training had fully normal speech compared to only 19% from the control group.

Amplified Auditory Stimulation

As mentioned previously, Hodson and Paden (1991) recommended this approach to perceptual training as part of their cycles phonological patterns approach, which is discussed in Chapter 11. It remains an integral part of more recent versions of that approach (Hodson, 2010a). Clinicians have also used it in conjunction with other treatment approaches, including motor-based treatments. This method is sometimes referred to as *auditory bombardment* (a term actually coined by Charles Van Riper). It is intended to be used concurrently with speech production training and involves presentation of lists of up to 20 words containing the target sound or sound pattern at the beginning and end of each treatment session. Similar to traditional ear training, a mild gain amplification device is used to ensure that the input is loud enough but not distorted (note that there is a natural tendency to distort speech when speaking louder than normal). The child merely listens; no production or judgment is required of the child.

Hodson and Paden (1991) described a variation on this perceptual training (referred to as *focused auditory input*) for a client who "... either has not been willing or was unable to produce a target at the time of initial contact (e.g., children functioning below the 3-year-old level)" (p. 107). In this case, initial treatment sessions are conducted in which no production is required of the child. A series of play activities is used in which the child is exposed to many models of specific target sounds or patterns (one or two specific targets per session) produced by the clinician or the parent during the natural course of the play activities. Hodson and Paden also suggested that word lists containing the target sounds be sent home for additional listening practice.

Summary of Perceptual Training

Many speech clinicians teach their clients to perceive the distinction between the target and error sounds or to identify phonemic contrasts as part of the establishment process. Such activities may precede and/or accompany production training. As stated earlier, routine discrimination/perceptual training in treatment has been questioned because many individuals with SSDs do not demonstrate discrimination problems. In addition, production training unaccompanied by direct perceptual training has been shown to modify phonologic errors and increase perception on target sounds. Perceptual training is justified in those specific cases where a perceptual problem accompanies a production problem.

Production Training

Motor-based intervention focuses on helping a client learn to correctly produce a target sound. Whether perceptual training is included, or whether it precedes or is interwoven with production training, the goal during this phase of training is to elicit a target sound from a client and stabilize it at a voluntary level. These procedures may also be used with linguistically based interventions (Chapter 11).

When a sound is not in a person's repertoire, it is sometimes taught in isolation or syllables rather than words. It should be remembered that some speech sounds, such as stops, are difficult to teach in isolation because stops by their physical nature are produced in combination with vowels or vowel approximations. Glides, likewise, involve production of more than the glide when they are produced. Continuant sounds such as fricatives can be taught in isolation because they are sounds that can be sustained (e.g., s-s-s-s-s). Stops and glides are usually taught in CV contexts (e.g., stop + schwa = /gə/).

Whether sounds should be taught initially in isolation, syllables, or words is a matter of some controversy. McDonald (1964a) urged that syllables be used in production training because the syllable is the basic unit of motor speech production. Some clinicians (e.g., Van Riper & Emerick, 1984) have argued that because isolated sounds are the least complex units of production and afford the least interference between the client's habitual speech sound error and the learning of a correct (adult) production, they should be taught first. Words sometimes elicit interference from old error patterns and, in such cases, may not be a good place to initiate instruction.

Others advocate words (lexical items) as the best place to begin instruction because the client can benefit from contextual influences in meaningful productions and because of the communicative benefits that accrue from the use of real words. The clinician can determine the level of production that is most facilitative for correct production and then determine whether interference from previous learning (i.e., long-established habits) is a problem. As a general rule, we recommend beginning at the highest level possible where production is correct.

Speech-language clinicians commonly employ one or more of four methods to establish the production of a target sound: imitation, phonetic placement, successive approximation (shaping), and contextual utilization. Each of these is discussed next.

Imitation

We recommend that the clinician attempt to elicit responses through imitation as an initial instructional method for production training. Usually, the clinician presents several auditory models of the desired behavior (typically a sound in isolation, syllables, or words), instructs the client to watch their mouth and listen to the sound that is being said, and then asks the client to repeat the target behavior. Sometimes, the clinician may amplify the model through some type of mild gain amplification device.

Eliciting /θ/ with Imitation. Consider the following example of a clinician eliciting /θ/ with imitation:

Clinician: Watch my mouth and listen while I say this sound—/θ/ [repeat it several times]. Now you say it.

Clinician: That's right, I heard the /θ/ sound. Now say this—/θɑ/ [repeat it several times].

Clinician: Good, now say /θi/ [proceed to have the client combine /θ/ and a couple of other vowels].

Clinician: Now say *thumb* [repeat it several times].

Sometimes the clinician tape records productions to play them back for the client's self-evaluation. Clients may also be asked to focus on how a sound feels during correct production and to modify their productions to maintain this kinesthetic awareness.

When an individual can imitate a target sound, the goal during establishment is simply to stabilize target productions. Subsequent instruction usually begins at the most complex linguistic level at which the client is able to imitate, whether it be isolation, syllables, or words. The level at which a client can imitate may already have been determined during stimulability testing, but it should be rechecked at the initiation of instruction. Even if the client was not stimulable on a sound during assessment, it is recommended that the clinician begin remediation by asking the client to imitate target productions using auditory, visual, and tactile cues.

Phonetic Placement

When the client is unable to imitate a target sound, the clinician typically begins to cue or instruct the client regarding where to place their articulators. (Chapter 2 offers a bit of a refresher if you feel your knowledge of phonetics is a bit rusty.) This type of instruction is called *phonetic placement.*

1. Instruct the client where to place the articulators to produce a specific speech sound (e.g., for /f/, tell the client to place their upper teeth on their lower lip and blow air over the lip; for /ʃ/, tell the client to pull the tongue back from the upper teeth past the rough part of the palate, make a groove in the tongue, round the lips, and blow air).

2. Provide visual and tactile cues to supplement verbal description (e.g., model the correct sound and provide verbal cueing as the client attempts the sounds: "Remember to lightly touch your lower lip as you blow air for /f/; remember the groove as you blow air for the /ʃ/.").

3. It may be helpful, depending on the client's maturity level, to analyze and describe differences between the error production and the target production. Sometimes clinicians like to use pictures or drawings reflecting placement of the articulators as part of the instruction.

The phonetic placement method has probably been used as long as anyone has attempted to modify speech patterns. Over 85 years ago, Scripture and Jackson (1927) published *A Manual of Exercises for the Correction of Speech Disorders,* which included phonetic placement techniques for speech instruction. These authors suggested:

1. Mirror work

2. Drawings designed to show the position of the articulators for the production of specific sounds

3. Mouth gymnastics; that is, movements of the articulators (lips and tongue) in response to models and verbal cues and instructions (note that we will discuss why these might not be advisable later)

4. The use of tongue blades to teach placement of sounds and straws to help direct the air stream

The tablet-based (and smart-phone based) application Sounds of Speech developed at the University of Iowa may also be of value for phonetic placement instruction. It shows both consonant and vowel production both statically and in motion. It includes sounds for English, Korean, Spanish, and both simplified and traditional Chinese. The sounds are simultaneously produced providing a direct connection between the placement and the resulting output. The website Seeing Speech (https://www.seeingspeech.ac.uk/) developed in the United Kingdom may also be useful as it provides additional images. The electronic format of these two tools may be especially motivating for some clients.

The phonetic placement approach involves explanations and descriptions of idealized phoneme productions. The verbal explanations provided to the client include descriptions of motor gestures or movements and the appropriate points of articulatory contact (tongue, jaw, lip, and velum) involved in producing the target segments. This approach to teaching sounds frequently is used alone or in combination with imitation plus successive approximation and context utilization (described in the following discussion).

Phonetic Placement for Teaching /s/.   To teach /s/ for example, the clinician would instruct the client to:

1. Raise the tongue so that its sides are firmly in contact with the inner surface of the upper back teeth.

2. Slightly groove the tongue along the midline. Insert a straw along the midline of the tongue to provide the client a tactile cue as to the place to form the groove.

3. Place the tip of the tongue immediately behind the upper or lower teeth. Show the client in a mirror where to place the tongue tip.

4. Bring the front teeth (central incisors) into alignment (as much as possible) so that a narrow small space between the rows of teeth is formed.

5. Direct the air stream along the groove of the tongue toward the cutting edges of the teeth.

Successive Approximation (Shaping)

Another procedure for teaching sounds that is, in some respects, an extension of using phonetic placement cues, involves shaping a new sound from one that is already in a client's repertoire, or even a behavior the client can perform, such as elevating the tongue. This is sometimes referred to as *shaping*. The first step in shaping is to identify an initial response that the client can produce that is related to the terminal goal. Instruction moves through a series of graded steps or approximations, each progressively closer to the target behavior.

Shaping /s/.   For instance, shaping /s/ would involve the following cues:

1. Make [t] (the alveolar place of constriction is similar for both /t/ and /s/).

2. Make [t] with a strong aspiration on the release, prior to the onset of the vowel.

3. Prolong the strongly aspirated release.

4. Remove the tip of the tongue slowly during the release from the alveolar ridge to make a [ts] cluster.

5. Prolong the [s] portion of the [ts] cluster in a word such as *oats*.

6. Practice prolonging the last portion of the [ts] production.

7. Practice sneaking up quietly on the /s/ (delete /t/).

8. Produce /s/.

Shaping /ɝ/.   An example of shaping /ɝ/ was described by Shriberg (1975):

1. Stick your tongue out (model provided).

2. Stick your tongue out and touch the tip of your finger (model provided).

3. Put your finger on the bumpy place right behind your top teeth (model provided).

4. Now put the tip of your tongue lightly on that bumpy place (model provided).

5. Now put your tongue tip there again and say [l] (model provided).

6. Say [l] each time I hold up my finger (clinician holds up finger).

7. Now say [l] for as long as I hold my finger up like this (model provided for 5 seconds). Ready. Go.

8. Say a long [l], but this time as you are saying it, drag the tip of your tongue slowly back along the roof of your mouth—so far back that you have to drop it. (Accompany instructions with hand gestures of moving fingertips back slowly, palm up.) (p. 104)

These examples for /s/ and /ɝ/ reflect ways that clinicians capitalize on successive approximations: by shaping behavior from a sound in the client's repertoire (e.g., /t/) and by shaping from a nonphonetic behavior in the client's repertoire (e.g., protruded tongue). Once the client produces a sound that is close to the target, the clinician can use other techniques, such as auditory stimulation, imitation, and phonetic placement cues, to reach the target production.

Appendix A includes descriptions of some additional ways to elicit various sounds. A more comprehensive list of various ways to elicit sounds can also be found in Secord and colleagues (2007).

Contextual Utilization

A final general procedure used to establish a sound involves isolating a target sound from a particular phonetic context in which a client may happen to produce a sound correctly, even though they typically produce the sound in error. As indicated in Chapter 6, correct sound productions can sometimes be elicited through contextual testing because sounds are affected by phonetic and positional context, and some contexts may facilitate the correct production of a particular sound. Contextual testing may also be used as a way to elicit productions for clients selected for remediation.

Specific contexts within words are the most common way to facilitate correct production. The following examples of these *facilitating contexts* were drawn from Curtis and Hardy (1959), Kent (1982), and Hodson and Paden (1991):

1. Word-initial /r/ may be easier to produce correctly in the clusters /tr/, /dr/, or /gr/.

2. Word-initial /r/ and /l/ may be easier to produce correctly before front vowels (e.g., /i/ or /e/) rather than before back vowels (e.g., /u/ or /o/). This is particularly true if the child's error sound is /w/.

3. The phoneme /ʃ/ may be easier to produce correctly before back vowels (e.g., /u/ or /o/) rather than before front vowels (e.g., /i/ or /e/).

4. Singleton /s/, /k/, and /g/ may be easier to produce correctly in word-final position rather than word-initial position.

5. The phoneme /s/ may be easier to produce correctly in clusters rather than as a singleton consonant. For some children, the word-initial clusters /sp/, /st/, and /sk/ may be easier, whereas for other children the word-final clusters /ps/, /ts/, and /ks/ may be easier.

6. For polysyllabic words, sounds tend to be easier to produce correctly in stressed syllables compared to unstressed syllables.

The idea of teaching clusters before singletons (item 5) is counterintuitive to typical assumptions about speech sound learning, but is consistent with the complexity approach to selecting targets discussed in Chapters 7 and 11. They both rely on the assumption that mastery of more complex targets will stimulate generalization to simpler targets. It is also consistent with data on teaching /s/ in clusters before singletons as reported by A. L. Williams (1991).

The context of sounds in adjoining words may also offer facilitation of correct production (McDonald, 1964a). The following example of contextual facilitation with /s/ illustrates this:

If /s/ is produced correctly in the context of the word pair *bright–sun,* the /t/ preceding the /s/ may be viewed as a facilitating context.

1. Ask the client to say *bright sun* slowly and prolong the /s/. Demonstrate what you mean by saying the two words and extending the duration of /s/ (e.g., *bright— ssssssssun*).

2. Next, ask the client to repeat *bright—ssssssink,* then *hot—sssssssea.* Other facilitating pairs may be used to extend and stabilize the /s/ production.

3. Ask the client to only say /s/ by itself.

Using phonetic/linguistic context as a method to establish a sound allows the clinician to capitalize on a behavior that could already be in the client's repertoire. This procedure also represents a form of shaping because one is using context to help the client isolate and stabilize production of an individual phoneme.

Motor Establishment Guidelines

Individual variations among clients preclude a detailed set of specific instructions applicable to all clients; however, the following are general guidelines for establishment:

1. Perceptual training, particularly contrast training employing minimal pairs, is suggested as part of establishment of those sounds when there is evidence that the production errors are due to problems perceiving appropriate phonologic contrasts.

2. When teaching production of a target sound, look for the target sound in the client's response repertoire through stimulability (imitation) testing, contextual testing (including consonant clusters, other word positions, and phonetic contexts), and observation of a connected speech sample. Our recommended hierarchy for eliciting sounds that cannot be produced on demand is a) imitation, b) phonetic placement, c) successive approximation (shaping), and d) contextual utilization. Once stable correct productions are obtained, they can be used as a starting point for more complex linguistic units and contexts.

BEYOND INDIVIDUAL SOUNDS

Teaching a sound (establishment) is typically the first step in motor-based intervention, and it may be used in linguistically based interventions as well. But correction of speech sound errors goes beyond establishment. Several motor-based treatment approaches include procedures designed to move a client through a multistep process from establishment through correct production of target sounds in conversational speech (the treatment continuum). The most frequently employed method for doing this is labeled the traditional approach and is described next.

Traditional Approach

The *traditional approach* (also called *traditional articulation* therapy) was formulated during the early decades of the 1900s by pioneering clinicians of the field. By the late 1930s, Charles Van Riper had assimilated these treatment techniques into an overall plan for treating articulation disorders and published them in his text titled *Speech Correction: Principles and Methods* (originally published in 1939 and modified in several subsequent editions). As an outgrowth of his writings, the traditional approach is sometimes referred to as the *Van Riper method*.

The traditional approach is motor oriented and was developed at a time when those receiving treatment were typically school-age clients, often with persistent or residual errors. At that time, clinicians were seeing few children with language disorders (the profession had not yet acknowledged that language disorders in children were an appropriate area of practice for speech therapists), and caseloads included more children with mild SSDs than at present. However, the traditional approach was successfully used with clients representing a range of severity. The traditional approach to articulation therapy is still widely used and is particularly appropriate for individuals with errors considered to be articulatory or motor in nature, including those identified as residual or persistent errors.

The traditional approach progresses from the speaker's identification of error productions in ear training, to the establishment of correct productions, and then moves on to generalization and, finally, to maintenance. As Van Riper and Emerick (1984) stated:

> The hallmark of traditional articulation therapy lies in its sequencing of activities for (1) sensory-perceptual training, which concentrates on identifying the standard sound and discriminating it from its error through scanning and comparing; (2) varying and correcting the various productions of the sound until it is produced correctly; (3) strengthening and stabilizing the correct production; and finally (4) transferring the new speech skill to everyday communication situations. This process is usually carried out first for the standard sound in isolation, then in syllables, then in words, and finally in sentences. (p. 206)

A characteristic of this approach is its emphasis on sensory-perceptual or ear training (described in detail earlier), which was originally seen as a necessary precursor to production training. In most cases, the primary ingredient of traditional instruction is production training, with the focus on helping a client learn to produce a sound on demand. Production training usually includes a series of sequential instructional steps described here.

Instructional steps for traditional production training (Secord, 1989; Van Riper & Erickson, 1996):

1. *Isolation.* The first step in the traditional method is to teach a client to produce a sound in isolation (i.e., by itself). An explanation for beginning with production of the target sound in isolation is the assumption that the articulatory gestures of a sound are most easily learned when the sound is highly identifiable and in the least complex context. The goal at this level is to develop a consistently correct response. Specific techniques for teaching sounds were discussed earlier under the establishment phase and are included in Appendix A (see also Secord et al., 2007). It should be pointed out that training should begin at whatever level of sound complexity a child can produce—isolation, sound clusters, syllables, or words.

2. *Nonsense syllables.* The second step involves teaching the client to produce a sound in a syllable. The goal at this step is consistently correct productions in a variety of nonsense syllable contexts. A suggested sequence for syllable practice is CV, VC, VCV, and CVC. It is also suggested that the transition from the consonant to the vowel should initially be accomplished with sounds that are similar in place of articulation. For example, an alveolar consonant such as /s/ should be facilitated in a high front vowel context, as in [sɪ]. The clinician might also wish to use the target sound in nonsense clusters. The value of the nonsense syllable level is that it provides for practice in different contexts, and (because such syllables are not likely to have been practiced before) it minimizes the possibility of old (incorrect) habits emerging.

3. *Words.* The third step involves having a client produce a sound in meaningful units; that is, words. This step begins once the client can consistently produce

Table 10.1. Substages of word level stabilization training

Substage	Syllables	Examples for /s/
1. Initial prevocalic words	1	*sun, sign, say*
2. Final postvocalic words	1	*glass, miss, pass*
3. Medial intervocalic words	2	*kissing, lassie, racer*
4. Initial blends/clusters	1	*star, spoon, skate*
5. Final blends/clusters	1	*lost, lips, rocks*
6. Medial blends/clusters	2	*whisper, outside, ice-skate*
7. All word positions	1–2	(any of the above)
8. All word positions	Any	*signaling, eraser, therapist*
9. All word positions; multiple targets	Any	*necessary, successful*

Source: Secord (1989).

the target sound in nonsense syllables. Instructions at this level should begin with monosyllabic words with the target consonant (assuming instruction is focusing on consonants as opposed to vowels) in the prevocalic position (CV). Instruction then moves to VC, CVC, CVCV, monosyllabic words with clusters, and more complex word forms. Table 10.1 reflects a hierarchy of phoneme production complexity at the word level as presented by Secord (1989).

Once a core group of words in which the client is readily able to produce the target sound is established, the clinician seeks to expand the small set of core words into a somewhat larger set of training words. Usually, target words are selected on the basis of meaningfulness to the client (e.g., family names, places, social expressions, words from the academic curriculum), but other factors, such as phonetic context and syllable complexity, should also be considered, just as they were for the initial set of core words.

4. *Phrases.* Once the client can produce a target sound in words on demand, instruction shifts from single-word productions to practicing a target sound in two- to four-word phrases. This level of production represents a complexity level between single words and sentence-level productions. This is especially true if carrier phrases are employed. *Carrier phrases* are phrases in which only a single word is changed with each repetition (e.g., I see the *car;* I see the *cup;* I see the *cane.*). In phrase-level productions, one should begin with phrases in which only one word contains the target sound. As the client produces a target sound in a single word, the clinician might wish to add a second word in the phrase that contains the target sound.

5. *Sentences.* An extension of phrase-level productions is sentence-level practice. Just as practice at other levels has involved sequencing of task complexity, this principle also holds at this level. Consideration should be given to factors such as phonetic context, syllable structure of words, and number of words in the sentence. The following sequence of sentence levels is suggested:

a. Simple short sentence with one instance of the target sound

b. Sentences of various lengths with one instance of the target sound

     c. Simple short sentences with two or more instances of the target sound

     d. Sentences of various lengths with two or more instances of the target sound

6. *Conversation.* The final step in production training involves using a target sound in everyday speech. At this point, the clinician is seeking to facilitate generalization of productions that have already proceeded through more structured production tasks. Initially, generalization situations are structured so that the client produces their sound correctly in situations in which the speech is monitored. Activities such as role-playing, talking about future plans, attempting to get information, interviewing, and oral reading can be used at this level. Following structured conversations, subsequent activities are more spontaneous and free and are sometimes characterized as off-guard type conversations. The intent is to provide activities to facilitate transfer that approximates real-life situations. Activities should include speaking situations in which the client focuses not on self-monitoring but on what they say.

    Telling about personal experiences, talking about topics that evoke strong feelings, and taking part in group discussions are used at this stage of instruction. Some clinicians include negative practice to help to stabilize a new response. In negative practice, a client deliberately produces a target sound incorrectly and then contrasts it to a correct production. Van Riper and Erickson (1996) stated that such deliberate productions of the error increased the rate of learning.

At this point, the clinician also seeks to facilitate the carryover of conversation to situations beyond the therapy environment. It is suggested that such situational generalization be encouraged once the client can produce a target sound at the word level. By encouraging transfer in earlier stages of instruction, it is assumed that generalization beyond the word level will be significantly enhanced and will perhaps decrease the amount of time needed at the phrase, sentence, and conversational levels.

Summary of the Traditional Approach

Background Statement. The underlying assumptions of the traditional approach to remediation include the following: 1) Faulty perception of speech sounds may be a factor in speech sound errors and 2) speech sound errors are viewed as an inadequate or incomplete learning of the motor production of the sounds. Thus, the traditional approach relies heavily on motor production practice combined with activities related to perceptual training.

Unique Features. Until the 1980s, the traditional approach to speech sound remediation constituted the basic methodology employed by most clinicians for instruction and treatment of speech sound errors and is still widely used today (see Brumbaugh & Smit, 2013). The traditional method focuses on motor learning of individual speech sounds and provides a complete instructional sequence for correcting articulatory errors. It can be modified to fit the needs of clients of all ages. Perceptual training is recommended as a precursor to or an accompaniment of direct work on sounds when perceptual difficulty is identified.

Strengths and Limitations. This approach has been widely used over time and forms the basis of several current treatment approaches. Its widespread usage is likely related to the logical sequence of training tasks, the success that accrues through motor practice, and the adaptability and applicability of the approach. The value of perceptual training has been questioned and studied with the suggestion that it not be required as a routine procedure. There is, however, some evidence for its use when there is a documented perceptual problem.

In addition, the traditional approach may not be the most efficient approach for clients with multiple errors, including those whose errors are linguistic rather than motor based (recall the study by Klein [1996] that was mentioned previously, in which children with multiple speech sound errors who received a traditional approach spent more time in therapy and were less likely to be dismissed with normal speech than were children who received a more linguistically based approach).

Research Support. The traditional approach has stood the test of time and continues to be widely used because it has worked for many clinicians with many clients. A review by Preston and Leece (2021) identified at least 63 studies (most peer-reviewed) supporting its effectiveness. Another five studies have suggested that other approaches may be more effective. By way of specific examples, an evidence level IIa study by Helmick (1976) compared 26 second-grade children receiving traditional articulation therapy to 23 second grade children receiving no treatment. Prior to treatment the two groups produced similar numbers of errors (averaging 7.46 and 7.26 sounds in error, respectively). After one school year the no treatment group averaged 5.3 sounds in error, whereas the treatment group produced a significantly lower average of 0.86 sounds in error.

Two randomized controlled trials (evidence level Ib) also illustrated the effectiveness of this approach. Note that in both cases, prerecorded stimuli were used for perceptual training rather than live voice presentations. Rvachew (1994) used concurrent perceptual training and traditional therapy with three groups of children. Groups 1 and 2 (with 10 and 9 children, respectively) did discrimination tasks with minimal pairs (either correct vs. distorted versions of /ʃ/ in *shoe* or correct vs. another phoneme—*shoe* vs. *moo*), whereas Group 3 (with 8 children) did discrimination tasks with a nonminimal word pair (*shoe* vs. *Pete*). Across 8 weeks of therapy, Group 3 made on average no gains on either production or perception of /ʃ/, whereas Groups 1 and 2 made significant improvement on both production and perception. None of the children had been stimulable for /ʃ/ at the beginning of the study.

Another level Ib study by Wolfe and colleagues (2003) compared traditional therapy with concurrent perceptual training (four children) to traditional therapy without perceptual training (five children). Treatment targets were specific to each child. All targets were stimulable prior to treatment. Overall, after an average of 11 treatment sessions, both groups made similar amounts of improvement in production skill. There was also no difference between the groups for progress on target sounds that had been well perceived correctly prior to therapy. However, the children who received the concurrent perceptual training achieved significantly better production outcomes on those target sounds that were not well perceived prior to therapy. This latter finding also supports the notion that the addition of perceptual training is appropriate only for those targets wherein the child is also having difficulty with perception.

Modifications to the Traditional Approach

Although it remains the most frequently used approach to remediating SSDs, the traditional approach has long been criticized as being somewhat inefficient. In recent years, several attempts have been proposed to remedy that. These are discussed next.

Speech Motor Chaining

Background Statement.   The principles of motor learning and the challenge point framework discussed earlier were intended to make traditional therapy more efficient (i.e., they optimize practice and feedback, as well as provide clear guidance for when to progress to the next step in treatment). However, for many clinicians they may only serve to make therapy more complicated. To try to reduce the practical burden, Jonathan Preston and his colleagues introduced a highly structured approach to treatment called *speech motor chaining (SMC)*. This approach is described in a tutorial (see Preston et al., 2019) as appropriate for both older children with persistent or residual speech sound errors as well as for those with CAS (see Chapter 12). A free version of the Preston and colleagues (2019) tutorial is available at https://osf.io/5jmf9/. That same site includes a fillable online form so that the stimuli and feedback can be customized to each child. Also included is a video tutorial for using the form and the approach.

Unique Features.   In brief, SMC aims to teach the child to generate complex speech by combining core movements with principles of motor learning. Feedback, variability, and complexity of the stimuli are varied systematically. During pre-practice the child is taught to produce the target sound in isolation and then in sound sequences (CV, VC, CCV). Thus, different word positions and both consonant singletons and clusters can all be targeted. Practice then begins at the syllable level. Complexity is slowly built up via a chain, which is a concept that appears to have been first introduced by Chappell (1973). A chain is a series of five steps, each consisting of progressively longer stimuli with the target sequence embedded within it. By doing this, SMC adds efficiency to traditional therapy by compressing much of the therapy hierarchy into a much shorter period. Some examples of chains might include:

/gʌ/ – gum – gumball – small gumball – [self-generated: "I can see the small gumball."]

/ɪs/ - miss – missing – missing link – [self-generated: "They found the missing link."]

/sti/ - steam – steaming – steaming bowl – [self-generated: "He ate a steaming bowl of soup."]

Each step in the chain is attempted six times. If the child is correct on five or six of the trials (i.e., is at least 80% correct), they move up to the next step in the chain. If fewer trials are correct, they attempt that step again. Changes in rate of production (faster or slower), loudness (softer or louder), or intonation (say it as question vs. as a statement) are introduced randomly. As they progress up the chain, less and less feedback is provided. As one chain is completed another is introduced to slowly expand the different contexts being practiced and encourage generalization.

Strengths and Limitations.   This approach offers a high level of structure and potentially allows for more rapid progression through the therapy sequence. It incorporates principles of motor learning as well as generalization from the beginning. Although it may appear somewhat complicated to keep track of all of the components, the scoring form provided at https://osf.io/5jmf9/ provides a structure to make SMC more manageable.

Research Support.   It was suggested that SMC is appropriate for both children with CAS and those with residual and persistent errors. Relative to CAS, several studies have been conducted. All involved older children and adolescents, and in each case SMC was used in combination with ultrasound feedback (to be discussed in

Chapter 12). In each study treatment sessions began with 8–10 minutes of auditory perceptual training using the SAILS program (Rvachew & Herbay, 2017). This was followed by treatment blocks of 10–13 minutes each alternating between ultrasound biofeedback and SMC training.

In the first study, Preston and colleagues (2016) treated three males aged 10–14 years using a level IIb design. Two participants were producing derhotacized versions of /r/, whereas the other was producing lateralized sibilants. Each received 16 hours of intervention (10 sessions) over a 2-week period. Findings were mixed. One participant showed improvement on /r/ accuracy and maintained most of the gains at post-testing. The second participant made little to no gain on /r/. The third participant showed gains on sibilant productions within the treatment sessions but did not retain the gains at post-testing.

A second study by Preston, Maas, and colleagues (2016) used a multiple baseline across behaviors design (level IIa evidence) with three males aged 10–13 years who were all producing derhotacized /r/. Both initial and final /r/ were targeted directly for each child. Each received 14 hours of treatment over a 2-week period. Two of the three participants increased /r/ accuracy within the treatment sessions but no generalization to untreated words was observed for any of the participants.

The third study by Preston, Leece, McNamara, and Maas (2017) was intended to examine the value of the prosodic variations used in SMC. In this case there were six participants (four males, two females) aged 8;2 to 16;8. It involved an alternating treatments design (level IIa evidence) with each participant receiving 14, 1-hour treatment sessions. The focus of treatment was on /r/ for five participants and both /s/ and /r/ for the other participant. One target in one word position was treated using variations in prosody in half the session, whereas the other word position (or the other target sound) was treated without prosodic variations in the other half of the session. Change was observed for all participants, though only two of six participants achieved at least 70% correct on generalization probes on any target. Overall, greater change was observed with the prosodic variations (mean change 38.1%) than without (mean change 31.0%).

Relative to children with persistent and residual speech sound errors, at least two studies have been published that indicate the effectiveness of SMC. As with the studies of CAS, both involved its use in combination with ultrasound feedback One study by Sjolie and colleagues (2016) involved four children aged 7–9 years who were treated for /r/ errors. A randomized block design (level Ib evidence) was used in which half the sessions included ultrasound feedback and half did not. The two treatments were randomly alternated every session. Each participant received a total of 14 1-hour treatment sessions. Two participants showed no improvement in accuracy of treated targets. For the other two participants, change began as soon as treatment was initiated and accuracy improved from 0% to approximately 50% correct in both cases. For one participant, greater progress was achieved with ultrasound, but there was no difference for the other participant.

A final study by Preston and colleagues (2017) included 12 children aged 10–16 years with /r/ errors. A single case multiple baseline design repeated across participants was used (level IIa evidence). All received 7 hours of treatment with ultrasound feedback and 7 hours of treatment without ultrasound feedback. Half received the ultrasound feedback first and half received it second. The phonetic context for /r/ differed in the two treatment conditions. Overall, there was an average improvement of about 30% on untreated target words. The two conditions yielded similar levels of improvement (defined as <15% difference in improvement between the conditions) for five participants. The addition of ultrasound resulted in greater improvement for four participants but less improvement for three participants. Together, findings from these two studies suggest that for some individuals SMC can be used to successfully remediate /r/. Further study is indicated. They also suggest that SMC can be effective for children with residual or persistent speech errors.

Two tentative conclusions may be drawn from these studies. First, considering the relatively small amount of treatment provided, the findings suggest that when used in combination with ultrasound feedback SMC can lead to improvement in speech sound production in at least some children with CAS, as well as some children with persistent and residual speech errors. Larger treatment doses (i.e., longer treatment periods) are likely required to ensure more substantial and sustained improvement. The inclusion of prosodic variations appears to be of value in bringing about the change. Findings from the last two studies in particular lead to a second tentative conclusion. Both studies showed some gains during periods when only SMC was used. This suggests that SMC may be a viable intervention approach by itself (i.e., without any ultrasound feedback). This is of considerable importance given the cost barriers currently associated with ultrasound feedback. Further study is clearly needed.

Concurrent Treatment

The second modification to traditional therapy involves a radical approach to the therapy hierarchy itself.

Background Statement.   Traditional articulation therapy follows a predictable bottom-up order of treatment. The sound is taught successively in isolation, syllables, words, phrases, sentences, and finally in conversation. Intuitively, the bottom-up approach makes sense, as it slowly builds from simpler to more complex tasks. And as discussed previously, there is certainly evidence that it can be effective. One modification to traditional therapy that was developed by Steven Skelton (2004) challenges the assumption that only this treatment order can be effective.

Unique Features.   As with traditional therapy, Skelton's *concurrent treatment* begins with establishment of the sound using any of the available elicitation procedures. However, the rest of the therapy sequence is then completely randomized. Each target sound is taught in a different random order. An example of a randomized treatment sequence for /k/ is shown in Table 10.2. For reference, the numbers in the left-hand column reflect the order of the steps as they would have occurred in the traditional sequence.

To apply this approach, a single trial of each step is presented to the child. If it is produced correctly, the next step is presented. If the attempt is incorrect, a second trial is presented. Regardless of success on the second attempt the next step is presented. If the end of the sequence is reached before the session ends, treatment begins again at the start of the sequence. During his 2004 study using this approach, Skelton (personal communication, 2020) determined that across the four participants in each 30-minute session the list of tasks was completed an average of 1.65 times.

Strengths and Limitations.   An obvious strength of this approach is that by randomizing the therapy sequence, generalization is built in from the very beginning.

Table 10.2. Example of randomized treatment order for concurrent treatment of /k/

Number[a]	Task
17	Evoked initial /k/ singleton in 2- to 4-word phrases
25	Evoked initial /k/ singleton in single sentences
14	Imitation of initial /k/ cluster in 2- to 4-word phrases
10	Evoked initial /k/ cluster in single words
5	Imitation of initial /k/ singleton in single words
21	Imitation of initial /k/ singleton in single sentences
13	Imitation of initial /k/ singleton in 2- to 4-word phrases
12	Evoked intervocalic /k/in single words
29	Evoked /k/ in any position in conversation
6	Imitation of initial /k/ cluster in single words
27	Evoked final /k/ singleton in single sentences
15	Imitation of final /k/ singleton in 2- to 4-word phrases
7	Imitation of final /k/ singleton in single words
11	Evoked final /k/ singleton in single words
24	Imitation of intervocalic /k/ in single sentences
18	Evoked initial /k/ cluster in 2- to 4-word phrases
23	Imitation of final /k/ singleton in single sentences
16	Imitation of intervocalic /k/ in 2- to 4-word phrases
9	Evoked initial /k/ singleton in single words
8	Imitation of intervocalic /k/ in single words
19	Evoked final /k/ singleton in 2- to 4-word phrases
22	Imitation of initial /k/ cluster in single sentences
1	Imitation of initial /k/ singleton in single syllables
3	Imitation of final /k/ singleton in single syllables
28	Evoked intervocalic /k/in single sentences
2	Imitation of initial /k/ cluster in single syllables
26	Evoked initial /k/ cluster in single sentences
4	Imitation of final /k/ cluster in single syllables
20	Evoked intervocalic /k/ in 2- to 4-word phrases

[a] Values represent placement in order that would be used in traditional articulation therapy.
Source: Skelton (2004).

The format also provides the child with considerable practice at generating a variety of motor plans for speech. Thus, it also teaches complex motor planning from the beginning.

As for limitations, the rapid switching of task demands that this approach requires may be very confusing for some younger children or for those with comorbid cognitive or language impairments. As well, although the available evidence suggests that the randomized order can work, it is not clear if it is actually more efficient than the traditional order. One study (Skelton & Price, 2006) involved a direct comparison with the traditional therapy sequence. It was not, however, a fully peer-reviewed study (i.e., it was presented at a professional conference). Although findings suggested that the randomized order was superior, generalization of those findings is difficult, as it only included two participants.

Research Support.   Evidence supporting the efficacy of this approach is beginning to accumulate. Skelton (2004) used a multiple baseline across participants design (level IIa evidence) involving four children aged 7 years who were producing /s/ distortions. For each participant, change only started once treatment began and, in each case, quickly improved from 0% to 90%+ correct. Two of the four participants generalized to over 80% correct in conversation in post-treatment probes. Skelton and Funk (2004) used the approach with three children aged 4–6 years with multiple errors. One child was treated for /k/ and two for /s/. Using an AB design repeated across the participants (level IIb evidence), the children improved from 0% to 30%–50% correct in conversation after five to eight sessions of treatment.

The highest level evidence available for concurrent treatment was from a randomized controlled trial (level Ib) by Skelton and Richard (2016). It included 28 6–9 year olds with errors on one to three speech sounds. Sixteen children were randomly assigned to the treatment group, whereas the remaining 12 were placed in a delayed treatment control group (who received treatment later). Treatment was provided in groups of four children. Targets included /k, r, s, z, ʃ/. After 20 weeks the treatment group improved their target sound accuracy on untreated words by an average of 61%. The control (untreated) group only improved by an average of 26% during that same period.

Systematic Articulation Training Program Accessing Computers

A third modification to the traditional approach involves modification to the stimuli that are used to establish the target.

Background Statement.   Systematic Articulation Training Program Accessing Computers (SATPAC) is a context utilization approach developed by Sacks and Shine (2004). It makes use of the traditional therapy sequence. Correct production of the target sound in SATPAC can be elicited using any one of the procedures discussed previously or in Appendix A, although the starting point is always a CV or VC context. Some additional elicitation procedures have also been developed by its primary creator (Stephen Sacks). A procedure for /s/ is described in Sacks and associates (2013), and a procedure for /r/ is described in Flipsen and Sacks (2015).

Unique Features.   Perhaps the most unique feature of SATPAC is its use of nonwords (also called nonsense words) to establish the target sounds. Nonwords are sound sequences that follow the phonotactic rules of English but have no meaning. Many clinicians use simple CV or CVC versions of these as an intermediate or transitional step between the isolation level and the real-word level. SATPAC uses complex two-syllable forms (e.g. /bitsik/, which is a CVCCVC). In addition, these nonwords are specifically structured to take advantage of coarticulation and facilitating contexts. Perhaps most important is that the use of the nonwords is extended up to the sentence level to establish and automatize new motor habits. Real words containing the target sound are introduced at that point.

Another unique feature of SATPAC is that output rate is monitored with practice beginning at slightly slower than normal rate. As treatment progresses, rate is slowly increased to normal rate. Normal prosody is infused using contrastive stress activities at the sentence level. Finally, to ensure development of the required motor skills, extensive drill is utilized.

As the name implies, the approach is managed via computer software, which generates the stimuli to help the clinician stay on track. If the child has other speech errors beyond the target sound, those can be entered into the software so they can be eliminated from the stimuli to avoid reinforcing error sounds. Sounds that potentially could interfere with the target (e.g., /θ/ when working on dentalized /s/) are also eliminated. Additional details regarding the approach and the software can be obtained at https://satpac.com/.

Strengths and Limitations. SATPAC offers a high level of structure to keep therapy focused and moving forward. Its use of nonwords avoids the practice of over-learned bad habits; the use of facilitating contexts helps ensure a high level of success. The software can also be used to prevent reinforcing other errors. Generalization to normal conversational speech is built in with its emphasis on normal rate and natural prosody. One limitation for some clinicians or clients may be its focus on drill, which some children may resist. Another potential limitation for some settings may be cost of the computer software.

Research Support. Two peer-reviewed studies supporting the efficacy of SATPAC have been published. The study by Sacks and colleagues (2013) involved a delayed treatment control design using 18 children aged 6–11 years with errors on /s/. It was a quasi-randomized controlled trial (level IIa evidence) with nine children at one school receiving treatment while a second group at another school served as a delayed treatment control group. After 15 weeks of treatment (once per week for 10 minutes) the groups were reversed. Change largely happened only when treatment was applied. Group 1 improved from 0% to 77% correct in conversation by the end of their treatment period and averaged 59% correct 2 years later. Group 2 showed minimal change while waiting for treatment and then improved from 11% to 74% correct in conversation by the end of their treatment period. They averaged 82% correct 2 years later. The other study (Flipsen & Sacks, 2015) was a single case (level III evidence) of a 12-year-old boy who had previously been discharged from therapy without remediating his /r/ errors. He received seven 30-minute SATPAC treatment sessions and improved from 0% correct in conversation at baseline to 90% correct at a 6-month follow-up evaluation.

Context Utilization Approaches

As mentioned in the previous discussion on establishment, certain phonetic contexts appear to facilitate the correct production of some sounds. Some investigators (Hoffman et al., 1989; McDonald, 1964a) have advocated for extending this idea into other stages of therapy. McDonald suggested that instruction for articulatory errors be initiated in a context(s) in which the error sound can be produced correctly. He provided an example of a child with an /s/ distortion who produced [s] correctly in the context of *watchsun*. He suggested the following sequence of instructions after *watchsun* was identified as a context when /s/ was correctly produced: 1) say *watchsun* with slow-motion speed; 2) say *watchsun* with equal stress on both syllables, then with primary stress on the first syllable, and then with primary stress on the second syllable; 3) say *watchs* and prolong [s] until a signal is given to complete the bisyllable with [ʌn]; and

4) say short sentences with the same facilitating context, such as "Watch, sun will burn you." The sequence is repeated with other sentences and stress patterns. The meaningfulness of the sentence is not important because the primary focus of the activity is the movement sequences.

Following these steps, the client is instructed to alter the movement patterns associated with the correct /s/ by changing the vowel following the segment in a suggested sequence, such as:

watch – sun	*watch – sat*
watch – sea	*watch – soon*
watch – sit	*watch – sew*
watch – send	*watch – saw*

The next step is to practice words that include a second context using words such as *teach, reach, pitch, catch,* and *beach,* that would be used in combination with one-syllable words beginning with /s/ and followed by a variety of vowels (such as *sand, sun, said, soon*). Various sound combinations are practiced with different rates and stress patterns and should eventually be practiced in sentence contexts.

Hoffman and colleagues (1989) described another variation of the contextual approach that involves a sequenced set of production-based training tasks designed to facilitate the automatization of articulator performance. The basic assumption behind their suggestions is that "revision of over learned, highly automatic behavior is possible through carefully planned and executed performance rehearsal" (p. 248). Intervention is seen as involving instruction and practice of motor articulatory adjustments to replace previously learned (incorrect) productions. The following paragraphs present the sequence of tasks and instructional activities these authors suggest.

Prior to working directly on error targets, the clinician elicits, via imitation, sound segments that the client can produce correctly. Such stimulability tasks provide the client with an opportunity to experience success in a speech task, as well as the opportunity to observe and imitate the clinician's productions. It is suggested that the clinician not only model the correct form of sounds in the child's repertoire, but also distort such productions through excessive movements (e.g., lip rounding for /m, p, f/) for the purpose of giving the client the opportunity to practice manipulation of the articulators in response to the clinician's model. It is hoped that such activity will facilitate the client's skill at identifying, comparing, and discriminating the clinician's and their own sound productions.

Following practice on stimulability tasks, the client needs to learn the articulatory adjustments necessary for correct target sound production. It is suggested that the clinician be able to repeat sentences using error productions similar to those of the client in order to be aware of the motoric acts involved in the client's misarticulations. The emphasis at this point is on doing interesting things with the speech mechanism (e.g., view their productions in the mirror or listen to recordings of themself).

Production practice (or rehearsal) then progresses through four levels of complexity: nonsymbolic units or nonsense syllables, words and word pairs, rehearsal sentences, and narratives. Once the narrative level has been reached, the four levels can be practiced randomly. Each of the rehearsal levels is discussed next.

Practice with nonsense syllables provides practice with articulatory gestures that were begun during pretraining. Nonsymbolic instruction focuses on target productions in VC, CV, VCV, and VCCV syllables. It is asserted that production of nonsymbolic units imposes minimal constraints on the speaker by allowing them to focus on the speech task rather than morphology, syntax, and semantics. The emphasis on nonsense words is also supported by findings from Gierut and associates (2010), who reported greater and more rapid generalization with practice on nonsense words compared to real words.

Word and word-pair practice is the next step in the program. Initial targets should reflect a transition from nonsymbolic units to meaningful units that encompass the nonsymbolic syllables already practiced. Practice activities at this level are designed to encourage the client to assume responsibility for recognizing and judging the adequacy of their performance. Table 10.3 reflects a list of words and word pairs by word position that might be used at this level.

The next step in the program involves rehearsal sentences. At this stage, the client repeats the clinician's model of sentences that include words practiced at the word level followed by practice on a word containing the target segment and then embedding it in a spontaneously generated sentence. For example, using key words from Table 10.3, sentences such as the following could be practiced:

> Jerry was very sad today.
>
> The sky was very cloudy on Tuesday.
>
> Toss me the red ball.
>
> Bison is another word for buffalo.
>
> Don't drink all the juice.
>
> His niece came to visit.

The final step in this program involves using a target sound in narratives that can be illustrated, acted out, or read. A series of clinician-generated narratives are employed; for example, for a preschool client, "This is Poky the turtle. Today is his birthday. He is 6 years old. He says, 'It's my birthday.' What does he say?" This is followed by the client saying, "It's my birthday." Through such narratives, practice of the target sound is embedded in communicative tasks. The clinician may have a client practice individual sentences from these narratives for additional practice at the sentence level.

Table 10.3. Word and word pair list for [s]

Prevocalic		Intervocalic		Postvocalic
Initial	Cluster	Medial	Final	Word pair
sad	scat	passing	pass	Jack sat
seed	ski	receive	niece	jeep seat
soup	scooter	loosen	juice	room soon
saw	scar	bossy	toss	cop saw
sit	skit	kissing	miss	lip sip
sign	sky	bison	mice	right side

Although this program has been presented as a series of steps or levels, the authors point out that these steps frequently overlap. Throughout the program, the client is the primary judge of adequacy of productions, describing the movement patterns and articulatory contacts.

The previously discussed SATPAC approach is another variation on the context utilization approach. As noted, it uses both facilitating contexts and systematic progression through the treatment continuum. The SATPAC approach also puts a heavy emphasis on the use of nonsense words as a means to overcome strongly ingrained error habits.

Summary of Contextually Based Approaches

Background Statement.   The theoretical concept underlying contextual approaches is that articulatory (i.e., motor-based) errors can be corrected by motor practice of articulatory behaviors, with syllabic units as a basic building block for later motor practice at more complex levels. To employ this approach, a sound must be in the client's repertoire.

Unique Features.   The emphasis on imitated, repetitive productions is a unique aspect of this approach. The systematic variation of phonetic contexts in productions of both sounds produced correctly and error sounds targeted for remediation sets this approach apart from others. A major value of context testing is to identify contexts that may be useful in different therapy approaches.

Strengths and Limitations.   A major strength of this approach is that it builds on behaviors (segmental productions in particular phonetic contexts) that are in a client's repertoire and capitalizes on syllables plus auditory, tactile, and kinesthetic awareness of motor movements. It may be particularly useful for clients who use a sound inconsistently and need methodology to facilitate consistent production in other contexts. The concept of syllable practice and systematic variation of phonetic contexts and stress may be useful to any training method that includes syllable productions. An often-cited limitation of this approach is the difficulty in motivating many children to engage in the extensive imitation and drill that this approach uses.

Research Support.   See also the previous discussion of research support for SATPAC. Contextual testing designed to locate facilitating contexts can be used to identify correct contexts with clients who are not stimulable in their attempts to produce the target. Published clinical investigations that provide support for the efficacy of using a context facilitation approach to intervention are available, although most are of a relatively low level. One report by Stringfellow and McLeod (1991) involved a case study (evidence level III) in which a facilitating context was used successfully to teach a child to produce distinctive versions of /l/ and /j/. Dunn and Barron (1982) also reported moderate improvement in another case study (level III) when word-final /z/ was targeted. One phase of their mixed approach (i.e., it was not purely a context utilization approach) involved the use of two-word sequences for which the context was systematically modified by changing the word immediately following the target.

Masterson and Daniels (1991) reported a case study (level III evidence) of a child aged 3;8 who exhibited both dentalized distortions of sibilants and /w/ for /r/ substitutions. Three semesters of therapy using a linguistically based approach resulted in complete correction of the /r/ errors. The sibilant errors were corrected in therapy sessions but did not generalize to conversational speech. Within 1 month of introducing the Hoffman and colleagues (1989) context-based approach described previously, generalization of correct production of the sibilants occurred and was maintained at the 100% correct level at a 3-month follow-up visit.

Summary of Motor Approaches to Remediation

The treatment approaches described previously focus on the development and habituation of the motor skills necessary for target sound productions. An underlying assumption is that motor practice leads to generalization of correct productions to untrained contexts and to automatization of behaviors. Motor approaches to remediation are especially appropriate for phonetically (motor) based errors but are frequently employed in combination with procedures described in Chapter 11 under linguistically based approaches and/or alternate feedback approaches described in Chapter 12.

Remediation Guidelines for Motor Approaches

1. A motor approach to remediation is recommended as a teaching procedure for clients who evidence motor production problems. One group of individuals who frequently are candidates for motor approaches includes those with persistent (residual) errors. This subpopulation will be discussed further in Chapter 12.

2. A motor approach can also be incorporated into treatment programs for clients reflecting linguistically based errors. Instruction should be initiated at the highest linguistic unit level (isolation, syllable, word) at which a client can produce target sounds.

3. Perceptual training for those clients who evidence perceptual problems related to their error sounds is recommended as part of a motor remediation program.

REMEDIATION OF VOWELS

Historically, most speech sound intervention in English has focused on consonants. This appears to reflect both a long-standing emphasis on working with school-age children and adults, as well as the fact that most typically developing children have mastered most vowels by age 3 years (see Chapter 3). The net result has been that other than errors on the rhotic vowels (i.e., /ɝ, ɚ/), most clinicians pay scant attention to vowel targets. Another reason for the neglect of vowels may be from the fact that differences among English dialects are reflected mostly in vowel differences; this may lead some clinicians to ignore vowel differences on the assumption that they do not reflect disorders. Finally, it has been suggested that in our preoccupation with consonant errors, which are clearly more common, vowels have simply been forgotten (Hargrove, 1982).

The publication of at least two books on vowel disorders (Ball & Gibbon, 2002, 2013) has refocused attention on vowels. This refocus has reminded us that at least four different clinical populations are likely to present with difficulty with vowels. These include 1) the birth–3 population, 2) second-language learners (see Chapter 14),

3) individuals with significant hearing impairment (Ertmer et al., 1996; Levitt & Stromberg, 1983), and 4) individuals with CAS (Jacks et al. 2013). Beyond these specific populations, our failure to attend to vowels may also mean that vowel errors are more common than once thought (Hargrove, 1982; Pollock, 2002).

Gibbon (2013) has suggested that targeting vowel errors (where present) may provide significant therapeutic benefits. For example, it may improve overall message intelligibility, improve speech acceptability (i.e., make it sound more similar to the intended dialect), potentially accelerate therapy progress, and make the child's overall speech system more consistent with the normal developmental pattern (i.e., given that vowels are typically mastered before consonants). Assessment of vowels was outlined in Chapter 6.

Treatment Approaches for Vowels

Baldwin and colleagues (2018) have suggested that vowel errors may reflect a variety of underlying conditions, including delayed language learning, structural anomalies, and motor impairments. Further, in some cases, perceptual problems cannot be ruled out (Kent & Rountrey, 2020). Thus, any number of intervention approaches (perceptual, motor, or linguistic in nature) may be appropriate and effective.

Several of the therapy approaches developed for consonants (discussed here and in Chapters 11 and 12) could be adapted for intervention for vowels (Gibbon, 2013). Relative to establishment, Secord and associates (2007) provide a series of suggestions for teaching vowels that use general procedures that are very similar to those used for consonants (i.e., phonetic placement, successive approximation, etc.). Beyond the individual sound level, findings from several case studies provide some support for the idea that the frameworks used for consonants may be equally effective for vowels. Hargrove and colleagues (1989), for example, presented findings from treatment of a pair of twin boys age 4;2 who both presented with abnormal prolongations of vowels and final consonants. Intervention involved a traditional therapy sequence with both imitation and spontaneous production tasks at each linguistic level and the provision of both visual and auditory cues as needed. After approximately 8 months of therapy, they reported a reduction in the proportion of words in spontaneous conversation containing prolongations from approximately 40% to 1%–2%.

Another case study by Gibbon and colleagues (1992) involved a boy age 4;0 who (in addition to numerous consonant errors) lacked any diphthongs in his vowel system and failed to produce consistent contrasts among many mid and high vowels. Intervention for vowels included six weekly sessions and focused on the missing diphthongs using a combination of perceptual, motor, and linguistic tasks. Eight months later the child's vowel system was largely complete, including all of the targeted diphthongs.

Pollock (1994) presented findings from a case study of a boy age 4;9 who presented with an overall percentage vowels correct (PVC) of 41% and only two vowels consistently correct. Four vowels/diphthongs were 33%–67% correct, and another nine were never correct. Two vowels and two diphthongs were targeted, and intervention occurred three times per week for two academic semesters. Procedures used included both auditory and visual cues with drill and drill-play activities. "Minimal pair contrasts were used whenever possible to facilitate the concept of a contrast between correct and error productions" (p. 34). After 9 months of therapy, his PVC improved to 54% and four vowels and two diphthongs were at least 80% accurate. Although limited in size and scope (and representing relatively low-level evidence) the findings from these studies suggest that intervention for vowels can be successful.

Summary

Vowels and potential vowel disorders have received limited attention, although there appears to be a greater need to assess vowel errors than has previously been thought. The field's understanding of both the acquisition and remediation for vowels remains limited. Approaches and techniques typically applied to consonants may offer a useful treatment starting point. Clearly, additional study is needed.

THE USE OF NONSPEECH ORAL-MOTOR ACTIVITIES

Some clinicians continue to use nonspeech oral-motor training (NSOMT) as a precursor to teaching sounds or to supplement speech sound instruction (Lof & Watson, 2008), although a recent survey by Brumbaugh and Smit (2013) suggested that the use of such procedures may be declining. These activities include horn or whistle blowing, sucking through straws, and tongue wagging for which no speech sounds are produced. These may also be what Scripture and Jackson (1927) referred to as mouth gymnastics. Such exercises differ from any activity that includes the production of speech sounds (even if just a single phoneme), which would be better described as speech motor training.

Despite their use, NSOMT activities have long been questioned. Until recently, the case against them was largely made philosophically (i.e., using indirect logic rather than direct evidence). Forrest (2002) argued in a rebuttal that addressed the four justifications that clinicians have historically used in support of NSOMT activities in therapy:

Justification	Rebuttal
1. They simplify the task.	Forrest pointed out that evidence from studies of complex motor skills other than speech suggests that mastery of such skills requires performance of the entire task rather than what are perceived as the individual components of the task. Brief discussion of components used in speaking for production of an individual sound may be helpful, but extensive practice of individual components is not sufficient to learn the overall skill.
2. They strengthen the articulators.	Forrest noted that a) most of the nonspeech oral-motor activities used are not practiced with sufficient frequency or against enough resistance to actually enhance strength and b) studies indicate that we usually need only 15%–20% of our strength capacity for speech. Recall also the discussion in Chapter 4 which indicated that, as a group, children with SSDs do not appear to differ significantly from their typically developing peers in terms of tongue strength.

3. They enhance the sensi-   Forrest noted (as we did in Chapter 4) that there is
    tivity of the articulators.   no clear relationship between oral-motor sensitiv-
                                  ity and SSDs.

4. They replicate normal   Although it seems counterintuitive, Forrest cited
    development.   considerable evidence that suggests that speech
                                  does not normally develop from nonspeech behav-
                                  iors; the latter just happen to emerge earlier in
                                  development. Nonspeech activities such as suck-
                                  ing, blowing, chewing, and swallowing are quite
                                  different from speech in terms of the types of move-
                                  ments, level of muscle activity, and coordination
                                  among the muscles. This is true even in very young
                                  children in whom speech is just emerging (Moore
                                  & Ruark, 1996; Ruark & Moore 1997). Put another
                                  way, speech and nonspeech activities may share
                                  structure, but they differ greatly in how those struc-
                                  tures are used, and they appear to develop indepen-
                                  dently.

Direct evidence regarding the value of NSOMT activities has begun to accumulate. Lass and Pannbacker (2008) identified 11 studies that examined speech outcomes
following nonspeech oral-motor treatments. Only 2 of the 11 studies showed significant change that could be attributed to the use of nonspeech oral-motor activities. One
of these (Fields & Polmanteer, 2002) was a level Ib study that has been criticized on
methodological grounds (e.g., inappropriate statistical analysis) and has never been
published in a peer-reviewed journal. The other was a level III study by A. McAllister (2003) that examined only voice quality and did not report outcomes for speech
sounds.

Additional evidence can be found in a level Ib study by Forrest and Iuzzini (2008),
which used an alternating treatments design with nine children aged 3;3 to 6;3 (eight
males). Each participant received NSOMT for one speech sound and traditional articulation therapy for another sound. For 8/9 participants a third untreated sound served
as a control. About half of the children received NSOMT first whereas the rest received
traditional therapy first. Results indicated an average improvement of 30% for sounds
treated with traditional therapy versus 3% improvement for sounds treated with
NSOMT. The superior result for traditional therapy was obtained for 8/9 participants.

Taken together, these research findings point in the same direction as the review
by Lee and Gibbon (2015), who concluded that "currently no strong evidence suggests
that NSOMTs are an effective treatment or an effective adjunctive treatment for children with developmental speech sound disorders" (p. 2).

Although NSOMT may not be generally effective, some might suggest that they
are of value for treating specific subpopulations of children with SSDs. The limited
evidence to date does not appear to support this. A systematic review by Ruscello and
Vallino (2020), for example, concluded that NSOMT is of no value for improving velopharyngeal function or correcting compensatory articulation errors in children with
cleft palate.

In summary, the logical arguments and the research evidence point to the same
conclusion; they support the long-held dictum that "if you want to improve speech,

you should focus on speech." We recommend against the use of nonspeech oral-motor activities for speech sound intervention and treatment.

CASE STUDY REVISITED: MOTOR PERSPECTIVE

In Chapter 7, we discussed the speech samples obtained from Kirk (a pseudonym), with an analysis and interpretation of his test data. We now discuss how one might proceed in developing an intervention plan based on that interpretation. In this chapter, we take a motor-based perspective. In Chapter 11, we assume a linguistic perspective.

Intervention Recommendations

As you recall, Kirk is a 3-year-old child with multiple errors who needs intervention because of poor speech intelligibility. You might wish to review the case study report at the end of Chapter 7 at this time. As you move through the discussion that follows, bear in mind that the steps involved and the variables considered are applicable to many clients with speech sound impairments.

Kirk is stimulable for most error sounds, but there are exceptions: /ʃ/, /tʃ/, /θ/, /r/, and /ɝ/. Intervention for these exceptions could readily be seen as needing a motor-based approach. Likewise, some of the stimulable sounds were more easily imitated than others, so instruction must also include teaching or stabilization of the motor production of sounds that he does not consistently imitate on demand.

First Consideration: How Many Targets Should I Address in a Session?

As noted in Chapter 7, Kirk has multiple error sounds, suggesting that a focus on several targets is more appropriate either within a single lesson or across lessons within a 3- or 4-week time frame (cycles or horizontal approach). This could include targets in which a motor-based approach is appropriate, as well as targets in which a linguistically based approach makes more sense (i.e., those sounds that are readily stimulable).

Second Consideration: How Should I Conceptualize the Overall Treatment Program?

Because Kirk has so many sounds in error and some are not stabilized at an imitative level, it is suggested that the clinician begin a session by spending about 5 minutes engaged in what has been identified as sound stimulation/practice, an activity designed to enhance Kirk's stimulability for all error sounds. Kirk is young and still acquiring phonemes, so it seems advisable to provide him with the opportunity to produce a variety of sounds that are not produced correctly in his conversational speech. Sound stimulation can include practice not only on error sounds (e.g., /ɝ/, /s/) but also on sounds that he does say correctly (/p/, /h/, /f/). Successful production of such sounds might facilitate his willingness to try other sounds he has made in error.

Kirk should make five attempts to produce each sound target during sound stimulation, using a cueing hierarchy for those in error, based on the level of support necessary to produce a sound (e.g., modeling, phonetic placement, or selected contexts). After five attempts, another sound is practiced. With only five attempts, the client is not overwhelmed with repeated failures if they cannot produce a sound. It is hoped that by briefly focusing in each session on production of a variety of sounds and levels of complexity (i.e., isolation, syllables, words), a child will acquire the skill to imitate the sound when given an auditory and/or visual model. Production in this type of activity is a building block for focusing on phonological contrasts and for facilitating generalization when a child is stimulable. Following sound stimulation/production practice, the treatment program focuses on those errors for which more linguistically based interventions, such as one of the contrast approaches, are more applicable.

Third Consideration: How Do Instructional Goals Relate to the Treatment Continuum and Specific Instructional Steps?

The treatment continuum, including establishment, generalization, and maintenance—which provides the focus for much of what we do in therapy—was discussed earlier. In the case of Kirk, the /ɝ/ and other nonstimulable sounds require an establishment activity, such as the sound stimulation mentioned previously. His other error patterns (i.e., initial consonant deletion, stopping, final consonant deletion) fit into the generalization phase of the continuum because he is stimulable on many of the sounds required to eliminate these patterns. Earlier, we discussed that in each stage of the treatment, the continuum of therapy comprises a sequence of steps and activities that include antecedent events from the clinician, responses from the client, and consequent events from the clinician based on client responses. One of the initial planning tasks is to determine how one is going to sequence antecedent events (e.g., verbal instruction, pictures, printed symbols, game activity) and consequent events (e.g., verbal reinforcement, tokens, back-up reinforcers).

A more complete outline of the overall treatment plan for Kirk is presented at the end of Chapter 11.

QUESTIONS FOR CHAPTER 10

1. How would one assess auditory perception in a child who is suspected of having difficulty with sound contrasts?

2. Outline a traditional approach to articulation therapy and specify for whom it is appropriate.

3. Outline a shaping procedure for teaching /tʃ/.

4. Discuss how traditional articulation therapy might be modified to make it more efficient.

5. What is meant by nonspeech oral motor activities? Why are these often regarded as not worthwhile?

11

Linguistically Based Treatment Approaches

PETER FLIPSEN JR., NICHOLAS W. BANKSON, AND JOHN E. BERNTHAL

LEARNING OBJECTIVES

This chapter discusses linguistically based approaches to treating speech sound disorders (SSDs). By the end of this chapter, the reader should be able to:

- Describe the difference between motor-based and linguistically based approaches.
- Discuss three basic elements of linguistically based approaches.
- Distinguish among the terms minimal pair, near minimal pair, minimal contrast, minimal opposition, and maximal opposition.
- Outline the basic protocol for contrast training.
- Discuss how minimal pairs can differ based on articulatory versus distinctive features.
- Contrast a conventional minimal pairs approach with a complexity approach, and a multiple oppositions approach.
- Define the three underlying concepts of the complexity approach.
- List examples to illustrate a phoneme collapse.
- Outline the basic phases of a multiple oppositions approach.
- List and describe three unique features of the cycles phonological patterns approach (CPPA).
- Discuss different options for conducting amplified auditory stimulation.
- Discuss the two basic premises underlying broader-based language approaches.
- Outline the basic storytelling procedure for the whole-language approach.
- Define a recast and discuss how they are used in the naturalistic recast approach.

Now we turn our attention to the second broad category of treatment approaches for SSDs, linguistically or phonologically based instruction. Whereas the motor approaches discussed in Chapter 10 may be described as phonetically based and focus on teaching the motor aspects of speech sound production, linguistic approaches are focused more on the rules of the language, including sound contrasts and appropriate phonological patterns. Although a linguistically based approach is generally considered to be most suitable for a child with multiple speech sound errors, aspects of these approaches can and are used in combination with more traditional, or motor-based approaches, including instances where one or just a few sounds are in error.

As in Chapter 10, we provide Background Statement, Unique Features, Strengths and Limitations, and Research Support sections for each approach discussed. Also, as done in Chapter 10, the evidence will be framed based on the levels of evidence that the American Speech-Language-Hearing Association (ASHA) has adopted, as outlined in Chapter 8. The emphasis, once again, will be on the best available (i.e., peer-reviewed) evidence.

The primary focus of linguistic approaches to remediation is the establishment of the adult phonological system, including the inventory of phonemes (i.e., sounds used to contrast meaning), allophonic rules (i.e., use of different allophones in different contexts), and phonotactic rules (i.e., how sounds are combined to form syllables and words).

Treatment programs designed to facilitate acquisition of the phonological system are not associated with a single unified method, but they—for the most part—include three basic elements. First, the focus is on meaning (function/communication) rather than form. In other words, the goal is to demonstrate which speech sounds may be used within the language to signal a change in meaning. Although form or physical production of the sound may occasionally be taught (using one or more of the elicitation methods discussed previously), this will be the exception rather than the rule. As a consequence, the focus of treatment will be largely at the word level and higher.

A second element included in linguistically based programs is that selection of the target behaviors is usually based on patterns that are reflected in the child's sound errors. These patterns often extend across groups of sounds. Following identification of the patterns used by the child, individual sounds, called *exemplars,* are chosen that are likely to facilitate generalization from the exemplar to other sounds that share similar features within each particular error pattern. There is, therefore, an expectation of generalization of the features taught in the exemplars to other sounds that have similar or the same features. For example, in targeting final consonant deletion, teaching one or several final consonants is assumed to facilitate generalization to other final consonants that are also deleted. As a consequence, not all of the sounds affected by the pattern of errors would need to be treated individually.

The third element of linguistically based programs relates to the instructional procedures being used. In order to demonstrate that a change in the sound being produced results in a change in meaning, naturalistic contexts (or at least naturalistic consequences) are typically used. If the incorrect sound is produced, an incorrect consequence is the likely result. This can include the clinician simply repeating the child's error back to them with corrective feedback (e.g., "No, this is *key,* not *tea.*") or the clinician continuing to point to the wrong picture until the child changes what they say. It can also include games where the clinician responds to what the child actually says rather than what they likely intended. For example, if the child points to a picture of *tea* and says "please give me the *key,*" the clinician gives them the picture for *tea* instead. A story retell format might also be used where the clinician pretends to misunderstand when the wrong word is produced (e.g., Child: "The big bad wolf will blow the /haʊt/ down? Clinician: What's a /haʊt/?").

Broadly speaking, linguistically based programs can be characterized as either using contrasts or not, and are focused on accurate communication. Several examples of each of those categories will be discussed here.

CONTRAST APPROACHES

Similar to traditional motor-based therapy, most linguistically based approaches follow bottom-up logic. Because training in the physical production of the sound is not often required, they frequently begin at the word level and then progress up through the various levels of linguistic complexity. Instead of using words by themselves, however, most of these approaches employ pairs of words. The word pairs usually include examples of the adult target (e.g., *key* for word-initial /k/), along with something else that provides a comparison. The comparison or contrast between the two words provides the child with an opportunity to learn something about the sound system (i.e., that a difference in sounds results in a difference in meaning). This explains why these approaches are referred to as *contrast approaches*. In most, but not all cases, the contrast is made between the adult target and the child's error (e.g., *tea–key* for the child who substitutes /t/ for /k/).

The specific focus of contrast approaches is to replace error patterns with appropriate phonological patterns. The error patterns often result in production of homonyms (one word being mistakenly used for two or more referents; e.g., *shoe* used for both *chew* and *shoe*). The goal is to eliminate the homonyms by establishing new sounds or sound classes in the child's language (phonological) system.

In addition to introducing new sounds or sound classes, contrast approaches may also target error patterns that limit the syllable and word shapes that a child uses. As an example, consider a client who deletes final consonants. Such a client might produce stops correctly in word-initial position but delete them in word-final position (resulting in an open syllable, which is one that ends in a vowel). For example, the words *two* and *tooth* might both be produced as *two,* and the words *bee* and *beet* might both be produced as *bee.* Because the client is able to produce stops correctly in initial position, the motoric production of stops (and /b/ and /t/ in particular) is assumed to be within a client's productive repertoire and, thus, motor production of the sound is not the focus of instruction. Rather, it appears that the child has a conceptual problem (i.e., they assume that only open syllables are permitted). The emphasis in therapy would be on developing cognitive awareness of final consonant contrasts/syllable closure. Treatment would involve engaging the child with the contrasts (*two–tooth* and *bee–beet*) in ways that demonstrate the need for the syllable closure to convey the correct meaning.

The contrast approach, or what Gierut (1990) termed a *phonological oppositions* approach, is the signature form of linguistically based remediation. Its underlying basis is that the client learns that different sounds or different word shapes signal different meanings. Over the years, a number of investigators have reported changes in children's phonological systems (Elbert & Gierut, 1986; Gierut, 1989, 1990; Weiner, 1981b; A. L. Williams, 1991) following training with word-pair contrasts. It should be noted that although contrast therapy emerged from a linguistic orientation, it is occasionally used with motor-based approaches.

From the examples cited, it is obvious that contrast training is appropriate in cases of a substituted or deleted sound versus the target sound. For example, if a client substitutes /t/ for /k/ in word-initial position, contrast training words might include

---

BOX 11.1   Contrast Terminology

The following terms appear frequently in the literature related to linguistically based approaches to treating SSDs. In addition to the following discussion of *Different Kinds of Contrasts*, we offer the following definitions:

Minimal pair—two words that differ in meaning and only differ by a single sound. This may include pairs with the same number of sounds (e.g., *son–ton*); may also include pairs where one word contains an additional sound (e.g., *bow–boat* or *tick–stick*).

Near minimal pair—a combination of a word and a nonword (or invented word) that differ by a single sound (e.g., *hat–/gæt/*).

Minimal contrast—same as minimal pair.[a]

Minimal opposition—same as minimal pair.[a, b]

Maximal opposition—specific kind of minimal pair in which the sounds that differ do so by the highest possible number of features. For example, the pair *have–hatch* differ on /v/ and /tʃ/, which differ on place, manner, and voicing.

[a]Authors have used this as a specific kind of minimal pair in which the sounds that differ do so by the fewest possible number of features. For example, the pair bet–pet differ on /b/ and /p/, which only differ in terms of voicing.
[b]May be used as a point of comparison for maximal opposition.

---

tea–key and *top–cop*. Similarly, if a child deletes the final /t/, contrast pairs might include *bow–boat* and *see–seat*. However, such instruction would typically not be appropriate for distortion errors, as the contrast between a distorted sound and a non-distorted version of the same sound usually does not result in a change in meaning.

Contrast Training

In applying contrast approaches, instruction typically focuses first on perception and then on production. LaRiviere and colleagues (1974) proposed a training task that focused on perceptual training using contrast pairs. In this procedure, the child was taught to identify words where the target sounds and errors were presented in word pairs. For example, if a child deletes /s/ in /s/ clusters (cluster reduction), the clinician names several pictures representing minimal pair words, such as *spool–pool* or *spill–pill* to the client. As each item is named, the client is required to either pick each word image up or perhaps sort the images into one or two categories (/p/ singletons or /sp/ clusters). In the same way, if the child substitutes /t/ for /s/, the clinician would name pictures representing pairs such as *tea–see, toe–so,* and *tie–sigh.*

Although many linguistically based treatments employ such perception training, the majority of the focus is on production. A production-based contrast pair task requires the client to produce both words as recognizably different words. For example, a client who deletes final consonants might ask the clinician to give them the picture of either a *bee* or a *beet* and then be reinforced by the clinician for the appropriate production. In this task, the client must be able to produce the distinction between *bee* and *beet.* If they produce the wrong word, the clinician would pick up the wrong picture (i.e., the picture representing what the client said, not what they may have intended). This creates a communication problem or mismatch for the client that must be resolved by a change in the production.

To illustrate, in a study by Weiner (1981b), a game was used to teach final /t/ in a minimal contrast format. For a contrast, such as *bow* and *boat*, stimuli would include several pictures of *bow* and several pictures of *boat*. The instructions for the game were as follows:

> "We are going to play a game. The object of the game is to get me to pick up all the pictures of the *boat*. Every time you say *boat*, I will pick one up. When I have all five, you may paste a star on your paper." If the child said *bow*, the clinician picked up the *bow* picture. At times he would provide an instruction, e.g., "You keep saying *bow*. If you want me to pick up the *boat* picture, you must say the [t] sound at the end. Listen, *boat*, *boat*, *boat*. You try it. Okay. Let's begin again." (p. 98)

Weiner (1981b) reported that such training established additional phonological contrasts in the child's repertoire and then generalized to untrained words. A variety of word lists (e.g., Bleile, 1995) and treatment materials (e.g., Bird & Higgins, 1990; Palin, 1992; Price & Scarry-Larkin, 1999) are available commercially to assist clinicians in finding contrasting word pairs and pictures for treatment. The tablet-based application Sound Contrasts in Phonology (SCIP; A. L. Williams, 2016; available at https://scipapp.com/) provides stimuli for a number of contrasting words and nonword pairs that can be used for sound contrast instruction.

Basic Protocol for Contrast Training

A sample protocol for contrast training follows:

1. Select a sound contrast to be trained. The specific contrast selected will depend on the contrast approach being followed (variations to be discussed next). For example, if the contrast is /t/ - /ʃ/, one might select *tea–she, toe–show,* and *tape–shape* as contrasting words. Select five pictures for each of the contrast words. Familiarize the child with the target items to ensure they understand the meaning associated with each.

2. Engage the client in contrast training at a perceptual level (e.g., "I want you to pick up the pictures that I name. Pick up _____.").

3. Pretest the client's motor production of each of the target words containing the error sound, and, if necessary, instruct them in production of the target phoneme. Such instruction usually only needs to be brief in duration; when more intensive instruction becomes necessary, treatment with a more motor-based approach (see Chapter 10) might need to be carried out before linguistic instruction proceeds.

4. Have the client produce each target word at least once by imitating your models.

5. Engage the client in contrast training at a production level (e.g., "I want you to tell me which picture to pick up. Every time you say *show,* I will pick up this picture.").

6. Engage the client in a task that requires them to incorporate each of the contrast words in a carrier phrase (e.g., "I want you to point to a picture and name it by saying 'I found a _____.'").

7. Continue the carrier phrase task by asking the child to incorporate each of the contrasting words into the phrase (e.g., "Pick up two pictures at a time. Then tell me about both together by saying, 'I found a _____ and a _____.'").

Clinicians can use their creativity and clinical knowledge to modify this protocol. For example, for those instances when meaningful contrast pairs cannot be found to reflect a particular contrast, near minimal pairs, in which one word might not have meaning, are sometimes used (e.g., *van–shan*). In this instance, the clinician may point to an abstract drawing and, as in the preceding example, say, "This is a picture of a thing with a funny name. It's called a *shan*." Thus, the child is taught a nonsensical but contrasting word to use in the contrast activity.

Different Kinds of Contrasts

As described previously, contrasts are typically selected in order to teach the difference between either two different sounds or the presence and absence of a sound. This is done either on the basis of individual phonemes (e.g., /t/ vs. /s/) or some type of phonological patterns analysis (e.g., absence vs. presence of a final consonant in a child who exhibits frequent final consonant deletion). Such words meet the conventional definition of a minimal pair (two words which differ in meaning and differ on a single sound). Historically, clinicians have created such pairs based on the child's error pattern; that is, the contrast is between the adult target and what the child currently uses in its place.

As the application of linguistics to clinical treatment has increased, however, it has become apparent that minimal pairs differ, and these differences may influence treatment decisions and perhaps treatment outcomes. If we compare the contrasting sounds in the pairs, sometimes the sounds differ on only a single articulatory feature. For example, in the pair *sun–ton* the /s/ and /t/ are contrasted, and they differ only on manner of articulation (fricative vs. stop). By comparison, in the word pair *lick–limb* the /k/ and /m/ are contrasted, and they differ on three articulatory features (place–velar vs. bilabial; manner–stop vs. nasal; and voicing–voiceless vs. voiced). Some additional examples are shown in Table 11.1.

The use of articulatory features (place, manner, voicing) to create contrasts is the most common approach used in treatment and reflects our long-standing emphasis on the motor aspects of production. However, in Chapter 2, it was noted that in studying the world's languages, linguists have long described phonemes as consisting of many more features. Table 2.1 for example, highlights nine possible vowel features and Table 2.4 highlights 15 possible consonant features. Linguists refer to these as *distinctive features,* where each phoneme is specified as either having the feature (+) or not having the feature (-). With so many more features available, contrasts described

Table 11.1. Contrast pairs illustrating articulatory feature differences

Word pair	Articulatory feature differences
time–dime	One-feature difference: voicing (voiceless vs. voiced)
lab–lad	One-feature difference: place of articulation (bilabial vs. alveolar)
lean–teen	Two-feature differences: manner of articulation (lateral vs. stop); voicing (voiced vs. voiceless)
path–pat	Two-feature differences: manner of articulation (fricative vs. stop); place of articulation (interdental vs. alveolar)
can–man	Three-feature differences: manner of articulation (stop vs. nasal); voicing (voiceless vs. voiced); place of articulation (velar vs. bilabial).
grab–grass	Three-feature differences: manner of articulation (stop vs. fricative); voicing (voiced vs. voiceless); place of articulation (bilabial vs. alveolar)

Table 11.2. Contrast pairs illustrating distinctive feature differences

Word pair	Distinctive feature differences
time–dime	One-feature difference: voiced (– vs +)
lab–lad	Two-feature differences: coronal (– vs +); distributed (+ vs –)
lean–teen	Five-feature differences: sonorant (+ vs –); interrupted (– vs +); coronal (+ vs –); lateral (+ vs –); voiced (+ vs –)
path–pat	Two-feature differences: interrupted (– vs +); distributed (+ vs –)
can–man	Eight-feature differences: sonorant (– vs +); interrupted (+ vs –); high (+ vs –); back (+ vs –); anterior (– vs. +); distributed (– vs +); nasal (- vs +); voiced (– vs +)
grab–grass	Five-feature differences: interrupted (+ vs –); strident (– vs +); coronal (– vs +); distributed (+ vs –); voiced (+ vs –)

using this perspective may differ in many more ways. To illustrate, the same word pairs from Table 11.1 are shown again in Table 11.2 with the contrasts defined using distinctive features.

Comparing Tables 11.1 and 11.2, notice that the number of feature differences does not change for some of the pairs (e.g., path–pat), although the specific features may be different. Yet, for other pairs, the number of features is quite different. The pair *lean–teen* differs on two articulatory features but differs on five distinctive features. The most extreme example shown is the word pair *can–man,* which only differs on three articulatory features but differs on eight distinctive features. As will be discussed later, this wider range of possible differences may be exploited in treatment.

With that background, several different variations on the contrast approach have been developed over the years and three more commonly used versions will now each be discussed.

Conventional Minimal Pairs Approach

Background Statement.   The use of minimal pairs in the treatment of SSDs appears to have been advocated since at least the late 1960s (see Baker, 2010b, for a discussion). It appears to have gained more widespread use in the 1980s and continues to be used by many clinicians. In the survey of 366 clinicians by Brumbaugh and Smit (2013) it was the third most widely used approach, with 65% of speech-language pathologists (SLPs) reporting that they used it sometimes, often, or always. Another 31% said they used it at least occasionally. Over the years this approach has gone by several names, including the method of meaningful minimal contrasts (Weiner, 1981b), minimal opposition contrast treatment (Gierut, 1990), or conventional minimal pair treatment (Barlow & Gierut, 2002).

Unique Features.   This approach was the first true linguistically based approach to emerge; it was therefore the first to be based on the premise that the problem for many children with SSDs is based on a poorly developed sound system rather than inadequate speech motor learning. The word pairs are typically chosen to reflect the contrast between the child's error and the adult target. Treatment often begins with those contrasts that differ by the smallest number of articulatory features possible (hence, the label minimal oppositions). It also usually involves working on stimulable sounds.

Strengths and Limitations.   One obvious strength of this approach is that focusing on contrasts between the child's error and the adult target makes identifying the contrast targets fairly straightforward. It also directly targets the use of homonyms (i.e., one word used for two or more others) that are common in the speech of children with linguistically based SSDs. Thus, it has the potential to immediately improve speech intelligibility. One limitation of this approach is that it may not be well suited for children whose error patterns are not consistent across word positions (Forrest et al., 1997).

Research Support.   A review by Baker (2021) identified 49 studies, representing 287 participants, which have examined the efficacy of this approach. Although the vast majority of these studies represented lower level evidence (Level IIb or III), Baker reported that "... the majority [all but six studies] reported that the approach was effective" (p. 41). The earliest published study using this approach appears to be that of Weiner (1981b). It involved a multiple baseline across behaviors design (Level IIb evidence) with two boys aged 4;10 and 4;4. For both children, change only began to occur on a target pattern once treatment was applied, suggesting that only the treatment was responsible for the change. Generalization to untreated probe words occurred for all three patterns for both children. For participant A, final consonant deletion, stopping, and fronting dropped from over 90% occurrence to 50%, 15%, and 10%, respectively, after a total of eight 1-hour treatment sessions. For participant B, the corresponding values dropped from 100% to 20%, 45%, and 70%, respectively, after 16 sessions.

The highest level of available evidence for conventional minimal pairs is found in two randomized controlled trials (Level Ib evidence). Ruscello and colleagues (1993) compared this approach when administered by clinicians with the same approach that included parents administering half of the therapy sessions at home. After 16 1-hour individual sessions, both groups improved from near 0% correct on untreated probe words to an average of over 60% correct. Neither group achieved more gains than the other. In the other study, Dodd and colleagues (2008) randomly assigned 19 children to either a minimal contrast group (words pairs contrasted the child's error with the target and differed on a single articulatory feature) or a nonminimal contrast group (word pairs differed on three articulatory features). Overall, after a total of 12 individual 30-minute sessions, the average percentage consonants correct (PCC) improved from 58% to 74%. There was no significant difference in progress between the two groups.

Complexity Approach

Background Statement.   There has been an evolution over time in this approach. According to Baker and Williams (2010), this approach was first introduced by Elbert and Gierut (1986) as the maximal oppositions approach. A variation emerged from a series of studies, which became known as the empty set approach, and then it finally evolved into what is now known as the complexity approach.

Unique Features.   Fundamental to this approach is that the specific choice of the therapy targets (i.e., contrasts) is more important than any specific intervention style or organization. Taking a strong linguistic orientation, contrast descriptions using distinctive features (see Table 11.2) are typically used.

Underlying the selection of the specific contrasts to be used with this approach are three concepts. The first is the need to maximize *learnability*. As Gierut (1989) points out:

Young normally developing children initially seem to attempt and to maintain maximal distinctions and contrasts among sounds and sound classes. With development and experience, sound contrasts progress from major oppositions, such as oral-nasal or obstruent-sonorant, to more finely differentiated distinctions . . . These observations suggest that children may first concentrate on wide extremes of sound contrasts, rather than on fine-grained minimal distinctions. (p. 10)

This perspective on normal language learning led to the idea that larger and more obvious (i.e., maximal) contrasts would be preferable to minimal contrasts and may lead to greater gains in therapy. And, more particularly, unlike articulatory features, not all distinctive features are considered equal. The use of certain features (termed *major class features*) may lead to even greater gains.

As an extension of learnability and generalization, the second concept underlying the complexity approach is the notion of the *empty set*. With a conventional minimal pairs approach, the target (i.e., an unknown sound) is contrasted with whatever the child produces in its place (a known sound). Advocates of the complexity approach propose that for children with multiple sounds missing from their sound system, targeting a contrast between two unknown sounds (i.e., an empty set) may be more efficient.

The third concept underlying the complexity approach is that selection of the contrasts to be targeted should also consider *implicational relationships*. These are patterns within languages wherein, if a language includes a complex form, it also always includes related simpler forms. Some examples include:

- Fricatives imply stops—languages that include fricatives include stops

- Liquids imply nasals—languages that include liquids include nasals

- Clusters imply singletons—languages that allow consonant clusters include singleton consonants within syllables

From an intervention perspective, proponents of the complexity approach assume that these implicational relationships extend to an individual language-learning child. Thus, teaching a child to produce a more complex form (e.g., a later developing sound rather than an earlier developing sound, or a consonant in a cluster prior to as a singleton) should generalize to the simpler forms. For example, if we teach a child an unknown fricative, any related stops would be more likely to be acquired without being directly treated. This results in the notion of ignoring development logic and focusing therapy on the most complex targets, which explains the use of the term complexity in this approach.

To further illustrate the very different perspective here, recall from Chapter 3 that most children master consonant clusters after they acquire the sounds in those clusters as singletons. From a complexity perspective, however, therapy should follow the opposite pattern. Teaching consonants in cluster contexts before singletons is considered at least appropriate, if not desirable. Mastering the cluster should simultaneously lead to mastery of the corresponding singletons. Targets in the complexity approach are usually not stimulable. See also our discussion of complexity relative to target selection in Chapter 7.

In addition to these concepts, there are several other considerations governing the creation of specific contrasts when using this approach. The details are beyond the scope of the current text, but the interested reader is referred to a clinical tutorial by

Storkel (2018a). A range of application materials based on that tutorial are available for free download at https://kuscholarworks.ku.edu/handle/1808/24767.

One final somewhat unique aspect of the complexity approach is that unlike most other linguistically based approaches, nonsense words (or nonwords) are considered quite acceptable for teaching contrasts. A retrospective analysis of previous studies by Gierut and colleagues (2010) suggested that using nonwords may result in greater generalization. The use of nonwords is assumed to make it easier to create the needed contrast pairs and it may limit the possible effect of experience (i.e., some children may have heard or attempted certain real words more often than other children). In clinical application of this approach, experience with the target words would not likely be an issue.

Strengths and Limitations. One strength of the complexity approach is that it is one of the more theoretically grounded approaches that is available. It has also been the subject of much investigation. One obvious limitation is that as originally described it does not involve the use of naturalistic activities or consequences. Studies of this approach have usually involved the clinician asking the child to produce the two sounds in response to a model or in response to words or pictures (i.e., simple imitative and spontaneous drill). As such, it may not offer the opportunity for the child to recognize the communicative breakdown that occurs when they produce their error sound. Including opportunities for resolving these breakdowns would appear to be an appropriate addition to using this approach.

Research Support. Morrisette (2021) identified at least 14 peer-reviewed studies that have examined the efficacy of this approach. As one example, Gierut (1990) used a multiple-baseline design with alternating treatments (Level IIa evidence) with three boys aged 4 years who were each producing errors on at least six sounds. For each child, one error was targeted with minimal oppositions (e.g., /s/ vs. /t/) in which the contrast was a single articulatory feature. The second sound was targeted with maximal oppositions (e.g., /g/ vs. /f/), where one of the sounds was already known to the child but the contrasting sound differed on three articulatory features. A total of 15 1-hour long treatment sessions were provided to each child. Improvement occurred for all participants on all of the targets. Change did not begin on a target until treatment was introduced, suggesting that the treatment was responsible for the change. Data presented suggested average gains in accuracy of approximately 62% for maximal oppositions targets but only 35% for minimal oppositions targets.

A study by Gierut (1991) specifically examined whether there is any advantage to targeting contrasts of two unknown sounds (i.e., an empty set). Again a multiple-baseline design with alternating treatments (Level IIa evidence) was used and included two 5-year-old boys and a 4-year-old girl. Each child received 10 1-hour treatment sessions for each of two contrasts. One was a conventional minimal pair contrast of an unknown sound and the error sound the child used in its place. The other included two unknown sounds. In both cases, the targeted sounds differed by two or fewer features, thus, neither was a maximal opposition. In each case, change did not begin on the contrasts until treatment was introduced. All three children showed greater gains in accuracy on untreated probes for the empty set targets (43%–86%) compared to the minimal pair targets (25%–50%).

Dodd and colleagues (2008) used a modified version of this approach to study different types of contrasts with 19 children aged 3;11 to 6;5 with SSDs. The children were randomly assigned to two groups. Targets for the minimal contrasts group (n=9) were conventional minimal pairs differing on one articulatory feature (or the presence/absence of a sound in the case of cluster targets; e.g., stop–top). Targets for the nonminimal contrast group (n=10) differed by all three articulatory features (for cluster targets neither of the targets were included in the contrasting word; e.g., stop–mop). Targets were always real words. All children received 12 treatment sessions (30 minutes each). Findings indicated no significant difference in the gains made by the two groups. Average consonant accuracy improved by 16.56% for the minimal contrast group and by 16.10% for the nonminimal contrast group. Neither group generalized to a greater extent; the minimal contrast group added an average of four consonants and seven clusters to their sound inventories, whereas the nonminimal contrast group added an average of four consonants and six clusters.

The complexity approach works on the assumption that there is an advantage to using later-developing rather than early-developing targets. This assumption (i.e., developmental logic vs. complexity logic) was evaluated by Rvachew and Nowak (2001). They treated 48 children with SSDs averaging just over 4 years of age. The children were randomly assigned to either the early-developing (most knowledge) target group or the later-developing (least knowledge) target group. All targets were stimulable. Each received two blocks of six weekly treatment sessions (30–40 minutes each) that involved motor practice of real words containing the target through a 7-step therapy hierarchy. No contrasts were used. Two different targets were treated in each block. For the early target group, 38.0% of the targets progressed to Step 7 in the hierarchy (spontaneous sentences), whereas 11.5% failed to progress past the first step (imitated syllables). Corresponding numbers for the later target group were 17.0% and 34.4%, respectively. This represented significantly greater progress for the early target group. Relative to individual targets "... treatment progress was generally better for earlier-developing than later-developing phonemes ..." (p. 617). No significant differences were observed between the two groups on generalization.

Together, findings from these studies suggest that the complexity approach may be effective for some children with SSDs. Some studies suggest it may be at least as effective as using conventional minimal pairs. Given some contradictory evidence, it is not clear whether choosing more complex targets leads to more rapid success or results in greater generalization compared to choosing targets using developmental logic. Further study is needed.

Multiple Oppositions Approach

Background Statement.   A different sense of complexity was proposed by A. L. Williams when she developed her *multiple oppositions approach* (A. L. Williams, 1993, 2000a, 2000b, 2003). While this is another variation on the contrast approach, the intent of therapy is to address the complexity of the child's overall sound system. A foundational observation for this approach is that multiple errors produced by children with SSDs are often collapsed into a single sound (i.e., one sound is used in place of two or more other sounds; also called a *phoneme collapse*). For example, if a child substitutes /t/ in the initial word position for each of the following sounds—/θ/, /tʃ/, /s/—the words *thick, chick, sick,* and *tick* would all be produced as *tick.* One sound is being used in place of four sounds. Such collapses result in both frequent production of homonyms and, by extension, significantly reduced intelligibility. Some additional examples of collapses are shown in each of the three boxes in Figure 11.1.

A. L. Williams (1993) was not the first to notice this phenomenon. Weiner (1981a) noted that reports of these had existed for some time. He referred to them as a *systematic sound preference,* which he considered its own form of phonological pattern

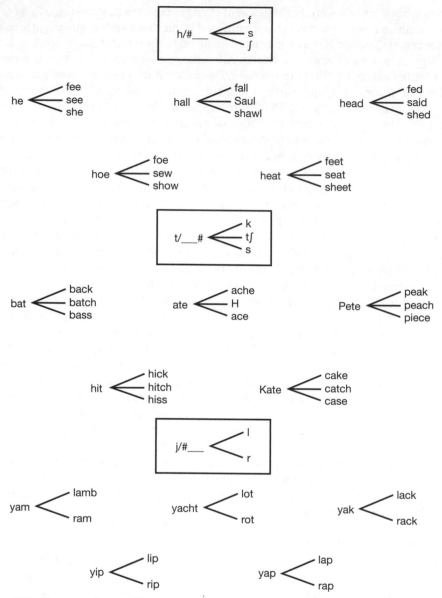

Figure 11.1. Phoneme collapses with related minimal pair treatment sets focusing on multiple oppositions. From Williams, A. L. (1999). *A systemic approach to phonological assessment and intervention.* Used with permission.

(i.e., process). Weiner studied 14 preschool children with highly unintelligible speech and identified 8 of them as engaging in such behavior.

Clinical Vignette 11.1

Systematic Sound Preference

Recall the child, Priscilla, described in Clinical Vignette 4.1 who substituted /j/ for /r/. Using phonological pattern labels, her error would be described as *gliding* (a prevocalic liquid being replaced by a glide). But it was also noted that Priscilla used /j/ in place of many other sounds in prevocalic position. It appeared that she preferred to use /j/ rather than other continuant consonants in that position. For example, the words *sip, ship, zip, rip,* and *lip* would all be produced as /jɪp/. This is entirely consistent with Weiner's (1981a) notion of a systematic sound preference.

Interestingly, in other word positions, Priscilla produced different errors. For example, postvocalic fricatives were usually replaced by stops, thus, she actually had more than one collapse. The combination of collapses likely explained why her speech was unintelligible. To illustrate (although at age 4 she would not have used all of these words), the words *use, lose, ruse, sues, zoos,* and *shoes* would all have been produced as /jut/. Although not available at the time, a system-wide approach such as multiple oppositions might have been helpful.

Advocates of other types of contrast approaches would likely address the problem of a phoneme collapse by treating each contrast independently. A. L. Williams (2000a) saw such a strategy as highly inefficient and perhaps counter-productive, as each contrast is isolated from the child's overall sound system. She saw the need for a more system-wide approach.

Unique Features.   The major innovation of the multiple oppositions approach is the treatment of several of the contrasts within a collapse simultaneously within the same activity. By doing so, each child's unique sound system is being treated in a broader way. Each collapse is thought to represent the child's unique attempt to understand how the sound system of the language is organized. The goal is to help the child recognize the relationships among several speech sounds at the same time and make their system more consistent with adult usage. A. L. Williams (2000a) hypothesized that through such an approach, the greatest change would occur in the smallest amount of time with the least effort.

In addition to illustrating sound collapses, Figure 11.1 also shows sets of contrasting training items that could be used in therapy activities for each collapse with this approach (A. L. Williams, 2000a, 2000b). Each collapse becomes a separate therapy target. Treatment sessions could either focus on a single collapse or might include instructional activities related to several phoneme collapses. Collapses affecting the most phonemes or unusual collapses (e.g., the first collapse shown in Figure 11.1) would be given priority because of their potentially higher impact on intelligibility (A. L. Williams, personal communication, 2020).

A. L. Williams and Sugden (2021) note that collapses have been observed where up to 17 phonemes (or clusters) are replaced by a single sound. Depending on the size of the collapse, two to four phonemes are selected to represent each collapse. As with other linguistically based approaches, generalization to other sounds within the collapse is expected. Specific application of what is termed a distance metric process for choosing contrasts is illustrated in A. L. Williams (2005). Essentially, priority for selection of the specific contrasts to work on is given to those contrasts that are maximally different from each other within the collapse. To assist with the process, A. L. Williams (2016) developed a tablet-based software program called Sound Contrasts in Phonology (SCIP), which includes contrasting vocabulary items available for multiple oppositions therapy and several other contrast approaches. More specific details are available at https://scipapp.com/.

Although the initial emphasis in multiple oppositions is on word-level production, eventually instruction moves to using the sounds in increasingly complex linguistic structures. This is seen in the four different treatment phases, which have been suggested for multiple oppositions (Williams, A. L., & Sugden, 2021). Phase 1 involves familiarizing the child with the target items. This includes pointing out the sound differences and how the different productions yield different meanings. Phase 2 involves focused practice of the individual items in interactive play. This typically begins with imitative productions and then transitions to spontaneous production. Phase 3 involves production of the contrasts in structured games at the word and phrase level. Phase 4 involves practice in natural conversation. For the last two phases, corrective recasts are provided to the child whenever errors occur. For example, "Oh, you wanted *sip*, but I heard you say *tip*. Remember, the /s/ in *sip* is a long sound, not a short sound."

Strengths and Limitations.   The potential to remediate multiple speech sound targets all at the same time is perhaps the most notable strength of this approach. Another strength is that the four planned phases include specific planning for generalization. One possible limitation is that presenting multiple contrasts at the same time may be confusing for some children, particularly those with significant comorbid cognitive or language impairments.

Research Support.   A summary of research findings for the multiple oppositions approach is presented by A. L. Williams and Sugden (2021). They reported that at least 10 peer-reviewed studies have examined the efficacy of the multiple oppositions approach. Findings from several of the studies will highlight the outcomes observed. A. L. Williams (2005) used a multiple baseline across behaviors design (Level IIa evidence) with a girl aged 6;5 who exhibited several phoneme collapses in her speech. Four contrasts were treated using a multiple oppositions approach and three different contrasts were treated using a conventional minimal pairs approach. Multiple oppositions treatment was provided first, followed by conventional minimal pairs. Both approaches were applied for 21 sessions (30 minutes each). Findings indicated that three of the four multiple oppositions contrasts met the success criterion (70% correct in conversation during treatment activities); none of three conventional minimal pairs targets did so, although one contrast was no longer in error on the generalization word probe. This suggested that the multiple oppositions approach was more effective than conventional minimal pairs.

A second paper by A. L. Williams (2012) included three separate studies, with one providing outcome data that could allow multiple oppositions itself to be evaluated. That study was a multiple baseline design (Level IIa evidence) which included 14 children aged 4;0 to 6;0. Each child received up to 21 (30 minutes) treatment sessions for each of two collapses (up to 42 total sessions). Using a 245 single-word generalization probe, gains in percentage correct on the target sounds ranged from 6%–64% (average 32.1%). Eight of the children showed gains of at least 20%.

A Brazilian study by Pagliarin and colleagues (2009) was a nonrandomized controlled trial (Level IIa evidence), which included nine children aged 4;2 to 6;6. Three children each received treatment with minimal oppositions, empty set (complexity), and multiple oppositions approaches. Treatment included 15–25 sessions (45 minutes each; twice weekly). Although all three approaches resulted in improvement, the children treated with multiple oppositions added the most sounds to their phoneme inventories (average of 6.3 vs. 2.7 and 2.7 for the minimal opposition and empty set groups, respectively) and added the most distinctive features to their sound systems (average of 12 vs. 4 and 6, respectively).

The highest available level of evidence supporting multiple oppositions comes from a randomized controlled trial (Level Ib evidence) by Allen (2013). Its main goal was to evaluate treatment intensity. A group of 54 children aged 3;0 to 5;5 were randomly assigned to one of three treatment conditions: 1) once per week for 24 weeks, 2) three times per week for 8 weeks, or 3) active control. The last group received 8 weeks of a print awareness intervention. A single collapse was targeted for each child. All sessions were 30 minutes long. After the first 8 weeks, group 2 outperformed the other two groups, which were not significantly different from each other. After 24 weeks, Group 2 continued to outperform the other two groups. Six weeks after their respective treatment periods ended, the groups were tested for maintenance using items from a single word articulation test. Group 1 had gained an average of 4.4% PCC, compared to 5.6% gained for Group 2. This suggested that an 8-week schedule would yield superior outcomes compared to the 24-week schedule when the same amount of treatment is provided.

Most of the studies using this approach showed success when treatment was provided for 3 hours per week. This level of intensity may be impractical in many settings, so the use of parents to assist with the delivery of multiple oppositions was explored by Sugden et al. (2020). Five children, aged 3;3 to 5;11, each received 8 weeks of clinician-provided therapy once per week for 60 minutes. At the same time, parents were trained in the approach and completed home practice activities twice per week. A multiple baseline across participants design (Level IIa evidence) was used. A single collapse was targeted for each child. In each case, change on treated words was not observed until treatment began for each participant. Clear evidence of generalization (achievement of 60%+ correct) to untreated target words was observed for some targets for three of the five participants, with a small amount of generalization (20%+ correct) for a fourth child.

Taken together, findings from these studies suggest that a multiple oppositions approach can be effective for remediation of some children with multiple speech sound errors. It may be more effective than conventional minimal pairs and the empty set approach. Training parents to assist with the approach may make its application more efficient.

Summary of Contrast Training

Contrast training is among the most commonly used linguistically based treatments for SSDs in children with multiple errors. Several versions of it have been developed and there is peer-reviewed evidence supporting the use of each version. The key elements of each of the contrast approaches are compared in Table 11.3.

NONCONTRAST APPROACHES

In addition to the contrast approaches, there are at least two other broad options to address linguistically based SSDs. These include continuing with a bottom-up approach but not using contrasts, or taking a top-down approach. Examples of both of these options are presented next.

Cycles Phonological Patterns Approach

The CPPA is a bottom-up approach, but it does not use contrasts except in a peripheral way. It is often simply called the *cycles approach*. Findings from Brumbaugh and Smit (2013) indicated that 52% of the 366 clinicians surveyed used it sometimes, often, or always. This made it the fourth most commonly used approach (after traditional therapy, phonological awareness, and minimal pairs). As such, it deserves to be discussed and summarized.

Table 11.3.   Comparison among the key elements of three contrast approaches

	Conventional minimal pairs	Complexity approach	Multiple oppositions
Targets	Earliest developed sounds	Most complex sounds or clusters[a]	Phoneme collapses
Stimulability of targets?	Yes	Not required	Not required
Use of nonwords?	No	Okay	Okay
What to contrast	Target sound versus child's error	Two targets not in child's inventory that create maximal contrast[a]	Child's error versus sounds within each phoneme collapse that are maximally distant[b]
Approach to treating contrasts	Each contrast separately	Each contrast separately	Two to four contrasts from within each collapse simultaneously

[a] See also Storkel (2018a).
[b] See A. L. Williams (2005) for distance metric.

Background Statement.   The CPPA is intended for children with multiple speech error patterns and highly unintelligible speech. It was developed by Barbara Hodson and Elaine Paden in the 1980s, building on several theoretical perspectives that had appeared at that time. These include *natural phonology* (Stampe, 1969), which captured the tendency of young children to simplify their speech output to match their limited capabilities. It also includes a heavy emphasis on the auditory channel as being crucial to speech sound acquisition (Van Riper, 1939) and the need for children to make a strong connection between the auditory channel and kinesthetic feedback from their articulators (Fairbanks, 1954). The confluence of these perspectives led to an approach that uses both focused auditory input and repeated practice of correct productions to help the child make strong connections between what a word feels like, what it sounds like, and what it means.

The CPPA was also built on the principle of gradualness in acquisition, which led to the development of the cyclical goal attack strategy. This strategy gives the child some concentrated exposure to and practice producing the correct forms related to each of their error patterns. It then allows the child's cognitive-linguistic system to reorganize itself on its own. Later versions of the approach added phonological awareness activities to facilitate the child making the proper connections between oral and written language forms.

Unique Features.   The signature element of the CPPA is in the name of this approach. The remediation plan for CPPA is organized around a cyclical or cycles goal attack strategy, which was outlined in Chapter 9. In fact, Hodson and Paden (1991) were the first to introduce such a strategy. Treatment cycles may range from 5–16 weeks, depending on the client's number of deficient patterns and the number of stimulable phonemes within each pattern. Hodson's (2010a) suggestions for treating behaviors through a cycles approach include the following:

> Each phoneme (or consonant cluster) within a pattern is targeted for approximately 60 minutes per cycle (i.e., one 60-minute, two 30-minute, or three 20-minute sessions) before progressing to the next phoneme in that pattern and then on to other deficient phonological patterns. Furthermore, it is desirable to provide stimulation for

two or more target *phonemes* (in successive weeks) within a pattern before changing to the next target *pattern* (i.e., each deficient phonological pattern is stimulated for two hours or more within each cycle). Only one phonological pattern is targeted during a beginning cycles session allowing the child to focus. Patterns are not intermingled (e.g., final /k/ in the same session as initial /st/) until the third or fourth cycle. (pp. 90–91, italics added)

A cycle is complete when all phonological patterns selected for remediation at a given point in time have been treated. Following completion of one cycle, a second cycle is initiated that will again cover those patterns not yet emerging and that need further instruction. Phonological patterns are recycled until the targeted patterns emerge in spontaneous utterances. Hodson (1989) indicated that 3–6 cycles of phonological remediation, involving 30–40 hours of instruction (40–60 minutes per week) are usually required for a client with a disordered phonological system to become intelligible. Practice in the first cycle is at the word level but is elevated to the structured phrase level by the second or third cycle to help facilitate generalization.

Another unique feature of the CPPA is the idea of not practicing errors, or what some have termed *errorless learning.* This leads to only targeting stimulable sounds (not unique to the CPPA) and only practicing those specific words containing the target that can be produced correctly. When only a few words are available, multiple examples of each word can be used to increase practice variety. Contrasting real words may be used in discussing the target words or in providing feedback on occasion, but this is not considered a major part of the approach (hence, we refer to the CPPA as a noncontrast approach).

A third unique feature of the approach is use of *amplified auditory stimulation,* which was introduced in Chapter 10. This involves spending a few minutes near the beginning and near the end of every therapy session where the child listens to lists of words containing the target sound or target pattern. The child should not repeat the words but, rather, just listen. Hodson (2010a) suggested two possible variations on such stimulation. The first is simply reading the words, whereas the second involves presenting each word followed by a contrast with the child's error. A third possible variation used by the third author of the current text (Peter Flipsen Jr.) is to bracket the child's error with the correct version (e.g., *key–tea–key* when working on velar fronting). Amplified auditory stimulation is intended to be used with a mild gain assistive listening device. Hodson and Paden (1991) have noted that it may be tempting to simply speak louder, but there is a common tendency to distort productions when doing so. Such a distorted signal is clearly something to be avoided.

A formal assessment protocol is available that was designed, in part, to be used with the CPPA. In the *Hodson Assessment of Phonological Patterns* (3rd ed.) (HAPP-3; Hodson, 2004), the author recommended that patterns (deviations or processes) targeted for remediation should include those occurring in at least 40% of the opportunities on the test words. For example, if there are 10 words on the test with opportunities for a specific pattern to occur, it would need to occur at least four times for it to be a viable remediation target. Phonological patterns targeted for remediation are also those patterns for which the client is stimulable.

Hodson (2010b) has identified "optimal primary target patterns for beginning cycles" and "potential secondary target patterns," a sequence that is generally consistent with our knowledge of normal speech sound acquisition. The potential primary targets are: 1) syllableness (omission of the syllabi nuclei: vowels, diphthongs, vocalic/syllabic consonants); 2) singleton consonants when consistently omitted in a word position (i.e., in CV, VC, CVC, or VCV); 3) /s/ clusters either in word-initial or word-final position; 4) anterior/posterior contrasts where the child lacks either velars or alveolars/labials and either fronts or backs sounds; and 5) liquids /l/, /r/, /kr/, /gr/, and /l/ clusters all in word-initial positions.

Potential secondary target patterns are not targeted until the child has acquired the following patterns in spontaneous speech: 1) syllableness; 2) basic word structure; 3) anterior/posterior contrasts; and 4) some evidence of stridency, suppression of gliding, and substitution for liquids in spontaneous utterances. Secondary target patterns are: 1) palatals (i.e., /j/, /ʃ/, /ʒ/, /tʃ/, /dʒ/), /ɚ/, /ɝ/, and word-medial /r/; 2) other consonant sequences (some of which may be primary targets), such as /s/ cluster in word-final position, /s/ plus stop in word-medial position (basket), glide clusters (tw, kj), liquid clusters /tr/, and CCC /skw, skr/; and 3) singleton stridents, such as /f, s/ and voicing contrasts (prevocalic, vowel contrasts, assimilations, and any other deviations).

The instructional sequence for each CPPA session is as follows:

1. *Review.* At the beginning of each session, the prior week's production practice word cards are reviewed.

2. *Listening activity.* This is amplified auditory stimulation and requires listening for about 30 seconds while the clinician reads approximately 20 words containing the target pattern.

3. *Target word cards.* The client draws, colors, or pastes pictures of three to five carefully selected target words based on phonetic environment of the words on 5-inch by 8-inch index cards. The name of the picture is written on each card, and the child says each word prior to its selection as a target word to evaluate it for difficulty.

4. *Production practice.* The client participates in experiential play production practice activities (i.e., games). The client is expected to have a very high success rate in terms of correct productions. Shifting activities every 5–7 minutes helps maintain a child's interest in production practice. The client is also given the opportunity to use target words in conversation. Production practice incorporates auditory, tactual, and visual stimulation and cues as needed for correct production at the word level. Usually, five words per target sound are used in a single session. The client must produce the target pattern in words in order to get their turn in the activity.

5. *Stimulability probing.* The target phoneme in the next session for a given pattern is selected based on stimulability probing (checking to see what words a child can imitate), which occurs at this point in the treatment session.

6. *Listening activity.* Auditory stimulation with amplification is repeated using the word list from the beginning of the session.

7. *Phonological awareness activities.* Activities such as rhyming and syllable segmentation are incorporated for a few minutes each session because many children with SSDs are at risk for later problems with literacy skills. See Chapter 13 for a review of the relationship among children with SSDs, phonological awareness skills, and literacy skills.

8. *Home program.* Parents are instructed to read a word list (5–10 words) to the child at least once a day and then have the child name the words on the picture

cards used in the listening activity. The five cards used during the session for production practice are also sent home for the child to practice daily. This activity should take only about 2 minutes each day.

Strengths and Limitations.   Many clinicians are attracted to the straightforward structure of the CPPA. Its emphasis on practice in game-like activities is also quite appealing to many young children. Another strength has been its adaptability. Unlike many other linguistically based approaches that have been developed and tested only with children who have no other difficulties, the CPPA has been adapted for use with other populations. This includes children with cleft palate (Hodson et al., 1983), developmental dyspraxia (Hodson & Paden, 1991), and recurrent otitis media and hearing impairments (Gordon-Brannan et al., 1992), as well as developmental delay.

Relative to limitations, the CPPA includes many elements and there has been limited study of which elements are crucial to the success of the approach. In particular, many clinicians have questioned whether amplified auditory stimulation is needed for all children and whether it is essential to use mild gain amplification.

Research Support.   At least 10 peer-reviewed papers provide evidence supporting the effectiveness of the CPPA. Findings from four reports will illustrate. The highest level evidence comes from a systematic review by Hassink and Wendt (2010; Level Ia evidence), who reviewed a total of six studies representing a total of 90 participants. They concluded that the available evidence ". . . indicated that it is plausible that the Cycles Approach results in improved consonant production in conversational contexts . . ." (p. 4).

As for specific studies, a randomized controlled trial (Level Ib) by Almost and Rosenbaum (1998) included 26 preschool-age children. Half were randomly assigned to a 4-month block of immediate treatment, and treatment for the other half was delayed. Treatment involved a modified version of the cycles approach. One significant modification involved the use of minimal pairs (not a required component of cycles) to teach the contrast between the child's error and the adult pattern. At the end of 4 months, the groups were reversed (the first group received no treatment, while the second entered treatment). Speech production accuracy improved for both groups, with significantly more change occurring during the treatment periods (PCC gains of 17%–18%) compared to the periods of no treatment (PCC gains of 2%–5%). Both groups improved to the same extent on a control measure (mean length of utterance) over the 8-month period.

A third report was a Level IIa investigation by Tyler and colleagues (1987) involving four preschool children. Two children received a minimal pairs treatment approach, while two received the cycles approach. After 2 months of treatment (twice weekly, 1-hour sessions), across the four children there was an average reduction of 87% in the use of the treated phonological patterns and little or no change in untreated (control) patterns. The two treatments were judged to be equally effective.

More recently, Rudolph and Wendt (2014) reported on a multiple-baseline study (Level IIa evidence) that included three children aged 4;3 to 5;3. Intervention involved 18 sessions of 60 minutes each using the cycles approach. Findings indicated significant improvement for two of the three children, which was maintained at follow-up 2 months later. Improvement relative to baseline performance was observed at follow-up for the third child.

Broader-Based Language Approaches

Another alternative to a contrast approach for remediating linguistically based SSDs is to take a top-down perspective. One of these (whole language) was reportedly used sometimes, often, or always by 41% of 366 clinicians surveyed by Brumbaugh and Smit (2013), making it the fifth most widely used approach.

These approaches are founded on two basic premises: 1) phonology is a part of the overall language system and should be treated in a language/communication context and 2) improvement in phonologic behaviors co-occurs when instruction is focused on higher levels of language (morphosyntax, semantics). Put another way, these approaches emphasize the communicative context and focus on the interactive nature of communication. In so doing, they attempt to reproduce the normal language learning context.

As discussed in Chapter 5, children with severe phonologic disorders frequently have difficulty with other aspects of language (Camarata & Schwartz, 1985; Fey et al., 1994; Hoffman et al., 1989; Panagos & Prelock, 1982; Paul & Shriberg, 1982; Tyler et al., 2002; Tyler & Watterson, 1991). The relationship between phonology and other language impairments has been shown to be high, and this close relationship impacts clinical practice. Such coexisting impairments suggest that many children with SSDs have difficulty with the overall process of language learning.

Although the precise nature of the relationship between phonology and other aspects of language is unknown, it has been suggested that phonologic delay, especially when it coincides with other language impairments, can be at least partially remediated by employing a language-based intervention approach (Gray & Ryan, 1973; Hoffman et al., 1990; Matheny & Panagos, 1978; Tyler et al., 2002). Because higher-level language organization likely has an effect on speech sound production (recall the discussion in both Chapters 2 and 4), Hoffman and colleagues suggest that remediation of SSDs outside the broader context of overall language development may not be the most efficacious way to treat children with SSDs.

As with contrast approaches, these broader-based language approaches may be most appropriate for individuals where a SSD is secondary to other difficulties or disorders. In addition to those with comorbid language impairments, Camarata (2021) has identified three such populations. For children with autism, these approaches offer the benefit of simultaneously working on social interactive skills, which are a common deficit area for those individuals. They may also be appropriate for children with comorbid fluency disorders, as the focus is on the interaction and less on the fine details of speech production; thus, it may be less likely to induce anxiety that may trigger dysfluency. Finally, for children with Down syndrome, the initial focus on intelligibility targets a major area of concern for most parents (Kumin, 1994). Recall also from Chapter 5 that some of the structural and physiological features of Down syndrome likely have a significant impact on speech. Fully accurate speech may not be achievable with some members of this population and a focus on overall message intelligibility may be more appropriate.

Others have indicated that the efficacy of a language-based approach for treating SSDs may be related to the degree of severity of the impairment (Fey et al., 1994; Tyler & Watterson, 1991), although results reported by Tyler and colleagues (2002) did not support this view. However, many clinicians use a language-based approach to remediation for children with mild phonological problems and language delay/disorders. For those with more severe phonological disorders, instruction may need to be focused specifically on phonology in addition to specific instruction related to the language problem. It may be that as children with severe SSDs progress in treatment, instruction may need to become more language based. Indeed, these approaches may be useful when a client is at the point in treatment at which carryover to connected speech is the goal. Regardless of when it is introduced, the following two approaches delineate possible ways to use language-based therapy to ameliorate an SSD.

Whole-Language Intervention

Background Statement.   This approach was developed and published by Norris and Hoffman (1990, 2005), who noted that learning the sound system should not be isolated from the rest of language. They suggested that intervention should be language-oriented, as well as naturalistic and interactive. In so doing, the clinician seeks to simultaneously improve semantics, syntax, morphology, pragmatics, and phonology. Such an approach puts the perceptual and motor cues of speech sound production into a broader communication context and integrates all aspects of communication, which speakers must ultimately do.

Unique Features.   For this approach, in terms of treatment priorities, phonology is the last component emphasized because intelligibility is a concern only after children have expressive language. Child–clinician interactions should be based on spontaneous events or utterances and communicative situations that arise in the context of daily play routines and instructional activities. Norris and Hoffman (1990) outline three steps for this intervention:

1. Provide appropriate organization of the environment/stimulus materials for the child to attend to, which enables the clinician to alter language complexity systematically throughout the course of therapy.

2. Provide a communicative opportunity, including scaffolding strategies that consist of various types of prompts, questions, information, and restatements that provide support to the child who is actively engaging in the process of communicating a message.

3. Provide consequences or feedback directly related to the effectiveness of the child's communication.

Application of these principles was described by Norris and Hoffman (1990) in the context of stories. Preschool children construct verbal stories in response to pictures from action-oriented children's stories and share them with a listener (another child, a parent, or a puppet). The clinician's primary role is to engage the children in constructing and talking about the pictures. The goal for each child is to produce meaningful linguistic units, syllable shapes, phonemes, and gestures to be shared with a listener. The clinician seeks to expand each child's language-processing ability by asking the child to produce utterances that exceed their current level of language use.

In this interactive storytelling technique, the clinician points to a picture, models language for the child, and then gives the child an opportunity to talk about the event. If the child miscommunicates the idea, the clinician can use one of three primary responses designed to help them reformulate the message:

1. *Clarification.* When the child's explanation is unclear, inaccurate, or poorly stated, the clinician asks for a clarification. The clinician then supplies relevant information to be incorporated in the child's response, restates the event using a variety of language forms, and asks the child to recommunicate the event. Hoffman and colleagues (1990) presented the following example of this type of response: If a child described a picture of a man cooking at a grill by saying, "Him eating," the clinician might say:

   "No, that's not what I see happening. The man isn't eating yet, he's cooking the food. See his fork, he is using it to turn the food. I see him—he is cooking the food. He will eat when he's done cooking, but right now the food is cooking on the grill. He is cooking the food so that they can eat." (p. 105)

   Then the clinician provides an opportunity for the child to restate the information (e.g., ". . . so tell that part of the story again"). Thus, feedback is based on meaning within the context rather than structure.

2. *Adding events.* If the child adequately reports an event, the clinician points out another event to incorporate in the story. This is done by presenting the child with a variety of language models. The child is then given the opportunity to retell the story. In an example from Hoffman and colleagues (1990), the clinician points to specific features in the picture and says something like:

   "That's right, the man is cooking. He is the dad and he is cooking the hamburgers for lunch. Mom is putting plates on the table. Dad will put the hamburgers on the plates. So you explain the story to the puppet." (p. 105)

3. *Increasing complexity.* If the child adequately describes a series of events, the clinician seeks to increase the complexity of the child's story by pointing out relationships among events, such as motives of the characters, cause-and-effect relationships among the individual events, time and space relationships, and predictions. The child is given the opportunity again to reformulate their own version of the story. Another example from these authors is:

   If the child said, "The daddy is cooking hamburgers and the mommy is setting the table," the clinician might prompt the child to link these two events in time and space by saying: "That's right, mommy and daddy are making lunch for the family. When daddy finishes cooking the hamburgers he will put them on the plates, so tell that part of the story to the puppet." (p. 105)

Although such interactive storytelling focuses on syntax, semantics, and narrative language skills, correct phonological models and feedback are also being provided to the child. More recently, Hoffman and Norris (2010) began to include a significant emphasis on written language in their approach. They have developed three visual tools to assist in this regard. This first is called Phonic Faces, which includes alphabet letters overlaid on a face drawing to help make the association between the speech sound and the letter usually associated with it. MorphoPhonic Faces presents a Phonic Face for the first letter of a word, along with drawings to illustrate the meaning of the intended word. Phonic Faces storybooks incorporate Phonic Faces and other images along with text to help solidify the association among speech sounds, letters, words, and meanings.

Strengths and Limitations.   One strength of this approach is the opportunity to target several aspects of communication simultaneously. This focus makes it worth consideration for children with comorbid language impairments. Another strength is that the interactive nature of the activities and the incorporation of stories may be very appealing to many young children. The limited evidence base supporting it is the biggest limitation. One additional limitation is that the informal structure of the treatment sessions may limit opportunities for practice. A final limitation is that the skill of the SLP to interact and engage the client is crucial to successful implantion.

Research Support. Although Hoffman and Norris (2010) identified six studies providing some efficacy for the whole-language approach, none of those were peer-reviewed. Some support for this approach can be found in two peer-reviewed studies, which utilized storytelling (although they did not include the Phonic Faces materials). In the first study, Hoffman and colleagues (1990) used an AB comparison design (Level IIb evidence) with a pair of identical twins aged 4;1 with SSDs and comorbid language delays. One twin received the whole-language intervention, while the other received conventional minimal pairs treatment. Treatment intensity was three 50-minute sessions per week for 6 weeks. Results indicated comparable improvements for both children in speech sound accuracy, with gains in PCC of 16% and 19%, respectively. The child who received the whole-language treatment showed significantly greater improvement in language skills. This supports the notion that the top-down approach can improve both speech and language skills when both are a part of the treatmet approach.

The second study was a multiple baseline design across groups (Level IIa evidence) study conducted by Lawrence (2014). Six children aged 3;11 to 5;4 were seen in three groups (each group also included a normal-speaking peer). The groups were defined by the speech error patterns being targeted (cluster reduction, fronting of velars, final consonant deletion). The stories were structured with many opportunities to focus on the particular error pattern. As each word containing the target pattern was encountered, the clinician asked the child to attempt to produce the word. If a child produced an error, a hierarchy of cues was provided to assist with production (direct imitation, placement cues), starting at the word level. Failure at the word level led to the use of the cues at the isolated sound level. Each session lasted 30 minutes and included at least 15 opportunities for each child to attempt the target. Group A completed three baseline sessions followed by 33 treatment sessions. Groups B and C completed 9 and 18 baseline sessions followed by 27 and 18 treatment sessions, respectively. In each case, change did not begin to occur until treatment began for the group. Significant change in target accuracy was observed for five of the six children, with data reported suggesting average gains from baseline of 56%, 57%, 65%, 38%, and 71%. Accuracy levels were maintained 2 weeks after the end of the study. The one exception was a child who saw essentially no gains during the treatment period; that child was not stimulable for the targeted error (velar fronting) at the beginning of the study. This same child then demonstrated progress in a second round of therapy that incorporated more direct motor-based techniques.

Together, these findings suggest that interactive storytelling can be effective at remediating speech production errors for some children.

Naturalistic Recast Intervention

Background Statement. A second top-down approach to improving speech sound skill is intended to improve speech sound production by initially targeting improvement of overall speech intelligibility. It is based on two ideas: 1) the primary presenting symptom for many children with SSDs is reduced intelligibility (problems making themselves understood by others) and 2) as discussed in Chapter 7, accuracy of production of speech sounds is not the only factor influencing how well speech is understood. Camarata (2021) proposed that the initial step for these children should be to increase the proportion of messages that are being understood by the listener. This would allow their conversations to move beyond what are often brief, unproductive encounters. By focusing on intelligibility first, the child obtains feedback about their messages, which is intended to enhance learning by encouraging both more speech attempts and more practice. From this perspective, speech and language development are seen as highly interactive processes that are stimulated in natural interactions. Once intelligibility has improved, attention can turn to accuracy of production of individual speech sounds.

Unique Features. Similar to the whole-language approach, naturalistic recast intervention is a child-centered approach in which the clinician arranges the therapy environment in ways that encourage communication attempts. In this case, toys and activities of interest to the child are made available, and the clinician (or a parent or other caregiver) engages naturally with the child. The activities can include requiring the child to ask for assistance and may involve more than one participant. The clinician and child interact in natural ways, with the clinician providing facilitating feedback referred to as *recasts*. The environment is organized so that most of the target words the child attempts are known, and the clinician provides both confirmation of the communicative attempt and a correct model of the target (e.g., Child: "A wemon"; Clinician: "Yes, it's a lemon."). The conversation can continue, and the child can learn to improve their speech from the feedback received. Providing good speech and language models and ensuring that the conversation between the child and the clinician continues are both critical to the process (Camarata, 1993). By presenting the feedback within a normal communicative context, it:

> "... may make it easier for the child with unintelligible speech to unconsciously compare their utterance to the adult's recast ... [and] increase the probability that the child will develop more accurate representations of the way words are produced ..." (Camarata, 2021; p. 341)

Strengths and Limitations. This approach shares many of the strengths of the whole-language approach described earlier. Its potential to target other deficit areas within the therapy activities is an obvious strength. This, again, makes it appropriate for children with comorbid language impairments. In such cases, once intelligibility improves, specific language targets may also be incorporated. The playlike nature of the activities is also likely to be appealing to many young children. And, as with whole language, one possible limitation is that the informal structure of the treatment sessions may limit opportunities for practice.

Research Support. At least three peer-reviewed studies provide some evidence for this approach. The highest level available evidence is from two randomized controlled trials (Level Ib evidence). The first (Yoder et al., 2005) included 52 preschool children with both speech and language impairments. Half of the children received the naturalistic intervention and the other half (control group) did not. Those in the control group were free to seek out whatever other treatment to which they might have access. The naturalistic treatment group received three 30-minute treatment sessions per week for 6 months. Parents of the control group participants documented how much treatment they received and data indicated that they actually received more treatment than those in the naturalistic intervention group. Intelligibility improved in both groups, but there were no overall differences between the groups. However, the naturalistic treatment resulted in significantly more intelligibility gains for the children with the poorest pretreatment accuracy. This suggested that a focus on overall intelligibility might be particularly helpful for children with the most severe SSDs, and possibly those with coexisting language disorders.

The second randomized control trial was conducted by Yoder and associates (2016) and included 51 children with Down syndrome, aged 5–12 years. Half of the children received the recast treatment and half received a structured bottom-up approach called Easy Does It for Articulation (Drake, 2002). All sessions were delivered twice per week (60 minutes) for 6 months. Overall, both groups improved the comprehensibility (how much listeners understood) of their speech by the same amount. However, gains were significantly greater for those with greater pretreatment ability to imitate speech if they had received the naturalistic approach. Post-hoc analysis did indicate that those children with better imitation skills also received more recasts during treatment. This only serves to reinforce the value of the recast procedure in making speech easier to understand.

The third study supporting the effectiveness of the naturalistic recast approach was that of Camarata (1993). This involved two children (aged 3;10 and 4;3) with SSDs, and used a multiple baseline across behaviors and participants design (Level IIa evidence). Sessions involved conversational interactions in which the clinician responded to any errors on the target sound with a correct model. For example, if the child said /wɛd/ for *red,* the clinician would say, "Yes, *red.*" Results indicated that accuracy of the target sound began to improve only after the recasts were introduced. Participant 1 achieved greater than 90% accuracy on his four speech sound targets within 5–16 sessions (15 minutes working on each target). Accuracy was maintained 9 months later. Participant 2 achieved that accuracy level for her one speech sound target within seven sessions and maintained that level for an additional four sessions (no follow-up data were available).

Together, these findings suggest that recasts can be a successful tool for remediating speech sound errors when used in naturalistic contexts.

Summary of Noncontrast Approaches

Although contrast approaches appear to be more commonly used than noncontrast approaches, the available evidence suggests that noncontrast approaches may also be effective for remediating linguistically based SSDs. They may be of particular value for milder cases or as a means to encourage generalization in the later stages of intervention. Broader-based language approaches may be of greater value for children with comorbid language impairments.

REMEDIATION GUIDELINES FOR LINGUISTICALLY BASED APPROACHES

1. A linguistic approach is recommended when there are multiple sound errors that reflect one or more phonologic error patterns. These approaches are particularly useful with young children who are unintelligible.

2. Once error patterns have been identified, a review of the child's phonetic inventory assists in the identification of target sounds (exemplars) to facilitate correct usage. This review usually includes examination for stimulability and may include phonetic contexts that facilitate correct production of a target, frequency of occurrence of potential target sounds, and the developmental appropriateness of targets.

3. Selection of training words should reflect the syllabic word shapes the child uses. For example, if the child uses only CV and CVC shapes, multisyllabic target words would not be targeted. This guideline is obviously inappropriate if the focus on remediation is on syllable structure simplifications and/or word structure complexity.

4. Selecting target words that facilitate the reduction of two or more patterns simultaneously could increase treatment efficiency. For example, if a child uses stopping and deletes final fricatives, the selection of a final fricative for training could aid in the simultaneous reduction of the patterns of stopping and final consonant deletion.

5. When errors cross several sound classes (e.g., final consonant deletion affecting stops, fricatives, and nasals), exemplars that reflect different sound classes or possibly the most complex (production) sound class should be selected.

6. Instruction related to phonologic patterns may focus on the broader pattern and less on the phonetic accuracy of individual sounds used in treatment. For example, if a child deletes final consonants but learns to say [dɔd] for [dɔg], the /d/ for /g/ replacement might be overlooked during the initial stage of instruction because the child has begun to change their phonologic system to incorporate final consonant productions.

7. Instruction focused on both perception and production of contrasts is commonly used and would appear appropriate in many cases.

8. When using contrast approaches, clinicians may wish to probe each client's response to both minimal and maximal oppositions contrasts.

9. For children with many sound collapses, a multiple oppositions approach might be an efficient way to impact the child's overall sound system.

10. Noncontrast approaches should be considered, especially in cases where the child is not responsive to the more structured contrast approaches.

11. For children with coexisting language impairments, a broader-based language (top-down) approach might be appropriate. Although this approach may work best with children evidencing milder phonological impairments, for those who are more severely involved, direct instruction related to production of speech sounds will likely be necessary. This may be approached either by beginning with work on language and introducing specific work on speech sounds later, or by working on both language and speech sounds concurrently.

CASE STUDY REVISITED: LINGUISTIC PERSPECTIVE

This section revisits the case of Kirk, that we introduced in Chapter 7, and also discussed in Chapter 10.

Intervention Recommendations

Kirk was stimulable for many of his errors, suggesting that motor-based treatment would be unnecessary for those errors that are stimulable. Some of the stimulable sounds were more easily imitated than others. Because he could imitate most of his error sounds, a major goal of instruction was to help Kirk learn to use sounds contrastively or, in other words, diminish his sound collapses by using sounds appropriately to ensure word contrasts.

First Consideration: How Many Targets Should I Address in a Session?

Because Kirk has multiple error sounds, a focus on several targets is suggested, either within a single lesson or across lessons within a 3- or 4-week time frame (cycles or horizontal approach). It is suggested that treatment sessions for Kirk should address error patterns, beginning with stopping and the sound collapses reflected in that pattern (i.e., /d/ replacing several other sounds and clusters such as /s, z, tʃ, θ/ and clusters /sl, sn, fl/).

Second Consideration: How Should I Conceptualize the Treatment Program?

One treatment option for addressing Kirk's errors is to use a cycles phonological pattern approach in which one or more sounds are targeted in a given lesson to help him learn to use a particular phonological pattern (e.g., frication because he currently substitutes stops for most fricatives). In a subsequent lesson within the same cycle, other fricatives related to that pattern would be the focus, continuing until most of the fricatives have been practiced. At that point, another pattern would be targeted, including one or more sounds in a given lesson (e.g., use of final consonants).

An alternative treatment approach that specifically addresses sound contrasts is to use a multiple oppositions approach that simultaneously addresses the collapse of numerous sounds to /d/. Instruction might initially focus on sound collapses that include sounds in Kirk's repertoire and then, as other sounds are established, expand to other sound collapses. In the following example, solid lines indicate initial collapses to focus on because the sounds are in Kirk's repertoire; broken lines reflect targets that can be addressed as additional sounds are added to Kirk's repertoire.

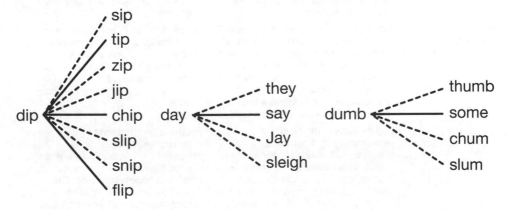

Another way to approach Kirk's stopping pattern is the use of a complexity approach rather than the multiple oppositions approach. This focuses on a single contrast and then progresses to other contrasts in his system. Instruction would begin with a pair evidencing the greatest difference between a target sound and a contrasting sound. For example, instruction might first focus on the word pair *seal–meal,* and once Kirk can produce that pair, go to *seal–veal,* and finally, *deal–seal.* The hope is that by initially contrasting /s/ with /m/ (sounds that evidence several feature differences from /d/), such practice will facilitate more rapid acquisition of other sound contrasts.

Overall Treatment Plan

As indicated by our preceding discussion and that in Chapter 10, the nature of Kirk's errors suggests an overall mixed approach, with some targets being treated with a more motor-based approach, but the remainder with a more linguistic approach. For either group of targets, several different options have been outlined. One possible general plan for his overall treatment is presented in Table 11.4.

Table 11.4. Possible intervention sequencing for Kirk

Component	Procedure	Rationale
Sound stimulation /practice	Ask the client to produce a variety of sounds five times each (both incorrect and correct sounds). Provide auditory models and cueing as necessary.	Stimulability has been shown to highly influence generalization. Therefore, we must help Kirk acquire all the sounds at a motor level. Brief practice periods serve to encourage continued attempts at sounds that may be difficult for Kirk to produce.
Production activities	Focus on teaching frication and final consonant usage. Focus on one or two sounds per session, moving from /f/ to /m/ to /s/ and other stimulable sounds. Use minimal pairs at a perceptual level before practicing on pairs at a production level. Drilling/ playing games and activities are recommended. Use a listening task to introduce each sound. Consider using multiple opposition contrasts for the /d/ collapses.	Cycling across patterns and sounds is helpful for children with multiple errors. Kirk is young and still developing his sound system, and he has a good attention span; therefore, he could benefit from shifting focus from week to week. Multiple oppositions may be helpful for phoneme collapses and are recommended because Kirk is stimulable on many of the collapses.
Increasing linguistic complexity	When Kirk can produce word targets accurately, including minimal pairs, shift production to phrases and then sentences. In addition, progress from targets occurring only once in a word or phrase to more complex productions involving more than one occurrence and competing sounds.	To reach the terminal objective of spontaneous use of appropriate speech sounds and patterns, Kirk must be able to use his new speech sounds and patterns in increasingly complex linguistic units.
Situational generalization	Bring persons in the child's environment into activities to reinforce Kirk's new speech skills. Using target names, preschool vocabulary, and frequently used words as a focus could be helpful. Monitor Kirk's use of his new speech in the classroom and home.	Focusing on situational generalization as early as possible will help this young client generalize the new language skills to his environment. The environment will very likely reinforce increased intelligibility.

QUESTIONS FOR CHAPTER 11

1. What is the difference between a motor-based treatment and a linguistically based treatment?

2. Outline a linguistic approach to speech sound intervention for a child with many error productions and specify for whom it is appropriate.

3. Discuss how and why one would use minimal pairs in phonological treatment.

4. What is the difference between conventional minimal pairs, the complexity approach, and multiple oppositions?

5. Describe multiple opposition treatment and when it might be appropriate to use with a child.

6. Outline the procedures for a cycles phonological patterns approach to therapy.

7. Describe how a whole-language or naturalistic recast approach differs from most other treatment approaches.

12

Treating Specific Populations: Childhood Apraxia and Older Children

PETER FLIPSEN JR., JOHN E. BERNTHAL, AND NICHOLAS W. BANKSON

LEARNING OBJECTIVES

This chapter discusses treatment of speech sound disorders (SSDs) in older children and adolescents. By the end of this chapter, the reader should be able to:

- Discuss how assessment of childhood apraxia of speech (CAS) differs from assessment for other types of SSDs.

- Differentiate among different treatment options for CAS.

- Discuss some ways in which traditional therapy might be modified for use with older children.

- Describe several different approaches to providing extra external feedback in speech sound intervention.

CHILDHOOD APRAXIA OF SPEECH

The topic of CAS was introduced in Chapter 5 in the discussion of classification of SSDs. This section addresses issues relevant to clinical assessment and intervention with this subpopulation.

As noted in Chapter 5, we do not yet have a clear sense of how CAS differs from other SSDs. The ASHA position statement (2007a), however, provides a starting point for such differentiation. From that perspective, CAS is generally viewed as primarily a problem of motor planning for speech sound production that manifests itself in errors of both precision and consistency of production. Children with CAS have difficulty producing precise speech sound targets on a consistent basis and may produce the same word in different ways on multiple attempts. Children with CAS can also have associated (comorbid) neuromuscular problems (i.e., dysarthria) and/or other types of apraxia, such as oral or limb apraxia (i.e., problems with nonspeech movements). The position statement also indicates that CAS is likely a disorder that is neurological in nature and might result from known neurological impairments, such as cerebral palsy. It may also be associated with complex neurobehavioral disorders, such as fragile X syndrome or Rett syndrome. However, the origin of any neurological limitations is in many cases unknown (idiopathic).

Consistent with the idea of problems with motor planning (transcoding) of speech output, Velleman and Strand (1994) have stated that children with CAS may be capable of producing the individual aspects of speech production (i.e., articulatory postures, phonemes, words) but have great difficulty "bridging among the various elements that constitute language performance" (p. 120). Put another way, CAS likely includes difficulty not only with phonology but also with other aspects of language.

In regard to higher levels of language, Velleman (2003) noted that many of these children often demonstrate receptive language skills that are superior to their expressive abilities. When the gap between receptive and expressive language skills is absent, a comorbid diagnosis such as specific language impairment might be appropriate. Gillon and Moriarty (2007) also suggested the possibility of a higher level of language problems in children with CAS, reporting an increased risk for reading and spelling difficulty in this population. It should also be noted that many children with CAS also manifest social and behavioral problems (Ball, 1999). This may be a consequence of the significant difficulty that many of these children appear to have in making themselves understood (i.e., they have greatly reduced intelligibility, which may lead to significant frustration and even social acceptance issues).

ASSESSMENT OF CHILDHOOD APRAXIA OF SPEECH

Assessment of this population is not unlike the process used with any child with any other SSD. In addition to a standard articulation/phonological battery, it typically includes a case history, hearing screening, and screening of other areas of communication (language, voice, fluency). However, additional specific aspects of the CAS population warrant elaboration. Given the challenges of identifying the diagnostic features for CAS discussed in Chapter 5, the following is offered as a starting point.

The oral mechanism examination should be particularly thorough to determine whether comorbid dysarthria or oral apraxia is present. It should include an assessment of strength, tone, and stability of the oral structures (e.g., Can the child move the tongue independently of the mandible? Does the child do anything special to stabilize the mandible, such as thrust it forward?). A review of the child's feeding history may be of interest in this regard. Young children in particular might exhibit uncoordinated feeding patterns without dysphagia (swallowing problems). Overall motor skills, both automatic and volitional, including the ability to perform imitative and rapidly alternating tongue movements, should be part of the assessment. Early speech history may also be informative. A retrospective study of home videos by Overby and colleagues (2020) compared eight infants later diagnosed with CAS, six typically developing infants, and six infants later diagnosed with (non-CAS) SSDs. Findings indicated those later diagnosed with CAS had later onset of canonical babbling, and produced both fewer canonical babbles and fewer syllables per minute compared to the other two groups.

Given the neurological basis now attributed to CAS, it may be prudent to refer more seriously impaired children with suspected CAS with or without dysarthria to a pediatric neurologist to determine the status of current neurological functioning. Seizure history, associated limb apraxia, presence of oral apraxia, and general knowledge of neurological functioning could influence the overall management program for a given child and, thus, warrant such a referral.

The main focus of the speech-language pathologist's (SLP's) assessment should be on speech, and speech motor skill in particular. In doing so, the clinician must keep in mind the nature of CAS as a disorder involving hierarchical levels of speech and language in which motor planning for syllable sequencing may be a challenge at many levels. Therefore, movements, transitions, and timing should be observed as speech is produced at a variety of linguistic levels, from simple to complex. A comprehensive procedure, such as the Dynamic Evaluation of Motor Speech Skill (DEMSS; Strand & McCauley, 2019) might be appropriate. It includes speech sound productions in a variety of utterance types; for example, assessing connected speech through conversation, picture description, and narrative. It employs diadochokinetic (DDK) tasks, as well as imitative utterances that include vowels (V), consonant-vowels (CV), vowel-consonant (VC) combinations, and CVC productions. It assesses repetition of single words of increasing length, multisyllabic words, plus words in phrases and sentences of increasing length.

Difficulty with planning and programming the required movement sequences for speech may be manifest in the emerging diagnostic features of CAS. One of these is difficulty with transitions between sounds and syllables. A challenge for assessing such transitions with young children is that many with both typical speech development and other types of SSDs (including CAS) have not yet mastered the production of many speech sounds. Using real-word tasks would yield errors that might not be unique to children with CAS. To bypass this problem, the use of simple sounds and nonword stimuli is frequently suggested. The classic approach is to examine performance on specific types of DDK tasks. Children with CAS without any comorbid dysarthria would likely have greater difficulty with tasks involving a changing place of articulation (e.g., puh-tuh-tuh, tuh-kuh-kuh, puh-tuh-kuh) compared to those where place of articulation does not change (e.g., tuh-tuh-tuh).

Individuals with both CAS and dysarthria would have difficulty with both kinds of tasks; however, DDK tasks may not be sufficient for at least two reasons. First, some young children have not mastered /k/, which then limits the number of sounds and movement combinations that can be evaluated with DDKs. Second, DDK tasks only test strings of up to three syllables long, which may not be a sufficient test of motor planning and programming. Shriberg and colleagues (2009) proposed an alternative called the Syllable Repetition Task (SRT), which uses four early-developing consonants (/b, d, m, n/) and the vowel /ɑ/. The 18 stimuli (shown in Table 12.1) contain 2–4 syllables and a total of 50 consonant targets. (Note: The SRT has other applications [see Shriberg et al., 2009] besides CAS. More complete instructions for administration and scoring, along with a PowerPoint presentation demonstrating the stimuli, can be found at https://phonology.waisman.wisc.edu/administration-scoring-materials/.)

In the SRT, each stimulus is presented once and the child is asked to repeat it. Two additional presentations of each item may be provided, but only one response is scored. Responses are transcribed phonetically. Several different scores can be

Table 12.1.   Stimuli for the Syllable Repetition Task (SRT)

/bada/	/nada/	/banada/
/dama/	/maba/	/manaba/
/bama/	/bamana/	/bamadana/
/mada/	/damana/	/danabama/
/naba/	/madaba/	/manabada/
/daba/	/nabada/	/nadamaba/

Source: Shriberg et al. (2009).

generated (see website link), but for application to CAS a transcoding score is of greatest interest. This score focuses on addition errors (e.g., producing [banda] or [babada] instead of [bada]). It is generated by dividing the number of items that included any addition errors by 18 and multiplying the resulting proportion by 100. For example, if there were two items with addition errors $2/18 \times 100 = 11.1$. This value is then subtracted from 100 (yielding 88.9 in this example) to yield the transcoding score. On the other hand, a child with seven items with addition errors on the SRT would have a transcoding score of 61.1 $(100 - (7/18 \times 100))$.

To examine the value of this tool with CAS, Shriberg and colleagues (2012) administered the SRT to a total of 379 children, including 40 with CAS (the remainder had either typical speech or other types of SSDs). They found that the children with CAS were 8.3 times more likely to have a transcoding score below 80. Using that cutoff, the first child in the fictitious examples previously mentioned would be unlikely to have CAS, wheras the second very likely would have CAS. The diagnosis then would need to be confirmed with other measures.

A second emerging diagnostic feature of CAS is inconsistency. As noted in Chapter 5, this is particularly manifest in CAS across multiple attempts at the same word. Therefore, particular attention should be paid to how words that occur multiple times in conversational speech are produced. Alternatively (or perhaps in addition), the consistency subtest of the Diagnostic Evaluation of Articulation and Phonology (DEAP; Dodd, Hua, et al., 2006) could be administered as it was in the CAS treatment studies by McCabe and associates (2014, 2016); it offers the advantages of a consistent set of target words and the availability of normative data. Another manifestation of inconsistency may be intermittent hypernasality in connected speech (Sealey & Giddens, 2010). Such output would be seen as speech that goes from sounding like the person has a head cold (denasal speech) to sounding like the person has a cleft palate (hypernasal speech) all in the same conversation or even within the same speaking turn. This could be evaluated either informally by perceptual judgements of connected speech samples or using acoustic analysis.

The third of the emerging diagnostic features of CAS is problems with the suprasegmental aspects of speech. These problems represent the challenge of coordinating the laryngeal and respiratory systems with the oral mechanism. This may result in difficulty with varying intonation contours, modulation of loudness, and maintenance of proper resonance. Vowels may be prolonged because the child needs time to organize coordination for the next series of speech sound movements. It may also be manifest in the presence of inappropriate pauses (Maassen et al., 2001; Shriberg et al., 2017a,b). Recall also that the ASHA (2007a) position statement specifically identified excessive and equal stress as a particularly notable error in CAS. This would be manifest, for example, in the production of two-syllable words where one syllable is normally stressed and the other is unstressed, as if both syllables were equally stressed. For example, the word proVIDE would be produced as PROVIDE and the word DAddy would be produced as DADDY. This can be evaluated by listening to samples of connected speech

Finally, it was noted in Chapter 5 that children with CAS may also present with difficulty with reading and spelling that may reflect problems with the underlying representation for speech sounds. As such, assessment of phonological awareness (see Chapter 13) would be appropriate.

Clinical Vignette 12.1

Does Slow Progress in Therapy Mean the Child has Childhood Apraxia of Speech?

Author Nicholas Bankson was once called by a clinician to visit her school and evaluate a 7-year-old boy with multiple speech errors and almost unintelligible speech. The boy was in all other respects a typical second-grade child. The SLP had been working with him for 1.5 years and was not making any progress using a traditional sound-by-sound therapy approach. This lack of progress was creating great concern for the parents and his teacher, as well as serious communication concerns for the child (who, fortunately, was a skilled baseball player and had a high level of social acceptance by his peers). But the lack of progress was of particular concern for the clinician.

This situation occurred well before the ASHA position statement on CAS was published and before the profession had firmly accepted such a diagnosis. Some suggestions were beginning to appear in the literature regarding the characteristics of CAS and how intervention needed to be modified to accommodate this type of speech disorder. It was noted that many of these children were slow to respond to therapy. Did this child have CAS? Could this be the key to a CAS diagnosis?

This question continues to arise. Oh, that it could be so easy! The problem with assuming that slow therapy progress equals a diagnosis of CAS is that there is another equally valid reason why a child might not be making progress in therapy. Perhaps we simply have not identified the precise nature of the problem and, thus, have not yet found the best therapy approach for the child. Traditional therapy (the default approach for many clinicians) does not work for all children with SSDs and there are now a variety of other therapy options available to us for children without CAS.

Recommended Assessment Battery for Childhood Apraxia of Speech

To assess for CAS, clinicians may use the following battery:

1. Case history (including review of feeding history)

2. Hearing screening/testing

3. Screening of voice and fluency characteristics

4. Speech mechanism examination

    a. Structure and function

    b. Strength, tone, stability

5. Motor speech evaluation including DDK tasks and the SRT

6. Connected speech sample

    a. Segmental productions

    b. Syllable and word shape productions

    c. Phonologic patterns present

    d. Intonation, vocal loudness, resonance

    e. Analysis of consistency (words occurring more than once)

7. Segmental productions (single-word testing; independent analysis for those with a limited phonological repertoire)

    a. Consonants, vowels, and diphthongs used

    b. Syllable shapes used

8. Intelligibility (how well the acoustic signal is understood with and without context)

9. Stimulability testing (include multiple opportunities)

    a. Segments

    b. Syllables

    c. Words with increasing number of syllables

10. Phonological awareness assessment

11. Interpersonal skills

    a. Social interaction

    b. Behavioral interactions

    c. Academic/community interactions

12. Language evaluation

    a. Comprehension and production

    b. Sound productions at various semantic and syntactic levels

Given the complexity of this process, it may be tempting to administer one or more of the published tests that are specifically intended for the assessment of children with suspected CAS. However, a review of six such tests by McCauley and Strand (2008) indicated that ". . . the items varied considerably in complexity, task requirements, and type of judgment made by the tester" (p. 85). This is not surprising given the previously discussed lack of agreement about the unique features of CAS. It is perhaps just as important to note McCauley and Strand's conclusion that developers of these tests also appeared to be attempting to assess too broadly, and they generally did not adequately develop the psychometric properties of the tests. Put another way, to date, the available published tests for CAS appear to be inadequate for the task. Such tools cannot, therefore, be recommended at this time.

TREATMENT FOR CHILDHOOD APRAXIA OF SPEECH

Over the years, many approaches to treating CAS have been proposed. Until recently, evaluating the evidence for those approaches has been a challenge, as much of the evidence predated the creation of the ASHA position statement on CAS. As such, they may not have all defined CAS the same way. Consequently, newer evidence continues to emerge and several reviews (e.g., Maas et al., 2014; Murray et al., 2014) have concluded that multiple approaches appear to be successful at remediating CAS. The following discussion includes those approaches where peer-reviewed evidence is beginning to accumulate.

Approaches to Improving Functional Communication in Childhood Apraxia of Speech

Although it is tempting to immediately focus on approaches that have the potential to completely solve the problem, young children with CAS and their families face an initial practical issue—the speech of these children is often highly unintelligible. This can create a significant challenge for them to meet their basic needs. Given the long-standing concern about slow progress in therapy with this population, these children need an immediate means of functional communication. Two possible approaches may be appropriate for this purpose. Both can be used in isolation as an initial step or alongside other longer-term solutions.

Core Vocabulary Approach

The first approach that might be considered is the *core vocabulary approach,* which has as its specific goal the improvement of consistency (one of the emerging diagnostic features of CAS). By selecting target words that are functionally powerful for the child and making their productions more consistent, it improves the chances that the child's intended message will be understood by the listener. Recall from the discussion of intelligibility in Chapter 6 that consistency of errors can have a significant impact on intelligibility. Some research has suggested that familiar listeners, like parents, appear to be able to translate their child's error patterns (Flipsen, 1995), but for children with CAS, inconsistency of production means the child's errors are less predictable. Improving consistency would, therefore, improve predictability and, by extension, improve intelligibility.

Background Statement.   The core vocabulary procedure focuses on functional outcomes in which a consistent (even if not fully correct) output is targeted. An underlying assumption of this approach appears to be that if the child changes what they do to make the outcomes more consistent, listeners will be better able to understand the intended message. The child will then receive consistent feedback, which will allow them to either make system-wide changes or modify their speech motor programs.

The core vocabulary approach was originally intended for children with severe but inconsistent speech sound productions (i.e., different sound substitutions across productions and ≥40% variable productions; Dodd et al., 2004). Children with inconsistent speech disorders are one of the four symptomatology subgroups described in Chapter 5. Inconsistent speech disorders are characterized by variable productions of words or variable phonological features across contexts, and also within the same context. Dodd and colleagues hypothesize that such children's unstable phonological system reflects a deficit in phonological planning (i.e., phoneme selection and sequencing). The authors differentiate this subgroup of children with inconsistent SSDs from those with CAS, although similar forms of inconsistency are present in both types of disorders. Dodd and colleagues state that the core vocabulary approach is the treatment of choice for children with inconsistent speech sound productions who may be resistant to contrast treatment or traditional therapy. A similar lack of responsiveness is often also seen in those with CAS; as such, the core vocabulary approach may be appropriate for both groups. Regardless of the population targeted, Dodd and colleagues suggest that this treatment results in a system-wide change by improving the consistency of whole-word production and at the same time addressing speech processing deficits.

Unique Features.   This approach does not dictate any specific teaching approach, but rather assumes that with the assistance of the clinician, the child will do whatever they need to do to modify the output. Likewise, the focus is on making the child more consistent and, thus, more understandable (intelligible). The core vocabulary procedure includes the following steps:

1. The child, parents, and teacher select a list of approximately 50 words that are functionally powerful for the child and that includes names (family, friends, teachers, pets), places (*school, library, shops, toilet*), function words (*please, sorry, thank you*), foods (*drinks, soda, hamburger, cereal*), and the child's favorite things (*games, Batman, sports*). Words are chosen because they are used frequently in the child's functional communication.

2. Each week, 10 of the functional 50 words are selected for treatment. The clinician teaches the child their best production using cues or teaching the word sound by sound. If the child is unable to produce a correct production of the word, developmental errors are permissible. The child is required to practice the 10 words during the week and during therapy sessions, with a high number of responses per session. Teachers and parents are instructed to reinforce and praise the child for best word production in communication situations. The intent is to make sure that the 10 words are said the same way each time; consistency is seen as slightly more important than fully correct productions at this stage of therapy. If a child produces a word differently from their best production, the clinician imitates the child's production of the word and explains that the word was said differently, as well as how it differed from the child's best production. However, the clinician does not ask the child to imitate the target word; rather, they provide information about the best production, because when a child imitates, they can produce it "without having to assemble/generate their own plan for the word" (Dodd, Holm, et al., 2006, p. 228).

3. At the end of the twice-weekly sessions, the child is asked to produce the entire set of words three times. Words produced consistently are then removed from the list of 50 words. Inconsistently produced words remain on the list, and the next week's words are randomly chosen from the 50-word list. Once every 2 weeks, untreated words from the 50-word list are selected as probe words. The probe words are elicited three times each to monitor generalization.

Strengths and Limitations.   Because intelligibility is the overriding goal of all communication, a clear strength of this approach is that, unlike most other approaches, it focuses on that important goal. By making the child more consistent, they should be more easily understood. One limitation is that the approach is intended only for those with inconsistent speech, which constitutes a small percentage of children with SSDs. Another limitation is that the lack of detail on how to achieve consistency may be frustrating for some clinicians.

Research Support.   Dodd and colleagues have conducted a number of studies to validate this approach (Crosbie et al., 2005, 2006; Dodd et al., 2004, 2006). The highest level of treatment study available (Level IIb) appears to be that of Crosbie and colleagues (2005). These authors compared treatment using a phonological contrast approach (discrimination with either minimal pairs or multiple oppositions; the specific approach depended on the child) with a core vocabulary treatment approach. Eighteen children aged 4;8 to 6;5 with severe speech disorders received two 8-week blocks of both of the intervention treatments. All of the children increased their accuracy of percent consonants correct, as well as their consistency of production. They reported that core vocabulary intervention resulted in more positive change in children with inconsistent SSDs and that contrast therapy resulted in improved changes in children with consistent speech disorders.

Augmentative and Alternative Communication

Background Statement.   *Augmentative and alternative communication (AAC)* has long been suggested as a temporary bridge to speech in this population (Strand & Skinder, 1999). One concern that parents and some clinicians may have with using AAC systems with children who have CAS is that the child will become dependent on the system and will not be motivated to learn speech. However, Silverman (1989) cites numerous studies that suggest exactly the opposite. Even the most technologically advanced voice output systems offer slower communication than real speech because complex messages often must be preprogrammed into the system. The available evidence suggests that where speech is possible, most children will be significantly motivated to learn to use the much more efficient (i.e., faster) mode of speech.

Unique Features.   Although any number of AAC options might be proposed, the most commonly considered options in cases of CAS are electronic, voice output devices, and sign language.

Strengths and Limitations.   One obvious strength of using AAC is that it has the potential to immediately provide clear and direct communication. Intelligibility would generally not be a concern. As for limitations, electronic devices pose the challenge of cost, as well as the need for both parents and the child to learn their operation. Gestural systems such as sign language take time to learn and are only useful where the communication partner understands the system.

Research Support.   Relative to evidence for AAC in children with CAS, Murray and colleagues (2014) identified several relevant studies in their systematic review. Although Murray and colleagues concluded that, overall, the evidence for using AAC with this population was still only suggestive of positive effects, it is worth examining the specific studies. Doing so supports the notion of AAC as a bridge to real speech, since most of the studies involved teaching other aspects of language or improving communication in general.

For example, Binger and colleagues (2011) used a multiple probe design (Level IIa evidence) to study a 6-year-old child with CAS. Findings indicated that the child successfully mastered the use of her AAC device to produce the possessive, regular past, and regular plural morphemes. The data reported revealed that change on each target only began to occur once treatment of the specific morpheme was introduced. Bornman and associates (2001) presented a case study (Level III evidence) involving a voice output device and a child age 6;5 with CAS. The findings indicated an increase in both communication attempts and in the number of appropriate responses to questions over the treatment period. Three case studies (Level III evidence) involving the use of AAC for children with CAS (aged 2;7, 3;4, 12;9) were presented by Cumley and Swanson (1999), who concluded that AAC:

> ... provided them with greater opportunities for communicative success and flexibility for initiating, participating in, and repairing their communication breakdowns ... [and] afforded greater opportunities for supporting and facilitating the language development, communicative interaction, and academic success of these children. (p. 121)

Motor Approaches

CAS has been classically considered a motor-based disorder and, thus, it should not be surprising that the largest group of proposed treatment approaches focus on motor skills. However, given that traditional articulation therapy is the default motor approach of most clinicians, it is somewhat surprising that traditional articulation therapy does not appear to have been directly evaluated in the research literature (see Murray et al., 2014). On the other hand, the frequent comment that children with CAS are slow to progress in therapy may be a direct reflection of a lack of success with traditional therapy (but see also Clinical Vignette 12.1). Slow progress with traditional therapy for the child who has CAS may also reflect insufficient intensity (dose). In their systematic review of the intensity literature, Kaipa and Peterson (2016) specifically noted that children with CAS appear to require much higher doses of treatment than those with other SSDs (see also Namasivayam et al., 2015). Thus, traditional articulation therapy provided at much higher than typical intensity would be worth considering for children with CAS. For example, rather than the widely used two 30-minute sessions per week, one might provide 3–4 sessions of 1 hour long per week.

Assuming greater treatment intensity may not be practical in many situations, several other motor approaches should be considered. These include speech motor chaining (SMC), Systematic Articulation Training Program Accessing Computers (SATPAC), and concurrent treatment (each discussed in Chapter 10), as well as the following options. There is published evidence available specifically demonstrating the efficacy of both SMC (Preston, Brick, & Landi, 2013; Preston, Leece, & Maas, 2016) and concurrent treatment (Skelton & Hagiopan, 2014) in cases of CAS.

Rapid Syllable Transition Treatment

Background Statement.   A second motor approach that has research support for use with children who have CAS is called *rapid syllable transition treatment (ReST)*. In their tutorial on this approach, McCabe and colleagues (2020) describe ReST as having been developed in direct response to the ASHA position statement on CAS. The intent was to target the three emerging features of CAS (inconsistency, transitions, prosody) simultaneously, while incorporating as many of the principles of motor learning as possible. With this approach, multisyllabic nonwords are presented randomly to encourage consistent planning and practice with transitions. Nonwords (e.g., /batigu/) are used to avoid the emergence of previously stored linguistic and motor representations. Variations in syllable stress (e.g., BAtigu vs. baTIgu vs. batiGU) are used to encourage the development of normal prosody. Imitative drill is used to encourage consistency.

Unique Features.   This approach was specifically designed for use with children with CAS and is based on our understanding of this disorder. ReST also appears to be the one approach that specifically targets the inappropriate use of stress seen in many children with CAS.

According to McCabe and colleagues (2020), to begin therapy with ReST the child must have at least four different consonants and three different vowels (or diphthongs) in their phoneme inventory and be capable of combining two syllables within words. The productions need not be fully correct, but the child must at least be producing two vowels to mark the presence of the syllables. If the child is capable of producing five three-syllable word strings (again, full accuracy not required), the starting point for therapy would be three-syllable nonwords; otherwise, therapy should begin with two-syllable nonwords.

A set of 20 target nonwords are created using a combination of sounds in the child's inventory that are fully correct and others that are emerging (correct at least 10% of the time). As much as can be managed, the sounds chosen should be as different from each other as possible (e.g., consonants that differ in place, manner, and/or voicing, and vowels from different parts of the vowel space). Word-initial consonant clusters are permissible. Ten of the words would follow either a stressed-unstressed-unstressed pattern (e.g., /vatəgɚ/) or a stressed-unstressed-stressed pattern (e.g., /glɑfəbi/). The other 10 would follow either an unstressed-stressed-unstressed pattern (e.g., /təkoobə/) or an unstressed-stressed-stressed pattern (e.g., /bəgooti). Additional details on creating the nonwords can be found at https://ReST .sydney.edu.au.

During the teaching or pre-practice phase, any number of prompts, models, and feedback can be used to help the child understand the task. In this phase the child is also taught that the individual sounds must be correct, the stress must be correct, and the overall production must be smooth. The practice phase begins once the child can correctly produce any five of the target nonwords. Correctness requires accuracy of the sounds, appropriate use of stress, and smooth transitions through the entire nonword. Practice sessions include 100 imitative trials (five times through the set of 20 nonwords) at each of the following complexity levels:

> Two-syllable nonwords (if necessary)
> Three-syllable nonwords
> Carrier phrases with a single three-syllable nonword
> Carrier phrases with two different three-syllable nonwords

Progression to the next level up occurs when the child achieves 80% correct at a level over two consecutive sessions. Progress down a level occurs when the child achieves 10% correct or less over two consecutive sessions. At the carrier phrase levels all elements of the phrase must be produced correctly. Data collection for this approach should include scoring of each in terms of accuracy of the sounds, appropriateness of the use of stress, and smoothness of the production. This allows subsequent pre-practice sessions to focus on any particular aspect that is causing difficulty for the child.

Strengths and Limitations.   The main strength of this approach appears to be its goal of integrating the learning of stress along with practicing syllable transitions and motor planning. Studies of the approach have included children between 4–12 years of age, indicating it can be used with children as young as 4. The emphasis on multisyllabic targets suggests, however, that it may not be appropriate for children with CAS who are more severely involved and/or who have very limited production capabilities.

Research Support.   Several published studies have used this approach with children with CAS and three are highlighted here. Ballard and associates (2010) used it in a multiple baseline across behaviors design (Level IIa evidence) with three children aged 7;8 to 10;10 with CAS from the same family. Their speech contained few speech sound errors but was described as robotic, with limited stress variation. After the children received four 60-minute treatment sessions per week for 3 weeks, the accuracy of their productions improved from 0% correct for all three children to 38%–80% correct for the treatment targets (the youngest child had the poorest performance). Some generalization to untrained four-syllable nonwords was observed, but little change was seen in the children's production of real words.

In a second study, McCabe and colleagues (2014) presented data from an AB treatment design (Level IIb evidence) replicated across four boys aged 5;5 to 8;6 with CAS. Following 12 one-hour treatment sessions over 3 weeks, accuracy of the speech sounds and the use of stress improved on the treated nonwords for all of the children. At follow-up all four improved their correct use of stress patterns in connected real speech, but very limited change in speech sound accuracy was observed.

The highest available level evidence for ReST appears to be from a randomized controlled trial (Level Ib) by Murray, McCabe, and Ballard (2015). It involved a comparison of ReST with the *Nuffield Centre Dyspraxia Programme* (3rd ed.) (NDP3; more details in next section). A group of 26 children with CAS (aged 4–12 years) were randomly assigned to the two treatments. Each treatment was delivered via 12 1-hour sessions over a 3-week period. Results indicated that both groups made large and significant gains (from 0% up to an average of 30%–35% correct) in accuracy of the treated nonword targets, but the NDP3 group made greater gains. Both groups also showed modest but significant increases in accuracy of real words, and small but significant gains in word accuracy in connected speech. At follow-up 4 months later the ReST group showed greater maintenance of their treatment gains compared to the NDP3 group.

Together, these studies demonstrate that the ReST approach can result in improvement in speech production skill in children with CAS. Similar to the studies of SMC, the gains observed were modest but noteworthy, given the relatively small amount of treatment that had been provided. Larger doses (i.e., longer treatment periods) would likely be needed to ensure more substantial and sustained gains.

Nuffield Centre Dyspraxia Programme

Background Statement.   NDP3 was developed in Britain and first published commercially in 1985. It includes both a testing protocol and a comprehensive set of therapy stimuli (black and white drawings). The third edition of the program (NDP3) was developed by P. Williams and Stephens (2004) and is intended ". . . for children 3–7 years of age with severe SSD, particularly CAS" (P. Williams, 2021, p. 448). The primary focus is on the motor planning and programming challenge of CAS, although its authors recommend teaching discrimination and phonological awareness simultaneously. Broadly speaking, therapy with NDP3 follows a similar gradual, bottom-up treatment hierarchy to that used in traditional articulation therapy.

Unique Features.   The therapy sequence for NDP3 differs from traditional articulation therapy in at least two respects. First, nonsense syllables are not used, although contrastive sequencing of individual sounds is often used once correct production in isolation is achieved. For example, if the child can produce /p/ and has now just learned /t/, the clinician might ask them to drill sequences such as /pə, tə, pə, tə, pə, tə, pə, tə/. Therapy then moves to the word level. The often troublesome transition to the word level is managed with the second unique aspect of the NDP3 therapy sequence. The word level is specifically subdivided into several very distinct smaller steps: CV words, CVCV words, CVC words, multisyllabic words, and consonant cluster words.

As with many other motor approaches, therapy at each step begins with imitation and progresses to spontaneous production. One-hour sessions once or twice a week are recommended. The picture stimuli are typically copied and sent home for practice outside the therapy situation; thus, generalization is begun early in the therapy. Additional details on the approach can be found in P. Williams (2021).

Strengths and Limitations.   The clear structure to the therapy progression and the availability of a large bank of premade therapy stimuli are strengths of this approach. Its most obvious limitation is the limited amount of research support.

Research Support.   At least two peer-reviewed randomized controlled trials (Level Ib evidence) involving children with CAS have been published that examined NDP3. The first was the study by Murray, McCabe, and Ballard (2015), discussed previously, which compared it to ReST. As noted, the findings indicated that 12 hours of treatment with NDP3 over a 3-week period resulted in noticeable speech sound improvement.

The second study was a matched group design by McKechnie and colleagues (2020). It included 14 children with CAS aged 4–10 years who were first matched by age and sex and the resulting matched pairs were then randomly assigned to two groups. Both groups received the intervention via a tablet-based version of NDP3; one group received only knowledge of performance (KP) feedback, whereas the other received only knowledge of results (KR) feedback. All attended 12-hour long sessions spread over 3 weeks. Both groups improved significantly, with average gains of 13.9% and 9.0% accuracy on generalization (untreated) items by the end of treatment. Gains were also not significantly different from findings obtained with the table-top version of the approach (average gains of 10.3%), as reported by Murray, McCabe, and Ballard (2015). Together, these studies suggest that both versions of the NDP3 approach can be effective for children with CAS.

Dynamic Temporal and Tactile Cueing

Background Statement.   This motor-based approach is what has been historically called *integral stimulation.* According to Strand (2020), *dynamic temporal and tactile cueing (DTTC)* uses repeated practice trials and . . . aids the development and refinement of motor programming by providing auditory and visual models, shaping the movement through slowed rate and visual and tactile cues as needed, providing feedback about the movement . . . to facilitate learning and retention (pp. 31–32).

Unique Features.   DTTC uses principles of motor learning and is based on the child watching, listening to, and imitating the clinician. The approach makes no specific assumptions about the underlying deficit (language formulation, motor planning, articulation), but is thought to be appropriate for children with severe forms of SSDs and/or if there is evidence that motor planning difficulties are involved (i.e., CAS). The term temporal in the name is derived from the timing between clinician input and the child's response. It assumes a temporal hierarchy ranging from simultaneous (choral) production through direct imitation to delayed imitation and finally, to spontaneous production. Tactile cueing is incorporated if needed. The overall goal is to eventually transition to other treatment methods for SSDs (Strand, 2020). These might include traditional articulation therapy or SMC.

As for treatment targets, coarticulation and motor planning are incorporated from the beginning. Strand (2020) notes that "DTTC does not focus on the production of a consonant or the linguistic elements of the phoneme but rather on the movement and prosodic accuracy of the syllable as a whole" (p. 40). Early targets could include vowels, particularly where they are being distorted. The sounds should be targeted in functional real words wherever possible. Treatment begins with direct imitation at a slightly slower than normal rate. If the child is not producing the correct response, simultaneous (choral) productions are introduced. Failure at this level would mean the clinician should slow the rate of the production even further and, if necessary, add tactile cues.

According to Strand and colleagues (2006), the tactile cues (if used) involve the clinician physically helping the child achieve the correct lip and jaw positions to begin the movements. After holding that position for a few moments to experience self-feedback, the child and clinician produce the target simultaneously. An additional substep that may be required is to have the child and clinician produce the movements (without any sound) simultaneously, then whispered versions and, eventually, fully voiced versions of the target can be introduced. Once the child achieves consistently correct versions of the targets in simultaneous production, the clinician reverts to direct imitation. Rate is then slowly increased to normal, and variations in prosody (e.g., application of different syllable or word stress) and rate are added. As the child achieves success, delayed imitation is added (delays of up to 3 seconds). Spontaneous production is then gradually introduced. It is worth noting that DTTC is not intended for long-term use (i.e., less than a year of treatment sessions 3–4 times per week). Additional details of the approach are outlined in tutorial form in Strand (2020).

Strengths and Limitations. Similar to traditional articulation therapy, DTTC offers considerable structure for the clinician in the treatment of CAS. It also takes advantage of the fact that many children with CAS (like individuals who stutter) may initially do better in choral activities than spontaneously. This offers the potential for immediate success with children whose poor communication skills may have led to considerable frustration. The heavy reliance on imitation, however, may not be particularly attractive to clinicians or parents who prefer more client-centered approaches. Likewise, some children may balk at engaging in direct imitation activities.

Research Support. At least six published studies support the use of DTTC with children who have CAS. Four examples here will illustrate. Strand and Debertine (2000) (Level IIb evidence) presented a multiple baseline across behaviors study of a 5-year-old girl with CAS. Her speech was described as roughly 10% understandable when context was known. Two years of previous treatment had produced little progress. Targets and control probes included functional words and phrases (e.g., "Hi dad," "I don't know."). Each was rated on a 3-point scale (0 = unintelligible, 1 = intelligible but containing errors, 2 = no errors). As treatment was introduced, performance on targeted items improved rapidly from 0 to an average of 1.5 or above. Performance on control items improved but never averaged higher than 1.0, suggesting that the treatment was working. No generalization data were provided.

Edeal and Gildersleeve-Neumann (2011) used DTTC in an AB design (Level IIb) repeated across two children (aged 6 and 3 years, respectively) with CAS. For each child, four or five different consonants were targeted in simple word shapes (CV, VC, CVCV, CVC). One child received 32 treatment sessions (40 minutes each) and his percentage correct on the treated targets improved from 25% to 73%. Some generalization to untrained words containing the target sounds. The other child received 12 treatment sessions and improved his percentage correct from 21% to 32%. For both children, change did not begin until the introduction of treatment. Some generalization to untreated target words was observed for both. No control data were reported.

Two additional Level IIb studies (Maas et al., 2012; Maas & Farinella, 2012) demonstrated the successful application of DTTC with four children with CAS (aged 5–8 years). Both examined aspects of motor-learning principles for treating this population. In the first study, contrary to findings from the motor-learning literature, Maas and Farinella showed no clear advantage for random presentation (i.e., where stimuli are practiced in random order) over blocked practice (i.e., where a single stimulus is repeated a specified number of times in a row). Two of the children responded better to blocked practice, one responded better to random practice, and one did not respond well to either practice schedule. The second study (Maas et al.) reported findings for feedback frequency that, again, did not fully support what is reported from research on motor learning.

As mentioned earlier in this chapter, using feedback that is not continuous offers the potential advantage that children are able to internally reflect on their own feedback (i.e., what they felt and what they heard) to facilitate their own learning. However, in the Maas and colleagues (2012) study, one child showed an advantage (i.e., appeared to progress more) under high frequency continuous feedback (feedback provided for every attempt), two children showed an advantage with less frequent feedback (randomly provided for 60% of attempts; a variable ratio schedule), and one showed no advantage under either condition. It is not clear at this point where the conflicting findings for these aspects of motor learning are specific to CAS or might apply to other types of speech and language disorders.

Together, findings from these studies, along with findings in Baas and colleagues (2008) and Strand and colleagues (2006), suggest that DTTC can be used to improve speech production in children with CAS. Additional study is warranted, with a particular eye to looking at long-term outcomes.

PROMPTS for Restructuring Oral Muscular Phonetic Targets

Background Statement.   A therapy approach that has long been suggested for CAS (but has been the subject of limited formal study) is the motor approach known as *PROMPTS for Restructuring Oral Muscular Phonetic Targets (PROMPT)*. It draws on several theoretical perspectives, including dynamic systems theory, neuronal group selection theory, and motor-learning theories. Detailed elaboration of how these theories relate to PROMPT is beyond the scope of this text, but can be found in Hayden and colleagues (2021).

Unique Features.   The PROMPT approach was originally developed by Chumpelik (1984) and is quite unique in its focus on jaw height, facial-labial contraction, tongue height and advancement, muscular tension, duration of contractions, and air stream management for phoneme production. It also includes various hands-on prompts or physical stimulation cues made on the client's face that are reminiscent of aspects of the moto-kinesthetic approach of Young and Hawk (1955). The use of such stimulation is shared with DTTC, but it is more central to the PROMPT approach (i.e., it is used only as an additional layer of support in DTTC when other aspects of the approach are not successful). Another unique aspect of PROMPT is that the complexity of the approach has motivated its proponents to develop highly structured clinician training programs for its implementation.

Strengths and Limitations.   With its emphasis on tactile and kinesthetic feedback, this approach has the potential to refocus the attention of both the clinician and the child onto aspects of production not often considered in much detail. This refocus may be particularly important because (as noted earlier) children with CAS appear to be less able to take advantage of their own tactile or kinesthetic feedback (see Iuzzini-Seigal et al., 2015) and/or the support provided with more traditional approaches. Relative to limitations, as it is described, PROMPT is a complex approach that may be difficult for some busy clinicians to implement. Perhaps its most significant limitation is the requirement for clinicians to participate in relatively elaborate training regimes. This may present serious financial and/or scheduling barriers for many school-based clinicians. It also makes it more difficult for independent researchers to fully evaluate the approach's details.

Research Support.   A summary presented in Hayden and colleagues (2021) suggests that this approach may be effective for other types of SSDs. Relative to CAS, only one peer-reviewed study (Dale & Hayden, 2013) appears to have been published. These investigators evaluated whether the overall PROMPT approach was effective and whether the specific inclusion of ". . . tactile-kinesthetic-proprioceptive (TKP) cues to support and shape movements of the oral articulators" (p. 644) was particularly beneficial. Four children with CAS aged 3;6 to 4;8 were randomly assigned to two groups (Level Ib evidence). Following initial baseline sessions, two children received 8 weeks of the full PROMPT approach, while the other two children received 4 weeks of PROMPT without the use of the TKP cues, followed by 4 weeks of the full PROMPT treatment. Single word intelligibility improved from 36% to 58%, 37% to 55%, 22% to 53%, and 5% to 24% for the four participants across the 8 weeks of the study. The speech of the children who did not receive TKP cues in the first 4 weeks appeared to improve to a greater extent following the introduction of the cues. Dale and Hayden suggested this was ". . . modest evidence for an additional effect of TKP cues" (p. 658). It is difficult to make strong conclusions based on a single study, but the findings are interesting. PROMPT may be useful for treating CAS, but more study is needed.

Phonological Approaches

The challenge with planning and programming for higher levels of speech and language that has been suggested for children with CAS would justify considering linguistically based treatment approaches that target the speech sound system. At least one such approach has been proposed and is discussed here.

Integrated Phonological Awareness Intervention

Background Statement.   The review by Murray and colleagues (2014) suggested that there was sufficient evidence to support the use of one linguistic approach, the *integrated phonological awareness intervention (IPAI),* for children with CAS (Moriarty

& Gillon, 2006). The main focus of this approach is phoneme-level phonological awareness activities (e.g., segmentation and blending, letter naming). There is also a simultaneous focus on production, as the specific words used in treatment are selected to
represent one or more of a client's speech production error patterns. When production
errors occur during the awareness activities, Moriarty and Gillon reported that:

> ...the researcher aided the child to identify the error and then used the coloured block or
> letter block as a prompt for speech production. For example, if Katie said "top" instead of
> "stop," it would be cued via the following method. "You said 'top' but I can see a /s/ sound
> at the start of the word (pointing to the s letter block). Try the word again with a /s/ sound
> at the start." The children did not receive any articulatory prompts regarding place or
> manner of production of the target sounds. (p. 723)

Unique Features.   The most unique aspect of IPAI is the linkage between the language system and the speech motor system by combining phonological awareness
with child-specific production targets. Thus, the child is learning about the phonological functions of the sounds in the language, while at the same time practicing and
receiving feedback about their productions. Additional details about the approach are
available in McNeill and Gillon (2021).

Strengths and Limitations.   Addressing the underlying foundations of written
language is a particular strength of IPAI, given children with CAS are at risk for difficulty with reading and spelling (Gillon & Moriarty, 2007). The descriptions provided,
however, suggest that (like ReST) it might be not be appropriate for the most severely
involved children who have very limited production skills.

Research Support.   Evidence supporting the use of IPAI in general is summarized in McNeill and Gillon (2021). Evidence for its use with CAS comes from
at least two published studies. Moriarty and Gillon (2006) used an AB design
repeated across three children with CAS aged 6;3 to 7;3 (Level IIb evidence). Treatment included three 45-minute treatment sessions per week for 3 weeks. Two of
the children showed improved percentage phonemes correct in conversation (53%
to 92%, 60% to 100%). The third child showed limited improvement (20% to 32%).
All three showed significant improvement in phonological awareness skills.
Generalization to untrained items was observed, as was improved nonword reading performance.

A second study by McNeill and colleagues (2009) used similar procedures but
included 12 children with CAS aged 4–7 years (Level IIb evidence). Two different speech
production error patterns were targeted for each child. Treatment sessions were twice a
week for 45 minutes, with 6 weeks focused on target 1 followed by 6 weeks of no treatment
and then 6 weeks focused on target 2. Nine of the 12 children improved their production of
treatment words for both targets, and 6/12 generalized to untrained words. Nine children
generalized from the first target to connected speech, and four children also generalized
from the second target to connected speech. Nine of the 12 children showed significant
gains in phonological awareness for at least one of the error targets.

Treatment Recommendations for Childhood Apraxia of Speech

Although the treatment literature for children with CAS has been expanding in
recent years, it is still too early to make specific recommendations. As noted previously, there is now published evidence to support several promising approaches.

Choosing which particular approach to use remains a significant challenge because few direct comparison studies of the different treatments have been conducted.

Preliminary suggestions are possible. The previous discussion suggests that some of the available approaches may be more appropriate for particular subsets of the CAS population. For example, perhaps highly structured approaches such as NDP3, DTTC, or PROMPT may be better suited to younger children and/or those with the most severe CAS involvement (i.e., those with the most limited production abilities). Approaches such as more intensive traditional therapy, SMC, ReST, or IPAI may then be more appropriate for older children and/or for milder cases of CAS.

TREATING OLDER CHILDREN

The second specific population to be discussed is older children (or those with residual or persistent errors). Recall from Chapter 9 that this includes children aged 7 years and older. Despite making many of the adjustments discussed for this group in Chapter 9, clinicians continue to report ongoing frustration with progress in therapy. Let us consider this age group more closely. Whether as a result of normal speech development, SLP intervention, or some combination thereof, it has been shown that the speech production skill of children with SSDs improves as they get older. Recall from Chapter 1 how the prevalence of SSDs declines from 15.6% at age 3 years to 11% at age 4 years and 3.8% at age 6 years. While progress continues well into middle and high school for most of these children, a review by Flipsen (2015) suggested that by adulthood, 1%–2% of the population continues to produce distortion errors on one or two sounds in their everyday speech.

Two perspectives are possible to explain these outcome data. First, approximately 90% of SSDs appear to resolve (i.e., normalize) between age 3 years and adulthood. This represents a substantial amount of change. On the other hand, it is worth asking why some children with SSDs never fully normalize their speech. The nature of the errors being produced may offer some insight. Data on 8-year-olds from the United Kingdom (Wren et al., 2016) indicate that of those children who are still producing errors, about 69% are only producing common distortions (e.g., dentalized /s, z/, derhotacized /r/). For those children, at least two reasons for a failure to normalize speech sound productions might be proposed. First, there is likely to be little or no communicative impact because distortions of a single speech sound rarely interfere with message intelligibility. Second, a single distortion error is unlikely to have a negative impact on academic performance or social acceptance. The net result may be limited motivation for these children to change their speech behavior. They may also not want to participate in therapy in order to avoid being singled out for attending speech services. Finally, some of these children may have attended therapy for a long time. As such, they may be suffering from therapy fatigue and, quite understandably, may simply want it to be over.

On the other hand, some children with only common distortion errors may be quite motivated to attend therapy because of the social stigma associated with the errors themselves. Studies of peer reactions to such errors in teenagers (Crowe-Hall, 1991; Silverman & Paulus, 1989) indicate that such a stigma may be significant. Findings from a survey by Hitchcock and McAllister Byun (2015b) suggests that social stigma toward a child may be sufficient to motivate parental referrals for extra services. Parents who had requested treatment for 91 children with residual or persistent

/r/ errors made such referrals primarily on the basis of concern about a negative social stigma related to such errors. Parents may also be motivated by an appreciation or awareness that some adults have reduced expectations for their children and do not want them to be in that category. Such differences in expectations have been documented in at least one study (Overby et al., 2007).

Data from the remaining 31% of 8-year-olds studied by Wren and colleagues (2016) indicate a more significant problem. These children continued to produce omissions, substitutions, additions, or atypical distortions significantly more often than their peers. For these children, the reasons for failure to normalize their errors are more difficult to ascertain. Reduced motivation may or may not be an issue. It should be pointed out, however, that both intelligibility and academics may well be impacted by their continuing sound errors.

Regardless of their level of motivation, a failure to normalize speech sound productions may relate to the fact that by age 7 years many of the errors being produced have become well-established habits. Breaking such habits likely requires focus and a willingness to engage in a lot of practice. The failure to normalize may also reflect the nature of the services being provided. Perhaps our current approaches are not as efficient as they might be with older children. This suggests the need for either a higher level of treatment intensity or some sort of alternative approach. These options will be addressed next.

SPECIFIC TREATMENT OPTIONS FOR OLDER CHILDREN

According to Brumbaugh and Smit (2013), traditional articulation therapy is the most common therapy approach used for SSDs. It is therefore likely the most common approach used not only with younger children, but for older children as well. However, there are at least two reasons to suggest a change in the approach for older children. First, the fact that many of these children are still in therapy after a prolonged period suggests that what has been done so far is not the optimum treatment approach. Second, as noted earlier, the errors being produced at this age have now become long-established habits. Breaking such habits may also require doing something different.

As with younger children, the nature of the problem needs to be considered. Recall that approximately 31% of 8-year-olds who have not yet normalized their speech continue to produce omission, substitution, addition, and uncommon distortion errors (Wren et al., 2016). Recall also that Shriberg, Kwiatkowski, et al. (2019) suggested that omission errors in particular may reflect a cognitive-linguistic problem. Assuming that is true, one or more of the linguistically based approaches described in Chapter 11 may be appropriate for such errors. For children who are producing distortion errors (whether common or uncommon), it is generally assumed that distortion errors reflect motor-learning issues. Thus, in addition to options from Chapter 10, one or more of the motor approaches discussed in this chapter may be appropriate for those errors. For children with both kinds of errors, both motor-based and linguistically based approaches may be used, with each approach focused on particular types of sound errors.

It should be noted that some of the approaches or aids to be discussed next need not be limited to older children and may be applied to other populations. Heng and colleagues (2016), for example, have demonstrated that ultrasound can be used effectively with preschool children. Further, Cleland and associates (2009) provided findings suggesting that electropalatography (EPG) can be used with individuals with Down syndrome.

Modifications to Traditional Therapy

Several different modifications are possible with traditional therapy that may make it more effective with older children. The first, which was mentioned earlier, is an increase in treatment intensity. This might include providing more sessions per week or having longer sessions. Another approach would be to condense therapy duration into a shorter period of time, as is sometimes done with adults who stutter. Preston and Leece (2017) explored the potential benefit of condensing 14 hours of treatment into a single week in a series of case studies (Level III evidence). Four participants aged 13–22 years with /r/ errors received a combination of auditory perceptual training, structured motor practice, and ultrasound feedback in a 1-week block. They reported that average accuracy improved from 35% to 83% at the word level and from 11% to 66% at the sentence level. Such rapid results suggest that short-term intensive treatment may be worth considering.

Given the busy caseloads of many clinicians serving school-age children, an increase in intensity may not be practical. The alternative would be to use the current service delivery pace, but consider modifications to the way traditional therapy is organized or delivered to make it more efficient. Several possible modifications (speech motor chaining, concurrent treatment, SATPAC) were discussed in Chapter 10.

Modified Feedback Approaches

Another option for older children may be to make changes to the feedback provided to them. As discussed in Chapter 2, speakers receive various kinds of feedback, including feedback from themselves (tactile, proprioceptive, kinesthetic, auditory) while they are speaking, and external feedback from others about whether the intended message or targets were understood. Speakers might also get negative external feedback about specific errors they produce. In therapy, clients also receive external feedback from the clinician regarding the accuracy of production (KR), what they might be doing wrong (KP), and/or what they might do to produce the target correctly (corrective feedback). The following approaches include those in which the client would receive a different kind of feedback, namely that from a mechanical or electronic device or system.

The use of instrumental support creates additional clinical challenges. First, the child must spend time becoming oriented to the device or system. Second, and perhaps more importantly, these approaches represent only feedback and do not necessarily include any formal therapy structure per se. As such, they need to be incorporated into some other treatment framework. It is quite common for them to be paired with some form of motor-based intervention. A third challenge is a concern that the child will become overly reliant on the feedback. To avoid this, a plan to systematically fade out the use of the instrumentation must be created at the outset to ensure that the new skills being learned are transferred to everyday speech absent the feedback.

Tactile Feedback Approaches

In Chapter 4, we discussed some evidence suggesting that some children with SSDs have poorer tactile sensitivity inside their oral cavities compared to their typically speaking peers. Ruscello (1972) reported that such sensitivity improved in some of these children following treatment for their speech errors. This would suggest that there may be some benefit to therapy approaches that incorporate supplemental tactile feedback.

Speech Buddies®

Many clinicians employ tongue blades, cotton-tip applicators, tweezers with ice chips, and other such ad hoc aids to provide supplemental tactile feedback to their clients. Such aids may also be employed to generally increase intraoral awareness. However, the evidence for the efficacy of such aids remains anecdotal at best. Recently, however, a set of devices was specifically developed to provide supplemental tactile feedback during speech intervention.

Background Statement.   These devices were developed through the collaborative efforts of two friends; one was an SLP and the other was a medical device engineer. They created five separate devices, one for each of /s, ʃ, tʃ, l, r/ (available separately or as a set). Each Speech Buddy® has a handle that the clinician or the child holds onto and the opposite end is inserted into the mouth. Each device also has a dental stop on it that is placed against the teeth to ensure it is positioned correctly. For /s, ʃ, tʃ, l/, the portion of the device that extends into the mouth provides a consistent point of contact for the tongue to rest against and provide correct place of articulation. In the case of /r/ the portion in the mouth is a coil of flexible material that the child unrolls with the tongue tip to generate the correct movement and positioning for retroflex /r/. More information on the devices and their use is available at https://www.speechbuddy.com/.

Unique Features.   Unlike devices such as tongue depressors, cotton swabs, or straws that SLPs try to use to provide supplemental tactile input, Speech Buddies® were specifically designed for use in speech remediation. Each device was also specifically designed with one particular speech sound in mind. Parents can purchase them for use in home practice.

Strengths and Limitations.   The materials and manufacturing processes for Speech Buddies® have been evaluated and found to be safe to use with children. They are registered as Class I medical devices with the U.S. Food and Drug Administration. The fact that they were each designed for a specific speech sound means it also minimizes any potential confusion on the part of the child as to what is to be done. One potential limitation is cost, which may be a barrier in some settings. A more notable limitation is that each is only useful for one sound and there are currently no devices for other common error sounds such as /k/ or /f/.

Research Support.   Two peer-reviewed studies provide some support for the efficacy of Speech Buddies®. Rogers (2013) conducted a case study (Level III evidence) on an 8-year-old boy who had problems with /r/. After eight 25-minute sessions over 7 weeks he improved his accuracy in words and sentences from 20% to 90%. The second study was a randomized controlled trial (Level Ib evidence) conducted by Rogers and Chesin (2013), which included 15 children aged 5–8 years with /s/ errors. Eight children received Speech Buddies® treatment and seven received traditional articulation therapy. All children received eight 25-minute individual treatment sessions. At the end of treatment the gains for the two groups were significantly different. The average word accuracy for the Speech Buddies® group improved from 0% to 74%, whereas it only improved from 2% to 45% for the traditional therapy group.

Visual Feedback Approaches

For some children, putting a device into the mouth may be unacceptable. Also, in some cases, additional tactile feedback may be insufficient to generate change. Another alternative is visual feedback. This is already available in traditional therapy to a limited extent. Clinicians often ask clients to watch what they do or have clients observe themselves in a mirror. However, although such visual information is available for sounds involving the bilabial, labiodental, interdental (and perhaps alveolar) places of articulation, it is not available for most other speech sounds, such as those produced at the palate, velum, or glottis.

At least three treatment approaches are currently available that provide some type of visual feedback for sounds produced within the oral cavity. As with tactile feedback, the presence of novel feedback and/or the use of instrumentation may provide additional motivation to participate in therapy. It may also offer enough of a different perspective on what is happening to modify long-established habits. These instrumental visual approaches all share one major advantage over both tactile feedback and typical visual feedback. In contrast to brief tactile feedback or the transitory image on the clinician's face or in a mirror, they can provide a permanent visual record of what was produced. This allows the clinician to carefully review what happened with the child or a parent. These records can also be used as visual reminders about change that may or may not be occurring. In addition, all three of the following approaches allow clinician models to be generated and stored for comparison purposes.

Visual Acoustic Feedback

Background Statement.   The oldest of the visual feedback approaches, *acoustic feedback,* has been around since the 1940s. Until recently, its use was largely confined to research labs and university clinics; however, advances in computer software have meant that free software is now available that operates on most laptop computers (e.g., PRAAT; Boersma & Weenink, 2021), making their use much more clinically applicable. Numerous online demonstrations and websites are also now available to aid in interpretation.

Traditionally, acoustic feedback has taken the form of spectrograms, which present a display of frequency on the vertical axis and time on the horizontal axis. Amplitude (or loudness) is also represented by the degree of lightness or darkness of the image. There has been a long-standing concern, however, that such displays are somewhat crowded and difficult to interpret. They also are unable to show what is happening in real-time, but rather represent what has recently happened (i.e., there is always some time delay). More recently, linear predictive coding (LPC) displays have been utilized, which display amplitude on the vertical axis and frequency on the horizontal axis. There is a single line shown (i.e., it is far less busy than a spectrogram) and the image changes in real time as the articulators move.

Unique Features.   Both spectrograms and LPC displays provide a visual representation of the acoustic output of the speaker. Both are especially useful for visualizing resonant sounds like /r/ and /l/, which have clear formant structure. Spectrograms may also be used for obstruent target sounds like /s, tʃ, k/.

Strengths and Limitations.   A notable strength of spectrograms is that speech at several levels of linguistic complexity can be analyzed. LPC displays are usually most useful for sound-level productions. Unlike tactile approaches or EPG (to be discussed next), neither requires anything to be placed in the mouth that might interfere with normal articulation. Their major limitation, however, is the abstract nature of what is being displayed. With spectrograms in particular it may be difficult for some children to make a clear association between what they see on the display and what is happening inside their mouths. Because LPC displays offer real-time feedback, the child is able to immediately see the impact of any changes they make in their mouth. Clinicians unfamiliar with interpreting these displays may also need to revisit their training in basic speech science to learn to apply them in the clinic. Some online tutorials are available.

Research Support.   Several older studies have been conducted using spectrographic feedback. Reports for individuals who are deaf (e.g., Ertmer et al., 1996; Ertmer & Maki, 2000; Stark, 1971) have demonstrated its effectiveness. One of the larger studies was conducted by Stark (1972) (Level Ib), who included 16 children at a school for the deaf who were trained to make the voiced–voiceless distinction /ba-pa/. Half of the children were randomly assigned to receive spectrographic feedback and half were trained with conventional measures (no details were provided). Each received six 10–15 minute treatment sessions. Both groups improved, but the improvement was greater in the visual feedback group. Using voice onset time (VOT) measurements, production accuracy of /ba/ did not change for either group, but both improved their accuracy of /pa/. Testing at 6–8 weeks after the end of treatment showed that the visual feedback group average had improved from 10% to 59% correct, which was twice the change in the no visual feedback group, whose average improved from 15% to 35% correct. In addition, several older single cases (Level III evidence) have been published (Ruscello, Shuster, et al., 1991; Shuster et al., 1992; Shuster et al., 1995) showing that spectrographic feedback can result in speech sound improvement.

More recently, at least three studies using LPC displays have been reported. McAllister Byun and Hitchcock (2012) studied 11 children aged 6–11 years who had failed to resolve /r/ errors with traditional treatment. Using a multiple baseline across participants design with random assignment (Level Ib evidence), they received 4–6 weeks of traditional treatment followed by 4–6 weeks of visual acoustic (LPC) feedback. Only 2 of the 11 participants showed improvement following traditional treatment. Eight of the 11 showed improvement on treated words within the acoustic treatment sessions, and 4 of those generalized to untreated words.

In 2016, McAllister Byun and colleagues conducted a multiple baseline across participants study (Level IIa evidence) with nine children aged 6–13 years with /r/ errors. All received 8 weeks of visual acoustic (LPC) feedback (16 sessions) and six of the nine showed some improvement on at least one of /r, ɝ, ɚ/. Finally, McAllister Byun and Campbell (2016) reported on a multiple baseline across participants study with random assignment (Level Ib evidence). Eleven participants aged 9–15 years received both traditional and visual acoustic (LPC) treatment (20 total sessions). They were randomly assigned to receive either traditional treatment first or visual acoustic feedback first. Seven participants showed meaningful improvement overall; both treatment types resulted in change, but larger treatment effects were observed when visual acoustic feedback was provided first.

Together, these studies suggest that visual acoustic feedback using both spectrograms and LPC displays can be an effective aid for remediating speech sound errors.

Electropalatography

Background Statement.   This approach, also called palatography or EPG, involves creating images of how the tongue contacts the palate during speech. Although this has been of interest since at least 1803 (see Fletcher, 1992), work by Fletcher and others in the 1970s and 1980s led to the development of the modern version of this approach. It involves creating a custom mouthpiece that covers the palate called an *artificial palate* or *pseudopalate*. This appliance has a series of small pressure sensors embedded within it that are connected to small wires. The wires extend out one corner of the mouth and are connected to a computer. When the child speaks, their tongue contacts the sensors, and there is an image created on the computer screen showing the pattern of contact along the upper teeth and palate. The clinician can have an artificial palate created for themself that can then be used to generate a model of what the pattern of contact should look like for particular speech sounds. The child is instructed to move their tongue around to create the right pattern of contact, which will be shown on the computer screen.

Unique Features.   Unlike visual acoustic methods, which show only the acoustic effect of the child's production, EPG offers a more direct window into what the tongue is doing to create that acoustic effect. It allows the child and the clinician to see specifically where the tongue is as it creates constrictions in the oral cavity. Modern versions of these systems provide the feedback in real time. As a consequence, this type of feedback will likely be much easier to relate to for many children than spectrograms or LPC displays. At least two different manufacturers currently produce these devices (see Rose Medical at http://rose-medical.com/electropalatography.html and Complete Speech at https://completespeech.com/).

Strengths and Limitations.   Being able to directly see where the tongue is contacting the palate represents a huge advancement compared to either asking our clients to describe what is happening or trying to visualize from the outside. The most recent software developments also mean that (unlike older systems that allowed for single snapshots) the image changes in real time so the clinician and child can watch how the tongue moves from one position to another.

Cost may still be a limitation for many clinicians, but may be manageable in some settings. Previously, constructing a pseudopalate could cost $1,000 or more per patient; the cost is now often less than $300. At least one manufacturer then requires nominal monthly fees for access to cloud-based software that generates the images and can store client data. The biggest limitation remains the need to have something artificial in the mouth during speech, which has the potential to adversely affect production. Another limitation is that because it measures tongue to palate contact, it would have limited application for work on sounds that involve little to no palate contact, such as /r/. A final limitation is that the pseudopalates are custom made and, thus, can be used only for a single client.

Research Support.   EPG appears to have been the most frequently studied of the visual approaches. Gibbon and Wood (2010) suggest that at least 150 reports of EPG being applied to a variety of different speech-disordered populations are available. Until very recently none has been above Level III (i.e., all involved case studies). A few examples of EPG studies for children with SSDs are presented here to illustrate the findings with this approach.

Carter and Edwards (2004) conducted a post hoc review of 10 cases of children with SSDs of unknown origin, aged 7–14 years, who had been treated with EPG for a variety of speech sound targets. After 10 weeks of treatment, a significant improvement was found in overall consonant accuracy, as well as in specific target sound accuracy in a single-word probe task. McAuliffe and Cornwell (2008) reported findings for an 11-year-old girl treated with EPG for lateralized /s, z/. After 4 weeks of direct therapy with an SLP and 6 weeks of home practice (using a portable EPG unit), she was producing normal versions of the targets (without the artificial palate in place) as determined by listener ratings and acoustic analysis.

Despite the positive result, analysis of EPG displays suggested only minimal change in the pattern of tongue contact with the artificial palate in place. Dagenais and associates (1994) also reported a similar outcome of normal production of /s/ (previously lateralized), but abnormal tongue contact for an 8-year-old girl. This latter study also reported no noticeable improvement with EPG for a second child despite 28 treatment sessions. Thus, outcomes with EPG, although quite promising, are not universally positive.

The vast majority of studies using EPG have focused on obstruent errors. Owing to limited tongue-to-palate contact for /r/, there have been few studies for that sound. However, since tongue bracing along the upper back teeth does appear to occur for a bunched /r/ production, EPG feedback has been regarded as appropriate for such sound errors. Hitchcock and colleagues (2017) examined the use of EPG for /r/ remediation using a multiple baseline across participants design with random assignment (Level Ib evidence). Five children aged 6–9 years were included and they received 16, 30-minute sessions over 8 weeks. Four children were able to produce correct /r/ during the sessions and two generalized to untreated words.

Ultrasound Visual Feedback

Background Statement.   This is the newest of the alternative approaches and borrows directly from obstetrics and other branches of medicine in creating live (and recordable) images of the tongue moving within the mouth and pharynx. The probe is positioned under the chin and directed upward. Although discussion of the details is outside the scope of the current text, this technology has also allowed us to learn more about aspects of normal speech production not previously obtainable, such as constrictions within the pharynx (Boyce, 2015).

Unique Features.   Ultrasound provides by far the most direct visual feedback currently available by showing the tongue in motion during speech. Images can be observed in real time and saved for later review. Research and clinical activity using this instrumentation has largely been focused on the production of /r/. The ability to visualize the tongue during production of /r/ has been particularly appealing, given the challenges many clinicians report trying to remediate this sound. In addition, the fact that the tongue makes little contact with other structures during /r/ production would appear to offer an advantage for this approach over EPG. The probe can be positioned to provide a lateral view of the head, which provides the best image for /r/. Recently, researchers have realized that rotating the ultrasound probe 90 degrees yields a coronal view, whereby tongue shapes for /s/ can also be examined. A clinician resource manual has been developed by Cleland and colleagues (2018) and is available at https://strathprints.strath.ac.uk/63372/.

Strengths and Limitations.   The major strength of this approach is that, similar to EPG, the client can see directly what the tongue is doing while they are speaking. Another strength is that, similar to acoustic feedback, it works without the need to place anything inside the mouth that might interfere with normal speech production. The possibility of undesired side effects would represent a limitation for using ultrasound. However, a survey of 62 participants in ultrasound studies (and their parents) by Preston and colleagues (2018) found that all reported concerns were very minor (e.g., slight soreness of the chin, coldness of the gel used).

One major limitation that remains is cost, with portable units costing approximately $5,000, although there is some indication that pricing for such units is decreasing. One approach to the cost issue has been to have regional centers where such instrumentation is available, along with clinicians with specific training to use this technology. Centers presently available (e.g., University of Cincinnati, New York University) have focused on remediation of the difficult-to-teach /r/. Having instrumentation available at central locations that would offer supplemental sessions used in conjunction with ongoing therapy is a possible direction for the future. Such an approach might minimize part of the final limitation of ultrasound, which is that many clinicians have limited experience with using and/or interpreting the information provided.

Research Support.   Evidence is beginning to accumulate for the efficacy of ultrasound. A systematic review by Sugden and associates (2019) identified 29 different studies that have used this approach. Most of the studies involved small samples (almost half were single case studies) and consisted of lower level evidence. The review authors concluded that ultrasound feedback ". . . can facilitate acquisition of a range of lingual speech targets for some individuals with SSD but that it does not always lead to generalization" (p. 9). The challenges with generalization underscore the earlier comment that a specific plan for generalization is necessary when using all forms of instrumental feedback in therapy.

A few studies are highlighted here to illustrate the nature of the outcomes obtained with ultrasound feedback. One of the first studies was that of Adler-Bock and associates (2007), who treated two adolescents who had long-standing difficulty with /r/. Results of this Level III study showed significant improvement in the percentage of /r/ productions judged as accurate by uninvolved SLP listeners. Subjective judgments of the ultrasound images also suggested more accurate tongue shapes during /r/ production post-treatment. Bernhardt and colleagues (2008) (Level III evidence) provided supplemental sessions to traditional speech therapy sessions for 13 school-age children. The ultrasound images provided both the children and their treating clinicians with specific feedback about activity in the vocal tract. The investigators reported significantly improved /r/ accuracy for 11 of the children following the supplemental sessions.

A report by McAllister Byun and colleagues (2014; Level IIa evidence) included two studies of ultrasound, each involving four children (eight total). This is one of the few studies that included some children under age 10 years (age range 6;1 to 15;8). The first study attempted to teach the children to use a bunched /r/ target and showed limited change. In the second study, the four children (age range 7;8 to 15;8) were encouraged to explore various tongue movements to try to achieve a normal /r/. All four showed significantly improved /r/ productions. A study by Preston and colleagues (2014; Level IIa evidence) differed from the previous ones in one important respect.

It included some children with multiple errors, thus allowing for greater control over extraneous effects.

As mentioned earlier, one of the challenges for clinicians wanting to demonstrate that their treatment works with older children is that if there is only one error sound, there are no control sounds to use. Most participants in the Preston and colleagues (2014) study showed a positive response to the treatment and generalized to untreated words containing the target. Where available, there was little to no change on the untreated control sounds. The poorest outcome was reported for the oldest participant (age 20 years), whose errors would have been the most strongly habituated. This study was also one of the few reports that has successfully applied this technology to targets sounds beyond /r/ (e.g., /s/).

Finally, a 2019 study by Preston, McAllister, and colleagues compared traditional treatment with ultrasound in a multiple baseline across participants format (Level Ib evidence). Six children aged 9–14 years with /r/ errors received eight sessions of traditional therapy followed by 8 weeks of ultrasound therapy. Another six children received the two treatments in reverse order. For both groups, accuracy of /r/ improved to a greater extent with ultrasound therapy. Outcomes were also better for those who received ultrasound therapy first. It may be noteworthy that this outcome is similar to the findings discussed earlier from McAllister Byun and Campbell (2016), which showed superior outcomes when visual acoustic feedback was provided before traditional therapy.

SUMMARY

Working with older children and adolescents poses its own set of challenges. Thankfully, there is now specific evidence available for several different treatment alternatives that can assist with remediating their speech errors. Clinicians are no longer limited to using traditional articulation therapy or simply hoping these errors will resolve. Choosing among the various options remains a challenge, as relatively few comparison studies have been conducted.

QUESTIONS FOR CHAPTER 12

1. Contrast the typical assessment battery with the one suggested for CAS.

2. How does therapy for a client with CAS differ from more traditional therapy? Discuss three possible treatment options.

3. Discuss ways in which traditional therapy might be modified for older children.

4. Contrast the advantages and disadvantages of providing additional tactile versus visual feedback.

5. Identify how instrumentation can assist in treatment for SSDs, including limitations of this type of assistance.

13

Phonological Awareness: Description, Assessment, and Intervention

BRIGID C. McNEILL, LAURA M. JUSTICE, AND GAIL T. GILLON

LEARNING OBJECTIVES

The focus of this chapter is the role of phonological awareness in preventing and/or remediating reading and writing problems in children with speech sound disorders (SSDs). By the end of this chapter, the reader should be able to:

- Define phonological awareness.

- Identify components of phonological awareness that develop early and those that develop later, including how these components relate to literacy (reading and spelling) development.

- Describe the role of the speech-language pathologist (SLP) in assessment and intervention of phonological awareness in young and older children with speech and/or language disorders.

- Identify how reading specialists, classroom teachers, and SLPs can combine their skills to assist children with both speech and literacy development limitations.

- Propose SLP intervention activities specific to incorporating phonological awareness into speech sound therapy for preschool and for school-age children.

Running speech consists of varying types of linguistic units that range in size from larger (sentences, words, syllables) to smaller (morphemes, phonemes). Most adult speakers of a language can readily and consciously recognize that speech comprises sentences, words, syllables, morphemes, and phonemes, and that these units are discrete and recurring elements of language. One's ability to consciously analyze the sound structure of speech emerges in early childhood, and this ability is called *phonological awareness*. Young children's phonological awareness is apparent when they successfully perform tasks requiring them to generate rhymes, identify the beginning sounds in words, or segment the individual phonemes comprising words. Children's successful performance on such tasks is consistently associated with performance on reading tasks—particularly those measuring word recognition—indicating that there are integrative linkages between phonological awareness and acquisition of word-level reading skills.

Of particular importance to SLPs is evidence showing that children with speech sound difficulties often show lags in their development of phonological awareness, and that such lags may pose specific risks for their timely development of skilled reading and spelling. This chapter provides a framework for understanding phonological awareness, recognizing why children with speech difficulties often have challenges in this area, and considering how such challenges may be addressed through clinical interventions and educational support.

WHAT IS PHONOLOGICAL AWARENESS?

Phonological awareness refers to an individual's awareness of the sound (phonological) structure of spoken words (Gillon, 2019). Phonological awareness is an overarching term that includes syllable awareness, rhyme awareness, and phoneme awareness. Often, at relatively young ages (3–4 years), children become aware that spoken words contain syllables and that syllables within words contain smaller sound units. With increasing age, children become more aware of the sound structure of words, including onsets, rimes, and individual phonemes. Phonological awareness is *sublexical,* meaning that representation of these units occurs at a level distinct from meaning. This awareness is also viewed as being *metalinguistic* in nature, in that it requires an individual to focus on language as an object of thought. Phonological awareness is contingent on and mediated by the child's access to the phonology of their language (Wagner & Torgesen, 1987).

Shallow Levels of Phonological Awareness

At more shallow levels of phonological awareness, children show sensitivity to the sound patterns that recur across and within words. At these levels, children may recognize, for instance, that the words *bell* and *tell* demonstrate certain phonological similarities (i.e., these words rhyme), and that *bell* can be divided into two components (i.e., its onset and rime: *b + ell*). They are also likely to be able to blend and segment multisyllabic words (e.g., *doorbell, pancake*), and to identify when words share the same singleton onsets (e.g., *me* and *moon*).

Deep Levels of Phonological Awareness

At the opposite end of the continuum, representing deeper levels of sensitivity, children demonstrate more conscious levels of awareness regarding a word or syllable's phonological structure. With access to deeper levels of sensitivity, children are able to compare, contrast, and even manipulate phonological segments within and across syllables and words. For example, they can delete phonemes in words to create new words (such as deleting the first sound in the word *track* to create *rack*), and can count the number of sounds in individual words. Phoneme awareness is fully realized when children can recognize that each word or syllable consists of a series of discrete phonemes and can explicitly identify, blend, and segment these phonemes. The terms *phonemic* and *phoneme awareness* have been used by a number of scholars in reference to this sophisticated level of awareness.

A Developmental Perspective

Recognizing that the development of phonological awareness occurs along a continuum is consistent with the perspective that children's attainment of phonological awareness is developmental in nature (Stanovich, 2000). In general, children's development of phonological awareness follows a continuum along which they gain sensitivity first to words followed by syllables, onset/rimes, and then phonemes (Anthony et al., 2003; Lonigan et al., 2009).

A considerable body of research supports a developmental trajectory in the growth of phonological awareness in both English and other alphabetic languages (Anthony et al., 2003; Ziegler & Goswami, 2005). Some researchers use the term *quasi-parallel progression* to emphasize how children's sensitivity to words, syllables, onset/rimes, and phonemes emerges in overlapping rather than discrete stages (Anthony et al., 2003). Understanding the quasi-parallel nature of phonological-awareness development suggests that children need not master one ability (e.g., rhyming) before another (e.g., identifying initial sounds in words). Children's growth in phonological awareness is highly mediated by both language abilities and experiences (Lonigan et al., 1998; Stahl & Murray, 1994). In particular, growth in vocabulary development and letter knowledge are considered influential variables on children's early phonological awareness development during the preschool years (Burgess & Lonigan, 1998).

PHONOLOGICAL AWARENESS AS LITERACY DEVELOPMENT

Phonological awareness has often been studied within the context of children's literacy development. Although children's ability to represent and manipulate the phonological structure of words consciously is highly mediated by their linguistic abilities and experiences, the fundamental (and potentially causal) role that phonological awareness plays in reading development has encouraged many scientists and practitioners to study phonological awareness within the framework of literacy development. The term *literacy* is used here in a general sense to describe children's attainment of both emergent and conventional literacy skills; *emergent literacy* refers to skills and knowledge serving as prerequisites to reading and writing, whereas *conventional literacy* refers to fluent and skilled reading and writing.

More specifically, emergent literacy describes precursory reading and writing skills that are acquired by most children within the preschool and kindergarten period. These skills lay the foundation for later skilled and fluent reading (van Kleeck, 1998). The two primary domains of development within this preliterate period are print knowledge (knowledge about forms and functions of written language; Justice & Ezell, 2004) and phonological awareness. Children's development of both print knowledge and phonological awareness are viewed as legitimate and critical elements of literacy development (Whitehurst & Lonigan, 1998) and provide the foundation for their eventual attainment of conventional literacy. To this end, preschool children with sophisticated levels of print knowledge and phonological awareness are more likely to develop into proficient conventional readers and writers as compared to preschoolers with low levels of awareness (Suggate et al., 2018). Conventional literacy is typically acquired within the context of formal instruction, usually beginning in first grade, or at about 6–7 years of age.

Historical perspectives of literacy development took the viewpoint—in both theoretical and practical terms—that children's acquisition of literacy skills began only within the context of formal literacy instruction. Relatively recently, scientists began to study literacy development in very young children and found that preschool children as young as 2 and 3 years of age possess considerable knowledge about reading and writing. A substantial number of researchers in the last two decades have described what young children know about literacy, as well as determining how this knowledge is mediated by linguistic, cognitive, and environmental influences (e.g., Justice et al., 2006; Strang & Piasta, 2016). Across numerous studies of literacy development in young children, a single set of variables—those representing phonological awareness—has stood out in terms of its robust value in predicting reading achievement (e.g., Hogan et al., 2005). Awareness of the phonological structure of spoken language helps children decode printed text, recognize words in print, and spell words (see Gillon, 2019, for review).

THE DEVELOPMENT OF PHONOLOGICAL AWARENESS

As previously noted, children's development of phonological awareness occurs on a continuum representing a hierarchy of sensitivity to the linguistic units that compose words (see Gillon, 2019). Children's early sensitivity to larger units, such as syllables and rime units, represents shallow levels of awareness, whereas later sensitivity to phonemes represents deep or higher levels of awareness (Burgess & Lonigan, 1998). Evidence for this developmental continuum comes from a substantial literature base indicating that sensitivity to syllable structure occurs considerably earlier than sensitivity to phonemes (e.g., Anthony et al., 2003; Lonigan et al., 1998, 2009).

Boys and girls show similar patterns of early phonological awareness development, but children from middle-income backgrounds demonstrate stronger phonological awareness knowledge at 4 and 5 years of age compared to children from lower-income backgrounds (Lonigan et al., 1998). A plausible explanation for the socioeconomic differences observed is the quality of the language and literacy environments these children are exposed to in their early years.

Awareness of Rhyme

Sensitivity to rhyme is often viewed as one of the earliest benchmarks in the growth of phonological awareness, given that awareness of rhyme is contingent on one's ability to represent words as discrete units that can be analyzed on a distinctly phonological basis (Bryant et al., 1990). The ability to detect and produce patterns of rhyme across words, observed in children as young as 2 years of age, has been viewed as a critical entry point in the development of phonological awareness (Hempenstall, 1997).

Sensitivity to rhyme begins to emerge in some children not long after they exhibit productive use of oral language. Large-scale laboratory studies of early phonological awareness development suggest that some children can perform above chance level on tasks tapping rhyming knowledge as young as 2 years, and the percentage of children demonstrating rhyming knowledge rapidly increases with age. The majority of children from middle-income backgrounds can show competency on simple rhyming tasks by age 5. Table 13.1 provides examples of the performance of various age groups on some common tasks used to evaluate young children's awareness of or sensitivity to rhyming words.

Awareness of Syllables

Initially, children begin to recognize that multisyllabic words can be segmented at the level of the syllable (e.g., that *butterfly* can be broken into three parts). Usually around 4 years of age, children begin to exhibit explicit awareness of syllabic distinctions within multisyllabic words (i.e., that *hotdog* can be readily divided into *hot* and *dog,* or that *baby* can be segmented into *ba-by*) (see Table 13.1). Subsequently, children show

Table 13.1. Examples of research findings concerning phonological awareness proficiency in young children

Task	Example	Age group	Proficiency	Reference
Syllable counting	How many syllables are in the word *puppy?*	4 years 5 years	50% of children successful 90% of children successful	Moats, 2000
Rhyme matching	Which word rhymes with *sail: nail* or *boot?*	2 and 3 years 4 and 5 years	Average: 52% accuracy Average: 70% accuracy	Lonigan et al., 2009
Rhyme oddity	Which word does not rhyme: *sail, nail,* or *boot?*	2 and 3 years 4 and 5 years	Average: 38% accuracy Average: 48% accuracy	Lonigan et al., 2009
Rhyme production	What rhymes with *boot?*	3 years	35% could generate at least one rhyming word	Chaney, 1992
Alliteration oddity	Which word does not start the same: *bed, hair,* or *bell?*	3 years	Low- and middle-income groups: 9% scored above chance level[a]	Lonigan et al., 1998
		5 years	Middle income: 49% scored above chance[a] Low income: 13% scored above chance	
Phoneme elision (deletion)	Say *time* without saying /m/.	3 years	Low- and middle-income groups: Less than 11% scored above zero	Lonigan et al., 1998
		5 years	Middle income: 72% scored one or more correct Low income: Only 7% scored one or more correct	

[a]Indicates the percentage of children within that age group whose accuracy rate significantly exceeded that which would be expected by chance.

increased sensitivity to distinctions within intrasyllabic units. Specific patterns govern children's growth in sensitivity to intrasyllabic units within the syllable. In the early stages of sensitivity to syllable structure (when children are not yet perceiving phonemes as the basic linguistic unit), children show greater facility at segmenting syllables into onsets and rimes when onsets occur as singleton consonants rather than consonant clusters (Treiman, 1983). For instance, children are more likely to be able to segment *tar* into an onset and rime as compared to *star*. Sensitivity to the onset-rime distinction appears to facilitate children's phoneme awareness, providing the framework for word and syllable analyses at the level of the phoneme.

Awareness of Alliteration

Alliteration describes the sharing of a phoneme across two words or syllables, such as *bad* and *big*. Sensitivity to alliteration is also an early indicator of the advent of phonological awareness. By age 3, a few children will begin to show sensitivity to alliteration across words and, by age 5, many children from advantaged backgrounds will demonstrate this level of phonological awareness. Table 13.1 provides examples of growth in alliteration awareness during the preschool years.

The propensity toward alliteration by very young children was described by Dowker (1989) in a naturalistic study of phonological awareness of young children. Examining the elicited poems of children ranging from 2 to 6 years of age, Dowker found that even 2-year-old children used alliteration with some frequency in their poems (27% of her 2-year-old sample used alliterative devices).

Children are more proficient at comparing and contrasting initial phonemes across two words if the words share a common vowel, such as *cup–cut* versus *cup–cat*. The identification of a similarity across the latter pair would be more difficult (Kirtley et al., 1989). In addition, children show substantially greater performance at comparing and contrasting final phonemes across syllables or monosyllabic words if the two words share a common vowel (in other words, the two words share a rime or rhyme; Kirtley et al., 1989). For instance, children are much better at identifying a final phoneme commonality for *map* and *tap* than for *map* and *tip*.

Awareness of Phonemes

Phoneme awareness—the ability to identify phonemes as the units comprising syllables and words—is not exhibited with mastery by many children until about 6 or 7 years of age (E. Ball, 1993), although Lonigan and colleagues (1998) found that 5-year-old children from advantaged backgrounds could complete at least one item successfully on a phoneme-deletion task (see Table 13.1).

Phoneme awareness comprises two areas of growth: phoneme segmentation (analysis or elision) and phoneme blending (or synthesis). *Phoneme segmentation* is the ability to sequentially isolate all the individual sounds in a syllable or word, or to segment (elide) a sound from a word or syllable. *Phoneme blending* is the ability to take a sequence of phonemes and build them into a larger linguistic unit. Using the word *pond,* for example, a phoneme segmentation task requires that a child break the word into its component phonemes and express those four phonemes in sequence: /p/ ... /a/ ... /n/ ... /d/. In contrast, a phoneme blending task involves presenting a series of four phonemes to the child (in this case, /p/, /a/, /n/, and /d/) and asking the child to combine the sounds into a word. Skills in both phoneme segmentation and blending are critical requisites for learning to read.

There is a developmental trend in children's performance on phoneme segmentation and blending tasks. In general, performance on phoneme blending tasks is superior to that on segmentation and elision tasks (e.g., Lonigan et al., 2009). Phoneme segmentation and manipulation skills are highly mediated by the complexity of the linguistic units being analyzed. Segmenting simple consonant-vowel-consonant (CVC) words is much easier that segmenting words with blends (e.g., CCVC words) (Treiman, 1983).

Phoneme awareness requires children to have acquired adequate representations of phonemes as the discrete elements of syllables and words (Nittrouer, 1996); that is, to engage in phoneme awareness tasks, children must have a well-developed phonological system comprising robust representations of the phonemes within their language. In fact, examining children's abilities to manipulate phonemes demonstrates the depth and robustness of their phoneme representations.

Calfee and colleagues (1973), in their seminal work, examined the attainment of relatively sophisticated levels of phoneme awareness in a study of 660 children from kindergarten through 12th grade. These researchers asked children to manipulate colored blocks representing the phoneme arrangements of nonsense syllables.

Although children showed gradual improvement on phoneme manipulation across the grades, 12th-grade students showed only about 60% accuracy on complex tasks. Although these students undoubtedly were able to produce phonemes accurately, their receptive performance showed that mastery was elusive in more advanced tasks of phoneme awareness. Such findings indicate that although young children gradually increase their ability to represent words as discrete phonemes, the ability to manipulate words at the phoneme level requires more advanced representational skills. Some children (particularly if they are poor readers) may never acquire proficiency on complex phoneme manipulation tasks.

PHONOLOGICAL AWARENESS DEVELOPMENT AND READING

There is considerable overlap between children's development of phonological awareness and learning to read. However, we must note that there is controversy regarding the nature of the relationship between phonological awareness and reading instruction (Johnston et al., 1996; Vandervelden & Siegel, 1995). Some researchers contend that reading development is driven by phonological awareness, particularly at the phoneme level, a view that asserts a causal relationship between phoneme awareness and reading ability. Research demonstrating that performance on phoneme segmentation and phoneme blending tasks are strong predictors of early reading development supports this position (Melby-Lervåg et al., 2012).

Other researchers assert that phoneme awareness and reading skill develop in a reciprocal, rather than causal, manner. Evidence showing that phonological awareness increases reciprocally and concomitantly with reading proficiency provides support for this argument (see Stanovich, 2000). A position representing both perspectives is that a certain level of phonological awareness is required for the development of reading skill but that, subsequently, phoneme awareness and reading ability develop in a reciprocal and interrelated manner, as shown in Figure 13.1. Regardless of perspectives regarding causality, a large body of literature, including meta-analyses, has shown that phoneme awareness is a robust correlate of reading ability (see Melby-Lervåg et al., 2012).

Bradley and Bryant (1983) were among the first researchers to demonstrate a relationship between phonological awareness at preschool and subsequent reading performance. In their seminal work, they tested 403 children aged 4 and 5 in their

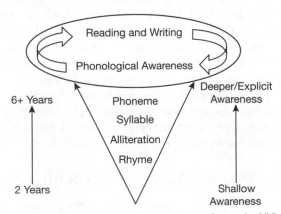

Figure 13.1. Developmental model of growth in phonological awareness from early childhood to school-age years.

ability to categorize sounds; that is, their skills in determining which word, of three or four words presented, did not share a common initial phoneme (e.g., *hill, pig, pen*). This measure of children's sensitivity to alliteration accounted for a significant and substantial proportion of variance in their reading skills 3 years later. These findings of a relationship between phonological sensitivity and reading performance have been replicated across multiple studies (see Gillon, 2019, for review).

The association between phonological awareness and reading is best understood by considering the skills that are most critical for the beginning reader. Faced with the task of decoding a novel word, the novice reader must know the distinctive features and names of alphabet letters in the word and must know its phoneme structure. In addition, and most importantly, the novice reader must bridge these two areas of knowledge by recognizing the systematic relationships between letters and phonemes (Hulme et al., 2007). Skill in recognizing and using the systematic correspondence between letters and phonemes is usually referred to as *phonological recoding* (Vandervelden & Siegel, 1995) or *phonological recoding in lexical access* (Wagner & Torgesen, 1987). The successful integration of these two areas of knowledge allows the child to decode novel words. Children with limited awareness of letter names and/ or deficits in phoneme awareness are prone to difficulties in reading (Stanovich, 2000).

Stahl and Murray (1994) sought to determine the amount of phonological awareness necessary for a beginning reader to negotiate novel words. These researchers found that the ability to represent onset-rime distinctions and to isolate phonemes at the beginning and end of words were prerequisites for beginning reading. In other words, children who did not have these requisite abilities were unable to achieve or surpass preprimer instructional levels. These findings emphasize the importance of intrasyllabic awareness over word and syllable awareness to reading development (see Gillon, 2019), and converge with other reports showing that phoneme awareness skills exhibit a stronger predictive relationship with reading than rhyme awareness skills (Muter et al., 2004). These findings are supported by intervention research, which has shown that therapy focused primarily on rhyme (rather than phoneme) awareness has limited transfer to improving children's reading skills (Nancollis et al., 2005).

For children who are already readers, abilities in phoneme awareness distinguish reliably between children who are proficient at reading and those who are struggling (Catts et al., 2001; Muter et al., 2004). In a classic study, Juel (1988) followed a group of 54 children from first through fourth grade. Juel found remarkable stability in reading achievement across these grades: "The probability that a child would remain a poor reader at the end of fourth grade, if the child was a poor reader at the end of first grade, was .88" (p. 440). In other words, children who experienced reading failure in first grade continued to experience failure in the next three grades. Deficits in phoneme awareness were important explanatory variables in distinguishing children who failed at reading from those who experienced success. At entry to first grade, children who subsequently experienced reading failure showed no skills in segmenting words into phonemes and analyzing words on the basis of phoneme properties. Such findings implicate the strong and reciprocal relationship between deficits in phonological awareness and the circumstances surrounding reading failure.

PHONOLOGICAL AWARENESS AND SPEECH SOUND DISORDERS

Let us now turn to considering the relationship between phonological awareness and SSDs. Among typically developing children, relationships exist between speech production performance and phonological awareness (Foy & Mann, 2001; Mann & Foy,

2007), with more articulation errors associated with lower scores on measures of phonological awareness. Neurocognitive research also supports this link, showing that reading utilizes areas of the brain that are initially developed for speech production during the preschool years (Frost et al., 2009). It makes sense, then, that children with SSDs face increased risks for experiencing difficulty in phonological awareness and subsequent reading and spelling impairment (for review, see Gillon, 2019).

This does not mean, however, that all children who exhibit speech problems will have literacy difficulties. Children with speech production problems specific to deficits in phonological rules are most prone to experiencing difficulties with phonological awareness and reading. We refer to these children as having a *phonological disorder (PD)*. Children with PDs have multiple speech sound production errors and compromised intelligibility. They may or may not have concomitant language difficulties in other domains (e.g., vocabulary, grammar). The speech sound difficulties of children with PDs tend to be more pronounced than the difficulties of children with articulation problems, who may exhibit distortions or substitutions of a relatively small set of sounds (e.g., substituting /w/ for /l/ and /r/ sounds). PD is often conceptualized as a cognitive-linguistic disorder rather than an articulatory or motoric disorder, resulting from underspecified or faulty phonological representations. For some children at least, difficulties with phonological development affect both expression (speech sound production problem) and reception (phonological awareness problem).

Children with PD, as a group, face an elevated risk for phonological awareness impairment, particularly when these are accompanied by more widespread language difficulties (Bird et al., 1995; Hayiou-Thomas et al., 2017; Overby et al., 2012; Peterson et al., 2009). However, even having a PD in isolation is linked with early reading difficulties (Nathan et al., 2004), and the presence of phonological awareness weakness in preschool children with SSDs is independent of whether these children have language impairment (Rvachew et al., 2003). Factors such as genetic risk and low socioeconomic status will further increase these children's risk for reading difficulties (Hayiou-Thomas et al., 2017).

Examination of longitudinal datasets highlighted the longer-term academic consequences for children identified with PD in the preschool years. McLeod and colleagues (2019) tracked the literacy achievement of 4,332 children whose parents had concerns about their speech and/or language at 4 years of age (preschool), as well as Grades, 3, 5, and 7. This cohort presented with significantly lower literacy skills at each timepoint than their peers without speech/language difficulties, even when other demographic and health influencers on literacy achievement were controlled. The two groups demonstrated parallel growth in literacy scores over time, suggesting that the gap in literacy performance was long-standing well into the schooling years.

Phonological awareness difficulty in preschool-age children with SSDs may interact with other important cognitive variables in determining their reading ability. Accurate speech production involves a complex array of perceptual, speech processing, linguistic, nonlinguistic, cognitive, and motor skills (Waring et al., 2019), many of which are also related to literacy acquisition. Peterson and associates (2009) concluded from their follow-up study of preschool children with SSDs that phonological awareness interacts with children's syntactic oral language ability and nonverbal IQ in determining reading performance at 8 years of age. The multiple deficit hypothesis that literacy outcome in children with SSDs is determined by a complex interaction between risk and protective factors is consistent with research evaluating potential genetic influences on comorbidity in SSDs (Lewis et al., 2011).

Understanding the nature of children's speech difficulties is also important for understanding their risk for literacy problems, including difficulties in phonological awareness (Dodd, 2005). Children with speech production problems that are articulatory rather than phonological in nature may not display difficulties in attaining phonological awareness (Bishop & Adams, 1990; Catts, 1993). Catts, for instance, found that first-graders with disorders of articulation performed similarly to a comparison group of typically developing peers on a variety of phonological awareness tasks. Children whose speech production problems are phonological in nature and accompanied by language difficulties (PD + language) face the greatest risks for failing to achieve good phonological awareness and, by extension, skilled reading (Lewis et al., 2000). By some estimates, nearly 50% of these children will fail to be good readers by third or fourth grade. These estimates suggest that growth in phonological awareness and reading achievement needs to be diligently tracked for children with PD, particularly those youngsters who also exhibit concomitant language problems.

The nature of children's speech errors has also been found to influence phonological awareness (and literacy) development within groups of children with PD (Hayiou-Thomas et al., 2017; Preston & Edwards, 2010; Preston, Hull, et al., 2013; Rvachew et al., 2007). Preston and Edwards found that the use of atypical speech errors predicted unique variance in phonological awareness (i.e., beyond that predicted by vocabulary and age) in 43 preschoolers with PD. Follow-up of this cohort 3 years later showed that children using more atypical errors at the preschool assessment presented with poorer phonological awareness, reading, and spelling performance at school age (Preston, Hull, et al., 2013). Other preschool speech measures were unrelated to school-age literacy performance. Masso, Baker, and colleagues (2017) highlighted speech accuracy during production of polysyllable words as an important indicator of children's propensity to experience phonological awareness and literacy difficulties. In particular, the type of speech error (frequency of deletion and phonotactic errors) was identified as an important indicator of literacy in children with PD.

Children with childhood apraxia of speech are an additional group of children who exhibit atypical speech errors, among other risk factors for literacy impairment, who are likely to experience phonological awareness deficits (Gillon & Moriarty, 2007; Marquardt et al., 2002; McNeill et al., 2009) and literacy difficulties into their school years (Lewis et al., 2004; Miller et al., 2019).

Bird and colleagues (1995) assert that problems in phonological awareness for children with PD can be attributed to their inability to master the phonological system, which translates into difficulties representing the phonological structure of language in both expression (i.e., speech intelligibility) and awareness tasks. This hypothesis is supported by a number of studies that have shown children with PD perform poorly on tasks designed to assess the strength of their phonological representations when compared to their typically developing peers (Anthony et al., 2011; Johnson et al., 2011; Sutherland & Gillon, 2005). The importance of access to distinct phonological representations to support early literacy development in children with PD exists irrespective of the presence of concomitant language delays (Anthony et al., 2011).

Collectively, the research on phonological awareness for children with PDs suggests several conclusions, although further research on this population is warranted to better understand the impact of speech production difficulties on phonological awareness and literacy. Those conclusions are:

1. Children with PDs are more likely than their peers with typical development to experience difficulties with phonological awareness and literacy achievement. Children who are most at risk for such problems are those whose speech difficulties are still pronounced at the onset of literacy instruction (e.g., kindergarten and first grade) and who have limited phoneme awareness (Burgoyne et al., 2019; Nathan et al., 2004).

2. Children with PDs who have concomitant receptive and/or expressive language difficulties are at greater risk than those with PDs alone (Hayiou-Thomas et al., 2017; Lewis et al., 2004; Peterson et al., 2009).

3. Some children with PDs may evidence problems in acquiring phonological awareness, but these problems do not present challenges to the early development of literacy (Peterson et al., 2009). However, as demands in the curriculum increase, and as predictors of reading ability change at different stages of literacy development, difficulties in inefficient word decoding as a result of poor phoneme awareness may become evident or more pronounced (Skebo et al., 2013).

4. Phonological awareness deficits may have their greatest impact on spelling, particularly around third grade and beyond (Lewis et al., 2000). There is evidence to suggest that children with PDs may have particular difficulty with spelling in comparison with their reading and phonological awareness performance (e.g., McNeill et al., 2017).

THE ROLE OF THE SPEECH-LANGUAGE PATHOLOGIST

At an international level, professional associations of speech-language pathology endorse the important and critical role SLPs should play in promoting phonological awareness (and literacy skills in general), particularly for children who experience communication disorders (ASHA, 2001; New Zealand Speech-language Therapists' Association, 2012; Royal College of Speech and Language Therapists, 2006; Speech-Language and Audiology Canada, 2016; Speech Pathology Association of Australia, 2011).

We must recognize that language consists of both written and oral dimensions, and that the role of SLPs does not stop with oral language. Moreover, we must also recognize that phonological abilities represent an important bridge between written and oral language because of the alphabetic principle, which relies on systematic relationships between sounds and letters. Children who experience problems with phonology—whether it manifests itself as a speech production problem or not—are more likely than other children to struggle with reading. Consequently, if SLPs are to promote children's success in schooling and in life, we must take a broadened view toward identifying specific goals for treatment so that we expand beyond the traditional dimensions that look at children's production of individual speech sounds or use of specific phonological processes patterns. We must look carefully at children's underlying sensitivities to the way in which spoken language is organized, to ensure that children are developing phonological awareness in a timely manner.

SLPs have been encouraged by ASHA (2001) to play a "critical and direct role in the development of literacy for children and adolescents with communication disorders" (p. 3). Primary roles and responsibilities include 1) prevention, 2) identification, 3) assessment, and 4) intervention. Cabbage and colleagues' (2018) clinical tutorial focused on SLPs' role in the early identification of children with dyslexia is also an excellent resource in this area. The next sections discuss in further detail the SLP's role in assessment and intervention.

ASSESSMENT

Phonological awareness should be routinely assessed in children with suspected or identified PDs as part of a comprehensive assessment battery. Assessment materials will vary depending on the developmental stage of the child. The aim of phonological awareness assessment in a 3-year-old child with a PD, for example, is not to diagnose the child with a phonological awareness deficit. The wide variability in phonological awareness development in children with typical development in this young age group would suggest such an assessment aim is inappropriate. Rather, phonological awareness assessment is required in young children with PDs to establish their current levels of awareness and to monitor their growth in phonological awareness over time in response to home and preschool language experiences or specific therapy interventions. In contrast, the assessment aim of a school-age child with a PD is to profile their strengths and needs in phonological awareness. Assessment is also used to ascertain whether deficits in phonological awareness, particularly at the phoneme level, are contributing to any current reading or spelling difficulties and whether phonological awareness is sufficiently well developed for the current demands of the child's reading and spelling curriculum. A phonological awareness assessment is also necessary to track the effects of any explicit phonological awareness intervention so that its effects can be documented.

A range of phonological awareness assessment tasks may be implemented, including norm-referenced and criterion-referenced measures, as well as dynamic assessment.

Norm-Referenced Measures: Preschool Years

Several norm-referenced measures for assessing phonological awareness in preschool children are available. When considering use of such tools, the clinician needs to consider the normative sample used for developing the instrument and its relevance to the child being assessed. Early language and preschool experiences will influence a child's phonological awareness development. In some early education environments, children may receive extensive and explicit guidance in letter sound knowledge (e.g., the sound /g/ goes with the letter *G*), whereas in other educational facilities the focus may be on rhyme and letter naming, with little attention directed at facilitating other levels of phonological awareness or print knowledge. Thus, children's performance on phonological awareness tasks is likely to be influenced by early instructional methods that may vary across differing educational settings. The use of local norms for phonological awareness skill development may be one strategy to help reduce this problem. However, given the general pattern of consistency in phonological awareness development that is evident across countries and across alphabetic languages, norm-referenced assessments with strong psychometric properties will provide a useful guide against which to compare phonological awareness development in preschool and kindergarten children with PDs.

It is also important that the clinician considers the type of assessment task(s) included in measures designed for young children. Many measures were not designed with the child with speech production problems in mind. Consequently, measures that ask children to produce rhyming words, for instance, are nearly impossible to use with children with speech sound problems. For instance, a child with speech production problems who is asked to produce several words that rhyme with *cat* might say "tat, tat, and tat." For a child who represents many initial sounds (e.g., /g/, /k/, /d/, and /t/) with a single phoneme (e.g., /t/), this might be a correct answer, but it is impossible to know. Gillon (2019) provides a comprehensive examination of phonological awareness assessment instruments and their psychometric properties.

Norm-Referenced Measures: School-Age Children

Several norm-referenced instruments for evaluating phonological awareness in school-age children have been developed in recent years. Table 13.2 provides a summary of several instruments widely used to assess phonological awareness in school-age children. These measures use age norms rather than grade norms; thus, one should be cautious when applying these norms to children who are young or old for their grade, as their experiences may not be similar to that of age-matched peers. In addition, interpretation must consider that educational experiences in the early elementary years can vary widely across schools. Norm-referenced measures such as these may prove useful in delineating the extent to which a child exhibits phonological awareness difficulties compared to a cohort of age-matched peers. With some of these measures, information about potential intervention targets may be gleaned from careful analysis of a child's pattern of performance. However, such targets must also be educationally relevant and developmentally appropriate.

Criterion-Referenced Measures

Criterion-referenced measures are used to determine a child's performance against a specific criterion. The child's performance is not compared to a cohort of age-matched peers, but rather to a particular local or curriculum-based standard. The Dynamic Indicators of Basic Early Literacy Skills (DIBELS; Good & Kaminski, 2002) and Phonological Awareness and Literacy Screening (PALS: K; Invernizzi et al., 2001; PALS: 1–3; Invernizzi & Meier, 2002–2003) are frequently used measures in schools that include criterion-based measures of phonological awareness.

Computer-administered assessment is also a promising form of criterion-referenced phonological awareness assessment. Carson and colleagues (2014) examined the validity and reliability of computer-based phonological awareness assessment by evaluating the performance of 95 children (including 21 children with spoken

Table 13.2.   Examples of norm-referenced phonological awareness measures

Measure name	Age range
Clinical Evaluation of Language Fundamentals Preschool–3 (includes phonological awareness subtest) (Wiig et al., 2020)	3–6 years
Pre-reading Inventory of Phonological Awareness (Dodd, Crosbie, et al., 2003)	4–7 years
Test of Phonological Awareness (2nd ed.): *PLUS* (Torgesen & Bryant, 2004)	5–8 years
The Phonological Awareness Test 2 (Robertson & Salter, 2007)	5–9 years
Test of Phonological Awareness Skills (Newcomer & Barenbaum, 2003)	5–10 years
Clinical Evaluation of Language Fundamentals–5 (includes phonological awareness subtest) (Semel et al., 2013)	5–21 years
Comprehensive Test of Phonological Processing–2 (Wagner et al., 2013)	5–24 years

language impairment) at the beginning, middle, and end of the first year of literacy instruction. The computer-based tool took 30% less administration time and produced comparable scores to paper-based measures. Further, children's performance at the beginning and middle of the year predicted reading outcomes at the end of the year with 94% accuracy.

The goal of criterion-referenced measures is to determine children's competency in a specific area of phonological awareness, and clinicians can devise their own criterion-referenced tasks to use for screening and diagnostic purposes. These more informal tasks can be used to identify children who are deficient relative to an established criterion, describe children's current level of performance (strengths and needs), delineate intervention goals, document treatment progress, and determine when intervention is no longer warranted.

Dynamic Assessment

Dynamic assessment examines children's performance in response to varying types of cues or prompts provided by the clinician. It provides a method for obtaining a clearer picture of children's underlying competencies, as well as their potential for learning new skills (Bain & Olswang, 1995). Knowledge gained from dynamic assessments can identify children's underlying competencies and their short- and long-term propensity for change. An example of a dynamic assessment task is shown in Table 13.3

The use of dynamic assessment in combination with static screening measures may be an important approach to improve the accuracy of early identification of children with phoneme awareness and reading difficulty. Catts and colleagues (2009) reported floor effects at initial assessment points that led to the over-identification of children at risk of reading disability in an analysis of the performance of 18,667 children in the DIBELS assessment from kindergarten to third grade. The presence of floor effects during assessment that takes place in the early stages of formal liter-

Table 13.3. Dynamic assessment task

Prompt 1	*Listen. I'm going to say the word very slowly.* Model slow pronunciation. *Now can you tell me each sound?*
Prompt 2	*What's the first sound that you hear in _____?* If first sound is correct: *Now can you tell me each of the sounds?* If incorrect or no response: *Try to tell me just a little bit of the word.* If child still does not isolate first sound, skip Prompts 3 and 4. Go to Prompt 5.
Prompt 3	If they correctly identified the first sound but not the next sound(s): _____ *is the first sound in _____.* *What sound comes next?* *Now can you tell me each sound?*
Prompt 4	_____ *has two (or three) sounds in it. What are they?*
Prompt 5	*Watch me.* Model segmentation of the word: Place a token in a square as each sound is spoken. Then repeat the word as a whole. After demo, say the following: *Try to do what I just did.* Score response as correct if child can imitate correct segmentation.
Prompt 6	*Let's try it together.* Model segmentation of word with child. Work hand-over-hand with child and ask them to pronounce segments along with you. *Now you try it. Do what we just did together.*
Prompt 7	Model again with child (as in Prompt 6). *Now try again to do it yourself.*

Source: Spector (1992).

acy instruction is likely due to the limited instructional experience of children at this age. The addition of dynamic assessment measures is a preferable method to improve accuracy of screening measures than delaying administration until later in the school year, as the latter approach is likely to compromise the early intervention of children who are indeed at risk of reading disability. Cunningham and Carroll (2011) reported that a dynamic phoneme segmentation task provided a more sensitive measure than static assessment of phoneme segmentation and deletion when disentangling age and schooling effects in phoneme awareness development in the first year of schooling.

Children's responses to the various prompts may provide insights into teaching strategies for therapy. Dynamic assessment can, thus, be used in conjunction with more static evaluation strategies to derive more sensitive profiles of children's phonological awareness development and to determine therapy goals and strategies.

INTERVENTION

SLPs who work with preschool and school-age children should pay close attention to phonological awareness in both their assessment and intervention practices. Several effective practice guidelines for phonological awareness instruction can be gleaned from research over the last two decades (Ehri et al., 2001; Gillon, 2019; Torgesen & Mathes, 2000). These practice guidelines stem from findings showing only a small percentage of children (less than 5%) would struggle with reading if we rigorously supported literacy development from preschool forward (e.g., Carson et al., 2013; Moats, 2000). The SLP should play an integral role in promoting effective practice by collaborating with other specialists, including classroom teachers.

1. For preschoolers and kindergartners, clinicians should provide phonological awareness experiences (and literacy experiences in general) as an integral part of therapy. Attention to phonological awareness can be embedded within speech production activities, and clinicians should work collaboratively with classroom teachers and reading specialists to ensure that classroom curricula provide adequate classroom-based phonological awareness experiences.

2. Children who have not attained adequate levels of performance at the end of kindergarten or the beginning of first grade should be provided small-group intensive intervention that includes phonological awareness instruction as a core objective (Torgesen, 1999).

3. For children in which small-group instructional intervention is not sufficient, intensive one-on-one instruction should be provided; phonological awareness as well as other key reading objectives are addressed (e.g., vocabulary, reading fluency).

Promoting Phonological Awareness in Preschool Children With Phonological Disorders

SLPs need to ensure that young children with PDs whose assessment profile suggests that they are at risk for written language difficulties develop strong phonological awareness. Preliminary evidence suggests it is possible to simultaneously improve both speech and phonological awareness development in children with SSDs (Gillon, 2005; Major & Bernhardt, 1998) and children with concomitant speech and language impairment (for review, see Otaiba et al., 2009; Tyler et al., 2011).

In a longitudinal study, Gillon (2005; Kirk & Gillon, 2007) demonstrated significant benefits for later reading and spelling development by facilitating children's phonological awareness and letter knowledge from children as young as 3 years. In this study, 12 children (mean age 3.5 years) with moderate or severe SSDs commenced school at 5 years of age with strong phoneme awareness and emerging letter knowledge following approximately 25 hours of intervention between the ages of 3–5 years. The intervention aimed to improve speech intelligibility, phoneme awareness, and letter knowledge. Results showed that the children accelerated quickly in reading development and 80% of the group demonstrated above-average reading ability by the end of the first year. In contrast, 60% of children in a control group of children with SSDs who received intervention to improve speech intelligibility but who did not receive any explicit instruction in phonological awareness showed delayed reading development and poor spelling ability over time.

Other studies have also showed that phonological awareness can be readily facilitated in young children with PDs. Van Kleeck and associates (1998) evaluated the effectiveness of a 9-month classroom-based phonological awareness training program for preschool children. Of the 16 children participating in the experimental classrooms, 11 exhibited speech impairment (9 of these children also exhibited language impairment). Over the course of intervention, the children participated in approximately 45 minutes of phonological awareness activities daily; for the first 12 weeks of the program, rhyming skills were targeted, and in the final 12 weeks, initial and final phoneme awareness within and across words was targeted. The children in the intervention classrooms made significant gains on measures of phonological awareness (e.g., test scores on rhyme detection and production tasks nearly doubled) when compared to a control group over the 9-month period. Hesketh and colleagues (2007) showed phoneme awareness intervention stimulated superior growth in the early phoneme awareness skills of 4-year-old children with SSDs than intervention focused on general language stimulation. However, outcomes for reading and spelling development were not measured in these studies.

Intervention Aims

Although a primary goal of intervention for children with PDs is to improve their speech intelligibility, a secondary goal should aim to facilitate these children's phonological awareness, particularly at the phoneme level. Research evidence suggests that to give preschool children with PDs the optimum chance for reading success, intervention should aim to achieve the following prior to formal literacy instruction or at least by the end of the first year of schooling:

1. Resolve or significantly improve the child's SSD (and any co-occurring language impairment) (Nathan et al., 2004).

2. Facilitate strong phonological awareness, including early developing awareness of phonemes in words (Gillon, 2005; Kirk & Gillon, 2007).

3. Facilitate at least some letter sound knowledge and stimulate the child's understanding of the relationship between spoken and written words (Hulme et al., 2007).

Achieving these aims may require relatively intensive periods of intervention during the preschool years, particularly for children with severe SSDs. If such intervention is successful in preventing reading problems in addition to improving speech intelligibility, the intervention will prove both efficient and cost effective.

Intervention Models

Intervention models that involve collaboration between the SLP, teacher, and parents are considered best practice when attempting to improve the phonological awareness of children with speech or language impairment (Roth & Paul, 2006). Thus, literacy skills are addressed within clinical therapy, within the classroom, and within the home.

Phonological Awareness Experiences Embedded Into Therapy

A variety of activities that stimulate phonological awareness along with knowledge of letter sounds can be integrated into therapy for preschool children. There are many relatively inexpensive manuals that can be examined for activity suggestions. Also, there are some reputable Internet sites with useful resources, including the University of Virginia PALS website (http://pals.virginia.edu/) and the National Center for Learning Disabilities Get Ready to Read website (www.getreadytoread.org/). Gillon and McNeill's (2007) integrated phonological awareness programme and resources for preschoolers with SSDs can also be downloaded online at https://www.canterbury.ac.nz/education-and-health/research/phonological-awareness-resources/. See also Justice and colleagues (2005) and Ukrainetz and colleagues (2000) for details of intervention activities.

Some practical suggestions for embedding phonological awareness into therapy include:

1. Write words clearly and in a large font underneath stimulus pictures for speech production goals. Specifically draw children's attention to the printed word (rather than the picture) when practicing the speech target words.

2. Regularly employ alliteration activities that ask children to attend to the initial sounds in words; for instance, at the start of therapy, children might have to sort a pile of picture cards into those starting with one sound (e.g., /s/) and those starting with another (e.g., /t/).

3. Use an alphabet chart or letter cards to practice target speech sounds and make explicit for the child the link between the letter and the speech sound the letter represents.

4. Model segmentation of target speech words that have two or three phonemes, as in: "Let's break the word *key* into its two sounds: /key/. . ./k/. . ./i/. . . Now you say it just the way I did, /k/. . ./i/."

5. Read storybooks that feature rhyme and alliteration patterns and explicitly bring the child's attention to these phonological patterns.

6. Ask children to draw pictures associated with their speech production goals and write a word or sentence underneath their picture. Explicitly identify and discuss the letter sound relationships when writing the words.

Written letters and words can serve as visual prompts or reminders of particular speech targets for children. For example, if the child is attempting to say *sun* and says *tun*, the clinician can point to the written word under a picture of the sun and use the initial letter *s* to cue the child: "Oops. You forgot this /s/ sound at the beginning of the word (pointing to the letter *s*). Put the /s/ at the beginning." Such activities do not necessarily require that the child understand the alphabetic references in order to produce accurate speech. Rather, the comments clinicians make with reference to print and sound structure are provided alongside the typical cues and prompts used to elicit accurate speech production (e.g., target models, phonetic placement cues). The pairing of letters with their corresponding sounds can provide children extra exposure to the phonological structure of language. Astute clinicians take advantage of teachable moments to scaffold children's attainment of higher levels of phonological awareness.

Phonological Awareness Experiences
for Preschool Children at Preschool and at Home

The SLP can collaborate with children's teachers and parents/caregivers to help them identify methods they may use to stimulate phonological awareness across the full range of childhood education settings. Many of the same activities discussed for therapeutic techniques can be used by teachers and parents. For teachers, however, it might be most important to adopt a classroom pre-reading curriculum that includes systematic and explicit attention to phonological awareness development over the academic year.

Lonigan and associates (2011) evaluated the effectiveness of a literacy-focused curriculum in stimulating phonological awareness, vocabulary, and print knowledge in 739 children across 48 preschools. The success of two professional development models (i.e., workshop attendance and workshop attendance plus mentoring) to support teacher implementation of the curriculum was also examined. Findings showed children receiving the literacy-focused curriculum outperformed the comparison curriculum by about one-third of a standard deviation in emergent literacy measures. There was an additional effect of professional development model, with children attending mentored classrooms producing the best scores. Similarly, Justice and colleagues (2010) examined the effects of introducing a language and literacy focus (including phonological awareness) into the curriculum for preschoolers at risk. Immediately following the intervention, children receiving the additional language-literacy focus exhibited superior emergent literacy skills to the comparison group who received the established curriculum alone.

There is also growing support for the effectiveness of small-group intervention for preschoolers who have not responded to quality classroom instruction. Koutsoftas and colleagues (2009) reported that a small-group phoneme awareness intervention for 34 low-income preschoolers implemented over 6 weeks was effective for more than 71% of participants. Ukrainetz and associates (2009) compared concentrated and dispersed scheduling of small-group phoneme awareness intervention for at-risk kindergarteners. Results showed no difference across the conditions, with participants in both groups showing comparable growth in their response to the intervention. It is critical that the literacy development in at-risk preschoolers who participate in early phonological awareness intervention are followed closely, as gains made in preschool may not translate into successful acquisition of later literacy skills (e.g., O'Connor et al., 2009)

Parents and teachers can also benefit from understanding ways to build phonological awareness in a less formal manner. Suggestions include encouraging parents and teachers to:

1. Read storybooks with children regularly that include interesting sound patterns (e.g., rhyme, alliteration); draw children's attention to these patterns.

2. Engage children in reciting nursery rhymes together and clap out the beat in the rhymes.

3. Find toys or objects in the house or preschool that start with the same sound and comment on the sounds that are the same. For example: "*Light* and *lid* both start with the /l/ sound. Listen to the /l/ sound at the beginning of these words: *light, lid*. Hear the /l/ sound at the beginning?"

4. Identify the first phoneme in the child's name and family members' names.

5. Clap out the syllables in children's names or segment short names (e.g., *Kim*) into their respective phonemes (e.g., /k/ /ɪ/ /m/).

6. Say words as a series of sounds (e.g., /b/ /ɪ/ /g/) and ask children to guess the word being said.

It is important to remember that the aim of phonological awareness intervention during this preschool period is to facilitate awareness of the sound structure of spoken language, not to teach skills to mastery level. The process of learning to read and write following school entry will rapidly develop more advanced levels of phonological awareness and alphabetic knowledge (Perfetti et al., 1987). What is most important for preschool children with PDs is that their phonological awareness is stimulated to a level where they can readily respond to the rigors of formal reading instruction that begins in later kindergarten and early first grade for most children today.

Promoting Phonological Awareness in School-Age Children With Phonological Disorders

School-age children with PDs who are experiencing reading and spelling difficulties may require direct and intensive periods of intervention specifically focused at enhancing phonological awareness, with the greatest attention focused on facilitating phoneme awareness. Numerous studies indicate that intensive small-group or individual phonological awareness intervention results in improved phonological awareness and reading ability for school-age children who are at risk, children experiencing reading difficulties, and children with speech-language impairments (for review, see Gillon, 2019). Ehri and colleagues (2001) concluded from a meta-analysis of 52 controlled research studies that phonological awareness has a statistically significant effect on developing reading accuracy and reading comprehension for children with typical development and children at risk. Interventions that focus at the phoneme level and integrate instruction on letter knowledge show the best results for reading development. Hulme and colleagues (2012) reanalyzed the intervention effects of a randomized controlled trial that compared a phonology-based reading program to an oral language-based intervention using a mediation model. The analysis showed that gains in phoneme awareness and letter knowledge made during the intervention explained the gains in literacy measures following completion of the programs. This type of analysis provides strong evidence for the effectiveness of enhancing phoneme awareness and letter-sound knowledge in order to enhance reading and spelling development.

Some studies have looked specifically at the effectiveness of phonological awareness intervention for school-age children with PDs. Gillon (2000a) demonstrated that 20 hours of structured phonological awareness intervention (The Gillon Phonological Awareness Training Programme; Gillon, 2000b; https://www.canterbury.ac.nz/education-and-health/research/phonological-awareness-resources/) was successful in accelerating phonological awareness development in 5- to 7-year-old children with SSDs to the level of their peers. This intervention resulted in significantly superior reading and spelling development that was maintained over time (Gillon, 2002), compared to a control group of children who received other types of speech and language intervention.

The phonological awareness intervention also resulted in improvements in speech production. The intervention was administered by an SLP to the child individually twice weekly for a 10-week period, or until 20 hours of intervention had been implemented. The activities predominantly focused at the phoneme level (e.g., phoneme identification, phoneme segmentation, phoneme blending and manipulation) and used a variety of materials and games to help maintain the child's interest. The link between the spoken and written form of the word was made explicit for the child in each teaching session through the manipulation of letter blocks to form words.

The inclusion of adequate intervention time appears to be an important factor in determining the outcomes of children participating in therapy designed to simultaneously promote speech and phonological awareness development. Denne and associates (2005) evaluated the effects of 12 hours of the Gillon Phonological Awareness Training Programme in 5- to 7-year-old children with SSDs (vs. the recommended 20 hours of intervention). Although participants improved their phonological awareness skills, gains in speech and literacy skills were not exhibited. Further research is required to determine the optimal service delivery model for providing integrated phonological awareness therapy for children with SSDs.

Intervention Aims

The aims of phonological awareness intervention for school-age children with phonological disorders are to:

1. Enhance phonological awareness development to that of their peers with typical development.

2. Ensure children have strong phoneme awareness as demonstrated on tasks requiring phoneme segmentation, phoneme blending, and phoneme manipulation.

3. Enable children to use phonological knowledge to help understand the relationship between a spoken and written representation of a word.

4. Enhance transfer of phonological awareness to the reading and spelling process.

Intervention Models

For school-age children with PDs, the most prevalent models of phonological awareness intervention are small-group intensive intervention, classroom-based intervention, and integration of phonological awareness goals into conventional therapy.

Small-Group Intensive Phonological Awareness Intervention   Increasingly, elementary schools are organizing small-group instruction focused explicitly on phonological awareness for its kindergartners and first-graders who struggle in this area. Led by an SLP, reading specialist, or other member of the school, children who are identified as at risk for literacy problems meet in small groups of three to six children one or more times per week for small-group sessions. These sessions may focus exclusively on phonological awareness or may include attention to other literacy goals as needed (e.g., reading fluency, vocabulary).

A number of available curricula exist for organizing small-group intensive phonological awareness programs. One option is to adopt a general instructional sequence and to increase the frequency and intensity of instruction within the highly individualized context provided by small-group instruction. Two commercially available small-group intensive intervention programs that provide explicit guidelines for implementation, and thus can be easily and efficiently implemented, are the following: *Road to the Code* (Blachman et al., 2000) and the *Intensive Phonological Awareness Program* (Schuele & Dayton, 2000). Torgesen and Mathes (2000) provide a description and critique of additional programs. These programs are recommended for 5- and 6-year-old children. Small groups of about six children are provided instruction several times weekly for an extended period of time (e.g., 4–5 months). Instruction can be provided by SLPs, reading specialists, and regular or special educators.

The program *Road to the Code* (Blachman et al., 2000) provides a detailed curriculum for intensive p instruction. Lessons are delivered four times weekly in 15-minute sessions for an 11-week period. The program was designed for children who are generally at risk for difficulties in early literacy achievement. The program consists of 44 detailed lesson plans, with scripts to guide implementation. Each lesson includes a phonological awareness (e.g., rhyme production), phoneme segmentation, and letter-sound correspondence activity. Investigators reported on the effectiveness of this program with kindergarten children (e.g., Ball & Blachman, 1991). They indicated that phonological awareness and word-decoding skills improved significantly.

The *Intensive Phonological Awareness Program* (Schuele & Dayton, 2000) was designed to meet the needs of children with language impairments. Intervention sessions are three times a week (30-minute sessions) for a 12-week period. Skills are targeted in 3-week blocks, and include rhyme, initial sounds, final sounds, and phoneme analysis and synthesis. Thirty-six lesson plans describe activities and provide detailed guidance on teaching strategies. Pilot studies (Dayton & Schuele, 1997; Schuele et al., 2008) have suggested that the program is effective in increasing phonological awareness and word-decoding skills in children with language impairment and also in a broad sample of kindergartners. However, the efficacy of this program for children with speech impairments still needs to be established.

Classroom-Based Phonological Awareness Instruction   Increasingly, explicit phonological awareness activities are found in the daily activities of kindergarten, first-grade, and second-grade classrooms. Providing phonological awareness instruction within the classroom can be an efficient and effective means for promoting these skills in all children, including those with speech difficulties (Carson et al., 2013; Fuchs et al., 2001; Shapiro & Solity, 2008).

SLPs have a dual role in ensuring the successful implementation of class-wide phonological awareness teaching. First, clinicians should review the school's curriculum to familiarize themselves with how phonological awareness is targeted. At school age, phonological awareness instruction should be based primarily at the phoneme level and explicitly connect speech and print (Gillon, 2004). SLPs may thus need to provide supplemental activities if the curriculum does not meet this requirement. Clinicians' second role lies in assisting with the successful implementation of an evidenced-based classroom program. There is now a large body of research showing that teachers tend to have a poor understanding of linguistic structure, including phonological awareness, that limits their ability to provide explicit instruction in these skills (e.g., Carroll et al., 2012). SLPs can provide professional development and ongoing coaching to support the use of explicit phonological awareness teaching. It is important that this is done in a collaborative manner whereby the teacher's knowledge of literacy development is acknowledged and links to other aspects of the classroom curriculum are emphasized (Wilson et al., 2016, 2017).

Preliminary evidence suggests that the implementation of quality literacy curricula by teachers with the appropriate professional support dramatically reduces the number of students who need specialist literacy support (Carson et al., 2013; Gillon et al., 2019). Carson and colleagues examined the effects of a 10-week phoneme awareness program delivered by teachers who were coached by an SLP for 34 children in their first year of schooling. A comparison group of 95 children was monitored while receiving their usual program. Decoding difficulty was reported for 6% of students in the intervention classrooms versus 26% for children who did not participate in the program. Similarly, Shapiro and Solity (2008) reported an incidence of reading difficulty of 5% in students receiving a classroom-based phoneme awareness program versus 20% in students receiving an established curriculum. Importantly, children with speech and/or language difficulty also benefit from classroom-based phoneme awareness instruction, but are likely to show a different pattern of response and should be monitored carefully to identify whether more intensive instruction is needed (Carson et al., 2013; Tyler et al., 2014). A summary of the classroom program and professional development support for the Carson and colleagues study is presented in Table 13.4.

More recent work has focused on classroom level (tier 1) intervention support in facilitating the early literacy development of children with lower levels of oral language (including children with SSDs). Gillon and colleagues (2019) investigated the impact of a 10-week (4 × 30-minute sessions per week) teacher-led phonological awareness and oral language intervention for 141 children entering school with low levels of oral language. A stepped wedge design was utilized where schools allocated to Strand A received the intervention first and schools allocated to Strand B received the intervention 10 weeks later. The results showed that the research intervention accelerated children's phoneme awareness, decoding, and vocabulary knowledge in comparison to the usual classroom curriculum.

Gillon and colleagues (2020) compared the impact of this teacher-led intervention for children with language difficulties alone (n=101), children with speech and language difficulties (n=40), and children with typical development (n=96). Children with speech and language difficulties showed a similar response to intervention in

Table 13.4. Example of classroom-based phonological awareness training

Timing	Activities
Weeks 1–3	Rhyme recognition; initial and final phoneme identity
Weeks 4–7	Phoneme segmentation and blending
Weeks 8–9	Phoneme manipulation
Week 10	Review
Weeks 1–10	Letter-sound knowledge was integrated into all activities
	Professional support: plenary sessions, modeling, and coaching in the classroom delivered by the speech-language pathologist during the program

Source: Carson et al. (2013).

phoneme awareness and vocabulary knowledge, but needed greater support than the comparison groups to transfer this knowledge to the word-decoding process. Comparison of the performance of the three groups at the reading and spelling scores at the end of the academic years showed a significant advantage for those who received the intervention earlier in the year (i.e., Strand A). A cornerstone of the Better Start to Literacy Approach (Gillon et al., 2019, 2020) is collaboration between teachers and SLPs in assessment, curriculum planning, and teaching.

Phonological Awareness Integrated Into Conventional Therapy   Children with PDs who appear not to have benefited from classroom or small-group phonological awareness programs, or for whom these programs are not available, may require explicit phonological awareness instruction embedded into their conventional speech therapy (one-on-one or small group). Clinicians can include activities in every session to stimulate children's awareness at the phoneme level and also facilitate their generalization of phonological awareness knowledge in reading and in spelling. Twenty hours of intervention (administered by an SLP twice weekly) has proven effective in ensuring long-term gains from phonological awareness to reading and spelling for children with speech impairment (Gillon, 2002). The phonological awareness intervention may be structured to simultaneously target speech goals and phonological awareness knowledge at the phoneme level. An example of integrating speech targets and phonological awareness for a 6-year-old child is provided next (see Gillon, 2019).

Intervention With Older Children

Research suggests that older children can increase their phonological awareness with direct instruction in phonological awareness (Gillon & Dodd, 1995; Swanson et al., 2005; Torgesen et al., 1997). Thus, older children experiencing reading difficulties in combination with PDs may benefit from explicit phonological awareness intervention delivered by the SLP; indeed, deficits in phonological awareness may contribute substantially to many of these children's problems with reading and writing (Preston & Edwards, 2007). In addition, some children who have moved beyond the early elementary grades may never have developed an adequate phonological awareness foundation. Other children may have rudimentary skills but fail to develop more complex phonological awareness skills (e.g., phoneme analysis and synthesis). For some children who have histories of phonologic impairment, this weakness may be most evident in poor spelling ability (McNeill et al., 2017). A thorough multidisciplinary evaluation of reading, writing, and phonological awareness will clarify children's needs. Subsequently, systematic instruction can be provided by clinicians, with specific goals and activities designed to meet the individual needs of these children.

We can expect that explicit phonological awareness intervention that facilitates children's awareness of phonemes in words and facilitates understanding of the link between spoken and written words will lead to improved phonological awareness, reading, and spelling for many children with disorders of speech production. However, continued research is necessary to more clearly understand the relationship among PDs, phonological awareness, and reading development. Of greatest need is identifying treatment approaches that are most effective and efficient for addressing speech difficulties simultaneously with phonological awareness challenges. Of particular importance is identifying a sufficient array of approaches so that children who do not respond adequately to one approach can be provided another. In this regard, the educational outcomes and literacy potential of children who exhibit developmental vulnerabilities in both speech and reading can be maximized.

Teaching Example

The following teaching example illustrates an activity for providing instruction with a goal of increasing phonological awareness:

Speech Goal: Reduce speech error pattern of cluster reduction for *st* cluster.

Phonological Awareness Goals: Increase awareness of phonemes in words and make explicit the link between phonemes and graphemes.

Target Speech Words for Lesson: *star, sty, stop, step, Stan*

Stimulus Items: Picture cards of target speech items with the words printed underneath in a large, clear font (e.g., font size 48).

Prompt: Prompt the correct articulation of the target cluster through integrating phonological awareness and letter knowledge. For example, the child articulates the word *star* as *tar* and the clinician prompts: "When you say *tar* I can't hear the /s/ sound at the beginning (pointing to the letter *s* in the word *star*). Listen to the /s/ sound at the beginning of the word *star*. Let's try again with the /s/ sound at the beginning of *star* (pointing to the letter *s* at the beginning of the word)."

Appendix B provides illustrations of various phoneme awareness activities that can be used to promote children's phoneme awareness. Activities such as these can be readily integrated into conventional therapies focused on speech intelligibility.

QUESTIONS FOR CHAPTER 13

1. What are some key indicators of phonological awareness that emerge during the preschool period?

2. What is the relationship between phonological awareness and reading ability?

3. Why are children with expressive PDs at increased risk for problems with phonological awareness?

4. What is the SLP's role with respect to phonological awareness?

5. What are specific strategies that the SLP can use to promote phonological awareness for preschool-age children?

6. What might a classroom-based or intensive small-group phonological awareness intervention program look like?

14

Language and Dialectal Variations

BRIAN A. GOLDSTEIN, LEAH FABIANO-SMITH, AND AQUILES IGLESIAS

LEARNING OBJECTIVES

This chapter focuses on how language and dialectal variations impact the assessment and treatment of speech sound disorders (SSDs). By the end of this chapter, the reader should be able to:

- Explain the term *dialect* and how it is involved in speech assessment and diagnosis.
- Compare and contrast General American English (GAE) with common non-mainstream English varieties.
- Explain the concept of speech disorder within a diverse society of speakers.
- List common phonological features of common nonmainstream dialects.
- Apply knowledge of nonmainstream dialects to the assessment and treatment process for possible SSDs.
- Demonstrate knowledge of best practices in speech pathology when working with bilingual speakers.
- Demonstrate knowledge of the phonologies of languages other than English commonly spoken in the United States.
- Apply knowledge of languages other than English to the assessment and treatment process of possible SSDs.

Speech patterns used by individuals in our society vary as a function of language, age, socioeconomic status, and geography. Speech patterns also vary as a function of an individual's ability to acquire and produce the speech patterns of their community. As speech-language pathologists (SLPs), it is our responsibility to sort out the array of patterns that are typical of a child's speech community from those that are indicative of an SSD (defined as including both segment- and pattern-based errors). Information on variations in speech patterns seen within and across particular speech communities is necessary to conduct least-biased phonological assessments that reflect the characteristics of the child's speech community. For example, if members of a child's speech community consist of individuals who are bilingual (e.g., speak Spanish and English) and the variety of English spoken in the child's community is African American English (AAE), then the child will most likely speak a variety of English that has been influenced by both AAE and Spanish. Assessment of such a child must take into account the influence that AAE and Spanish might have on the child's phonological patterns. Sensitivity to and knowledge of variation are also required to adequately serve those individuals who elect to modify the language variety that they speak. The following sections examine phonological variation within and across languages and show how this information can be used to conduct least-biased assessments and plan for intervention.

DIALECT

Dialects are mutually intelligible forms of a language associated with a particular region, social class, or ethnic group. GAE, Southern White Standard, Appalachian English, Caribbean English, AAE, Eastern American English, and Spanish-influenced English are just some of the dialects spoken in the United States. No dialect of any language is superior to any other because all thoughts can be expressed using any dialect of any language. This is not to say that all varieties of a language carry the same prestige. Some varieties of a language, specifically those used by the dominant groups in any socially stratified society, will be considered to have higher prestige (Wolfram, 1986), will be promulgated within the educational system (Adler, 1984), and will be valued by the private sector of that society (Shuy, 1972; Terrell & Terrell, 1983).

The promulgation of GAE (the prestige dialect in the United States) within the educational system and by contact through broadcast media between members of different regional dialects has decreased differences between dialects. This is referred to as *dialect leveling.* At the same time, lack of linguistic contact among groups due to geographical or socioeconomic reasons has resulted in a linguistic isolation that has increased the distance between dialects (Labov, 1991). In addition, the increased immigration and ethnic isolation that have occurred among some subgroups have further increased the number and pervasiveness of dialects. The courts' acknowledgment of the rights of linguistic minority populations has resulted in greater acceptance of varieties other than GAE. For example, *Martin Luther King Junior Elementary School Children et al. v. Ann Arbor School District* (1978) provided for the use of children's home language, including AAE, in the educational process. At least in terms of dialects, the melting pot hypothesis appears to be a myth for certain segments of our society.

Regardless of whether dialects are becoming more or less like each other, people hold many different myths about dialects. Wolfram and Schilling-Estes (1998) have identified a number of myths held about dialects and have countered those myths with corresponding facts (see Table 14.1).

Speakers of a particular dialect do not always use all of the features present in their dialect. A speaker's use of particular features depends on the context and interlocutors (register). *Registral varieties* are dependent on the participants, setting, and topic. For example, one would typically use one register when talking to friends about an enjoyable weekend and use another variety when giving an important presentation to colleagues at work.

The extent to which particular individuals use the available features of their dialect (*dialect density*) may depend on factors such as socioeconomic status and geography (e.g., Oetting & McDonald, 2002). Sometimes the differences in dialect density are associated with socioeconomic status, a sociolinguistic phenomenon referred to by Wolfram (1986) as *social diagnosticity.* Wolfram observed the frequency of occurrence of selected AAE features among the speech of individuals representing four socioeconomic groups: upper middle class, lower middle class, upper working class, and lower working class. His research revealed that certain AAE linguistic features

Table 14.1. Dialect myths and facts

Myth	Fact	Example
A dialect is a variety spoken by someone else.	Everyone speaks some dialect of a language.	Although there is a dialect form often referred to as the standard (e.g., Standard or GAE), it is usually a form not actually spoken by anyone in an invariable form. There is variation to one extent or another used by all speakers.
Dialectal features are always distinct and noticeable.	Some dialectal features are shared by many different dialects.	The weakening of postvocalic r (e.g., /moɚ/ → [moə]) is exhibited by speakers of AAE, Eastern American English, and Southern American English.
Dialects arise from ineffective tries at speaking the correct form of the language.	Speakers of dialects acquire those features by interacting with members of the speech community in which they live.	Some native speakers of Spanish often use characteristics of AAE because speakers of both varieties often live in the same community (Poplack, 1978).
Dialects are random changes from the standard.	Dialects are precise and show regular patterns.	In many dialects of the American South, /ɪ/ and /ɛ/ are pronounced as [ɪ] before nasals; /pɪn/; /pɛn/ → [pɪn].
Dialects are always viewed negatively.	Dialects are not inherently viewed negatively (or positively, for that matter); the prestige of any dialect is derived from the social prestige of its speakers.	Ramirez and Milk (1986) found that bilingual teachers rated the local Mexican dialect of Spanish as less prestigious than the general dialect of Spanish. The dialect of English spoken by the British monarchy, however, is often perceived as prestigious.

showed *gradient stratification* across the four groups. That is, individuals in lower socioeconomic groups used more of the available features of that dialect than individuals in higher socioeconomic groups.

Washington and Craig (1998) found this same effect for 5- and 6-year-old AAE-speaking boys. For example, the lack of realization of postvocalic r (e.g., /sɪstɚ/ → [sɪstə]) is an example of gradient stratification because all socioeconomic groups use this phonological feature, albeit with different levels of frequency. On the other hand, certain AAE features show a pattern of usage referred to as *sharp stratification,* which refers to linguistic features that more clearly differentiate socioeconomic groups, based on significant differences in frequency of usage. One example of this type of stratification is the substitution of [f] for /θ/. The use of this feature contrasts middle-class with working-class groups, as working-class groups use the feature much more frequently than middle-class speakers. Wolfram has indicated that features revealing sharp stratification are of greater social diagnosticity than those showing gradient stratification.

Geography may also play a role in the likelihood of a specific dialect feature being expressed. For example, Hinton and Pollock (1999) examined the occurrence of vocalic and postvocalic American English /ɪ/ in AAE speakers from two geographic regions (Davenport, Iowa, and Memphis, Tennessee). Overall, they found that speakers in Davenport were more likely than speakers in Memphis to maintain the rhotic quality of vocalic and postvocalic /ɪ/. (Note: For purposes of this chapter, the symbol /ɪ/ is used to represent the rhotic sound found in GAE and its dialects. The symbol /r/, as specified by the International Phonetic Alphabet Association, is used to designate the alveolar trill.) Hinton and Pollock accounted for these results largely in terms of the demographic characteristics of the two communities. The African American community in Memphis accounts for close to 50% of the city's population, compared to only 5% in Davenport. Moreover, African American children in Memphis are much more likely to be taught by African American teachers compared to those in Davenport.

DISORDER WITHIN DIALECT

The problem of misdiagnosis of speech and language disorders in children who are speakers of dialects other than GAE is well documented, both in terms of underdiagnosis (Washington et al., 2019) and overdiagnosis (Oetting et al., 2013). The categorization of dialect versus disorder in the diagnostic process has been the framework used until recently to avoid over-identifying children as language impaired. Oetting and colleagues (2016) reminded us that children who speak nonmainstream dialect varieties and also present with language impairment are often unidentified due to the perceived mutual exclusivity of dialect and disorder. They offered a new framework for considering how we can adjust this dichotomy to more accurately view language impairment within a diverse society.

Oetting and colleagues (2016) posited that all children in society are dialect speakers and that only a small proportion of children will present with language impairment. They also point out that children who are speakers of a dialect can also present with language impairment, therefore, the dialect versus disorder dichotomy falls short; it misses children who are dialect speakers and also present with language impairment. This leads clinicians to underdiagnose language impairment in children who speak nonmainstream dialect varieties. SLPs can avoid underdiagnosis of language impairment by focusing on the children with disorders as the clinical population in need of services. This chapter will detail dialect varieties of less common dialect varieties, but as we move toward accurate identification of children with language impairment, the Oetting and colleagues (2016) conceptualization of disorder within dialect will serve as our theoretical rationale.

It is important to note that dialects are often stigmatized, arbitrarily, based on the group of people who use a certain dialect (Wolfram, 2004). For example, AAE and Puerto Rican Spanish are often viewed as less prestigious dialects as compared to GAE and Standard Castilian Spanish (Wolfram, 2004). SLPs should take care in discussions of dialect with their clients. It is often helpful to ask clients themselves to identify the variety of language they use rather than labeling their language variety for them.

CHARACTERISTICS OF AMERICAN ENGLISH DIALECTS

In addition to GAE, there are a number of dialects of English spoken in the United States. This chapter focuses on five common dialects: AAE, Eastern American English, Southern American English, Appalachian English, and Ozark English. Most of the available literature on these dialects focuses on their characteristics rather than on their development.

African American English

AAE is a variety of American English that is spoken by many, but not all, African Americans. Other groups who have contact with AAE speakers also speak it. For example,

English-speaking Puerto Rican teenagers in East Harlem, New York, have been found to use features of AAE (Wolfram, 1974). Wolfram found that the degree of contact that the teenagers had with AAE speakers greatly influenced the number of AAE features in their speech. Those individuals with the most contact showed the greatest number of features in their speech. Poplack (1978) examined the use of AAE, Puerto Rican Spanish, and Philadelphia English variants in the speech of sixth-grade Puerto Rican boys and girls. She found that the Puerto Rican boys tended to use more features of AAE, and the girls used more features of Philadelphia English. Poplack concluded that the specific variants used by the children were more related to covert prestige than to their linguistic environment, with the boys assigning more prestige to AAE speakers and the girls assigning more prestige to Philadelphia English. The results of both of these studies support the notion that use of dialect features is influenced by patterns in the speech community and that speech patterns are greatly affected by peer interaction.

Children who are speakers of AAE learn very early on in child development how to code-switch between AAE and GAE. Craig and Washington (2004) examined AAE-speaking children from preschool through fifth grade and found that children started to shift their dialect use toward GAE in first grade. The ability to code-switch requires a metalinguistic skill set that takes into consideration pragmatics (e.g., the sociolinguistic consequences of switching from one dialect to another) and cognitive processes such as analysis and control (Bialystock, 2001); therefore, children may not demonstrate code-switching until they reach 6 or 7 years old, but from that point on, SLPs should not wonder if AAE-speaking children have the ability to code-switch or not. Whether or not AAE-speaking school-age children demonstrate code-switching is not a matter of GAE mastery, but rather, due to sociolinguistic variables.

Like all dialects, AAE is systematic, with rule-governed phonological, semantic, syntactic, pragmatic, and proxemic systems (Wolfram et al., 1999). There are two major hypotheses accounting for the origin of AAE (Poplack, 2000; Wolfram & Schilling-Estes, 1998). The Creole hypothesis assumes that AAE descended from Plantation Creole (Wolfram, 1994; Wolfram & Schilling-Estes, 1998), a language that developed from a mixture of languages brought into contact during the slave trade period. Plantation Creole was commonly used by Black people who were enslaved on plantations in the South but was not spoken by European Americans at the time.

Over time, AAE has further spread and changed. The exodus of African Americans from the Southeast to the Northeast and other parts of the United States in the early 1900s brought AAE to the urban areas of the North (Stewart, 1971). In many cases, individuals from a particular state tended to migrate to particular cities (e.g., many South Carolinians moved to Philadelphia). The restricted social environments in which many African Americans lived, in addition to the continued contact with their southern families and communities, reinforced the use of AAE. In its evolution, AAE has undergone a decreolization process, showing fewer links to its Creole past and acquiring features that are not traceable to the original Creole (e.g., stopping of interdental fricatives) (Wolfram & Schilling-Estes, 1998).

An alternative hypothesis, the (Neo-) Anglicist hypothesis, states that AAE is considered a dialect of English; that is, AAE can be traced to the varieties of English spoken in Britain (Wolfram & Schilling-Estes, 1998). Thus, enslaved peoples who were brought to the United States eventually "learned the regional and social varieties of surrounding white speakers" (p. 176). Although the exact origins of AAE are unsettled, the prevailing view seems to be that AAE owes its current form to influences of its dialect and Creole roots (Green, 2004).

A number of linguistic features distinguish AAE from GAE. The major phonological features that distinguish these two varieties are listed in Table 14.2. These features are always optional, are not used in each possible phonetic context, and are not produced by all AAE speakers. For example, the simplification of word-final clusters tends to occur when one of the consonants is an alveolar and the other (i.e., the deleted consonant) is a morphological marker (Stockman, 1996a). Hence, some AAE speakers may not differentiate between the present and past tense of the same verb (e.g., *miss* and *missed* are pronounced as [mɪs]), but would retain the cluster in a word such as *mist*. Moreover, the occurrence of phonological dialect features appears to change over time. Craig and Washington (2004) found a significant decline in the number of phonological dialect features produced between second and third grades in a group of 400 typically developing African American children from low- and middle-income households.

Features of AAE extend to suprasegmental phenomena as well (Hyter, 1996; Stockman, 1996a). For example, AAE speakers may place stress on the first rather than second syllable (*Detróit → Détroit*), use a wide range of intonation contours and vowel elongations, and produce more level and falling final contours than rising contours.

Table 14.2. Major phonological features distinguishing African American English and General American English

Pattern	Example(s)
Word-final consonant cluster reduction (particularly when one of the two consonants is an alveolar)	/tɛst/ → [tɛs]
Final /d/ glottalization	/mæd/ → [mæʔ]
Deletion of /ɹ/	/sɪstæ/ → [sɪstə]
	/kæɹəl/ → [kæəl]
	/pɹʌfɛsɚ/ → [pʌfɛsə]
Hyperarticulation of /ɹ/	/hɛɹ/ → [hɛɹə]
Deletion of /l/ in word-final abutting consonants	/ hɛlp/ → [hɛp]
Deletion of nasal consonant in word-final position with nasalization of preceding vowel	/mun/ → [mũ]
Substitution of [ɪ] for /ɛ/ before nasals	pin /pɪn/ and pen /pɛn/ pronounced as [pɪn]
Substitution of [k] for /t/ in initial /stɹ/ clusters	/stɹit/ → [skɹit]
Realization of /θɹ/ as [θ]	/θɹo/ → [θo]
Substitution of f/θ and v/ ð in intervocalic position	/nʌθɪŋ/ → [nʌfɪŋ]
	/beðɪŋ/ → [bevɪŋ]
Substitution of f/θ in word-final position	/saʊθ/ → [saʊf]
Realization of /v/ as [b] and /z/ as [d], in word-internal position before syllabic nasals	/sɛvən/ → [sɛbən]
Stopping of word-initial interdentals	/ðe/ → [de]
	/ðɑt/ → [dɑt]
Metathesis (might be lexically specific)	/æsk/ → [æks]
Omission of unstressed syllables in iambic words	/əɹaʊnd/ → [ɹaʊnd]
Omission of word internal, unstressed syllables	/mɪsɪsɪpi/ → [mɪsɪpi]
Stressing of initial weak syllables	/ɪnˈʃɚəns/ → [ˈɪnʃɚəns]

Sources: Compiled from Bailey & Thomas (1998); Craig et al. (2003); Hyter (1996); Pollock et al. (1998); Rickford (1999); Stockman (1996a); Velleman & Pearson (2010); Wolfram & Schilling-Estes (1998).

Moreover, phonotactics and suprasegmental phenomena tend to interact. For example, AAE-speaking children tend to produce /d/ less accurately in unstressed syllables versus stressed ones and to reduce clusters more often in unstressed versus stressed syllables (Burns et al., 2010).

Phonological Development in African American English

In comparison to the investigation of phonological skills in speakers of GAE, more research is needed on the development of AAE phonology. Existing studies have examined phonological development in typically developing AAE-speaking children and AAE-speaking children with SSDs. Major findings indicate that AAE-speaking children tend to produce the same phonetic inventory as speakers of GAE (Stockman, 1996a), show great intersubject variability, exhibit systematic error patterns, show increased consonant accuracy by age, and demonstrate differences in both the type and quantity of speech errors exhibited by typically developing speakers and those with SSDs (Stockman, 2010).

Preschoolers speaking AAE and GAE often exhibit similar phonological patterns, although with different frequencies. Bland-Stewart (2003) examined the phonological skills of eight AAE-speaking 2-year-olds. She found that their phonological skills were similar to those exhibited by GAE-speaking peers. Seymour and Seymour (1981) compared the performance of 4- and 5-year-old African American and white children. They reported that both groups evidenced phonological variations typically associated with AAE (e.g., f/' in medial and final positions; d/ð in initial and medial positions; b/v in initial and medial positions). The AAE features, however, occurred more frequently in the productions of the African American children. Thus, both groups produced the same type of substitutions, but the frequency of their use differed between the two groups. These results suggested that, for the children they studied, the contrast between AAE and GAE was qualitatively undifferentiated at this age. The same result has also been demonstrated for phonological processes (i.e., patterns) (Haynes & Moran, 1989). Differences across dialect groups, however, have been noted in the production of final consonants. In the speech of AAE-speaking children, final consonants are often absent (Stockman, 2010). These absences are rule governed. For example, nasal and oral stops are omitted less often if words that precede them begin with vowels (Stockman).

Stockman (2006a) examined the production of syllable-initial consonants in seven typically developing AAE-speaking children aged 2;8 to 3;0. All seven children produced 15 syllable-initial, singleton consonants (/m, n, p, b, t, d, k, g, w, j, l, ɹ, f, s, h/) at least four times in at least two different words. These 15 segments represent the minimal competence core (MCC) of phonemes that are invariant in both AAE and GAE (Stockman). Accuracy for the group of segments in the MCC exceeded 80% (range = 81%–99%) compared to less than 80% (range = 14%–76%) for sounds not in the MCC (i.e., the segments that vary between AAE and GAE). Error patterns included voicing errors, liquid gliding, stopping, and fronting. All seven children produced syllable-initial consonant clusters, totaling 19 types. Of the 19 types, 15 were of the oral stop + sonorant or fricative + sonorant variety. The children also produced /s/ + stop clusters and one three-member cluster, /skr-/. Results show that the phonetic skills of young AAE-speaking children are similar to those of same-aged children speaking GAE.

In a follow-up study with 120 African American children, Stockman (2008) corroborated findings from the earlier study. Results from this study also were commensurate with those examining the production of initial consonants in speakers of

Standard (i.e., General) American English (e.g., Smit et al., 1990) and Standard British English (e.g., Dodd, Holm et al., 2003). Finally, Stockman and associates (2013) found a relationship between the MCC for phonology and other aspects of language; for example, morphology.

Pearson and colleagues (2009) examined the phonological skills of 537 children aged 4–12 years acquiring AAE and 317 children of the same age acquiring Mainstream (i.e., General) American English (MAE). They found that children acquiring AAE and MAE showed commensurate mastery (accuracy greater than or equal to 90%) of most singleton consonants in initial position—(/b/, /t/, /k/, /g/, /m/, /n/, /h/, /j/, /w/, /dʒ/, /ʃ/, /tʃ/, /l/). However, children acquiring AAE mastered some initial segments (e.g., /ɪ/ and /s/), initial clusters (/kl-, pl-, kɹ-, gɹ-, pɹ-, sp-, st-, skɹ-/), and some final singletons (/s/ and /z/) earlier than did children acquiring MAE. Finally, acquisition of /d/ and /ð/ by AAE speakers occurred after that of MAE speakers. In final position results were similar, in that speakers of AAE and MAE generally showed comparable skills. By 6 years of age, AAE speakers had mastered all consonants except /t/, /d/, /θ/, and /ð/; MAE speakers had mastered all consonants except /θ/ and /ð/. It should be noted that MAE speakers mastered /ð/ at age 8 compared with age 12 for AAE speakers. However, AAE speakers mastered /s/ and /z/ by age 4 compared with age 6 for MAE speakers. Finally, speakers of AAE tended to master a number of initial clusters (e.g., /kl/, pɹ/) earlier than MAE speakers, but MAE speakers mastered final clusters (e.g., /ks/, /nt/) before AAE speakers.

In an examination of data from this same group of participants, Velleman and Pearson (2010) discussed the relationship between phonetic and phonotactic (e.g., syllable structure) development in AAE and MAE speakers. Results indicated that AAE speakers showed more advanced phonological skills related to segments than to phonotactics. The authors predicted this finding, given that AAE speakers have less overall exposure to structures, such as final singleton consonants, final clusters, and iambic words (i.e., words like *gi-RAFFE* that have a weak-strong stress pattern). Taken together, the results from these two studies indicate that AAE speakers may be placing greater emphasis on segmental rather than phonotactic learning, which, in turn, leads to mastery of some later-developing consonants by AAE speakers before MAE speakers. Consonant accuracy also has been examined in AAE. For typically developing children, Stockman (2008) found that consonant accuracy averaged 81%–82% in 3-year-olds on a spontaneous speech task. In elicited single words, it averaged 95%–98% for children aged 3;7 to 6;1 (Pollock & Berni, 1997, in Stockman, 2010).

Variability across children has been found to be a hallmark of AAE phonological development. Seymour and Seymour (1981) reported considerable interchild variability among AAE speakers. All of the target features were not present in each AAE speaker, nor were they equally distributed among the speakers. Although there is variability in phonological development between AAE-speaking children, the context for error patterns exhibited by these children has been found to be systematic. For example, although AAE-speaking children delete final consonants, they do not do so arbitrarily. Stockman (1996a, 2006b) noted that alveolar consonants were more likely than either labials or velars to be deleted, oral stops and nasals were more likely than fricatives to be deleted, and final consonants preceding a consonant were more likely to be deleted. In addition, the absence of final consonants may be marked by lengthening or nasalizing the vowel that precedes the absent consonant (Moran, 1993).

Bryant and associates (2001) found that AAE-speaking children were more likely to delete one element of a word-final cluster if a more sonorous element preceded a less sonorous element. For example, words ending in /sk/ clusters (more sonorous element preceding less sonorous element) were more likely to undergo deletion than those ending in /ks/ clusters (less sonorous element preceding more sonorous element). In addition, their results indicated that in the clusters in which a more sonorous element preceded a less sonorous one, the most sonorous element was preserved. For example, AAE-speaking children would produce *desk* /dɛsk/ as [dɛs] and not [dɛk].

Developmental differences between typically developing AAE speakers and those with SSDs have been found to be quantitatively and qualitatively different. Bleile and Wallach (1992) compared the articulation of typically developing and speech-delayed AAE-speaking children ranging in age from 3;6 to 5;5. Head Start teachers who shared the same racial and linguistic background as the children differentiated the two groups of children. Data analysis was based on non-AAE phonological patterns exhibited by the children in a picture-identification, single-word test. The delayed and typically developing groups demonstrated differences in the type and quantity of their speech errors. Speech-delayed children had a larger number of 1) stop errors (especially velars), 2) fricative errors in all positions (especially fricatives other than /θ/), and 3) affricate errors in all positions. Typically developing participants evidenced greater devoicing of final /d/, sonorant errors, and errors related to /ɹ/. Both groups of children produced a large number of consonant cluster errors, with the speech-delayed children exhibiting a larger number of cluster errors. Bleile and Wallach concluded that a combination of characteristics, rather than a single indicator, appears to be the most reliable index of speech delay in AAE speakers, just as it is with children who do not speak AAE.

Velleman and Pearson (2010) examined the phonological skills of 76 AAE speakers with SSDs and 72 GAE speakers with SSDs, aged 4–12 years. They found that the features exhibited by both groups were similar. Moreover, the children "did not differ by dialect with respect to their overall number of mismatches to GAE targets in any position" (p. 184), indicating that dialect was largely neutralized in these groups of children with SSDs. Finally, the AAE-speaking children with SSDs mastered some consonants before their GAE counterparts—/s, tʃ, dʒ, ɹ/. Results from this study show the similarity and differences in the phonological skills of AAE- and GAE-speaking children, and highlight the need to account for dialect features in children's speech.

Eastern American English and Southern American English

Eastern American English and Southern American English, described by Labov (1991) as northern and southern dialects, are two geographical variations of GAE. The Eastern American dialect runs generally from Vermont on the north, parts of Iowa and Minnesota to the west, and New Jersey to the south (Wolfram & Schilling-Estes, 1998). The Southern American dialect runs generally from Maryland on the north, Texas to the west, and Florida to the south (Wolfram & Schilling-Estes, 1998). Although these two dialects share many of the same features, they can also be differentiated from each other through differences in the production of both vowels and consonants (see Table 14.3).

Appalachian English and Ozark English

Two other common geographical dialects of English are Appalachian English (AE) and Ozark English (OE). Christian and colleagues (1988) indicate that AE and OE are related linguistically, with OE having many features that are similar to AE. Given the

Table 14.3. Common dialectal variations in English

Pattern	Example		Dialect
Vowels			
Tense → lax	/i/ → [ɪ]	/rili/ → [rɪlɪ]	SAE
	/u/ → [ʊ]	/rut/ → [rʊt]	EAE
Lax → tense	/ɪ/ → [i]	/fɪʃ/ → [fiʃ]	SAE
	/ɛ/ → [e]	/ɛg/ → [eg]	SAE
	/æ/ → [a]	/hæf/ → [haf]	EAE
Vowel neutralization	/ɪ/; /ɛ/ → [ɪ]	/pɪn/; /pɛn/ → [pɪn]	SAE
Diphthong reduction	/aɪ/ → [a]	/paɪ/ → [pa]	SAE
a/ɔ		[fɔt] → [fat]	SAE, EAE
Lowering	/ɔ/ → [a]	/fɔɚ/ → [faɚ]	SAE, EAE
Derhoticization	/ɚ/ → [ə]	/fɔɚ/ → [fɔə]	SAE, EAE
r deletion		/kaɚ/ → [ka]	SAE, EAE
r addition	/ə/ → [ɚ]	/lɪndə/ → [lɪndɚ]	EAE
Consonants			
Velar fronting	/ŋ/→ [n]	/ɹʌnɪŋ / → [ɹʌnɪn]	SAE
/j/ addition		/nu/ → [nju]	SAE, EAE
Voicing assimilation	/s/ → [z]	/gɹisi/ → [gɹizi]	SAE
Glottalization	/t/; /d/ → [ʔ]	/batəl/ → [baʔəl]	EAE
[t]; [d] for /θ/; /ð/	/θ/ → [t]	/θɪŋk/ → [tɪŋk]	EAE
	/ð/ → [d]	/ðɪs/ → [dɪs]	EAE

Key: SAE, Southern American English; EAE, Eastern American English.

Sources: Compiled from Bailey & Thomas, 1998; Craig, Thompson, Washington, & Potter, 2003; Hyter, 1996; Pollock, Bailey, Berni, Fletcher, Hinton, Johnson, & Weaver, 1998; Rickford, 1999; Stockman, 1996a; Velleman & Pearson, 2010; Wolfram & Schilling-Estes, 1998.

phonological similarities of these two dialects, they will be discussed together. Appalachian English is spoken generally in parts of Kentucky, Tennessee, Virginia, North Carolina, and West Virginia (parts of the Carolinas, Georgia, and Alabama may also be included). Ozark English is spoken in an area encompassing northern Arkansas, southern Missouri, and northwestern Oklahoma. Christian and colleagues (1988, pp. 153–159) have outlined the characteristics of AE and OE in Table 14.4. Only the most common features are shown (see also Flipsen, 2007, for more details).

As was the case for AAE in African American speakers, not all features of AE and OE are utilized by every speaker, used in every situation, or produced in every context. For example, the rule noted as *intrusive t*, in which [t] may be added to words ending in /s/ or /f/, is usually limited to a small set of words. Most commonly, the rule takes effect on the words *once* and *twice*. In addition, the number of words exhibiting this rule seems to be more extensive in AE than OE.

PHONOLOGY IN SPEAKERS OF LANGUAGE VARIETIES OTHER THAN ENGLISH

Prior to the arrival of Europeans, what is now the continental United States was a polyglot area with over 200 languages or dialects spoken (Leap, 1981). Over the past 600 years, immigrants to this area have brought their culture and language.

Table 14.4. Characteristics of Appalachian English and Ozark English

Rule	Example
Epenthesis following clusters	
CCC# → CC↔C#	/gosts/ → [gostəs]
Intrusive *t* (more common in AE)	
/s/# → [st]	/wʌns/ → [wʌnst]
/f/# → [ft]	/klɪf/ → [klɪft]
Stopping of fricatives	
/θ/ → [t]	/θɑt/ → [tɑt]
/ð/ → [d]	/ðe/ → [de]
Initial *w* reduction	
/w/ → Ø	/wɪl/ → [ɪl]
Initial unstressed syllables lost	
IUS → Ø	/əlaʊd/ → [laʊd]
h retention	
Ø → [h]	/ɪt/ → [hɪt]
Retroflex *r* lost	
/ɹ/ → Ø (postconsonantal)	/θɹo/ → [θo]
/ɹ/ → Ø (intervocalic)	/kæɹi/ → [kæi]
Lateral *l* lost	
/l/ → Ø before labials	/wʊlf/ → [wʊf]

Source: Christian et al., 1988.

Historically, the general trend for most immigrants to the United States was to use their home language as their primary language of communication. By the third generation, though, immigrants tended to lose their language of origin (Veltman, 1988). Some immigrant groups, however, have maintained the use of their home language (also termed *first* or *primary language*) from generation to generation, with reinforcement from new immigrants and travel to their country of origin.

In total, there are over 60 million individuals older than 5 years in the United States who speak a language other than or in addition to English, 42% of whom speak English less than very well (U.S. Census Bureau, 2011). Of those 60 million speakers, over 37 million speak Spanish, and there are over 1 million speakers of Chinese (including all dialects), French, German, Korean, Tagalog, and Vietnamese, with almost 1 million Arabic speakers as well. The number of individuals speaking a language other than English at home in the United States increased from over 23 million in 1980 to over 60 million in 2010—a 158% increase. The number of individuals speaking a language variety other than English in the United States is likely to continue to increase in the coming years.

There has been a realization that although English is the most common and dominant language spoken in the United States, other languages have a right to coexist in our linguistically plural society. For example, *Lau v. Nichols* (1974) and the Lau Remedies (1975) mandated that federally funded schools must eliminate language barriers in school programs that excluded nonnative English speakers. The Individuals with Disabilities Education Act (IDEA; 2004) required that the native language commonly used in the home or learning environment be utilized in all contact for a child with a disability.

The current number and future increase of individuals from culturally and linguistically diverse populations mean that SLPs will likely encounter even more speakers of languages and language varieties other than English. To complete appropriate phonological assessments that guide the intervention process for children whose home language is not English, SLPs need to gather segmental, prosodic, syllabic, and developmental information. In this section, the characteristics of pidgins, creoles, and Spanish and Asian languages, along with information about phonological acquisition and development in speakers of Spanish and Asian languages, will be described. Although languages other than Spanish and those of Asia are spoken in the United States (e.g., Arabic) (Amayreh & Dyson, 1998, 2000; Dyson & Amayreh, 2000), we focus on those languages because the majority of children in the schools use those languages (Kindler, 2001).

Pidgins and Creoles

Language is always changing. This change is represented in all areas of language—phonology, syntax, semantics, lexicon, and pragmatics. This change may take place because of a number of factors, such as geography, social prestige, and the introduction of new vocabulary (Crystal, 1997). Pidgins and creoles are two examples of language change.

A *pidgin* is a communication system used by groups of people who wish and need to communicate with each other but have no means to do so. They use a limited vocabulary and simplified syntactic structure compared with their two native languages (Crystal, 1997). Pidgins are not degraded natural languages but rather come to have rules all their own. In fact, some pidgins, for example, Tok Pisin in Papua New Guinea, have become the most widely used linguistic variety in the country. Crystal notes, however, that a pidgin often has a short life (perhaps a few years) and disappears when the need for a common communication system ceases to exist.

A *creole* is a pidgin that becomes the mother tongue of a community. Thus, pidgins and creoles are two points on the same language development continuum (Crystal, 1997). In essence, a creole is a pidgin that serves as primary input to the next generation of speakers. That is, a pidgin becomes a creole when it is passed on to child speakers. Compared with pidgins, creoles show increased complexity in syntax, phonology, lexicon, semantics, and pragmatics (Muyksen & Smith, 1995). Creoles tend to show rules that were not exhibited in their pidgin ancestor (Holm, 1988).

Common Creoles in the United States

There are four main creoles that SLPs may encounter in the U.S.: Gullah, Hawaiian Creole, Louisiana French Creole, and Haitian Creole. This section briefly outlines their phonological characteristics.

Gullah (or *Geechee* or *Sea Island Creole,* as it is sometimes called) is spoken by approximately 250,000–300,000 speakers, mostly on the barrier islands off the coasts of South Carolina and Georgia (Holm, 1989). This English creole is closely related to other creoles, such as Sierra Leone Krio, Cameroons Creole, Jamaican Creole, the Creole of British Guiana, and the Creoles of Surinam (Cunningham, 1992). The origin of this creole is debated. Some believe that Gullah arrived in the American colonies from the west coast of Africa as a fully developed creole (Nichols, 1981). Others link its development to a complex interaction of white British settlers, Africans, and Caribbeans

(Holm). Some phonological features of Gullah (compared with GAE) include the use of [a] for /æ/, [t] for /θ/, [d] for /ð/, [dʒ] for /z/, and deletion of postvocalic /ɹ/.

Hawaiian Creole arose in the 19th century and culminates from the influence of many sources, such as Polynesian, European, Asian, and pidgin languages (Holm, 1989). Some phonological features of Hawaiian Creole (compared with GAE) include [t] for /θ/, [d] for /ð/, backing in the environment of [ɹ] (/θɹ/ → [tʃɹ]; /tɹ/ → [tʃɹ]; /stɹ/ → [ʃɹ]), deletion of postvocalic /ɹ/, and deletion of the second member of word-final abutting consonants; for example, /nɛst/ → [nɛs] (Bleile, 1996).

Louisiana French Creole evolved as the native language of descendants of enslaved West African people brought to southern Louisiana by French colonists (Dubois & Horvath, 2003; Nichols, 1981). This creole has also been influenced by features of Cajun, a variety of regional French brought from Canada (Holm, 1989). It is estimated that there are 60,000–80,000 speakers of this creole, although the number of speakers of French Creole in the United States is estimated to be approximately 750,000 (U.S. Census Bureau, 2011). The vowel system consists of four front vowels /i, e, ɛ, a/, four back vowels /u, o, ɔ, ɑ/, schwa /ə/, and three nasalized vowels /ɛ̃, ɔ̃, ɑ̃/ (Morgan, 1959; Nichols, 1981; Oetting, 2007). The consonant system contains six oral stops /b, d, g, p, t, k/, three nasal stops /m, n, ŋ/, seven fricatives /f, s, ʃ, v, z, ʒ, h/, two liquids /l, ɹ/, and one glide /j/. Common phonological patterns (Nichols, 1981; Oetting and Garrity, 2006) are: 1) abutting consonants across word boundaries are often assimilated to the voicing of the second member of the consonant pair, for example, /pæsði/ → [pæzði]; 2) word-final consonants may be deleted; 3) word-final unstressed syllables are often weakened or deleted; 4) voiceless stops might be deaspirated; 5) [t, d] is substituted for /θ, ð/; 6) vowel raising may take place in which [i] is substituted for /ɛ/; and 7) /ɑɪ/ is monophthongized.

SLPs might also encounter speakers of *Haitian Creole*. This Caribbean creole, spoken in Haiti, has approximately 6 million speakers (Muyksen & Veenstra, 1995). There are three dialects of Haitian Creole: northern, central (including the capital Port-au-Prince), and southern. The Haitian Creole vowel system contains seven segments: five uncounted vowels /i, u, e, o, a/ and two front-rounded vowels /ø/ and /æ/. The creole also contains 17 consonants, 6 stops /b, d, g, p, t, k/, 6 fricatives /f, s, ʃ, v, z, ʒ/, 3 nasals /m, n, ŋ/, and 2 liquids /l/ and /ɹ/.

Spanish

Spanish has become the second most common language spoken in the United States, with approximately 38 million speakers, or 12.8% of the U.S. population over 5 years of age (U.S. Census Bureau, 2011). According to Hammond (2001), there are two main dialects of American Spanish: Highland Spanish and Coastal Spanish. Dialects are categorized by one of these two types based on the behavior of syllable- and word-final consonants. Dialects in which syllable- and word-final consonants are preserved are known as *conservative dialects;* and those in which final consonants tend to be deleted are known as *radical dialects* (Guitart, 1978, 1996). Mexican Spanish exemplifies a conservative dialect, and Puerto Rican Spanish is emblematic of a radical dialect. In the following sections, we will review Spanish phonology and phonological development in Spanish speakers. It is important to note that children and adults who arrive in the United States from Spanish-speaking countries may also speak indigenous languages, exclusively or in addition to Spanish, associated with their region of origin.

Spanish Phonology

A brief overview of the Spanish consonant and vowel system is presented here (for a more complete description, see Goldstein, 1995, 2007a; Hammond, 2001; and Lipski, 2008). There are five primary vowels in Spanish:

- Two front vowels /i/ and /e/
- Three back vowels /u/, /o/, and /a/

There are 18 consonants in General Spanish (Núñez-Cedeño & Morales-Front, 1999):

- Voiceless unaspirated stops /p/, /t/, /k/
- Voiced stops /b/, /d/, /g/
- Nasals /m/, /n/, /ɲ/
- Voiceless fricatives /f/, /x/, /s/
- Affricate /tʃ/
- Glides /w/, /j/
- Lateral /l/
- Flap /ɾ/
- Trill /r/

The existence of differences between Spanish dialects further complicates the process of characterizing phonological patterns in Spanish-speaking children. Unlike English, in which dialectal variations are generally defined by variations in vowels, Spanish dialectal differences primarily affect consonant sound classes rather than vowels or a few specific phonemes. These are summarized in Table 14.5.

The dialect differences primarily affect certain sound classes over others. Fricatives and liquids (in particular /s/, flap /ɾ/, and trill /r/) tend to show more variation than stops, glides, or the affricate. The differences between Spanish dialects make it paramount that SLPs be aware of the dialect the children are speaking; otherwise, the likelihood of misdiagnosis increases.

Spanish-speaking children living in the United States may or may not be members of a broader bilingual community. Children might be exposed to one dialect variety of Spanish or many dialect varieties. According to Khattab (2006), speech production characteristics in children will be influenced by the language, or languages, they speak, their communication partner, and the broader linguistic environment. Spanish-speaking children can be exposed to native speakers, nonnative speakers, and bilingual speakers. This variation in input can influence how a child produces their speech sounds. For this reason, comparing Spanish-speaking children in the United State to monolingual Spanish speakers in primarily Spanish-speaking countries is problematic and opens up the possibility of clinical error. It is of great clinical importance that SLPs gather information on a child's linguistic community so that misinterpretation of speech production characteristics does not occur.

Phonological Development in Spanish-Speaking Children

Normative data (summarized in detail in Goldstein, 1995, 2000, 2007a) show that typically developing Spanish-speaking infants will tend to produce CV syllables

Table 14.5. Phonemes and allophones and their variants in spoken Spanish

Phoneme	Allophones/Variants	Example
Stops		
/p/	[p]	[pato] duck
/b/	[b]	[beso] kiss
	[β]	[neβera] refrigerator
	[v]	[nevera] refrigerator
/t/	[t]	[pato] duck
/d/	[d]	[doce] twelve
	[ð]	[deðo] finger
	Ø (deletion)	[deo] finger/[ciuda] city
/k/	[k]	[bloke] block
/g/	[g]	[gato] cat
	[ɣ]	[laɣo] lake
Nasals		
/m/	[m]	[mono] monkey
/n/	[n]	[mono] monkey
	[ŋ]	[xamoŋ] ham
	Ø (deletion)	[xamo]/[xamõ] ham
/ɲ/	[ɲ]	[baɲo] bathroom
Fricatives		
/f/	[f]	[fasil]/[fácil] easy
	[ɸ]	[emɸermo] sick
/x/	[x]	[roxo] red
	[h]	[roho] red
/s/	[s]	[sapato] shoe
	vʰ	[doʰ] two
	Ø (deletion)	[do] two
Glides		
/w/	[w]	[weso] bone
	[u]	[ueso] bone
	[gu]	[gueso] bone
	[ɣu]	[ɣueso] bone
/j/	[j]	[amarijo] yellow
	[ʒ]	[amariʒo] yellow
	[dʒ]	[amaridʒo] yellow
Affricate		
/tʃ/	[tʃ]	[letʃe] milk
	[ʃ]	[leʃe] milk
Liquid		
/l/	[l]	[elefante] elephant

(continued)

Table 14.5.   *(continued)*

Phoneme	Allophones/Variants	Example
Flap/tap		
/ɾ/	[ɾ]	[kaɾa] face
	[l]	[maltijo] hammer/[seɲol] mister
Trill		
/r/	[r]	[pero] dog
	[ʀ]	[peʀo] dog
	[x]	[pexo] dog
	[h]	[peho] dog

Sources: Goldstein (1995, 2007a); Hammond (2001); Lipski (2008).

containing oral and nasal stops with front vowels (e.g., Oller & Eilers, 1982). By the time typically developing Spanish-speaking children reach 3.5 years of age, it is likely that they will use the dialect features of the community and will have mastered the vowel system and most of the consonant system (e.g., Anderson & Smith, 1987; Goldstein & Cintron, 2001; Pandolfi & Herrera, 1990). In terms of vowel development in Spanish-speaking children, Oller and Eilers found that the mean proportion occurrence of vowel-like productions in 12- to 14-month-old English- and Spanish-speaking children was remarkably similar. In general, they noted that the children were likely to produce more anterior-like vowels than posterior-like ones. The rank order of the first 10 vowels in Spanish-speaking infants was: 1) [ɛ], 2) [æ], 3) [e], 4) [i], 5) [a], 6) [ʌ], 7) [ʊ], 8) [u], 9) [ɪ], and 10) [o] (p. 573). Maez (1981) indicated that by 18 months the three children in the study had mastered (i.e., produced correctly at least 90% of the time) the five basic Spanish vowels, [i], [e], [u], [o], and [a]. Maez's study, however, focused on consonant development and did not indicate if any vowel errors occurred.

Goldstein and Pollock (2000) examined vowel productions in 23 Spanish-speaking children (10 were 3 years old; 13 were 4 years old) with SSDs. Of the 23 children in the study, 14 exhibited vowel errors. Only one child exhibited more than one vowel error (five errors). The other 13 children each exhibited only one vowel error. Across all children, the results indicated that there were only 18 total vowel errors. Almost half the errors were on the vowel /o/.

In terms of consonant production, typically developing children will exhibit some difficulty by the end of preschool with consonant clusters and a few phonemes, specifically /ð, x, s, ɲ, tʃ, ɾ, r, l/ (e.g., Acevedo, 1991; Jimenez, 1987). These children may exhibit low percentages of occurrence of the following phonological patterns: cluster reduction, unstressed syllable deletion, stridency deletion, and tap/trill deviation, but will likely have suppressed phonological patterns such as velar and palatal fronting, prevocalic singleton omission, stopping, and assimilation (e.g., Goldstein & Iglesias, 1996a; Stepanof, 1990). For some Spanish-speaking children, phonetic mastery will continue into the early elementary school years, when they continue to show some, although infrequent, errors on the fricatives [x] and [s], the affricate [tʃ], the flap [ɾ], the trill [r], the lateral [l], and consonant clusters (e.g., Bailey, 1982; De la Fuente, 1985).

Although there have been quite a number of studies describing phonological patterns in typically developing children, the data remain scarce for Spanish-speaking children with SSDs. Data indicate that the percentage of Spanish-speaking children with SSDs who exhibit specific phonological patterns is similar across studies (e.g., Bichotte et al., 1993; Goldstein & Iglesias, 1996b; Meza, 1983). Phonological patterns exhibited by a large percentage of children (>40%) included cluster reduction, unstressed syllable deletion, stopping, liquid simplification, and assimilation.

Finally, Goldstein (2007b) found that children speaking the Puerto Rican and Mexican dialects of Spanish show similar error types and error rates on complexity of the phonetic inventory, vowel accuracy, consonant accuracy, sound class accuracy, percentage of occurrence of phonological patterns, and frequency and types of substitutions.

Asian Languages

In 2013, there were approximately 9.5 million speakers of Asian languages in the United States, 3.3% of the total U.S. population over 5 years of age (U.S. Census Bureau, 2015b). There are three main families of languages spoken in Asia (Crystal, 1997). The first is the over 100 Austro-Asiatic languages, most of the languages spoken in Southeast Asia (the countries between China and Indonesia), including Khmer, Hmong, and Vietnamese. The second is the Tai languages centered in Thailand and extending into Laos, North Vietnam, and parts of China. The third branch is Sino-Tibetan, which contains the languages of Tibet, Burma, and China, including Mandarin (also termed Putonghua) and Cantonese. Combined, these families contain over 440 languages spoken by over 1 billion people. Two other families, Austronesian and Papuan, contain languages spoken in the Pacific Islands (Cheng, 1993). Austronesian contains languages such as Hawaiian, Chamorro, Ilocano, and Tagalog. Papuan contains languages of New Guinea.

There are a number of dialectal variations in Asian languages, just as there are within English (e.g., Wang, 1990). For example, there are two main dialects of Chinese spoken in the United States: Mandarin and Cantonese (Cheng, 1987). There are also a number of subdialects within those two main dialects. Japanese has a few dialects, but they are mutually unintelligible; however, Khmer's four dialects are mutually intelligible (Cheng, 1993). In the next two sections, Asian language phonology and phonological development in children speaking Asian languages will be described.

Asian Language Phonology

The phonological structure of Asian languages varies greatly. In general, there are few syllable-final segments and few consonant clusters. For example, 1) the only syllable-final consonants in Mandarin Chinese are /n/ and /ŋ/; 2) there are no labiodental, interdental, or palatal fricatives in Korean; 3) Hawaiian contains only five vowels and eight consonants; and 4) the only final consonant in Japanese is /n/. There are, however, segmental systems in Asian languages that are relatively complex. For example, Hmong (the language spoken by people living in mountainous areas of Indochina) contains 56 initial consonants, 13 or 14 vowels (depending on dialect), 7 tones, and 1 final consonant /ŋ/ (Cheng, 1993). For segmental information on specific languages and dialects, consult the following sources: Cheng (1987, 1993), Hwa-Froelich and colleagues (2002), Tipton (1975), and Wang (1989).

Syllable structure in Asian languages also shows considerable variation. For example, Laotian contains three syllable types (CVC, CVVC, and CVV). Khmer exhibits eight syllable types (CVC, CCVC, CCCVC, CVVC, CCVVC, CCCVVC, CVV, CCVV); however, there are few polysyllabic words in Khmer (Cheng, 1987). Many Asian languages also show restrictions on the types of segments that may appear in certain syllable positions. Vietnamese has a limited number of final consonants (voiceless stops and nasals); the only final consonant in Hmong is /ŋ/; and in Korean, there are no fricatives or affricates in word-final position. Stress also may be different in Asian languages compared with English. For example, there is no tonic word stress in Korean, so to native English speakers, native speakers of Korean may sound somewhat monotone when speaking English (Cheng, 1993).

Many, but not all, Asian languages are tone languages. For example, Cantonese is a tone language, but Japanese is not. *Tone languages* are ones in which differences in word meaning can be signified by differences in pitch. Tone languages are generally composed of register tones (typically two or three in a language) and contour tones (usually two or three per language) (O'Grady et al., 2010). *Register tones* are level tones, usually signaled by high, mid, and low tones. *Contour tones* are a combination of register tones over a single syllable. For example, in Mandarin Chinese, the phonetic string [ma] takes on different meanings depending on the tone or tone sequence that is applied. If produced with a high, level tone, [ma] means *mother*, but if that same phonetic form is produced with a high-fall, register tone (i.e., a high then low tone), it means *scold*. In contrast, Japanese places equal stress on each syllable and does not utilize tones for phonemic distinction (Cheng, 2001).

There have been few studies on tone acquisition in Asian languages. Existing studies have illustrated the developmental process of tone (Li & Thompson, 1977; So & Dodd, 1995; Tse, 1978; Zhu & Dodd, 2000a). For example, Tse found that perceptual discrimination of tone began as early as age 10 months. The results from all four studies found that 1) children acquired the correct tone system relatively quickly (in about 8 months), 2) mastery of tone occurred before segmental mastery, 3) high and falling tones were acquired earlier and more easily than rising and contour tones, and 4) substitution errors often exist for rising and contour tones during the two- and three-word stages.

Phonological Development in Speakers of Asian Languages

Major findings from studies focused on children acquiring the phonology of Asian languages are summarized here by language. Detail is included as well, when it is available. For most languages, the summary includes speech sound acquisition, consonant accuracy, and occurrence of phonological processes/patterns.

Cantonese.   So (2006, 2007) indicated that early-acquired speech sounds (typically by 2;6) in Cantonese are vowels, bilabial and alveolar stops, nasals, and glides. Aspirated stops are acquired around 3;6, followed by fricatives and affricates. Consonant accuracy is approximately 85% at age 2 years. By age 4;0, only cluster reduction and stopping are commonly occurring. So and Dodd (1994, 1995) investigated phonological development in typically developing Cantonese-speaking children and noted similar phoneme acquisition to English but at a more rapid rate. In general, anterior consonants were acquired before posterior ones, and oral and nasal stops and glides were acquired before fricatives and affricates. They also noted the presence of phonological processes and found that by age 4 years, no process was exhibited over 15% of the time. Between the ages of 2;0 and 4;0, these children showed processes similar in quantity (>15%) and type to English-speaking children: assimilation, cluster reduction, stopping, fronting, affrication, and final consonant deletion.

So and Dodd (1994) further provided increased detail on the phonological patterns exhibited by the 13 children labeled as either phonological delay or consistently disordered. Children with phonological delay tended to exhibit assimilation, cluster reduction, stopping, fronting, deaspiration, affrication, and final consonant deletion. Children with phonological disorders tended to exhibit final consonant deletion, final glide deletion, initial consonant deletion, aspiration, gliding, vowel rule, and backing.

Cheung and Abberton (2000) examined the phonological skills of 251 Cantonese-speaking children (aged 3;6 to 6;0) with SSDs. They found that tones and vowels were usually produced accurately, with consonants being most affected. The children showed most difficulty with /s/, aspirated consonants (e.g., /pʰ/), and labialized consonants (e.g., /kʷ/). Thus, deaspiration was a commonly occurring phonological pattern, as were stopping and fronting of velars.

Japanese (Ota & Ueda, 2007).   In Japanese, most consonants are acquired by 4;0, except [ɕ, s, ts, z, ɾ], with clusters being acquired by 4;6. Vowels are acquired by 3;0. There are few occurrences of any phonological process at age 5. By age 5 years, 94% of children produced syllables accurately (Sumio, 1978, in Ota & Ueda, 2007).

Korean (Kim & Pae, 2007).   By age 3 years, all consonants in Korean are typically acquired except [l], [ɾ], [s], [s*] (voiceless fortis). Bilabials are acquired before velars and affricates. Intersyllabic clusters are acquired by age 4. Few phonological processes are exhibited at age 6;5.

Putonghua (Modern Standard Chinese).   Hua (2006, 2007) indicated that consonants in Putonghua are acquired by age 4;6, with consonant accuracy being 92% by age 4;6. Vowels are acquired by age 2;0. The following phonological processes are still exhibited at age 4;6: fronting, backing, deaspiration, final /n/ deletion, and triphthong reduction. Zhu and Dodd (2000a) examined the phonological skills of 129 typically developing speakers of Putonghua aged 1;6 to 4;6. Their results indicated that tone was acquired first, followed by syllable-final consonants and vowels, and finally, syllable-initial consonants. By age 4;6, all the syllable-initial consonants were accurately produced by 90% of the children. Similar to typically developing children acquiring other languages, the Putonghua-speaking children exhibited syllabic and substitution phonological processes, such as unstressed syllable deletion, fronting, and gliding. The children also showed language-specific patterns, such as deaspiration and triphthong reduction of vowels.

A few studies have also investigated speakers of Asian languages with SSDs. Zhu and Dodd (2000b) assessed 33 children aged 2;8 to 7;6 with "atypical speech development" (p. 170). The largest subgroup of speakers (18 of 33 children) was characterized to have "delayed phonological development" ("use of non-age-appropriate processes and/or restricted phonetic or phonemic inventory" [p. 168]). The most commonly exhibited phonological processes included fronting and stopping. These children with SSDs had less difficulty with syllable components described as having more "phonological saliency" (p. 180). Phonological saliency, according to the authors, is based on syllable structure and is specific to each ambient language. In the case of Putonghua, tones, vowels, and syllable-final consonants are more salient, and syllable-initial consonants are less salient. As predicted, children with disorders had most difficulty with less salient features (e.g., syllable-initial consonants).

Using an early version of Dodd's classification scheme that was previously discussed in Chapter 5, So and Dodd (1994, pp. 238–240) outlined and defined four subgroups of children with SSDs: Delayed phonological development ("rules or processes used by more than 10% of children acquiring phonology normally"), consistent use of one or more unusual rules ("rules not used by more than 10 percent of children acquiring phonology normally"), articulation disorder ("consistent distortion of a phoneme"), and children who make inconsistent errors ("production of specific words or particular phonological segments"). So and Dodd applied these categories to 17 Cantonese-speaking children with SSDs aged 3;6 to 6;4. Their results revealed that 8/17 participants (47%) displayed delayed phonological development, 5/17 (30%) were categorized as consistent users of one or more unusual rules, 2/17 (12%) had an articulation disorder, and another 2/17 (12%) were defined as making inconsistent errors.

Thai (Lorwatanapongsa & Maroonroge, 2007). In Thai, consonants are acquired by age 5;0, except /s/ and /r/. Thai-speaking children exhibit many of the same phonological patterns exhibited by children speaking other languages: backing, cluster reduction, final consonant deletion, fronting, stopping, and stridency deletion.

Vietnamese (Tang & Barlow, 2006). Tang and Barlow investigated the phonological skills of four Vietnamese-speaking children (aged 4;4 to 5;5) with SSDs. They found that tone was adultlike for all four children. The four children also produced all vowels and the majority of stops, nasals, and glides in syllable-initial and syllable-final positions. Seven phonological patterns were exhibited by at least two of the children: gliding, fronting, glottal replacement, backing, velar assimilation, stopping, and final consonant deletion. Many of these patterns are common cross-linguistically (e.g., stopping, fronting, and final consonant deletion), although others are not (e.g., glottal replacement). Finally, final consonants were acquired before initial ones.

Arabic

Arabic is the second most commonly spoken language by bilingual children in 16 U.S. states and is among the top five languages spoken in 39 states (Pew Research Center, 2018). With an influx of refugees from countries such as Syria, American schools are serving increasing numbers of monolingual Arabic-speaking children as well as bilingual Arabic-English speakers. Two main points about Arabic that are important for those encountering this language for the first time are 1) there is a separate written form (standard form) and a spoken form (colloquial form) and 2) there are many dialects of Arabic, and not all are mutually intelligible (Sabri & Fabiano-Smith, 2018). It is important for SLPs to understand that all speakers of Arabic write using the standard form, but they might not understand one another using the spoken form. As a result, it is important to identify the dialect of Arabic a client speaks before requesting assistance from an interpreter to ensure that support personnel use the same variety of Arabic as the client. Khamis-Dakwar and Khattab (2014) provide a detailed overview of cultural and linguistic considerations within the Arab community that play a central role in cultural competence with this diverse population.

Arabic is a Semitic language that is spoken throughout the Middle East and parts of Africa. As explained by Sabri and Fabiano-Smith (2018), there are 28 consonants and 6 vowels (including two diphthongs) in Arabic. Vowel productions vary greatly based on phonetic context. Short vowels (/a, i, u/) and their longer counterparts (/aː, iː, uː/) have allophonic variations (/a, aː, e, eː/) when preceding or following emphatic phonemes. Emphatic phonemes are consonants that have both a primary and secondary place of articulation (Table 14.6, underlined). The secondary place of articulation involves retraction of the tongue root toward the pharyngeal wall,

Table 14.6. Comparison of English and Arabic consonant phonemes

Manner class	English phonemes	Arabic phonemes
Stops	p b t d k g	b t d k t̪ d q ʔ gᵃ
Fricatives	f v s z ʃ ʒ θ h ð	f s z z̪ ʃ θ ð ð̪ h χ ʁ ʕ ħ ʒᵃ
Affricates	dʒ tʃ	dʒ
Nasals	m n ŋ	m n
Glides	w j	w j
Liquids	l ɹ	l
Flap	N/A	ɾ
Trill	N/A	r
Emphatics	N/A	t d q z ð s χᵇ ʁᵇ rᵇ
Vowels	ɑ a æ ɪ i e ɛ ʊ u ʊ ɔ ʌ ɜ ɝ ɚ ʊ ɪə ɪc eɪ ɪɔ	a, aː, u, uː, i, iː ɑᶜ, ɑːᶜ, aj, aw

[a]Dialectal variation.
[b]Becomes emphatic in specific environments.
[c]Allophonic variation.
Source: Sabri & Fabiano-Smith (2018).

causing changes in production of surrounding vowels (Amayreh & Dyson, 1998). Consonant clusters are found in word-initial position, but are separated by epenthesis in word-final position. Syllable types allowed in Arabic include CV, CVV (CVVː), CVC, CVVC (CVːC), CVCC, and CVVCC (CVːCC).

Few studies on Arabic phonological development and disorders have been published to date; however, some studies are available to guide SLPs in diagnostic decision making and treatment goal selection (Amayreh, 2003; Amayreh & Dyson, 1998; Fokes et al., 1985; Khamis-Dakwar & Khattab, 2014; Khattab, 2006; Sabri & Fabiano-Smith, 2018). Table 14.6 illustrates consonant phoneme comparison between English and Arabic (Sabri & Fabiano-Smith). Amayreh and Dyson studied the phonological acquisition of 180 Jordanian-Arabic speaking children and identified developmental trends for the acquisition of consonant phonemes. Table 14.7 details developmental trends for Jordanian Arabic consonant production from ages 2;0 to 6;4.

As is observed across the world's languages, Arabic-speaking children acquire their phonological system in a simple to complex fashion, as early-developing sounds consist of stops, middle-developing sounds are fricatives and affricates, and late-developing sounds include emphatics and the trill /r/. It will be typical to observe vowel and syllable structure variation and cluster reduction in word-final consonant clusters in this population due to the influence of Arabic on English. It is essential that SLPs familiarize themselves with the similarities and differences between Arabic and English phonologies so that errors in diagnosis are not make.

PHONOLOGICAL DEVELOPMENT IN BILINGUAL CHILDREN

Although there is no doubt that SLPs will be assessing and providing intervention services to monolingual speakers of Spanish and Asian languages, it is more likely that SLPs in the United States will be delivering clinical services to bilingual children acquiring a language in addition to English. The historical view of phonological development in bilingual children is that it is slower than that of monolingual children; that is, bilingual children exhibit negative transfer. More recent studies of bilingual

Table 14.7. Early-, intermediate- (middle-) and late-developing consonant phonemes in Arabic by age

Early-developing phonemes	/b, t, d, k, f, ħ, m, n, w, j, l/
Middle-developing phonemes	/s, χ, ʃ ,ʁ ,h ,r /
Late-developing phonemes	/t̪, d̪, q, ð, ð̪, s̪, z, ħ, θ, ʔ, ʕ/

Source: Amayreh and Dyson (1998).

children indicate that phonological development in these children is similar, although not identical, to that of monolingual speakers of either language (Goldstein, 2004; Goldstein & Gildersleeve-Neumann, 2012; Morrow et al., 2014). For a detailed review, see Goldstein and McLeod (2012) as well as Grech and McLeod (2012).

Negative Transfer

Results from a number of studies of bilingual children have indicated that their phonological development is slower than that of monolingual peers. Dodd and colleagues (1996) examined the phonology of 16 typically developing Cantonese-speaking children who were acquiring English in preschool. The results indicated that the children differentiated the phonology of each language. They also found that the children's error patterns were atypical for monolingual speakers of either language, and that these children produced a higher number of atypical error patterns (e.g., initial consonant deletion), in an amount usually associated with children evidencing SSDs. Holm and Dodd (2000) examined the phonological skills of two Cantonese-English bilingual children from ages 2;3 to 3;1 and from ages 2;9 to 3;5. They found that the children maintained separate phonological systems of each language, and both children exhibited phonological patterns that were not typical for monolingual speakers (e.g., atypical aspiration); however, these patterns were exhibited by Cantonese-English bilingual speakers in other studies (e.g., Dodd et al., 1996).

In a group of typically developing Spanish–English bilingual preschoolers, Gildersleeve-Neumann and associates (2008) found that the bilingual children exhibited lower overall accuracy and a higher number of errors than their English and Spanish monolingual counterparts. Goldstein and Washington (2001) found that, compared with monolinguals, typically developing Spanish–English bilingual children exhibited significantly lower accuracy on some sound classes (e.g., spirants, flap, trill) but not on others (e.g., stops, nasals, fricatives).

Positive Transfer

In addition to findings indicating negative transfer of phonological skills in bilinguals relative to monolinguals, results from other studies show positive transfer. In these studies, positive transfer was defined as bilinguals exhibiting either more advanced skills or commensurate skills in comparison to monolingual peers.

Studies of German-Spanish (Lleó & Kehoe, 2002; Lleó et al., 2003) and Maltese-English (Grech & Dodd, 2008) bilingual children have indicated that they have more advanced skills than their monolingual counterparts. Gildersleeve-Neumann and Davis (1998) demonstrated that although bilingual speakers exhibited different developmental patterns than their monolingual peers and exhibited more errors initially than monolingual speakers, these differences faded over time.

A number of studies of bilingual children indicate that their phonological development is commensurate with that of monolinguals (e.g., Fabiano-Smith & Goldstein, 2010). The children in Holm and Dodd's (2000) investigation of two Cantonese-English bilingual children showed phonetic development that was similar to that of monolingual children. Similarities in phonological skills between monolingual and bilingual speakers are also supported by the work of Goldstein and Washington (2001) and Goldstein and colleagues (2005). These researchers examined the Spanish and English phonological skills in typically developing 4- and 5-year-old bilingual (Spanish–English) children, respectively. They largely found similarities in phonological skills between bilingual and monolingual children. Differences between groups were relegated to the accuracy of production of sounds in specific sound classes, especially in Spanish. Spirants, flap, and trill in Spanish were produced much less accurately in bilingual children than have been shown for monolingual Spanish-speaking children (Goldstein, 1988). In a group of Russian-English bilingual children aged 3;3 to 5;7, Gildersleeve-Neumann and Wright (2010) did not find differences across bilingual and monolingual children for syllable-level errors. Finally, in examining 4- and 5-year-old Spanish–English bilingual children, Prezas and colleagues (2014) found their phonological skills to be similar to those of monolinguals in both English and Spanish. Percentages of occurrence for some patterns were higher in bilinguals than in monolinguals. Conversely, percentages of occurrence for some patterns were higher in monolinguals than in the bilingual children.

The results of these studies indicate that bilingual phonological development appears to proceed along the same course as that for monolingual speakers. This trajectory, however, is not entirely the same as it is for monolingual speakers. Bilingual children might exhibit error types that are less common in monolingual speakers, are likely to show cross-linguistic effects, and may be less accurate on some aspects of the phonological system in comparison to their monolingual peers. Those differences seem to diminish over time, such that bilingual children are able to achieve adultlike phonological skills in both languages.

The Influence of One Language on Another

When there is contact between speakers of two or more languages, a tendency exists for one language to influence the other (Goldstein, 2007c; Goldstein & McLeod, 2012; Grech & McLeod, 2012). This influence is often bidirectional, with each language influencing the other. For example, a native Spanish speaker acquiring English will exhibit characteristics of Spanish-influenced English and English-influenced Spanish. In a group of bilingual (Spanish–English) children, Goldstein and Iglesias (1999) found that a few children substituted [tʃ] for /ʃ/; /ʃʌvəl/ (*shovel*) was produced as [tʃʌvəl] (Spanish-influenced English). The children also used the postvocalic *r* of GAE for the Spanish flap; /floɾ/ (*flower*) was produced as [floɚ] (English-influenced Spanish). In groups of Russian-English bilingual children and English-speaking children, Gildersleeve-Neumann and Wright (2010) found examples of Russian-influenced English. For example, the bilingual children produced palatalized consonants (e.g., /kʲ/) in their English.

For speakers acquiring more than one language, there are many ways that the phonology of one language may have an effect on the phonology of another language (Goldstein, 2007c). First, the specific phonemes and allophones in the inventories of each language will not be the same. For example, the palatal affricate [tʃ] found in English is not in the inventory of Cantonese (Cheng, 1993). A native Cantonese-speaking individual acquiring English might substitute [ts] for the palatal affricate because [ts] exists in the inventory of Cantonese and is close to the place of articulation of the English affricate. Second, differences in the distribution of sounds exist across languages. For example, [ŋ] might be the only word-final sound realized in English by a native Hmong speaker because it is the only word-final sound in Hmong (Cheng, 1993). Third, consonants may have different places of articulation in each language. For example, Spanish speakers acquiring English may produce /d/ with a dental place of articulation, as is common in Spanish, versus an alveolar place of articulation that is typical in English (Perez, 1994). Fourth, phonological rules may be different in each language. For example, the phrase, "Cómo se llama su niño?" (What is your child's name?), which would be produced as [komo se jama su niɲo] in Spanish, might be realized as [koʊmoʊ se jama su niɲoʊ] in English-influenced Spanish because the speaker is diphthongizing vowels, as is common in English. Finally, how and when pronunciation is acquired may contribute to the influence of one language on another. For some individuals learning English as a second language, their major exposure might be in school, where written language is being introduced. The lack of one-to-one correspondence between grapheme and phoneme in English may influence pronunciation (August et al., 2002). For example, the grapheme *s* in English is produced as [s] in *basin* and as [ʒ] in *measure,* causing a speaker of Spanish-influenced English to produce both as [s].

ASSESSMENT CONSIDERATIONS FOR CHILDREN FROM CULTURALLY AND LINGUISTICALLY DIVERSE POPULATIONS

In assessing the speech and language skills of children from culturally and linguistically diverse populations, the same types of information are gathered as for all children: case history, oral mechanism examination, hearing screening, language (e.g., syntax, semantics, pragmatics, and the lexicon), voice, fluency, and phonological patterns. In the case history section of culturally competent evaluations, it is especially important to ask if a family history of speech or language impairment exists (Oetting et al., 2016). Work by Oetting and colleagues and Grimm and Schulz (2014) observed that a positive family history of speech and language impairment paired with delay in achieving early speech and language milestones predicted speech and language impairment in children who are speakers of nonmainstream dialects and in bilingual children.

The analysis of phonological patterns in children from culturally and linguistically diverse populations requires a determination of whether the child's phonological system is within normal limits for their linguistic community (ASHA, 2004a; Horton-Ikard, 2010). Thus, the assessment must be approached with an understanding of the social, cultural, and linguistic characteristics of that community, always guarding against stereotyping (Taylor et al., 1987). One cannot assume that any individual from any geographical area or ethnic/racial group is a speaker of a particular dialect. For example, although one African American's production of f/θ in the word *mouth* may be regarded as a dialect feature of AAE, it would be inappropriate to make the same clinical judgment for another African American who also produces f/θ. The first speaker may be an AAE speaker, but the second speaker may not be, and therefore the production would be considered a true error.

SLPs must also differentiate dialect differences from SSDs. In ASHA's position papers on social dialects and communication disorders and variations, the association officially acknowledges the distinction between a speech-language difference and a speech-language disorder (ASHA, 1983, 1993). A few investigators have attempted to determine if scoring dialectal features as errors would penalize children for patterns that are, in effect, dialect features, thus artificially inflating their severity ratings. In their examination of 10 AAE-speaking children aged 5;11 to 6;11, Cole and Taylor (1990) found that not taking dialect into account resulted in the misdiagnosis of SSD for half the children, on average, across three phonological assessments. Two other studies, while advocating that dialect should be accounted for in phonological assessment, did not find the same significant results as Cole and Taylor. Fleming and Hartman (1989) used the Computer Assessment of Phonological Processes (CAPP; Hodson, 1985) to examine 72 speakers of AAE who were 4 years old. They determined that although some test items are influenced by "Black English phonological rules," the assessment as a whole is not invalidated (p. 28). Moreover, they indicated that no typically developing child was labeled as having a disorder based solely on the factor of dialect.

Washington and Craig (1992) examined 28 preschool Black English or AAE-speaking children aged 4;6 to 5;3. Their results indicated that dialect scoring changes did "not seem to penalize the BE-speaking preschooler to a degree that is clinically significant" (p. 23). Washington and Craig ascribed the contrast of their results to those of Cole and Taylor (1990) based on geographical location. The participants in Cole and Taylor's study were from Mississippi, whereas the children in Washington and Craig's study resided in Detroit.

Goldstein and Iglesias (2001) examined 54 typically developing Spanish-speaking children and 54 Spanish-speaking children with SSDs to determine if taking or not taking into account Puerto Rican Spanish dialect features altered the results of the analyses. The results indicated that if dialect features had not been taken into account, almost 75% of typically developing children might have been erroneously characterized as exhibiting SSDs. In addition, not taking dialect into account might have resulted in unnecessarily targeting for intervention phonological processes whose percentages of occurrence were inflated. Wing and Flipsen (2010) replicated the Goldstein and Iglesias study with speakers of a Mexican dialect of Spanish. Children in the study included 24 typically developing children (mean age = 5;0) and three children with phonological disorders (mean age = 4;10). Results from Goldstein and Iglesias were largely confirmed in that under-identification and over-identification occurred relative to the General Spanish Referent (i.e., not taking dialect into account). Accounting for dialect significantly increased classification accuracy.

Although the results of these studies led to somewhat different conclusions as to whether scoring dialectal features as errors affected the child's severity rating, these researchers all agreed that accounting for dialect features is a prime consideration in the assessment of children from culturally and linguistically diverse populations. Analysis of phonological information must be made while taking the child's dialect into account, especially given that SLPs with less familiarity with a dialect yield less comprehensibility of that dialect (e.g., Robinson & Stockman, 2009). Thus, errors can be counted as such only when they are in conflict with the child's dialect. For example, in the Puerto Rican dialect of Spanish, the production of /dos/ (two) as [do:] would not be scored as an error because syllable-final /s/ is often deleted. The production of /flor/ (flower) as [flo] would be scored as an error because syllable-final deletion of /r/ is not considered a typical feature of the dialect.

Thus, in order to minimize the possibility of misdiagnosis, all phonological analyses should take into account the features of that particular dialect and should not be scored as errors. To account for dialect features in any particular linguistic group, SLPs might 1) become thoroughly familiar with features of the dialects and language,

2) sample the adult speakers in the child's linguistic community, and 3) obtain information from interpreters/support personnel.

In order to minimize the effect that not accounting for dialect features might have on the phonological analysis of speakers from culturally and linguistically diverse populations, Stockman has suggested assessing a minimal competency core (MCC), developed to decrease bias in the assessment of AAE-speaking children (Stockman, 1996b). *Minimal competency core* is defined as "the *least* amount of knowledge that one must exhibit to be judged as normal in a given age range" (p. 358, emphasis in original). Stockman noted that MCC may best be used as a screening tool on a core subgroup of specific behaviors. The phonological features core includes the following word/syllable initial sounds that are invariable in GAE and AAE: /m, n, p, b, t, d, k, g, f, s, h, w, j, l, ɹ/. Wilcox and Anderson (1998) found that assessing these sounds along with clusters provided enough information to differentiate typical from atypical speech sound development in a group of AAE speakers.

Examiners must be aware of their own dialect and its effect on the assessment process. Seymour and Seymour (1977) noted that the client's perception of the formality of the situation affects dialect density. For example, casual speaking settings may increase dialect density by encouraging more frequent use of AAE, whereas a more formal setting may result in a decrease in dialect density by inhibiting and stigmatizing speech forms other than GAE. A similar issue may be encountered when a clinician uses Castilian Spanish (i.e., the dialect of Spanish spoken in some areas of Spain and taught in most educational systems in the United States) when conversing with a speaker of any of the other major Spanish dialects. This is not to say that one should force oneself to use the client's dialect. One must realize, however, the potential effect that one's particular dialect may have on a client and family.

The assessment of speakers of languages other than or in addition to English presents a challenge to the SLP. The SLP must determine the language or languages of assessment and then choose appropriate assessment tools. Even if the child seems to be a dominant English speaker, it is common practice to assess phonological skills in both languages, as the child's phonological knowledge will be distributed across the two languages (Goldstein, 2006). Analyses then should be completed in both languages. The SLP must differentiate true speech sound errors from developmental errors from atypical/disordered patterns from cross-linguistic effects (Yavaş & Goldstein, 1998).

A detailed phonological assessment would include both formal measures (instruments standardized on speakers from a particular language group) and informal measures (such as a spontaneous language sample). The formal assessment tool should be designed specifically to assess phonological patterns in that language. Unfortunately, there are few available formal measures covering a variety of languages. Using an assessment tool designed for any linguistic group other than the one for which it was intended will likely increase bias and lead to over-referral. In the absence of formal measures, the SLP might utilize informal client observations with siblings, peers, and/or parent(s), asking a series of questions designed to determine the adequacy of the child's phonological system (Yavaş & Goldstein, 1998):

- Does the child sound like other children in their peer group (i.e., like other members of their speech community)?

- What consonants does the child produce (front vs. back, syllable-initial vs. syllable-final)?

- Does the child make any vowel errors?

- If appropriate, does the child use tone accurately?

- What percentage of the time is the child intelligible?

- Is the child understood by their parents, family members, teachers, and friends all, some, or none of the time?

Clinical Vignette 14.1

Typical Bilingual Development or Speech Sound Disorder?

Carlos is a 4-year-old child who has been exposed to both English and Spanish in the home since birth. Carlos's teacher expressed concern about his English intelligibility in the classroom, but Carlos's mother is not concerned about his speech skills in either English or Spanish. Carlos was referred to the school SLP for a speech and language evaluation.

An oral mechanism examination showed structure and function of the articulators within normal limits and a referral to the audiologist yielded normal hearing. A parent interview with Carlos's mother indicated that mostly Spanish is spoken in the home and mostly English is used at school. Carlos was asked to engage in a single-word picture-naming task in both English and Spanish and provided a connected speech sample, in both English and Spanish, using the wordless picture book, *Frog Where Are You?* (Mayer, 1969). Single-word speech samples were phonetically transcribed and connected-speech samples were judged for intelligibility, in both languages. Results indicated a complete phonetic inventory in both English and Spanish, percent occurrence of phonological patterns that were age appropriate in Spanish, but a higher occurrence of cluster reduction, weak syllable deletion, and gliding in English than is age appropriate. Substitution errors and phonological transfer were within normal limits.

Carlos was not diagnosed with an SSD because he demonstrated age-appropriate phonological skills in Spanish. It was concluded that Carlos requires more experience with English in order to increase his intelligibility of speech in the classroom. The SLP recommended English enrichment activities to increase Carlos's English language proficiency.

Role of the Monolingual Speech-Language Pathologist

SLPs may have difficulty assessing children who speak more than one language because SLPs often are not bilingual themselves (Goldstein, 2001). Clinicians who do not speak the language of the individual they are assessing might consider alternatives such as hiring a bilingual consultant or bilingual diagnostician, training bilingual aides, or using interpreters/translators (I/Ts) (Langdon & Cheng, 2002). If I/Ts are used, SLPs should be sure the I/Ts are trained, have exemplary bilingual/bidialectal communication skills, understand their responsibilities, act professionally, and can relate to members of the cultural group (Kayser, 1995; Langdon & Cheng). I/Ts should assist the SLP in completing the assessment but not conduct the assessment themselves. It might be tempting for SLPs to use family members as I/Ts. Lynch (2004) advises against this practice because acting in this role may be burdensome to the family member, and family members may be reticent in discussing emotional matters, uncomfortable providing information to older or younger family members or to members of the opposite gender, and leave out information provided by the SLP.

In the absence of a bilingual SLP at the site, monolingual SLPs may also play a role in the assessment of children who do not speak English. If they have knowledge, skills, competencies, and training in providing services to individuals with limited or non-English proficiency, monolingual SLPs may assess in English, administer an oral mechanism examination, conduct a hearing screening, and administer nonverbal assessments (ASHA, 1985).

INTERVENTION FOR SPEECH SOUND DISORDERS IN CHILDREN FROM CULTURALLY AND LINGUISTICALLY DIVERSE POPULATIONS

Once the results of an assessment are gathered, SLPs must decide if intervention is warranted. The traditional role of the SLP is to provide clinical services for communication disorders but not for dialectal differences. However, ASHA's position paper on social dialects identifies the following expanded role for SLPs (ASHA, 1983):

> Aside from the traditionally recognized role, the SLP may also be available to provide *elective* clinical services to nonstandard English speakers who do not present a disorder. The role of the SLP for these individuals is to prepare the desired competency in Standard English without jeopardizing the integrity of the individual's first dialect. The approach must be functional and based on context-specific appropriateness of the given dialect. (p. 24)

If elective services are to take place, it is important to remember that elective therapy does not necessarily mean that the client wants to eliminate the first dialect (D1). More often, the client prefers to be bidialectal. Taylor (1986) suggested a number of principles for SLPs who seek to guide speakers who want to acquire a second dialect: 1) develop a positive attitude toward the home dialect of the speaker; 2) compare the features of the home dialect to the one being acquired; 3) select targets based on language acquisition norms, frequency of occurrence of the features, and the speaker's attitude toward the features; 4) know the rules of the speaker's home dialect and the ones to be acquired; 5) take the speaker's learning style into account; and 6) integrate language issues into the larger culture of the speaker. Taylor also proposed a series of steps to be followed in order to maintain both dialects. First, a positive attitude toward D1 must be established. Second, the client must learn to contrast the features of the first dialect and the second dialect (D2). Finally, the client uses D2 in controlled, structured, and eventually spontaneous situations with a focus on form, content, and use.

Modifying someone's dialect involves more than simply having the person produce consonants and vowels as a native speaker would pronounce them. Learning nonsegmental aspects of speech production such as stress, pitch, and intonation is equally important. There are likely to be differences between the person's home language/dialect and the variety being acquired as a second language/dialect. For example, stress in English is relatively more complicated than in other languages. Placement of stress depends on a number of factors, including syntactic category and weight of the syllable (i.e., whether the vowel is long or short and the number of consonants that follow the vowel) (Goodluck, 1991). Pitch also differs as a function of language. For example, pitch modulates less in Spanish than it does in English (Hadlich et al., 1968). Finally, intonational contours for statements, questions, and exclamations may be different in English than in other languages. For example, in English, utterances (statements, questions, and exclamations) may begin at an overall higher pitch than in other languages.

SLPs must also recognize how dialectal variation and SSDs interact (Wolfram, 1994). Wolfram has suggested the following guiding principles. He divided impairments into three types. Type I impairments are judged to be atypical patterns regardless of the speaker's dialect; for example, initial consonant deletion (e.g., [it] for /mit/) or velar fronting (e.g., [dot] for /got/). In Type II impairments, there is a cross-dialectal difference in the normative (or underlying) form. For example, the normative form for the word *bathing* would be /beðiŋ/ for speakers of GAE but /beviŋ/ for AAE speakers, even though speakers from both dialect groups might misarticulate that word as [beziŋ]. Type III impairments influence forms that are shared across dialects but are applied with different frequency. For example, syllable-final cluster reduction is exhibited in many dialects. In AAE, this pattern is observed more frequently than in other dialects. Wolfram noted that treating a Type I impairment would not necessitate gathering different norms across dialect groups. The treatment of Type II and Type III impairments, however, would involve taking into account both qualitative and quantitative differences between dialect groups.

Velleman and Pearson (2010) have compiled a number of suggestions relative to providing intervention to AAE-speaking children with SSDs (along with some based on their own experience):

- Early developing sounds (except /j/) will not likely be intervention targets, as AAE speakers with SSDs tend to produce them accurately.

- /ð/ is not likely to be an intervention targets, as its status as a phoneme in AAE is questionable (Stockman, 2006a).

- Syllable and word structure rules (i.e., phonotactics) need to be considered in the development of intervention targets and stimuli, in that obstruents and nasals are often optional in final position, clusters are typically reduced in final position, and initial, unstressed syllables are often omitted. Stress might also differ for AAE speakers (e.g., *inSURance* might be produced as *INsurance*) (Burns et al., 2010).

- Target /j, f, s, v, tʃ, dʒ, ɹ/ and /-ɹ/ clusters earlier in the intervention sequence and /t, g, k, ʃ, ð/ and /s/ + stop clusters later in the intervention sequence.

Intervention for Bilingual Children With Speech Sound Disorders

Relatively little information is available regarding direct intervention for individuals with SSDs who speak a language other than or in addition to English. Available data indicate that principles guiding intervention choices for these children are both similar to and different from those for monolingual children. As with all children, the intervention process begins with the completion of a comprehensively broad and deep assessment. Once this information is collected, SLPs need to compare those results with the appropriate comparison database. SLPs should remember that they should neither use normative data gathered from English-speaking children to assess children who speak a language other than or in addition to English, nor generalize developmental phonological data from one dialect group to another. That is, phonological skills in the bilingual child who is being assessed need to be compared to those of other, similar bilingual children.

Once the assessment is completed, the next step should be to determine the intervention goal and the intervention approach (Goldstein, 2006). Choosing the goal and approach will guide the SLP in determining the language of intervention. Kohnert and Derr (2012) and Kohnert and colleagues (2005) have proposed two main approaches for providing intervention to bilingual children. In the *bilingual approach,* they propose that SLPs should improve the child's skills common to both languages. For example, initial goals would focus on constructs common to both languages (e.g., the phoneme /s/, final consonant deletion). To extend that approach, Gildersleeve-Neumann and Goldstein (2012) and Yavaş and Goldstein (1998) suggested that for a bilingual child with at least a moderate SSD, SLPs should choose intervention targets based on the error rates in both languages. Initially, error patterns that were exhibited with similar error rates in both languages should be targeted. For example, a pattern such as unstressed syllable deletion would be an initial intervention target because it would likely show similar error rates in both languages and greatly affect intelligibility in both languages. Treating errors that occur frequently in both languages likely will improve intelligibility in both languages, rather than in only one of the bilingual child's languages.

Using this approach, however, requires frequent monitoring of generalization across both languages, although generalization across languages is not guaranteed. For example, Holm and colleagues (1997) found that intervention on one sound in English did generalize to Cantonese, but intervention on a phonological pattern did not. Subsequent to treating errors occurring with similar frequency in both languages, error patterns that are exhibited in both languages with unequal frequency should be treated. For example, final consonant deletion is a phonological pattern that is likely to be exhibited in English with a high percentage of occurrence but with a low percentage of occurrence in Spanish (Goldstein & Iglesias, 1996b). Finally, phonological patterns exhibited in only one language should be targeted. For example, final consonant devoicing may be exhibited in English but not in Spanish (Goldstein & Washington, 2001).

In the *cross-linguistic approach,* Kohnert and colleagues (2005) suggest that clinicians focus on skills distinct in each constituent language. This approach also will be necessary (likely in conjunction with the bilingual approach) because of the differences in the phonological structures of the two languages. For example, labialized consonants exist in Cantonese, but not in English, and thus can be remediated in only one language. As an adjunct, SLPs might utilize the cross-linguistic approach based on types of errors and/or error rates (Gildersleeve-Neumann & Goldstein, 2012; Yavaş & Goldstein, 1998). For example, the frequency of occurrence of final consonant deletion in Spanish–English bilingual children is higher in their English than in their Spanish (Goldstein et al., 2005). Thus, intervention to decrease the use of final consonant deletion likely will occur in English but not in Spanish. Finally, errors occurring in only one language would be targets for phonological intervention (e.g., final devoicing in language B but not in language A).

Adapting Intervention Approaches to Individuals From Culturally and Linguistically Diverse Populations

Although little specific information is available to guide the intervention of SSDs in speakers of languages other than or in addition to English, specific intervention approaches developed for English-speaking children might be adapted for use with those from culturally and linguistically diverse populations. A number of different methods for remediating speech sound errors have been categorized into two main types: phonetic and phonemic (Bauman-Waengler, 2008), which are described in Chapters 10 and 11 as motor-based and linguistically based, respectively. *Phonetic approaches,* such as the traditional approach (Van Riper, 1972) and the multiple phoneme approach (Bradley, 1985), and *phonemic approaches,* such as the cycles approach (Hodson & Paden, 1991) and language-based approaches (Hoffman et al., 1990), can be adapted for use with individuals from culturally and linguistically diverse populations. More recently, the *complexity approach* to target selection in phonological treatment has gained ground (Gierut, 2001; Gierut et al., 1996). In this approach, late-developing, more complex sounds are selected as initial treatment targets utilizing implicational hierarchies to encourage less complex sounds to be acquired without direct treatment (Barlow et al., 2010).

Utilizing a phonetic approach poses several difficulties, unless the SLP is a speaker of the child's native/home language. First, the SLP must be able to carry out the perceptual training phase of this approach. This includes the ability to produce an auditory model for the child. Second, the SLP must discern the segments in the child's home language, the segments in the child's repertoire, the order of acquisition of the sounds, the ease of production for the sounds, the frequency of occurrence of each phone in the language, and phonetic contexts that may facilitate production of the target sound (Stoel-Gammon & Dunn, 1985).

A phonemic approach also raises several issues for the SLP. First, each specific program would have to be adapted to the child's language and dialect. For example, English has about 25 consonants, but Hmong has about 60. Although English and Hmong both have affricates in their inventories, Hmong has a set of aspirated affricates, which English does not. Second, because this type of approach is based on patterns rather than individual sound segments, the SLP would need to differentiate a series of unrelated errors from a single phonological rule (A. L. Williams, 2001). Third, in order to apply this type of approach, the SLP should be able to identify errors most affecting intelligibility, errors that cut across sound classes, and errors that disappear at the earliest age from typically developing children (Stoel-Gammon & Dunn, 1985). In bilingual children, an error might occur in one language but not in the other (Gildersleeve-Neumann & Goldstein, 2012). Finally, the order of intervention advocated by the approach might need to be altered for a speaker of a language other than English. For example, Hodson and Paden (1991), in their cycles approach, suggest treating syllabicity early in the remediation process. That is, if the child does not use two-syllable words, then increasing the child's production of multisyllabic words might be warranted. In a language such as Khmer, for example, which has complex syllable types but few polysyllabic words, this might not be the initial target of choice.

A number of phonemic approaches advocate the use of contrastive word pairs (i.e., minimal opposition pairs [e.g., *so–toe*] or maximal opposition pairs [e.g., *beet–seat*]). Approaches using contrastive word pairs include the paired stimuli approach (Weston & Irwin, 1985), minimal phonemic contrast approach (Cooper, 1985), minimal triads (Nelson, 1995), metaphon (Howell & Dean, 1991), maximal opposition (Gierut, 1989), and multiple oppositions (A. L. Williams, 2000a, 2000b). Contrastive word pairs, however, may be difficult to adapt to speakers of languages other than English. English, unlike other languages, is replete with minimal pairs. It may be more difficult to apply this methodology to languages other than English if those languages lack a significant number of contrastive word pairs that are appropriate for children.

SUMMARY

To provide least-biased assessment and evidence-based intervention to linguistically diverse individuals, SLPs must carry out a number of steps. First, they should gather information about the cultural and linguistic norms of the individuals to whom they are providing service. These norms include the phonological rules of the dialects/languages spoken by the client, remembering that not all speakers of a particular dialect will show or use every characteristic of it. Second, SLPs should complete a comprehensive phonological assessment that includes a wide array of independent and relational analyses. For these analyses, they should take into account dialect features that occur in all the client's languages. Finally, extensive information collected from the assessment should be used to plan intervention, remembering that intervention for a dialect difference should not occur unless elected by the client. For children acquiring more than one language, it is likely that both the bilingual approach and the cross-linguistic approach will be required. Following these steps will aid in providing appropriate services to children from culturally and linguistically diverse populations.

QUESTIONS FOR CHAPTER 14

1. What dialect do you speak? How do you think you acquired your dialect? If your dialect were to change, what dialect would you most and least like to have? Provide reasons for your decisions.

2. Administer a formal assessment to a speaker with a dialect other than yours. Score the assessment while not taking into account the speaker's dialect features, then score it while taking into account the dialect features. How did the person's score change between each administration? Would the person have been labeled with an SSD if dialect features had not been taken into account?

3. How would you determine whether the phonological patterns exhibited by someone were characteristic of true errors or were dialect features?

4. Design a protocol that employs the services of support personnel in the assessment of a preschool child who is bilingual in English and Vietnamese. You might consult the following ASHA papers to aid in your planning:

    - American Speech-Language-Hearing Association. (2004a). Knowledge and skills needed by SLPs and audiologists to provide culturally and linguistically appropriate services. *ASHA* (Suppl. 24).

    - American Speech-Language-Hearing Association. (1996). Guidelines for the training, credentialing, use, and supervision of speech-language pathology assistants. *ASHA, 38* (Suppl. 16): 21–34.

    - American Speech-Language Hearing Association. (1994). ASHA policy regarding support personnel. *ASHA, 36* (Suppl. 13): 24.

5. Define *pidgin, creole, dialect,* and *language.* What are the similarities and differences between these language varieties?

6. Take an informal poll about myths and facts related to dialect. Ask individuals to give you their opinion on people's dialects and how they feel about certain

dialects. You might survey individuals who have a background in language studies and individuals who do not have such a background to compare their responses. Then write a paper listing those perceptions followed by facts that counter any myths that are mentioned by the people you interview.

7. Create a quick reference guide for phonological development in AAE, Spanish, Cantonese, Mandarin, and Hmong. You might list sounds in each of their inventories, age of acquisition for segments and tones (if appropriate), and age of suppression for phonological processes. Create a reference guide for a language or dialect not listed here.

8. Design a protocol for modifying the dialect of a native Spanish-speaking woman who wishes to sound more like a native English speaker. List at least 10 questions you would ask her during the case history, enumerate the ways in which you would assess her speech, and outline your short- and long-term goals, providing a rationale for each of those goals. What aspects of her speech do you think will be less difficult and which will be more difficult to modify? Why?

9. Do you think newcomers to the United States who do not speak English should maintain their home language? Provide a rationale for your response. What are the advantages and disadvantages of immigrants to the United States maintaining or losing their native language?

10. Define *dialect, accent,* and *idiolect.*

11. Based on the following productions from an African American-speaking child, age 4:5, indicate if the child's production is a dialect feature of AAE or a true error:

Gloss	Child's production	AAE feature	True error
soap	[top]	No	Yes
mother	[mʌðə]		
mouth	[maʊf]		
tell	[tɪl]		
self	[sɛf]		
cool	[ku]		
bell	[bɛ]		
cool	[kū]		
playing	[pejiŋ]		
fast	[fæs]		
stool	[tul]		

15

Accent Modification

CAROL TESSEL

LEARNING OBJECTIVES

This chapter discusses the articulatory and phonological aspects of second language (L2) acquisition, the neurobiological factors behind L2 acquisition, how to evaluate and treat L2 learners, and some tips on treating clients from specific language backgrounds. By the end of this chapter, the reader should be able to:

- Summarize the necessary background information needed when initiating a treatment program for accent modification.
- Explain why adult learners have the most difficulty with phonological aspects of language.
- Describe options for foreign accent assessment procedures.
- Formulate feasible and appropriate goals for accent modification clients.
- Demonstrate knowledge of common transfer patterns for a few common languages.

Although this book is focused on delays and disorders of speech sounds in children, it is important to note that the issues that L2 learners experience in developing accurate speech sound productions in their second language can often benefit from the procedures commonly used in treating speech sound disorders (SSDs). Although many university clinics provide accent modification services, most graduate speech pathology coursework includes only minimal information or instruction in this area. The current chapter is intended to fill that gap by providing brief descriptions of services, assessment, variables that effect accents, instructional suggestions, and information related to L2 learners in the United States.

Accent modification is more appropriately referred to as *English pronunciation training,* but as this book is dedicated to English pronunciation in general, it was important to distinguish between first language (L1) and L2 learner pronunciation treatment. In addition to the focus in this chapter on the speaker, it should also be noted that the communication issues that L2 learners may experience can also be eased by training the listeners. For example, listeners can be trained in cultural understanding as well as perception of accented speech (Derwing et al., 2002). Additionally, adult listeners can benefit from being exposed to multiple speakers from different language backgrounds, thus increasing their exposure and likely increasing their perception skills (Baese-Berk et al., 2020). Graduate students as well as seasoned clinicians should consider their own exposure to diverse speakers and provide themselves with more exposure through social interactions, online videos, and/or by visiting diverse communities.

This work represents a significant challenge for clinicians. It is widely recognized that L2 learners can be found throughout the United States, having immigrated from many different countries and geographic regions. The cities of New York, Los Angeles, Washington, D.C., Phoenix, and Dallas (U.S. Census Bureau, 2015a), for example, each have more than 150 different languages represented. It probably will not be a surprise that Spanish is the second most frequently spoken language in the United States (U.S. Census Bureau, 2015b). More people speak Spanish than the next five most frequent languages combined: Chinese, Tagalog, Vietnamese, French (including French Creole), and Korean (U.S. Census Bureau, 2015b).

English poses a number of challenges for L2 learners. Although English includes the consonants /m/ and /k/ and the vowel /i/, which are three of the most common phonemes across languages of the world (Maddieson & Precoda, 1991), it also includes sounds that are highly marked, or rare in the world's languages, such as the two interdental fricatives /θ, ð/ and the rhotic /ɹ/. In terms of phonotactics, English words often end in consonants, whereas many of the world's languages mainly have words that end in vowels. And lastly, although some languages have clusters of longer length than English, the frequent use of consonant clusters in English often creates difficulty for speakers from a variety of different language backgrounds. It is also vital to be cognizant that all languages have dialectal variations in which certain sounds may be more or less difficult to learn depending on a speaker's dialectal background.

FOREIGN ACCENT

All languages differ to varying degrees in terms of their phonological and phonotactic rules. Phonology, or the sound system, is the aspect of language that is the most frequent cause of difficulty for L2 learners. As a consequence, individuals who speak more than one language may have difficulty fully mastering the phonology of the second language, which may reduce their intelligibility to some extent in the second language. The net result is that at times they produce phonological forms that include aspects of each of their spoken languages. This transfer between a learner's two (or more) languages results in what may be perceived by native language users as a *foreign accent*. These interacting forms are also sometimes referred to as *interlanguage* (Sikorski, 2005). In addition to phonological transfers, foreign accent also includes differences in the prosody of the productions. For example, many L2 learners speak at a slower pace and use more pauses in their L2 than when speaking their first language (Cenoz, 2000; Guion et al., 2000; Munro & Derwing, 1995).

Differences in various speech production details by adult L2 learners allow others to perceive them as nonnative speakers. However, these same speech productions also allow them to maintain aspects of their native language identity within their communities, which may be important for many individuals.

Factors Influencing Foreign Accent

Age of first exposure to a language appears to be the single largest influence on the extent of foreign accent. Individuals who learn a second language as early as 7 years of age can show differences in phonological productions when compared to native speakers (Flege, Munro, et al., 1995); that is, they may display some degree of foreign accent. Most likely, there is a sensitive period where L2 phonology is more easily learned and this ease declines with age (Newport, 1990; Oyama, 1978). There is not a clear cutoff, but rather a gradual decrease of ability to gain native-like language skills, particularly in the area of phonology. The relationship between age of first exposure and degree of native-like skill with L2 likely follows what Birdsong (2006) has called a stretched Z shape pattern (see Figure 15.1).

Some discussion of the typical process of language learning is in order here. To understand and speak a language, you must first learn which phonological and phonetic cues are important in that language. For example, the child learning English must learn how nasalization occurs with vowels. English vowels are often produced with some nasal resonance (i.e., they are nasalized) when in the presence of a nasal consonant. The word *moon* would therefore contain a nasalized [ũ]. However, in English, whether or not this vowel is produced as a nasalized version does not change the meaning of the word. That is not the case in some other languages, such as French, where nasalization can be phonemic. This means that adding nasalization to a vowel in French has the power to change the meaning of the word.

In order to be a functional speaker of English, a speaker has to learn to ignore the distinction of nasal versus oral [u], as it is not phonemic in English. Another example is that most languages include bilabial stops, however, not all have voicing contrasts. English has a voicing contrast for each of its stop consonants (i.e., bilabials are both voiced /b/ and voiceless /p/). Arabic, however, only contains the voiced [b]. It does not include [p] as a separate phoneme. Because the b/p contrast is phonemic in English but not in Arabic, an Arabic learner of English may have difficulty perceiving and producing word pairs that differ only in the b/p voicing contrast (e.g., *pat–bat* or *pair–bear*).

Infants must essentially take note of the frequency and consistency of sound patterns and sound combinations in their native language in order to form accurate phonological representations in that language (Kuhl, 2000). This allows infants and toddlers to build language-specific phonological categories. By the time infants are 12 months of age, they typically have difficulty perceiving contrasts that are not phonemic in their native language. As this knowledge solidifies, infants begin to practice production of the phonemes contained in their native language(s) and make the initial link between perception and production (Vihman & de Boysson-Boudries, 1994). By adulthood, the brain has committed to these early-formed phonological categories. For example, English has a vowel category for /i/ and a separate one for /ɪ/, whereas other languages, like Spanish, have only an equivalent to /i/. In this situation, an

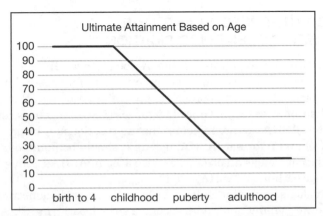

Figure 15.1. General relationship between age of acquisition of a second language and degree of native-like production skill. *Source:* Birdsong (2006).

adult's perception of the /ɪ/ might be assimilated into the /i/ category. This would place them at risk for perceiving and/or producing words like *sheep/ship* or *beet/bit* without the appropriate contrast. Reshaping such categories, even when fully immersed in a new language environment, is often difficult for an adult due to a decrease in the brain's flexibility and the early cerebral commitment (perception) to these phonological categories.

Parentese, which is the term frequently used to refer to the typical way in which adults speak and verbally interact with infants and young children, plays an important role in L1 acquisition. Parents, other adults, and older children speak to infants using such modifications as a slower rate of speech, a greater variety of prosodic patterns, simpler vocabulary and grammatical forms, and extra emphasis placed on new/target words. These changes appear to allow the infant to identify and master the fine details of the phonology of the language. One possible contributing factor in why foreign accent may manifest itself in those learning a second language as early as age 3 years is that the modifications of parentese are no longer available. It is interesting to note that L2 learners appear to benefit from similar modifications, such as speaker variability, when they are made available (Lively et al., 1993).

In addition to age of first exposure, there are other factors involved in the extent to which an individual displays a foreign accent. For example, length of residence (LOR) in a language environment and age when an individual first enters a new language environment has been studied and found to be a critical factor in a person's learning a second language. It is not uncommon for L2 speakers to show continued improvement (change) over time and the exposure they experience to the second language. Adult speakers with 20 years in a new language environment may demonstrate native-like productions, whereas those with less than 2 years of experience often struggle with nonnative consonant contrasts (Flege, Tagaki, et al., 1995).

However, most studies have shown that LOR is not a strong predictor for the strength of perceived foreign accent. Without specific instruction, there typically is minimal change in the accent after 1 or 2 years of residence in a new country (Flege et al., 1994; Munro, 1993; Munro & Derwing, 2008; Piske, MacKay, & Flege, 2001). There is, however, evidence of spontaneous improvement during the first year of residence without specific instruction (Munro & Derwing, 2008). In addition to LOR, individual motivation (Moyer, 1999) and amount of L1 usage (Flege, Frieda, et al., 1997) have also been shown to be significant factors in strength of perceived foreign accent.

THE ROLE OF THE SPEECH-LANGUAGE PATHOLOGIST IN ACCENT MODIFICATION

The American Speech-Language-Hearing Association (ASHA) considers accent modification services to be an appropriate practice area for speech-language pathologists (SLPs). It may also be an appropriate area of practice for other professionals, including English for Speakers of Other Languages (ESOL) teachers, and other types of speech coaches. ASHA further indicates that instruction may be provided in either individual and/or group format (ASHA, n.d.-a). It should be pointed out that accent modification is identified as an elective service area in ASHA's Scope of Practice in Speech-Language Pathology (ASHA, n.d.-c)

Some individuals, including SLPs, have been shown to demonstrate discriminative attitudes towards individuals with accented speech patterns (Chakraborty et al., 2017). Therefore, as SLPs, we must be mindful of how we interact with this population both in and out of therapy and recognize how their accent may affect their self-esteem and confidence. We must also be aware of their communication needs in their work and social lives.

GOALS OF ACCENT MODIFICATION

In working with young L1 learners who have SSDs, the goal is typically to help the child attain native-like mastery of the speech sound system. This is not always the case with accent modification clients. The goals for accent modification clients tend to be much more functional, with a focus on reducing accentedness and improving intelligibility, comprehensibility, and general communication ability. Skills learned through accent modification instruction also often provide clients with enhanced speaking confidence when speaking their second language.

The ASHA website includes the following definitions that relate to accent modification (ASHA, n.d.-a):

Accentedness is the perceived degree of an accent by a listener and refers to the perceived differences in comparison to the speech patterns of the listener's community.

Comprehensibility refers to the ease with which a listener understands the message and is based on the amount of time or the level of effort that it takes the listener to process an utterance (Derwing & Munro, 2009).

Intelligibility is "the extent to which a listener actually understands an utterance or message" (Celce-Murcia et al., 1996, p. 32).

On the other hand, there are some L2 learners who may have an end goal of sounding as native-like as possible. This includes those who have attained a relatively high level of intelligibility but have educational, social, or occupational reasons for achieving a higher level of proficiency. Clients, such as college instructors and psychological counselors, who are recipients of graduate degrees in their areas of study may still seek out services due to the high communication demands of their professions. Difficulty communicating in a second language and having to frequently repeat themselves can be a source of anxiety and may affect both their self-esteem and communication effectiveness (Brady et al., 2016; Carlson & McHenry, 2006).

UNDERSTANDING LANGUAGE INTERACTIONS

A clinician who wishes to provide services for accent modification should first learn about the native language of any potential client. One resource in this area is McLeod (2007a), who provides consonant and vowel inventories for many languages and dialects. Some of this information is also available through the ASHA website or through linguistic websites, such as https://phoible.org/inventories/view/1395. It is important to also learn about the morphology and syntax of the L1, as this can affect production of phonemes in an L2. For example, many languages have few (or no) final consonants. Therefore, L2 learners will often omit consonants in the final syllable or word position, indicating a difficulty with the phonotactic (word) structure rather than production of the phoneme.

Another well-known example of a structural issue is the difficulty that many L2 learners of English have producing consonant clusters. Depending on language background, L2 learners of English may be observed to reduce the cluster, substitute one or more sounds of the cluster, add a phoneme before the cluster, or insert a phoneme between the two consonant segments in the cluster. For example, a native Japanese speaker might pronounce the English word *ski* as /suki/, with an epenthetical vowel in between the two segments of the cluster. These phonological or phonotactic differences should not be considered errors, but rather transfers. Ellis (1997) defined transfers as "the influence that the learner's L1 exerts over the acquisition of an L2" (p. 51). The greater the difference between the structure of the L1 and L2, the greater the interference L1 may have on L2 acquisition/learning (Ellis, 1997).

ASSESSMENT

Assessment of foreign-accented speech must not only include phonological assessment, but also an in-depth analysis of how effective the person is as a communicator. For example, in what instances/situations is a speaker more or less intelligible? What is the individual's own perception of how well they are communicating? Sometimes a balance needs to be found between what the client desires and what the clinician believes to be most beneficial in terms of overall communication.

As mentioned earlier, foreign accent often includes differences in the prosodic aspects of speech. Assessment, therefore, should include analysis of suprasegmentals such as stress, intonation, and timing. In addition, some clinicians include assessments of grammar, vocabulary, and/or figurative language. One useful tool might be the Comprehensive Assessment of Spoken Language (2nd ed.) (CASL-2; Carrow-Woolfolk, 2017), which has an idiomatic language subtest that could be used informally as both comprehension and production of idioms, which are a frequent source of difficulty for L2 learners. There are other idioms tests available online, such as https://www.ereadingworksheets.com/figurative-language-worksheets/idiom-test-1.pdf.

Assessing the client's use of bound morphemes is also important. An example of a morphological challenge for many L2 learners of English is the lack of a third person -s marker. Careful examination of the use of this form is needed so as not to misinterpret this as a phonological problem, such as final consonant deletion or final cluster reduction, when it may actually be a morphological issue (ASHA, n.d.-a).

One commonly used assessment measure for use with accent modification clients is the Proficiency in Oral English Communication (POEC; Sikorski, 1991). The POEC assesses articulation, intonation, and auditory discrimination (perception). It typically takes 20–30 minutes to administer. Another assessment tool, the Compton Phonological Assessment of Foreign Language (Compton, 1983), includes a deck of 66 flash cards with English words for the client to produce in isolation and then in a self-made sentence. Each English phoneme is targeted two times in two different words. It also includes a passage to be read aloud and then in imitation after the clinician's model. This test can take up to 1 hour to administer but allows the clinician to also take note of deficiencies in vocabulary or grammar, as the client is required to form spontaneous sentences with the provided words.

If a test geared specifically for foreign-accented speech is not available, a test of articulation and phonology for English speakers can be used informally. When doing so, care should be taken that pictures and stimuli are age appropriate for the client. Typically, clinicians use a collection of smaller informal testing procedures that fit each individual client's needs. For example, word lists that target frequently challenging structures (i.e., final consonants) and phonemes (i.e., /ð/ or /dʒ/) that reflect the common issues with individuals with similar L1 issues can be useful.

Finally, detailed information regarding when and how each of the speaker's languages were learned should be obtained, as well as information regarding current and past language use. Given that there is evidence that the more an L1 is used, the greater the perceived foreign accent in the L2, current language usage information is crucial. If the client continues to use L1 to a much greater extent than L2, ways of increasing L2 immersion may be suggested. For example, socializing in L2, finding a conversation group in L2 (many public libraries have these), listening to music in L2, watching TV in L2, and reading in L2. Of course, it is preferable that the client speak their L2 as often as possible; however, increased media exposure has been observed to improve language outcomes in the L2 (Flege et al., 1999).

The Role of Speech Perception

Although the ability to produce new L2 phonemes has been linked to the ability to perceive them (Flege, Bohn, et al., 1997), the relationship between perception and production is not always clear (Tsukada et al., 2005). Some evidence indicates that training in perception alone can lead to improved production (Thomson, 2011). There is also evidence that, in some cases, the ability to produce a phoneme in a more native-like manner precedes the ability to perceive it in a more native-like manner (Flege, Bohn, et al., 1997). Care should be taken to assess the client's perception and make case-by-case decisions on whether perception tasks would be an appropriate activity for treatment and, when appropriate, to provide instruction for such skills as part of the production focus.

TREATMENT AND INSTRUCTION

Depending on the needs of the speaker, treatment plans might be focused on individual sound productions, phonological transfers from L1 to L2, prosodic issues, or all of these. Zhao and colleagues (2012) reported that prosody contributed more to accentedness for English learners from China and Vietnam, whereas it was segmental production that was the greatest contributor for English learners from India. It should also be noted that although some treatment approaches used with children with SSDs can also be effective with L2 learners, it is important to remember that foreign accents are not disorders and a large evidence base for use of these tactics for L2 learners is still lacking.

Pretreatment Training

As an initial step of phoneme instruction, it may be beneficial to give the client some basic information and instruction related to phonology and the International Phonetic Alphabet (IPA) (Tessel & Luque, 2020; Turner & Gutierrez, 2013). This could be in the form of contrasting differences that may be observed in consonant charts and vowel quadrilateral charts between L1 and L2 or instructing the client regarding differences in manner and place of phonemes used in English. A client who is able to understand differences in IPA symbols and distinguish between fricative consonants and stop consonants or rounded vowels and nonrounded vowels will likely have an easier time adjusting their articulators to the correct positions when instructed.

Segmental Instruction

The usual range of motor-based instructional activities for treating sounds (see Chapter 10) may be useful for instruction with L2 learners. Initial elicitation might include repeating a clinician's verbal model (i.e., imitation), providing articulatory/ placement cues, visual models of articulatory placement (using a mirror), digital animation of production movements, reading word lists with target phonemes, reading selected materials aloud, acting out a conversation with target vocabulary/phrases, and answering egocentric questions. It should be noted that while still at the isolated sound level, practice should include the consonant along with a variety of different vowels both before and after the target sound (Schmidt, 1997). Often, those who seek out accent modification are professionals and, therefore, target vocabulary that pertains to their profession should be included as instructional materials. A traditional progression through ever higher linguistic levels is commonly used. For purposes of teaching, both new motor movements and meaningful minimal contrasts may also be employed.

A brief warning is warranted for using activities that require reading, as this adds in another component of difficulty. English spelling may present problems for many clients, as the letters do not always match sounds in a one-to-one manner, which can cause phonological changes based on lack of familiarity with the word. For example, many words that are spelled with an *o* are actually produced as /ɑ/ or /ʌ/ (e.g., the vowels in *dog* or *ton*). Clinicians should be cautious of reading errors that may have an impact on speech production. If the client's productions reflect a completely different phoneme rather than the target phoneme, the change may cause semantic confusion, which can be pointed out with word contrasts (e.g., *sheep* vs. *ship*). To address an issue such as tensing of the /ɪ/, both segmental and contrast-based instruction can prove useful. For example, instructing the client to say an /ɪ/, and if the client has difficulty with this vowel and instead says /i/, then have them produce the sound with the jaw slightly more open and the tongue slightly lowered, which may result in a closer approximation. Similarly, a list of minimal pairs can help to point out the difference between the /ɪ/ and /i/. Minimal pairs such as *slip–sleep, beet–bit,* or *pit–Pete* can be used to show the contrasts. These words can eventually be used in simple carrier phrases such as, "Is it your turn to *sleep–slip*?" and eventually into novel phrases.

Another instructional approach that may be helpful is a go-to word for each phoneme being addressed. Often times a client will be able to produce a sound or sound combination correctly in one or more words. This strategy is based in using a stimulable production to assist in increasing the automaticity of the target sound, a common strategy used with children that have SSDs (McLeod & Baker, 2014; Weiss et al., 1987). For example, a client might say the /f/ correctly in the word *fan,* but often replaces it with a /p/, such as saying *pile* for *file.* The word *fan* can be used as a facilitator and reminder throughout. The client can be asked to say the word *fan* before each production of other words in order to cue them. This cueing system can be slowly removed as the client improves productions of the sound contrasts.

A related area is that of consonant clusters, which are a common area of difficulty for L2 learners. Depending on language background, learners might be more likely to engage in epenthesis by inserting a vowel between two consonant phonemes (Schmidt, 1997), inserting a vowel before the cluster (Tessel & Luque, 2020), or deleting a portion of the cluster (Altenberg, 2005; Franklin & McDaniel, 2016; Tessel & Luque, 2020). Although minimal research has been conducted as to best practices in instruction for L2 cluster acquisition, a few recent studies show promise for using current evidence-based methodologies for treating children with difficulties producing these sequences (Franklin & McDaniel, 2016; Tessel & Luque, 2020). Possibilities for instruction on production of English clusters include using a cycles-based phonological approach (Franklin & McDaniel, 2016) where clusters would be targeted in a weekly cycle and minimal pair contrasts would be utilized. There is also evidence that both phonological/contrast-based instruction and segmental/motor-based instruction can be effective for improving accuracy of consonant cluster production (Tessel & Luque, 2020). A contrast approach using pairs such as *rides–rise* can also be utilized (Mojsin, 2016).

Prosodic Instruction

In addition to the focus on the segmental aspects of the language, prosodic goals likely will need to be targeted. Prosodic goals can include both word- and sentence-level stress patterns, as both can change the meaning of a word/sentence. For example, the word *record* can be either a noun or a verb depending on the stress. Typically, nouns have first syllable stress whereas verbs have second syllable stress (e.g., 'record vs. re'cord). For sentence-level stress, clients can be reminded that declarative sentences and wh- questions have falling pitch and yes/no questions end with rising pitch. A list of sentences to rehearse for native-like intonation can be used with cues, such as underlining or bolding the words that require the most stress. Including prosodic targets such as speech rate, intonation, and rhythm may prove beneficial either as separate targets or in addition to segmental targets (Derwing et al., 1998).

Another prosody-focused instructional approach that has shown promise is the use of the *clear speech* method to decrease a speaker's level of perceived accentedness. This approach instructs the client to increase pausing, decrease speaking rate, and increase vowel duration in order to increase intelligibility (Ferguson & Kewley-Port, 2002, 2007). Smiljanić and Bradlow (2011) studied the effectiveness of the clear speech approach for both native and nonnative speakers. Findings revealed that clear speech strategies improved intelligibility for both groups. Another study by Behrman and colleagues (2017) included 5 weeks of clear speech-based accent modification training. At the conclusion of the 5 weeks the group of six native Spanish-speaking learners of English demonstrated improvement in both their accentedness ratings and ease of understanding as judged by native speakers of English.

Use of Biofeedback

As discussed in Chapter 12, biofeedback techniques can show the client a visual representation of their sound production and provide a comparison to the target production. Visual acoustic feedback using spectrograms is an example of a biofeedback technique. Spectrograms may be used to demonstrate differences in vowel formants, voice onset time, prosody, and differences in manner of articulation (e.g., stops vs. fricatives). Research has demonstrated that use of visual computer feedback programs with spectrograms can increase L2 learner's ability to perceive English vowel contrasts; however, the rate of carryover to production is still unclear (Wang & Munro, 2004).

Figure 15.2a (top) demonstrates a recording of a native speaker saying *that* and *dat*. Vertical rectangles indicate where a fricative versus a stop consonant can be visually demonstrated to a client. Figure 15.2b (bottom) demonstrates a native speaker saying *beet* and *bit*. Horizontal rectangles surrounding the formants can demonstrate the larger difference between F1 and F2 for the /i/ vowel (left) versus the /ɪ/ vowel (right), which can be a good visual demonstration for a client.

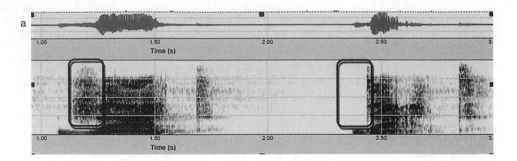

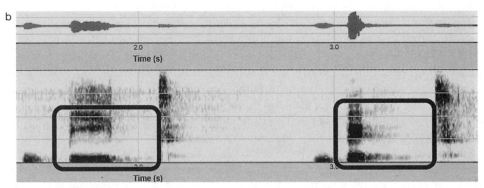

Figure 15.2. Examples of formants on a spectrogram using WASP, an acoustic analysis program. Figure 15.2a (*top*) demonstrates a recording of a native speaker saying *that* and *dat*. Figure 2b (*bottom*) demonstrates a native speaker saying *beet* and *bi.*

Several different acoustics programs are available. One of the more versatile programs is called Sona-Match, which operates on the Computerized Speech Lab (CSL) system (KayPentax). It will plot a speaker's vowel formants directly onto a vowel quadrilateral; however, vowels may not always be correctly identified. Unfortunately, the cost of the CSL system is a major drawback for most SLP's working outside of a university clinic or lab, even for someone who makes accent modification the primary focus of their practice. Another program often used in Europe is called lingWAVES (WEVOSYS; Forchheim, Germany). This system provides visual feedback for clients and can be programmed for the desired target phoneme. The PRAAT program (Boersma & Weenink, 2021) offers the most practical (i.e., free) visual feedback in the form of spectrograms and formant contours. WASP (Waveforms, Annotations, Spectrograms, and Pitch) at https://www.speechandhearing.net/laboratory/wasp/ (Huckvale, 2016) is a browser-based acoustic analysis program that can also be used without the need to download any content to your computer (see Figures 15.2a and 15.2b for examples of how WASP can be used as biofeedback). It does not show exact formant values but displays the formants on a spectrogram and tracks the fundamental frequency.

Group Treatment

Clinicians may come across situations where they are able provide accent modification services in a group setting. The group may contain clients of different language backgrounds. Reviewing the list of common transfer patterns for the languages represented in the group can facilitate determining instructional goals that relate to shared language needs. If the group includes a language not presented in this chapter, you can research the phonological repertoire of the first languages of the clients and try to find common ground for targets in the group. For example, many languages have fewer or no final consonants when compared to English and/or fewer consonant clusters than English, therefore, these two structures can lend themselves to being appropriate group treatment goals. Group instruction also lends itself to using students as a model for sounds that they produce well that others find challenging.

EVIDENCE OF SUCCESS OF ACCENT MODIFICATION

Multiple studies have shown that both segmental and prosodic based approaches can yield positive outcomes, but a combination of both has demonstrated the most success (Behrman, 2014; Derwing et al., 1998). Behrman and colleagues (2017) completed a single-subject multiple-baseline treatment program for native speakers of Hindi. The results demonstrated that a combination of both segmental and prosodic training resulted in improvements in increased accuracy of pronunciation of targets. Similarly, Derwing and colleagues (1998) compared programs that were segmental only, no specific pronunciation training, or global training that included both segmental and prosodic instruction. After the treatment programs, each group produced an extemporaneous narrative that was judged in terms of comprehensibility. Only the global group demonstrated true improvements in both comprehensibility and fluency.

Another study compared a segmental/motor-based approach with a phonological/contrast-based approach, with both reported to have positive outcomes for overall accuracy of production post-treatment (Tessel & Luque, 2020). Teaching students to recognize their own errors by playing recordings of their speech and discussing the differences in their speech and the target production, while using specific metalanguage to describe the phonological changes that need to be made, can also be effective for long-term change (Couper, 2006). Long-term changes were observed while focusing on epenthesis, consonant deletion, as well as grammatical aspects of English (Couper, 2006).

APPLICATION TO SPECIFIC LANGUAGES

Characteristics of five major languages, Spanish, Mandarin, Vietnamese, Russian, and Korean, are presented next. After each language description is a list of possible goals to be used for instruction in accent modification and higher-level linguistic skills, such as grammar or morphology. A rationale for each goal will also be provided. These goals can be intertwined in treatment. For example, sentences that contain a target phoneme may also contain a targeted syntactical structure.

Spanish

English and Spanish share a number of consonant and vowel phonemes. Consonants that are shared between the two languages include /b, p, d, t, k, g, m, n, s, f, tʃ, l, j, w/, whereas shared vowels are limited to /i, o, u, e, a/. It should be noted that shared phonemes may not always be produced in exactly the same manner in the two languages. For example, there are different average voice onset times for Spanish and English stop consonants, making a sound such as [p] have a slightly different quality across

Table 15.1. List of shared and nonshared sounds across English and Spanish

Consonants	Shared	English only	Spanish only
Stops	b, p, t, d, k, g		
Fricatives	s, f	θ, ð, z, v, ʃ, ʒ, h	x
Nasals	m, n	ŋ	ɲ
Affricates	tʃ	dʒ	
Approximants	l, w, j	ɹ	
Flap/trill			ɾ, r

Vowels	Shared	English only	Spanish only
High	i, u	ɪ, ʊ	
Mid	e, o	ɛ, ʌ	
Low		æ, ɑ	a

the two languages. The only fricative phonemes in Spanish are /f, x, s/, although many more serve as allophones of the voiced stop consonants. This often leads to confusion between English sound pairs, such as /b/ and /v/, which serve as separate phonemes in English. In Spanish, /b/ has a labial fricative allophone ([β]) that may sound similar to a /v/ to an English listener. The voiceless interdental fricative of English (/θ/) exists as a phoneme in some dialects of Spanish, whereas the voiced interdental fricative of English ([ð]) often exists as an allophone of the /d/ phoneme in Spanish.

Regarding vowels, Spanish has only five vowels /i, o, u, e, a/ and none are lax, nor are vowels typically reduced (i.e., produced closer to the center of the vowel space) in Spanish as they often are in English. Lax and central vowels such as [ɪ, ʊ, æ, ʌ] are often areas of great challenge for native Spanish speakers, as these vowels are not used in Spanish. See Table 15.1 for a list of shared and unique sound comparison in English and Spanish.

Some examples of typical cross-linguistic phonological transfers in Spanish-speaking learners of English include (see Table 15.2 for specific word examples):

- The /θ/ and /ð/ sounds are often difficult for many L2 learners, as they are rare outside of English. They may be substituted with either a stop consonant (i.e., /t, d/) or another fricative (i.e., /f, s/).

- Initial /s/ clusters are not allowable in Spanish and, therefore, are often produced with an added initial vowel (often /ɛ/).

Table 15.2. Examples of common phonological transfer patterns in adult Spanish-speaking learners of English

Phonological pattern	Target	Example transfer
Epenthesis	street–/strit/	estreet–/ɛstrit/
Stopping	this–/ðɪs/	dis–/dɪs/
Final consonant deletion	time–/taɪm/	tie–/taɪ/
Affrication	year–/jɪɹ/	jear–/dzɪɹ/
Tensing of lax vowels	bit–/bɪt/	beet–/bit/
/ɚ, ɝ/→ /ɛɹ/	her–/hɝ/	hair–/hɛɹ/

- A confusion will often arise between phoneme pairs, such as /b/ and /v/, making them interchangeable.

- Vowel assimilation patterns will often result in the merging of two English vowels into one Spanish vowel category and can result in semantic changes. For example, the /i/ and /ɪ/ vowels are often merged, rendering words like *ship* and *sheep* indistinguishable. A similar pattern occurs with the /ɑ/ and /æ/ vowels, which are often merged, rendering words such as *rocket* and *racket* indistinguishable. In addition, the rhotic /ɚ, ɝ/ sound is often produced as the rhotic diphthong /ɛɪ/.

- Other common transfer patterns include deletion of final consonants, reduction of final consonant clusters, affrication of /ʃ/ and /ʒ/, and deaffrication of /tʃ/ and /dʒ/.

- Native Spanish learners of English (L2) also tend to decentralize English central vowels, such as /ʌ/ or /ə/.

Examples of Segmental and Contrast Goals

Examples of segmental and contrast goals for Spanish-speaking learners of English include:

1. The client will produce the lax vowels /ɪ/ and /æ/ accurately at the word level.

   Rationale: As mentioned previously, the Spanish vowel system is smaller in number than English and lacks lax vowels; therefore, tense and lax vowels are often merged into one category. In order for clients to avoid transfer patterns that are influences from their L1, a client may need instruction to form new vowel categories. These additional vowel categories will allow speakers to accurately produce a greater variety of words and increase their overall intelligibility.

2. The client will produce the interdental fricatives /θ, ð/ accurately at the word level given an auditory and visual model.

   Rationale: Due to the lack of interdental fricatives in Spanish, as well as the general marked/difficult nature of interdental fricative productions, this is a common goal for L2 learners of English. The transfer pattern of substituting the interdental fricative with another fricative or stop doesn't often affect overall intelligibility; however, listeners and the clients themselves often readily notice these types of changes. For clients who may wish to sound more like a native speaker, production of interdental sounds may be an appropriate goal for L2 clients. Interdental sounds, though marked in some languages of the world, are fairly easy to teach as they are highly visual.

3. The client will produce the /b/ and /v/ phonemes accurately during a read-aloud activity.

   Rationale: Spanish contains the *b* and *v* as graphemes (letters), but they both phonetically are represented as the [b] phoneme. This phoneme often changes to a fricative allophone when in the intervocalic position. These two issues often cause confusion for the Spanish L2 speaker of English, wherein these sounds represent two distinct phonemes. Spending time reviewing these sounds as separate English phonemes and providing instruction on how the *b* and *v* graphemes consistently represent the /b/ and /v/ phonemes in English will assist in forming a [v] category. As with the interdental fricatives, these sounds can be demonstrated using visual cues, demonstrating how /b/ uses both lips together and /v/ requires the upper teeth to touch the bottom lips.

4. The client will demonstrate accurate sentence-level intonation in English after the clinician's model. For example, the client might engage in a paragraph reading exercise or question/answer exercise and the clinician would point out where the client used inaccurate stress. The clinician could model the correct use of intonation and then have the client repeat it.

   Rationale: Spanish is a syllable-timed language, where all syllables are produced with equal length, whereas English is a stress-timed language, where syllables can change length depending on context. Inaccurate use of suprasegmentals can lead to communication breakdowns.

Possible Higher-Level Linguistic Goals

Examples of higher-level linguistic goals for Spanish-speaking learners of English include:

1. The client will utilize the articles *a* and *the* appropriately in all obligatory contexts.

   Rationale: L2 learners often have difficulty using articles correctly in English. Omission of articles may not have a great impact on intelligibility, but they are an obvious production difference that most listeners will notice and can impact the client's ability to perform well in business or other speaking and writing situations.

2. The client will demonstrate appropriate use of third-person singular -s in all obligatory contexts. For example, a client might be asked to tell a story or retell a past event. They would be expected to utilize the third-person singular -s in their conjugation of verbs. An accurate sentence might include, "She runs home every day" or "He waits outside for his mother."

   Rationale: Use of third-person singular is a common area of difficulty for L2 leaners of English and can lead to listener confusion if omitted.

3. The client will demonstrate understanding of a variety of typical English idioms. First, a simple assessment could be used to see which idioms a client is familiar with (these are easily accessed online). Then the clinician could produce sentences using the unfamiliar idioms (e.g., "That test was a piece of cake") and ask the client to communicate what they thought the sentence was trying to convey. The clinician would give cues as necessary and eventually ask the client to use these idioms in their own sentence.

   Rationale: L2 learners often struggle with figurative language in English. This is often due to limited social exposure to English and the fact that they did not grow up learning the English language. Including figurative language as a goal can help the client to feel more comfortable in social situations and avoid misunderstandings.

Clinical Vignette 15.1

Accent Modification for a Spanish-English Bilingual Adult

Angela (a pseudonym) is a 40-year-old woman from Cuba. Her first language is Spanish, and she began speaking English when she moved to Miami, Florida in her late 20s. She is currently in graduate school for her master's of divinity degree and hopes to become a full-time minister/mission leader. She also works part-time as a tennis instructor to help pay for school. She is seeking out accent modification treatment to help her be better understood when she is preaching to an English-speaking audience, as well as to grow her client base for tennis lessons.

After completion of an in-depth interview and speech sample, administration of the POEC, recordings of the grandfather passage, and an informal assessment of grammar, Angela was found to have difficulty producing the interdental fricatives, the voiced affricate /dʒ/, the English /ɹ/, and English lax vowels such as /ɪ/. She also demonstrated difficulty with appropriate syllable stress in multisyllabic words and grammatical differences were noted in her use of prepositions and gender pronouns.

Angela attended 6 months of private accent modification services via teletherapy. Goals included production of the voiced affricate and the interdental fricatives using an articulation-based approach with coaching regarding articulator placement. The English lax vowels were addressed using a combination of phonetic placement cues as well as minimal pairs (e.g., *beat* vs. *bit*). Multisyllabic words were addressed using words taken from copies of Angela's sermons that she provided to the therapist. Grammar was addressed through informal conversation, with the therapist using recasting of the client's spoken sentences. In addition, Angela recorded some of her own sermons and the therapist reviewed them with her to point out any instances of atypical grammar or pronunciation.

Angela made a marked improvement in all areas of treatment, however, the interdental fricatives remained the most challenging aspect of pronunciation. The therapist counseled Angela on the limited impact that mispronunciation of the interdental fricatives had on her speech. The English /ɹ/ was not directly addressed in treatment, as the client and therapist agreed that it had limited impact on her intelligibility and that occasional substitution with the Spanish trill /r/ was an indication of her native language culture and she felt this was part of her identity and her heritage.

Mandarin

Mandarin is one of the official languages of mainland China. The Beijing dialect of Mandarin is also known as Pǔtōnghuà. It bears little similarity to English. It is a tone language, which means that it uses pitch changes rather than speaker intent or syllable stress to indicate semantic differences. Mandarin uses mostly single-syllable words and does not allow consonant clusters. There are only two phonemes that can legally occur in word-final position, therefore, production of English final consonants is often a challenge for L1 Mandarin speakers. In addition, Mandarin does not use the palatal fricatives or affricates that are present in English. A few common challenging forms for Mandarin speakers learning English include:

- There is difficulty producing the /v/ sound, which is often substituted with /f/ or /w/ or omitted, especially in the medial word position.

- Interdental fricatives /θ, ð/ are often produced as stop consonants or other fricatives.

- The phonemes /l/ and /ɹ/ are produced interchangeably and words such as *war* and *wall* may be indistinguishable. Words with more than one /l/ or /ɹ/ may prove even more difficult (e.g., *rarely*) (Mojsin, 2016).

- Final /n/ is often produced as /ŋ/ or deleted.

- Confusion with /n/ and /l/ frequently occurs.

- The lax /ɪ/ is often replaced by the tense /i/.

- There is confusion of /æ/ and /ɛ/ vowels.

- Consonant clusters are often reduced.

Mosjin (2016) suggests initially working on final consonants by linking them to a following word that begins in a vowel, effectively producing them as an intervocalic consonant. For the /v/ sound, she suggests working on common words in phrases such as, "I saw you have a bee hive."

Examples of Segmental and Contrast Goals

Examples of segmental and contrast goals for Mandarin-speaking learners of English include:

1. The client will use the /n/ phoneme accurately in phrases. A list of phrases that contain the /n/ phoneme in the final position can be used until the client reaches a targeted level of accuracy and can then be moved to spontaneous speech. Sentences like, "The man ran down to the station" could be utilized.

   Rationale: Substitution or deletion of /n/, especially in the final position, is common in Mandarin learners of English. These transfers can lead to confusion and misunderstanding on the part of the listener.

2. The client will produce words with /ɛ/ and /æ/ accurately while reading a word list (see Table 15.3 for examples).

   Rationale: As with many languages, Mandarin does not contain all of the English lax vowels and clients will often confuse them or produce them as the closest tense vowel. Confusion of these vowels can lead to misunderstandings due to their presence in minimal pairs.

3. The client will accurately produce words with consonant clusters following a model. High function words could be a focus here, specifically ones where the

Table 15.3. Example word list for minimal pair work with vowels /æ/ and /ɛ/

/æ/ words	/ɛ/ words
pan	pen
mat	met
bat	bet
can	Ken
man	men
gnat	net

transfer production causes a change in meaning. For example, in the word *best,* when the initial consonant in the cluster is deleted, it becomes the word *bet.* (See also information in the Treatment section regarding consonant clusters intervention.)

Rationale: Mandarin does not contain consonant clusters, whereas English contains a great number. Inability to produce two or three adjoining consonants will certainly affect intelligibility and lead to listener confusion.

Possible Higher-Level Linguistic Goals

Examples of higher-level linguistic goals for Mandarin-speaking learners of English include:

1. The client will use gender pronouns (he/she) appropriately in spontaneous speech. During discussion of someone known to the client, they will use that person's preferred gender pronoun accurately in the discussion.

   Rationale: Spoken Mandarin has only one third-person pronoun that represents *he, she,* and *it,* often causing Mandarin-speaking learners of English difficulty using these pronouns that require a gender distinction. Difficulty using gender pronouns correctly can lead to listener confusion and, therefore, is an appropriate goal for both newer as well as for more experienced Mandarin L1 speakers who are English L2 learners.

2. The client will use the plural -s in all obligatory contexts during a question-answering activity. For example, the clinician could ask the client questions like, "What is your favorite fruit?" with the client's hypothetical answer being, "I like apples." Other questions could take the form of, "How many miles did you run yesterday?" with the hypothetical answer being, "I ran 4 miles."

   Rationale: Mandarin does not require a plural marker in the way that English does, therefore plurals are often omitted. Omitting plurals will likely lead to listener confusion.

3. The client will correctly conjugate all verbs when answering questions about a preferred topic.

   Rationale: Mandarin does not use verb conjugation to indicate past, present, or future. Instead, the context provides the cues to timing. Verb conjugation is therefore a frequent area of difficulty for Mandarin speakers of English. Correct verb conjugation is an essential element in being a competent English speaker.

Vietnamese

Vietnamese is a tone language that shares many phonemes with English. However, the Vietnamese phoneme inventory does not include the fricatives /θ, ð/ or the affricates /tʃ, dʒ/. There are also many differences between Vietnamese and English in phonotactics. For example, Vietnamese does not allow for consonant clusters and most words are monosyllabic, though some multisyllabic words do exist (Hwa-Froelich et al., 2002). Vietnamese does not contain voiced consonants in the word-final position. In terms of syntactical transfers, Vietnamese speakers often have difficulty using plurals, auxiliary verbs, and the correct adjective-noun word order. They also have difficulty including obligatory verb tense endings, such as past tense -ed.

Some common patterns in Vietnamese that will influence English L2 speakers include:

- Consonant clusters are often reduced, omitted, or replaced by substitutions.

- Final consonants are often deleted or substituted, with /z, s, dʒ/ being three of the most challenging final consonants (Tuan, 2011).

- Medial consonant sounds are often deleted due to the limited number of multisyllabic words in Vietnamese.

- There are substitutions of /t/, /tr/, and /dʒ/ with /tʃ/.

- The fricative /ð/ is often replaced with /d/ or /z/.

- The following vowel pairs are often merged: /ɪ, i/, /ʊ, u/, /ɔ, ɑ/ (Cunningham, 2010).

- There is confusion of /n/ and /l/.

- There is difficulty with English stress patterns at the word and sentence level.

Examples of Segmental and Contrast Goals

Examples of segmental and contrast goals for Vietnamese-speaking learners of English include:

1. The client will produce word-final voiced consonants at the phrase level. Phrases containing common words such as *has, have, bed,* or *big* could be used. Words can be increased in complexity as the client improves.

   Rationale: Vietnamese does not have any word-final voiced consonants, which makes these forms difficult to pronounce for native Vietnamese speakers of English (L2). Sounds that could be used for initial teaching of final consonants could be /b, d, g, l, v, dʒ/. Demonstrating to the client how omission or substitution of a voiceless sound in word-final position will change the word meaning should be useful. For example, the word *bead* would be perceived as *beat* if a voiceless sound was substituted, or as the word *bee* if the final consonant was deleted.

2. The client will produce English vowels accurately at the single-word level when provided with a model.

   Rationale: Vietnamese speakers tend to merge English lax vowels into a tense vowel category. Sounds to start with include /ɪ, ʊ, ə/.

3. The client will produce /n/ and /l/ contrastively in conversational speech.

   Rationale: Vietnamese speakers often use the /n/ and /l/ phonemes interchangeably. This can cause confusion for the listener and learning to contrast these two phonemes may improve speech intelligibility.

Possible Higher-Level Linguistic Goals

Examples of higher-level linguistic goals for Vietnamese-speaking learners of English include:

1. The client will demonstrate use of the obligatory past tense -ed and present progressive -ing during a storytelling activity. The clinician could record the client telling the story and then review the recording with the client, pointing out any possible omissions of the -ed or -ing endings.

   Rationale: Vietnamese clients often have difficulty including English verb tense morphology, which can often lead to listener confusion.

2. The client will use correct word order during a picture-description activity. The clinician could provide the client with the picture scene and ask the client to describe the scene, analyzing the client's speech for proper subject-verb-object or modifier-noun word order.

   Rationale: Vietnamese speakers often have difficulty with accurate word order in English and will produce forms such as *the house big* instead of *the big house.*

Russian

The Russian phonological system includes only five vowels(/i, u, e, o, a/). Its consonant inventory does not include /θ, ð, w, ŋ/. Some common transfer patterns with Russian learners of English are:

- Interdental fricatives /θ, ð/ are often substituted with the /t/ or /d/ sounds.

- There is confusion of /v/ and /w/.

- Devoicing of final consonants occurs.

- The trill /r/ is used when rhotic /ɹ/ is in the initial position or following another consonant. It is often deleted in final position.

- Tensing of lax vowel (e.g., /ɪ/ →/i/) and decentralizing of central vowels (i.e., /ə/→/ɑ/) occurs.

Examples of Segmental and Contrast Goals

Examples of segmental and contrast goals for Russian-speaking learners of English include:

1. The client will accurately produce the /v/ and /w/ phonemes in a distinguishable manner during a structured sentence completion task. Sentences that need to be completed with common /v/ and /w/ words could be utilized. Words such as *very, water, vest, van, when, which, women,* and so on, could be a focus in treatment.

   Rationale: Russian does not contain a distinction between the phonemes /v/ and /w/, therefore, these sounds are often used interchangeably by Russian learners of English. Using word pairs or sentences containing phrases like *very wild* will assist the client in learning to distinguish these sounds. Use of visual cues to pronunciation, distinguishing the labial versus labiodental places of articulation may prove useful.

2. The client will produce the English /ɹ/ accurately during word list reading.

   Rationale: Russian speakers tend to delete the English /ɹ/ in final position or roll their /ɹ/ (i.e., produce a trill) in other positions, especially in consonant clusters. Accurate production of /ɹ/ is essential for intelligibility and decreasing the perception of a foreign accent.

3. The client will produce lax and central vowels accurately after a clinician model.

    Rationale: Due to the Russian vowel system being much smaller than that of English, Russian speakers will often assimilate English central and lax vowels into a tense category. For example, /ɪ/ is often produced as /i/ and /ə/ is often produced as /ɑ/. Due to the large number of minimal pairs in English that differ only by a vowel, accurate production of vowels in English will contribute to improved intelligibility.

Possible Higher-Level Linguistic Goals

Examples of higher-level linguistic goals for Russian-speaking learners of English include:

1. The client will use the prepositions *on, in,* and *from* accurately when answering simple ego-centric question prompts. Questions such as, "Tell me about how you decided on your major in college" or "Tell me one of your best childhood memories" would be good starting points.

    Rationale: The rules for use of English prepositions can be challenging, as Russian and English have many nonequivalent prepositions and do not require prepositions in the same circumstances. Mastering prepositions will improve the listener's ability to accurately understand the speaker's intent.

2. The client will use the plural -s correctly, distinguishing countable from noncountable nouns in a sentence completion activity. This activity could start by having pictures of multiple items, including both count and noncount nouns, and asking the client to label each plural group.

    Rationale: This is a common grammatical issue for Russian speakers and can certainly lead to confusion by the listener. It may be worthwhile to discuss how count nouns change, including examples of common count (e.g., *books, cars*) and noncount (e.g., *sugar, wood*) nouns. In addition, the clinician might point out nouns that can be both count and noncount (e.g., *danger(s)*).

3. The client will accurately produce sentences distinguishing between verb pairs such as *learn–teach* and *say–tell* during a structured activity. This goal could be initiated with a fill-in activity where a client is given a sentence such as, "The professor enjoys _____ history as his job" or "I need to ____ my mom that I will be late" and is asked to fill in the blank.

    Rationale: These verb pairs are commonly confused in Russian L2 learners and result in sentences such as, "Can you say me how to do that?" Instructing the client to distinguish these verbs using sentence pairs can assist them in learning their distinct functions. Although these transfers don't have a great effect on the listeners understanding of the message, they contribute to the listener's perception of the client's speech as nonnative.

Korean

Korean is an East Asian language and currently the sixth most widely spoken foreign language in the United States. Korean has a two- or three-way contrast for many of the stops, fricatives, and affricates that are not present in English because English lacks this type of consonant distinction (ASHA, n.d.-b). It should also be noted that due to these distinctions, although Korean and English do have shared phonemes, the pronunciation of these phonemes may differ to the point that there is an audible difference. Grammatical transfer patterns include omission of articles, prepositions, and auxiliary verbs (Yoon, 2012).

Some common transfer patterns in Korean learners of English are:

- Confusion of the English r/l occurs.

- Confusion of b/v and p/f occurs.

- There is difficulty producing the interdental fricatives.

- There is a tendency to delete the /w/ phoneme.

- Confusion of the /ɛ/ and /æ/ vowels occurs.

- Use of monotone stress occurs.

Examples of Segmental and Contrast Goals

Examples of segmental and contrast goals for Korean-speaking learners of English include:

1. The client will accurately produce the p/f and b/v phonemes contrastively during a minimal pair activity. Minimal pairs such as *pail–fail* or *best–vest* can be utilized.

   Rationale: Confusion of these stop and fricative phoneme pairs can lead to listener confusion and are a common transfer pattern demonstrated by Korean speakers. This can be addressed through the use of minimal pairs, such as *past–fast* or *bet–vet*.

2. The client will produce the /ɛ/ and /æ/ vowels contrastively in provided sentences (see Table 15.3).

   Rationale: Confusion of these two lax vowels is a common characteristic in the speech of Korean learners of English. A large number of minimal pairs exist in English using these phonemes (e.g., *bed–bad*) and the difference, although subtle, can also lead to listener confusion. The clinician can point out to the client that the /æ/ requires the jaw to be open further than when producing the /ɛ/. It should also be noted that one study found that Korean speakers benefited more from a contrast-based approach than from a segmental-based approach when addressing the production of vowels (Lee & Sancibrian, 2013).

3. The client will produce the /z/ phoneme accurately at the word level after a verbal model.

   Rationale: Korean does not include the /z/ phoneme, and Korean learners of English will often confuse the /z/ with the voiced affricate /dʒ/.

Possible Higher-Level Linguistic Goal

An example of a higher-level linguistic goal for Korean-speaking learners of English follows:

The client will include the obligatory article or preposition during a question answering task. A variety of different questions could be asked that require at least a sentence as a response. The clinician would then monitor the client's responses for the obligatory *the, a, on, in, at,* etc.

Rationale: Korean speakers often leave out words, such as the articles *the* and *a,* as well as prepositions, such as *about, for,* or *on.* Omission of these obligatory function words can cause confusion or change the meaning of a sentence.

Clinical Vignette 15.2

Accent Modification for a Multilingual Doctoral Candidate

Govind (a pseudonym) is a 30-year-old male from Nepal. His first language is Nepali, but he is also fluent in Urdu and another regional dialect. He sought out services from the university speech and hearing clinic for accent modification at the recommendation of his dissertation committee. He is a doctoral candidate in statistics and looking to begin the process of job applications and interviews as he approaches graduation.

After completion of an in-depth interview, the Compton assessment, a reading passage, and some informal conversation, Govind was found to have difficulty with interdental fricatives, affricates, /z/, and lax vowels. In addition, he demonstrated significant differences in his word- and sentence-level stress patterns and his use of certain colloquial phrases/figurative language. At times, he was observed to speak at a rapid pace that appeared to negatively impact his intelligibility.

Govind attended three semesters of treatment at the university clinic. The first semester was focused on segmental changes, where erred sounds were initially addressed in isolation, working up to the phrase level. The second semester focused on sounds at the sentence level, while also incorporating goals to address rate of speech and stress patterns. During the third semester there was a great emphasis placed on intelligibility at the conversational level and mock job interviews were used to assist the client in feeling more comfortable during his impending job interviews.

During these three semesters, the client also provided the clinician with a list of approximately 100 statistics-related words that the client used frequently in his academic and work life in order to ensure accurate production. During the first semester, Govind was required to reach an 80% accuracy point for each target sound at the isolation level before moving on to syllable, word, and phrase level. Typically, he took about 3 weeks to reach the 80% mark with most of the sounds, with /z/ being his most challenging production. After about 12 weeks of work on each of the sounds, he was then moved to sentence-level practice, where progress was a bit slower, as he needed to also attend to the production of the other sounds/words in the sentence and not only be focusing his energy on the target sound. Sentence-level stress was also a great challenge for Govind, as he required a clinician model for more than one semester to reach the 80% accuracy goal.

SUMMARY

Accent modification is an elective service sought by adults who want to modify their speech pattern. It can be an extremely interesting and rewarding aspect of the field of speech-language pathology. You will learn more than you ever knew you could about your own language and the language of your client, while helping highly motivated individuals to communicate more effectively and pursue their academic and occupational aspirations.

QUESTIONS FOR CHAPTER 15

1. Discuss some of the factors that influence foreign accent.

2. Differentiate between accentedness, comprehensibility, and intelligibility.

3. Describe some of the elements of a foreign accent assessment.

4. Discuss how biofeedback might be used on accent modification.

5. Contrast goals and approaches for accent modification across any two first languages.

A

Procedures for Teaching Sounds

SPECIFIC INSTRUCTIONAL TECHNIQUES

As a supplement to the establishment procedures presented in Chapter 10, the following methods for teaching sounds are presented. Clinicians must be familiar not only with general approaches to the establishment of phonemes, but also with specific suggestions for teaching sounds. What follows represents a potpourri of ideas that may be helpful to those who are beginning to develop a repertoire of techniques for evoking and establishing consonant sounds that are frequently in error. Sources such as Secord and colleagues (2007) include more extensive instruction related to sound teaching. Clinicians needing word lists, pictures, and/or treatment materials are referred to the following sources.

Printed Materials

- *Contrasts: The Use of Minimal Pairs in Articulation Training* (Elbert, Rockman, & Saltzman, 1980)

- *Manual of Articulation and Phonological Disorders* (Bleile, 1996)

- *Phonetic Context Drill Book* (Griffith & Miner, 1979)

- *Speech and Language Activities for Young Learners* (Lanza & Flahive, 2007)

- *Target Words for Contextual Training* (Secord & Shine, 1997b)

Online Software/Apps

- Web-Based Exercises (Scarry-Larkin) https://www.marnaslp.com/index.php?p =Software

- Sound Contrasts in Phonology (Williams) https://scipapp.com/

Instructions for Correction of an Interdental Lisp

It is important to remember that /s/ may be taught by having the client place their tongue behind either the upper teeth or the lower teeth.

1. Instruct the client to protrude the tongue between the teeth and produce a /θ/. Then push the tip of their tongue inward with a thin instrument, such as a tongue blade. As a variation, instruct the client to slowly and gradually withdraw the tongue while saying /θ/ and, while still attempting to make /θ/, scrape the tongue tip along the back of the front teeth and upward.

2. Instruct the client to produce /t/ in a word such as *tea*. Have them pronounce it with a strong aspiration after release of the /t/ prior to the vowel. Instruct the client to slowly slide the tip of the tongue backward from the alveolar ridge following a prolonged release. The result should be [ts]. Then have the client prolong the [s] portion of [ts].

3. Instruct the client to say the following word pairs, pointing out that the tongue is in a similar position for /t/ and /s/.

tea–sea	*teal–seal*	*tell–sell*	*told–sold*	*tame–same*	*tip–sip*
top–sop	*tight–sight*	*too–Sue*	*tub–sub*	*turf–surf*	*till–sill*

4. Instruct the client to open their mouth, put the tongue in position for /t/, drop the tip of the tongue slightly, and send the air stream through the passage. The client can sometimes feel the emission of air by placing a finger in front of their mouth.

5. Instruct the client to produce /ʃ/ and then retract their lips (smile) and push the tongue slightly forward.

6. Instruct the client to say /i/ and blow through the teeth to produce /s/.

7. Insert a straw in the groove of the tongue and have the client blow to produce /s/.

8. Instruct the client to use the following phonetic placement cues:

   a. Raise the tongue so that the sides are firmly in contact with the inner surface of the upper back teeth.

   b. Groove the tongue slightly along the midline.

   c. Place the tip of the tongue about a quarter of an inch behind the upper teeth.

   d. Bring the teeth together.

   e. Direct the air stream along the groove of the tongue toward the cutting edges of the lower teeth.

Instructions for Correction of a Lateral Lisp

1. Position a straw so that it protrudes from the side of the client's mouth. When a lateral [s] is made, the straw should resonate on the side of the mouth where the air stream is directed. When the straw is inserted into the front of the mouth and a correct /s/ is made, the straw will resonate in the front of the mouth.

2. Direct attention to a central emission of the air stream by holding a feather, a strip of paper, or a finger in front of the center of the client's mouth, or have the client tap the incisor gently with their forefinger while producing [s]. If the sound is being emitted through a central aperture, a break in continuity of the outflow of the breath will be noted. If the sound is being emitted laterally, no break in the continuity of the air stream will be noted. Instructing the client to inhale air and directing their attention to the cool sensation from the intake of air can also develop an awareness of central emission. Then instruct the client to exhale the air through the same aperture by which air entered upon inhalation.

3. Instruct the client to put a tongue blade down the midline of the tongue in order to establish a groove for the air stream.

4. Instruct the client to retract the lips sharply and push the tongue forward, attempting to say /s/.

5. Instruct the client to make /t/, holding the release position for a relatively long time, and then retract the lips and drop the jaw slightly. A [ts] should be heard if grooving was properly maintained. Then have the client extend the duration of the [ts], gradually decreasing the release phase of [t] until /s/ is approximated. Saying a word that ends with /ts/, such as /kæts/ or /lɛts/, might be useful.

6. Consider the butterfly technique described in the following link by Caroline Bowen: https://www.speech-language-therapy.com/index.php?option=com _content&view=article&id=48:butterfly&catid=11:admin

Instructions for Production of /ɝ/

1. Instruct the client to growl like a tiger (grrr), crow like a rooster (r-rr-rr), or sound like a race car (rrr).

2. Instruct the client to lower the jaw, say /l/, and push the tongue back until [ɝ] is produced. One can also move from [n] to [nɚ] or [d] to [dɚ].

3. Instruct the client to produce /l/. Then, using a tongue blade, gently push the tip of the tongue back until the depressor can be inserted between the tongue tip and teeth ridge so that an /ɝ/ is produced.

4. Instruct the client to imitate a trilled tongue plus /ɝ/ sound with the tongue tip on the alveolar ridge. Have the client stop the trill but continue producing /ɝ/.

5. Instruct the client to produce /ɑ/ as in the word *father*. As they produces the [ɑ], instruct them to raise the tongue tip and blade, arching the tongue toward the palate but not touching the palate.

6. Instruct the client to produce /i/ and then lift and retract the tongue tip to produce /ɝ/.

7. Instruct the client to place the tongue lightly between the incisors as in /θ/ and then retract the tip quickly into the /ɝ/. Instruct the client to keep the tip of the tongue near the alveolar ridge to avoid the intrusion of a vowel sound.

8. Instruct the client to say /z/ and to continue to do so while dropping the jaw and saying /ɝ/.

9. Instruct the client to position the tongue for /d/ and then retract it slightly, at the same time dropping the tongue tip and saying /ɝ/. Other clusters such as /tr/, /θr/, and /gr/ may also be used.

10. Have the client spread the sides of their mouth with their fingers and then ask them to produce a prolonged /n/ and then curl the tongue backward, continuing to make the sound. The clinician, with rubber gloves on their hands, could also take their fingers and spread the sides of the client's mouth if the client has difficulty spreading the sides of their mouth.

11. Contrast pairs of words beginning with /w/ and /r/. This task may make the distinction between these two sounds more obvious for the client who substitutes /w/ for /r/. Practice word pairs might include the following:

wipe–ripe	*woo–rue*	*wing–ring*	*way–ray*	*wake–rake*
wag–rag	*wail–rail*	*woe–roe*	*weep–reap*	*wed–red*

Instructions for Production of /l/

1. In front of a mirror, instruct the client to produce /l/ with the mouth open.

2. Instruct the client to position the tongue for /l/ and then lower it to produce /ɑ/. Alternate these movements. The result should be [lɑ], [lɑ], [lɑ]. This procedure can be varied by using /i/ and /u/ instead of /ɑ/.

3. Instruct the client to imitate the clinician's singing of the nonsense syllables [leɪ], [li], [laɪ].

4. Using a lollipop, peanut butter, or tongue blade, touch the place on the client's alveolar ridge where the tongue tip makes contact to produce a correct /l/, then tell the client to place the tongue at that point and say /l/.

5. Instruct the client to pretend that the tongue is one part of a bird's beak and the roof of the mouth is the other part of the beak. Tell them to put the tongue directly behind the teeth and move it up and down quickly, as a bird's beak might move when it is chirping, and say /ɑ/.

Instructions for Production of /f/ and /v/

1. Instruct the client to touch the lower lip with the upper front teeth and blow. The air stream may be directed by placing a feather or strip of paper in front of their mouth while /f/ or /v/ is being produced.

2. Instruct the client to say [ɑ], place the lower lip under the edge of the upper teeth, and blow the air stream between the lip and teeth so that frication is audible.

Instructions for Production of /k/ and /g/

1. Press underneath the posterior portion of the client's chin and ask them to say [kʌ] in a whisper as the pressure is suddenly released.

2. Hold the tongue tip behind the lower teeth, using a tongue blade if necessary. Instruct the client to hump the back of the tongue and build up oral pressure. The tongue contact should be released quickly, thus releasing the pressure built up behind the constriction.

3. Instruct the client to imitate the clinician as the clinician pretends to shoot a gun, producing a lingua-fricative, as in [kɑ].

4. Instruct the client to alternate the raising of the back and front of the tongue in a rocking movement from [k] to [t].

Instructions for Production of /t/ and /d/

1. Instruct the client to press the tongue tip firmly against the upper dental ridge in front of a mirror, then have them quickly lower the tongue; air pressure will be released, producing approximations of /t/ or /d/.

2. Instruct the client to make a /p/, then ask them to place the tongue tip between the lips and again try to say /p/. This gives the tactual sensation of a stop made with the tip of the tongue, but is not the correct position for /t/ or /d/. Finally, instruct the client to make a similar sound with the tongue tip in contact with the upper lip only. Repeat with the tongue tip touching the alveolar ridge.

B

Activities for Facilitating Phonemic Awareness in School-Age Children

PHONEME IDENTITY

Teach the child to identify the initial sounds in words. Find pictures (with words written clearly underneath) that start with /s/. Prompt the child as necessary to articulate each word by reading the word under the picture. Ask the child to identify those words that begin with the sound /s/. Initially, introduce distracter items that have wide initial phonological and visual contrasts. An initial set of words might include: star, moon, step, box, Stan, Carl, stop, go, sty, and barn.

After several experiences with this activity, repeat it but remove the picture stimuli and focus the child's attention on the print. Place words written in a large, clear font in front of the child or on a computer screen and ask the child to find the words that start with /s/. A fun alternative is putting the words on the floor (as shown in the figure) and asking the child to jump onto the words that start with /s/. As the child reads the words aloud, prompt for the correct articulation of the /s/ cluster.

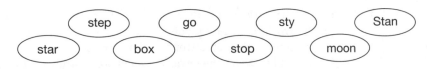

Use the same activity to teach any other initial sounds in words.

PHONEME SEGMENTATION

Teach the child that words can be segmented into phonemes. Use different-colored blocks to represent each sound in a word to help the child understand the concept of segmentation. Require the child to use colored blocks to articulate each phoneme; one block represents each color.

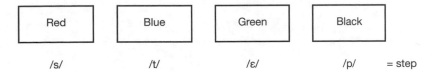

The child moves a colored block as they produce each sound in a word. This can be repeated for many different words, as in:

Stop: s- t- o- p (four different-colored blocks)

Star: s- t- a- r (three different-colored blocks)

Stan: s- t- a- n (four different-colored blocks)

Sty: s- t- y (three different-colored blocks)

PHONEME MANIPULATION

Similar to the previous activity, here the child is taught that the phonemes in words can be rearranged to make new words. Colored blocks or cards featuring individual letters can serve this purpose. The child is asked to manipulate phonemes in words to form new words using the blocks or cards. Encourage the child to articulate each new word and to reflect on the sound change that is being made. Prompt the child as necessary to ensure success and gradually reduce the prompts. Here is an example:

SLP: "If this word says 'top,' show me 'stop.'"

Child adds a new block to the beginning of the word and says, "stop."

SLP: "Now, then, turn 'stop' into 'tops.'"

Child moves the initial block to the end of the word and says, "tops."

SPELLING

Practice spelling target speech words by putting letters into boxes that represent the number of phonemes in the word. Begin by modeling the activity for the child and articulate the phonemes as you write each letter in a box for the child. Repeat the activity and encourage the child to write the letters in each box as they segment the word and articulate the phonemes. If the child is unable to write the letters easily, use letter cards or letter blocks to spell the word. Prompt as necessary to ensure success.

References

Aase, D., Hovre, C., Krause, K., Schelfhout, S., Smith, J., & Carpenter, L. (2000). *Contextual test of articulation*. Thinking Publications.

Abdel-Aziz, M., El-Fouly, M., Nassar, A., Kamel, A., & Kamel, A. (2019). The effect of hypertrophied tonsils on the velopharyngeal function in children with normal palate. *International Journal of Pediatric Otorhinolaryngology, 119*, 59–62.

Acevedo, M. (1991, November). *Spanish consonants among two groups of Head Start children* [Paper presentation]. ASHA 1991 Convention, Atlanta, GA, United States.

Acevedo, M. A. (1993). Development of Spanish consonants in preschool children. *Journal of Childhood Communication Disorders, 15*, 9–15.

Ackerman, J. L., Ackerman, A. L., & Ackerman, A. B. (1973). Taurodont, pyramidal and fused molar roots associated with other anomalies in a kindred. *American Journal of Physical Anthropology, 38*, 681–694.

Adams, P. F., & Benson, V. (1991). Current estimates from the National Health Interview Survey. *Vital Health Statistics, 10*, 184.

Adams, S. G., (1990) *Rate and clarity of speech: An x-ray microbeam study* [Unpublished doctoral dissertation]. University of Wisconsin–Madison.

Adams, S. G., Weismer, G., & Kent, R. D. (1993). Speaking rate and speech movement velocity profiles. *Journal of Speech and Hearing Research, 36*, 41–54.

Adler, S. (1984). *Cultural language differences: Their educational and clinical-professional implications*. Charles Thomas.

Adler-Bock, M., Bernhardt, B. M. Gick, B., & Bacsfalvi, P. (2007). The use of ultrasound in remediation of North American English /r/ in 2 adolescents. *American Journal of Speech-Language Pathology, 16*, 128–139.

Ahn, J. H., & Lee, K., -S. (2013). Outcomes of cochlear implantation in children with CHARGE syndrome. *Acta Oto-Laryngologica, 133*, 1148–1153.

Alaraifi, J. A., Kamal, S. M., Qa'dan, W. N., & Haj-Tas, M. A. (2014). Family history in patients who present with functional articulation disorders. *Education, 135*(1), 1–8.

Alfwaress, F., Maaitah, E. A., Al-Khateeb, S., & Zama, Z. A. (2015). The relationship of vocal tract dimensions and substitution of the palatal approximant /j/ for the alveolar trill /r/. *International Journal of Speech-Language Pathology, 17*, 518–526.

Allen, G., & Hawkins, S. (1980). Phonological rhythm: Definition and development. In G. Yeni-Komshian, J. Kavanagh, & C. Ferguson (Eds.), *Child phonology 1* (Vol. 1, pp. 227–256). Academic Press.

Allen, M. M. (2013). Intervention efficacy and intensity for children with speech sound disorder. *Journal of Speech, Language, and Hearing Research, 56*, 865–877.

Almost, D., & Rosenbaum, P. (1998). Effectiveness of speech intervention for phonological disorders: A randomized control trial. *Developmental Medicine & Child Neurology, 40*, 319–325.

Altenberg, E. P. (2005). The judgement, perception, and production of consonant clusters in a second language. *International Review of Applied Linguistics in Language Teaching, 43*(1), 53–80.

Amayreh, M. M. (2003). Completion of the consonant inventory of Arabic. *Journal of Speech, Language, and Hearing Research, 46*(3), 517–529.

Amayreh, M. M., & Dyson, A. (1998). The acquisition of Arabic consonants. *Journal of Speech, Language, and Hearing Research, 41*(3), 642–653.

Amayreh, M., & Dyson, A. (2000). Phonetic inventories of young Arabic-speaking children. *Clinical Linguistics and Phonetics, 14*, 193–215.

American Academy of Pediatrics. (2005). *The changing concept of sudden infant death syndrome: Diagnostic coding shifts, controversies regarding the sleeping environment, and new variables to consider in reducing risk* [Policy statement]. https://doi.org/10.1542/peds.2005-1499

American Speech-Language-Hearing Association. (1983). Social dialects: A position paper. *ASHA, 23*–27.

American Speech-Language Hearing Association. (1985). Clinical management of communicatively handicapped minority language populations. *ASHA, 29*–32.

American Speech-Language-Hearing Association. (1991). The role of the speech-language pathologist in management of oral myofunctional disorders. *ASHA, 33*(5), 7.

American Speech-Language-Hearing Association. (1993). Definitions of communication disorders and variations. *ASHA, 10*, 40–41.

American Speech-Language Hearing Association. (1994). ASHA policy regarding support personnel. *ASHA, 36* (Suppl. 13), 24.

American Speech-Language-Hearing Association. (1996). Guidelines for the training, credentialing, use, and supervision of speech-language pathology assistants. *ASHA, 38* (Suppl. 16), 21–34.

American Speech-Language-Hearing Association. (2001). Roles and responsibilities of speech-language pathologists with respect to reading and writing in children and adolescents [Position statement, executive summary of guidelines, technical report]. *ASHA, 21*, 17–27.

American Speech-Language Hearing Association. (2004a). Knowledge and skills needed by speech-language pathologists and audiologists to provide culturally and linguistically appropriate services. *ASHA*

American Speech-Language Hearing Association. (2004b). Evidence-based practice in communication disorders: An introduction [Technical report]. *ASHA*

American Speech-Language Hearing Association. (2005). Evidence-based practice in communication disorders [Position statement]. *ASHA*

American Speech-Language-Hearing Association. (2007a). Childhood apraxia of speech [Position statement]. *ASHA*

American Speech-Language-Hearing Association. (2007b). Childhood apraxia of speech [Technical report]. *ASHA*

American Speech-Language-Hearing Association. (2008). Schools survey: Caseload characteristics trends, 1995–2008. *ASHA*

American Speech-Language-Hearing Association. (2018). 2018 Schools Survey report: SLP caseload and workload characteristics. Retrieved from https://www.asha.org/siteassets/surveys/schools-2018-slp-caseload-and-workload-characteristics.pdf

American Speech-Language Hearing Association. (n.d.-a). Accent modification. Retrieved from https://www.asha.org/practice-portal/professional-issues/accent-modification/

American Speech-Language Hearing Association. (n.d.-b). Korean phonemic inventory. Retrieved from https://www.asha.org/uploadedFiles/KoreanPhonemicinventory.pdf

American Speech-Language Hearing Association. (n.d.-c). Practice portal. Retrieved from https://www.asha.org/PRPSpecificTopic.aspx?folderid=8589943199andsection=Overview

Anderson, E. E. (2011). *Examining conversational prosody and intelligibility in children with cochlear implants* [Unpublished master's thesis]. Idaho State University.

Anderson, R. (2000). *Onset clusters and the sonority sequencing principle in Spanish: A treatment efficacy study* [Poster presentation]. Eighth International Clinical Phonetics and Linguistics Association Conference, Edinburgh.

Anderson, R., & Smith, B. (1987). Phonological development of two-year-old monolingual Puerto Rican Spanish-speaking children. *Journal of Child Language, 14*, 57–78.

Anderson, R. T. (2004). Phonological acquisition in preschoolers learning a second language via immersion: A longitudinal study. *Clinical Linguistics & Phonetics, 18*, 183–210.

Anthony, A., Bogle, D., Ingram, T. T. S., & McIsaac, M. W. (1971). *The Edinburgh articulation test.* E. and S. Livingstone.

Anthony, J. L., Aghara, R. G., Dunkelberger, M. J., Anthony, T. I., Williams, J. M., & Zhang, Z. (2011). What factors place children with speech sound disorders at risk for reading problems? *American Journal of Speech-Language Pathology, 20,* 146–160.

Anthony, J. L., Lonigan, C. J., Driscoll, K., Phillips, B. M., & Burgess, S. R. (2003). Phonological sensitivity: A quasi-parallel progression of word structure units and cognitive operations. *Reading Research Quarterly, 38*(4), 470–487.

Aram, D. M., & Horwitz, S. J. (1983). Sequential and non-speech praxic abilities in developmental verbal apraxia. *Developmental Medicine and Child Neurology, 25,* 197–206.

Arlt, P. B., & Goodban, M. T. (1976). A comparative study of articulation acquisition as based on a study of 240 normals, aged three to six. *Language, Speech, and Hearing Services in Schools, 7,* 173–180.

Arndt, J., & Healey, E. C. (2001). Concomitant disorders in school-age children who stutter. *Language, Speech, and Hearing Services in Schools, 32,* 68–78.

Arndt, W., Elbert, M., & Shelton, R. (1970). Standardization of a test of oral stereognosis. In J. F. Bosma (Ed.), *Second symposium on oral sensation and perception* (pp. 363–378). Charles Thomas.

Arnst, D., & Fucci, D. (1975). Vibrotactile sensitivity of the tongue in hearing impaired subjects. *Journal of Auditory Research, 15,* 115–118.

Aslin, R. N., Pisoni, D. B., & Jusczyk, P. W. (1983). Auditory development and speech perception in infancy. In M. M. Haith & J. J. Campos (Eds.), *Infancy and psychobiology* (pp. 573–687). Wiley.

August, D., Calderón, M., & Carlo, M. (2002). *Transfer of skills from Spanish to English: A study of young learners.* Washington, DC: Center for Applied Linguistics.

Augustyn, M., & Zuckerman, B. (2007). From mother's mouth to infant's brain. *Archives of Disease in Childhood: Fetal & Neonatal, 92*(2), F82.

Aungst, L., & Frick, J. (1964). Auditory discrimination ability and consistency of articulation of /r/. *Journal of Speech and Hearing Disorders, 29,* 76–85.

Baas, B. S., Strand, E. A., Elmer, L. M., & Barbaresi, W. J. (2008). Treatment of severe childhood apraxia of speech in a 12-year-old male with CHARGE association. *Journal of Medical Speech-Language Pathology, 16*(4), 181–190.

Backus, O. (1940). Speech rehabilitation following excision of tip of the tongue. *American Journal of the Disabled Child, 60,* 368–370.

Baese-Berk, M. M., McLaughlin, D. J., & McGowan, K. B. (2020). Perception of non-native speech. *Language and Linguistics Compass, 14*(7), e12375.

Bailey, G., & Thomas, E. (1998). Some aspects of African-American vernacular English phonology. In S. Mufwene, J. Rickford, G. Bailey, & J. Baugh (Eds.), *African American English: History and use* (pp. 85–109). Routledge.

Bailey, S. (1982). *Normative data for Spanish articulatory skills of Mexican children between the ages of six and seven* [Unpublished master's thesis]. San Diego State University.

Bain, B., & Olswang, L. (1995). Examining readiness for learning two-word utterances by children with specific expressive language impairment: Dynamic assessment validation. *American Journal of Speech-Language Pathology, 4*(1), 81–91.

Baker, E. (2000). *Changing nail to snail: A treatment efficacy study of phonological impairment in children* [Unpublished doctoral thesis]. The University of Sydney.

Baker, E. (2002). The pros and cons of dummies. *Acquiring Knowledge in Speech, Language, and Hearing, 4,* 134–136.

Baker, E. (2010a). The experience of discharging children from phonological intervention. *International Journal of Speech-Language Pathology, 12,* 325–328.

Baker, E. (2010b). Minimal pair intervention. In A. L. Williams, S. McLeod, & R. J. McCauley (Eds.), *Interventions for speech sound disorders in children* (pp. 41–72). Paul H. Brookes Publishing Co.

Baker, E. (2021). Minimal pairs intervention. In A. L. Williams, S. McLeod, & R. J. McCauley (Eds.), *Interventions for speech sound disorders in children* (2nd ed., pp. 33–60). Paul H. Brookes Publishing Co.

Baker, E., Croot, K., McLeod, S., & Paul, R. (2001). Psycholinguistic models of speech development and their application to clinical practice. *Journal of Speech, Language, and Hearing Research, 44,* 685–702.

Baker, E., Masso, S., McLeod, S., & Wren, Y. (2018). Pacifiers, thumb sucking, breastfeeding, and bottle use: Oral sucking habits of children with and without phonological impairment. *Folia Phoniatrica et LogoPaedica, 70,* 165–173.

Baker, E., & McLeod, S. (2004). Evidence-based management of phonological impairment in children. *Child Language Teaching and Therapy, 20*, 261–285.

Baker, E., & McLeod, S. (2011a). Evidence-based practice for children with speech-sound disorders: Part 1. Narrative review. *Language, Speech, and Hearing Services in Schools, 42*, 102–139.

Baker, E., & McLeod, S. (2011b). Evidence-based practice for children with speech-sound disorders: Part 2. Application to clinical practice. *Language, Speech, and Hearing Services in Schools, 42*, 140–151.

Baker, E., & Williams, A. L. (2010). Complexity approaches to intervention. In A. L. Williams, S. McLeod, & R. J. McCauley (Eds.), *Interventions for speech sound disorders* (pp. 95–115). Paul H. Brookes Publishing Co.

Baldwin, R., Mason, S., & Holman, K. (2018, November). *Let's stop the one-size-fits-all approach to vowel errors* [Poster presentation]. ASHA 2018 Convention, Boston, MA, United States.

Ball, E. (1993). Assessing phoneme awareness. *Language, Speech, and Hearing Services in Schools, 24*, 130–139.

Ball, E., & Blachman, B. (1991). Does phoneme awareness training in kindergarten make a difference in early word recognition and developmental spelling? *Reading Research Quarterly, 26*, 49–66.

Ball, L. (1999). *Communication characteristics of children with developmental apraxia of speech* [Unpublished doctoral dissertation]. University of Nebraska–Lincoln.

Ball, M. J., & Gibbon, F. (Eds.). (2002). *Vowel disorders.* Butterworth Heineman.

Ball, M. J., & Gibbon, F. E. (2013). *Handbook of vowels and vowel disorders.* Psychology Press.

Ball, M. J., & Kent, R. D. (Eds.). (1997). *The new phonologies: Developments in clinical linguistics.* Singular Publishing.

Ball, M. J., & Müller, N. (2002). *Sonority as an explanation in clinical phonology* [Paper presentation]. Ninth Meeting of the International Clinical Phonetics and Linguistics Association, Hong Kong.

Ballard, K. J., Robin, D. A., McCabe, P., & McDonald, J. (2010). A treatment for dysprosody in childhood apraxia of speech. *Journal of Speech, Language, and Hearing Research, 53*, 1227–1245.

Bankson, N. W., & Bernthal, J. E. (1990). *Bankson-Bernthal test of phonology.* Special Press.

Bankson, N. W., & Bernthal, J. E. (2020). *Bankson-Bernthal test of phonology* (2nd ed.). Pro-Ed.

Bankson, N. W., & Byrne, M. (1962). The relationship between missing teeth and selected consonant sounds. *Journal of Speech and Hearing Disorders, 24*, 341–348.

Bankson, N. W., & Byrne, M. C. (1972). The effect of a timed correct sound production task on carryover. *Journal of Speech and Hearing Research, 15*, 160–168.

Barbosa, C., Vasquez, S., Parada, M. A., Gonzalez, J. C. V., Jackson, C., Yanez, N. D., Gelaye, B., & Fitzpatrick, A. L. (2009). The relationship of bottle feeding and other sucking behaviors with speech disorder in Patagonian preschoolers. *BMC Pediatrics, 9*, 66.

Barkovich, A. J., Kjos, B. O., Jackson, Jr., D. E., & Norman, D. (1988). Normal maturation of the neonatal and infant brain: MR imaging at 1.5 T. *Radiology, 166*, 173–180.

Barlow, J. A. (1996). Variability and phonological knowledge. In T. W. Powell (Ed.), *Pathologies of speech and language: Contributions of clinical phonetics and linguistics* (pp. 125–133). International Clinical Phonetics and Linguistics Association.

Barlow, J. A., & Gierut, J. A. (1999). Optimality theory in phonological acquisition. *Journal of Speech, Language, and Hearing Research, 42*, 1482–1498.

Barlow, J. A., & Gierut, J. A. (2002). Minimal pair approaches to phonological remediation. *Seminars in Speech and Language, 23*(1), 57–67.

Barlow, J. A., Taps, J., & Storkel, H. (2010). *Phonological assessment and treatment target (PATT) selection* [Assessment protocol]. https://slhs.sdsu.edu/phont/the-patt/

Barnes, E., Roberts, J., Long, S. H., Martin, G. E., Berni, M. C., Mandulak, K. C., & Sideris, J. (2009). Phonological accuracy and intelligibility in connected speech of boys with fragile X or Down syndrome. *Journal of Speech, Language, and Hearing Research, 52*, 1048–1061.

Barr, J., McLeod, S., & Daniel, G. (2008). Siblings of children with speech impairment: Cavalry on the hill. *Language, Speech, and Hearing Services in Schools, 29*, 21–32.

Bates, E., Dale, P. S., & Thal, D. (1995). Individual differences and their implications for theories of language development. In P. Fletcher & B. MacWhinney (Eds.), *The handbook of child language* (pp. 96–151). Blackwell.

Bauman-Waengler, J. (2008). *Articulatory and phonological impairments: A clinical focus* (3rd ed.). Allyn & Bacon.

Baylis, A. L., & Shriberg, L. D. (2019). Estimates of the prevalence of speech and motor speech disorders in youth with 22q11.2 deletion syndrome. *American Journal of Speech-Language Pathology, 28*(1), 53–82.

Behne, D. (1989). *Acoustic effects of focus and sentence position on stress in English and French* [Unpublished doctoral dissertation]. University of Wisconsin–Madison.

Behrman, A. (2014). Segmental and prosodic approaches to accent management. *American Journal of Speech-Language Pathology, 23*, 246–561.

Behrman, A., Ferguson, S. H., Akhund, A., & Moeyaert, M. (2017). The effect of clear speech on temporal metrics of rhythm in Spanish-accented speakers of English. *Language and Speech, 62*(1), 5–29.

Berg, T. (1995). Sound change in child language: A study of inter-word variation. *Language and Speech, 38*, 331–363.

Berko, J., & Brown, R. (1960). Psycholinguistic research methods. In P. H. Mussen (Ed.), *Handbook of research methods in child development* (pp. 517–557). Wiley.

Bernhardt, B. (1992a). Developmental implications of nonlinear phonological theory. *Clinical Linguistics & Phonetics, 6*, 259–281.

Bernhardt, B. (1992b). The application of nonlinear phonological theory to intervention with one phonologically disordered child. *Clinical Linguistics & Phonetics, 6*, 283–316.

Bernhardt, B. M., Bacsfalvi, P., Adler-Bock, M., Shimizu, R., Cheney, A., Giesbrecht, N., O'Connell, M., Sirianni, J., & Radanov, B. (2008). Ultrasound as visual feedback in speech habilitation: Exploring consultative use in rural British Columbia, Canada. *Clinical Linguistics & Phonetics, 22*, 149–162.

Bernhardt, B. M., Bopp, K. D., Daudlin, B., Edwards, S. M., & Wastie, S. E. (2010). Nonlinear phonological intervention. In A. L. Williams, S. McLeod, & R. J. McCauley (Eds.), *Interventions for speech sound disorders in children* (pp. 315–331). Paul H. Brookes Publishing Co.

Bernhardt, B. H., & Stemberger, J. (1998). *Handbook of phonological development from the perspective of constraint-based nonlinear phonology.* Academic Press.

Bernhardt, B. H., & Stemberger, J. P. (2000). *Workbook in nonlinear phonology for clinical application.* Pro-Ed.

Bernhardt, B. H., & Stoel-Gammon, C. (1994). Nonlinear phonology: Introduction and clinical application. *Journal of Speech and Hearing Research, 37*, 123–143.

Bernstein, M. (1954). The relation of speech defects and malocclusion. *American Journal of Orthodontia, 40*, 149–150.

Bernstein-Ratner, N. (1993). Interactive influences on phonological behaviour: A case study. *Journal of Child Language, 20*, 191–197.

Bernthal, J. E., & Bankson, N. W. (1998). *Articulation and phonological disorders* (4th ed.). Allyn & Bacon.

Bernthal, J. E., & Beukelman, D. R. (1978). Intraoral air pressures during the production of *p* and *b* by children, youths, and adults. *Journal of Speech and Hearing Research, 21*, 361–371.

Bertolini, M. M., & Paschoal, J. R. (2001). Prevalence of adapted swallowing in a population of school children. *International Journal of Orofacial Myology, 27*, 33–43.

Bialystock, E. (2001). Metalinguistic aspects of bilingual processing. *Annual Review of Applied Linguistics, 21*, 169–181.

Bichotte, M., Dunn, B., Gonzalez, L., Orpi, J., & Nye, C. (1993, November). *Assessing phonological performance of bilingual school-age Puerto Rican children* [Paper presentation]. ASHA 1993 Convention, Anaheim, CA, United States.

Biever, A., & Kelsall, D. (2007). *Impact of bilateral pediatric cochlear implantation on speech perception abilities in quiet and noise* [Paper presentation]. 11th International Conference on Cochlear Implants in Children, Charlotte, NC, United States.

Binger, C., Macguire-Marshall, M., & Kent-Walsh, J. (2011). Using aided AAC models, recasts, and contrastive targets to teach grammatical morphemes to children who use AAC. *Journal of Speech, Language, and Hearing Research, 54*, 160–176.

Bird, A., & Higgins, A. (1990). *Minimal pair cards.* Pro-Ed.

Bird, J., Bishop, D., & Freeman, N. H. (1995). Phonological awareness and literacy development in children with expressive phonological impairments. *Journal of Speech and Hearing Research, 38*, 446–462.

Birdsong, D. (2006). Age and second language acquisition and processing: A selective overview. *Language Learning, 56*(1), 9–49.

Bishop, D., & Adams, C. (1990). A prospective study of the relationship between specific language impairment, phonological disorders and reading retardation. *Journal of Child Psychology and Psychiatry, 31*, 1027–1050.

Bishop, M., Ringel, R., & House, H. (1973). Orosensory perception, speech production and deafness. *Journal of Speech and Hearing Research, 16*, 257–266.

Blachman, B., Ball, E., Black, R., & Tangel, D. (2000). *Road to the code: A phonological awareness program for young children.* Paul H. Brookes Publishing Co.

Bland-Stewart, L. (2003). Phonetic inventories and phonological patterns of African American two-year-olds: A preliminary investigation. *Communication Disorders Quarterly, 24*, 109–120.

Blanton, S. (1916). A survey of speech defects. *Journal of Educational Psychology, 7*, 581–592.

Bleile, K. (1982). Consonant ordering in Down's syndrome. *Journal of Communication Disorders, 15*, 275–285.

Bleile, K. M. (1991). Individual differences. In K. M. Bleile (Ed.), *Child phonology: A book of exercises for students* (pp. 57–71). Singular Publishing.

Bleile, K. M. (1995). *Manual of articulation and phonological disorders.* Singular Publishing.

Bleile, K. M. (1996). *Articulation and phonological disorders: A book of exercises* (2nd ed.). Singular Publishing.

Bleile, K. M. (2004). *Manual of articulation and phonological disorders: Infancy through adulthood* (2nd ed.). Thomson Delmar Learning.

Bleile, K. M. (2007). Neurological foundations of speech acquisition. In S. McLeod (Ed.), *The international guide to speech acquisition* (pp. 14–18). Thomson Delmar Learning.

Bleile, K. M. (2013). *The late eight* (2nd ed.). Plural Publishing.

Bleile, K. M., & Wallach, H. (1992). A sociolinguistic investigation of the speech of African-American preschoolers. *American Journal of Speech-Language Pathology, 1*, 44–52.

Bloch, R., & Goodstein, L. (1971). Functional speech disorders and personality: A decade of research. *Journal of Speech and Hearing Disorders, 36*, 295–314.

Blood, G. W., & Seider, R. (1981). The concomitant problems of young stutterers. *Journal of Speech and Hearing Disorders, 46*, 31–33.

Bloodstein, O. (2002). Early stuttering as a type of language difficulty. *Journal of Fluency Disorders, 27*, 163–167.

Blyth, K. M., McCabe, P., Madill, C., & Ballard, K. J. (2014). Speech and swallow rehabilitation following partial glossectomy: A systematic review. *International Journal of Speech-Language Pathology, 17*, 401–410.

Blyth, K. M., McCabe, P. Madill, C. & Ballard, K. J. (2016). Ultrasound visual feedback in articulation therapy following partial glossectomy. *Journal of Communication Disorders, 61*, 1–15.

Bock, J. K. (1982). Toward a cognitive psychology of syntax: Information processing contributions to sentence formulation. *Psychological Review, 89*, 1–47.

Boersma, P. & Weenink, D. (2021). *PRAAT: Doing Phonetics by Computer (Version 6.1.42);* [computer program] *Amsterdam, Institute of Phonetic Sciences.* http://www.praat.org

Bogusiak, K., Puch, A., & Arkuszewski, P. (2017). Goldenhar syndrome: Current perspectives. *World Journal of Pediatrics, 13*(5), 405–415.

Bordon, G. (1984). Consideration of motor-sensory targets and a problem of perception. In H. Winitz (Ed.), *Treating articulation disorders: For clinicians by clinicians* (pp. 51–65). Pro-Ed.

Bornman, J., Alant, E., & Meiring, E. (2001). The use of a digital voice output device to facilitate language development in a child with developmental apraxia of speech: A case study. *Disability and Rehabilitation, 23*(14), 623–634.

Bowen, C., & Cupples, L. (1999). Parents and children together (PACT): A collaborative approach to phonological therapy. *International Journal of Language & Communication Disorders, 34*, 35–83.

Boyce, S. E. (2015). The articulatory phonetics of /r/ for residual speech errors. *Seminars in Speech and Language, 36*, 257–270.

Bradford, A., Murdoch, B., Thompson, E., & Stokes, P. (1997). Lip and tongue function in children with developmental speech disorders: A preliminary investigation. *Clinical Linguistics & Phonetics, 11*, 363–387.

Bradley, D. (1985). A systematic multiple-phoneme approach to articulation treatment. In P. Newman, N. Creaghead, & W. Secord (Eds.), *Assessment and remediation of articulatory and phonological disorders* (pp. 315–335). Merrill.

Bradley, L., & Bryant, P. E. (1983). Categorizing sounds and learning to read: A causal connection. *Nature, 301*, 419–421.

Brady, K., Duewer, N., & King, A. (2016). The effectiveness of a multimodal vowel-targeted intervention in accent modification. *Contemporary Issues in Communication Science and Disorders, 43*, 23–34.

Braine, M. D. S. (1979). *On what might constitute learnable phonology.* College Hill.

Brandel, J., & Loeb, D. F. (2011). Program intensity and service delivery models in the schools: SLP survey results. *Language, Speech, and Hearing Services in Schools, 42*, 461–490.

Branigan, G. (1976). Syllabic structure and the acquisition of consonants: The great conspiracy in word formation. *Journal of Psycholinguistic Research, 5*, 117–133.

Bressmann, T. (2006). Speech adaptation to a self-inflicted cosmetic tongue split: Perceptual and ultrasonographic analysis. *Clinical Linguistics & Phonetics, 20*(2/3), 205–210.

Bressmann, T., Foltz, A., Zimmerman, J., & Irish, J. C. (2014). Production of tongue twisters by speakers with partial glossectomy. *Clinical Linguistics and Phonetics, 28*(12), 951–964.

Bressmann, T., Sader, R., Whitehill, T. L., & Samman, N. (2004). Consonant intelligibility and tongue mobility in patients with partial glossectomy. *Journal of Oral and Maxillofacial Surgery, 62*, 298–303.

Broomfield, J., & Dodd, B. (2004). The nature of referred subtypes of primary speech disability. *Child Language Teaching and Therapy, 20*, 135–151.

Bruce, L., Lynde, S., Weinhold, J., & Peter, B. (2018). A team approach to response to intervention for speech sound errors in the school setting. *Perspectives of the ASHA Special Interest Group, SIG 16, 3*(3), 110–119.

Brumbaugh, K. M., & Smit, A. B. (2013). Treating children ages 3–6 who have speech sound disorder: A survey. *Language, Speech, and Hearing Services in Schools, 44*, 306–319.

Brunner, J., Fuchs, S., & Perrier, P. (2009). On the relationship between palate shape and articulatory behavior. *Journal of the Acoustical Society of America, 125*, 3936–3949.

Bryan, A., & Howard, D. (1992). Frozen phonology thawed: The analysis and remediation of a developmental disorder of real word phonology. *European Journal of Disorders of Communication, 27*, 343–365.

Bryant, P., MacLean, M., & Bradley, L. (1990). Rhyme, language, and children's reading. *Applied Psycholinguistics, 11*, 237–252.

Bryant, T., Velleman, S., Abdulkarim, L., & Seymour, H. (2001). *A sonority account of consonant cluster reduction in AAE* [Paper presentation]. Child Phonology Conference, Boston, MA, United States.

Bunton, K. (2008). Speech versus nonspeech: Different tasks, different neural organization. *Seminars in Speech and Language, 29*, 267–275.

Bunton, K., & Leddy, M. (2011). An evaluation of articulatory working space area in vowel production of adults with Down syndrome. *Clinical Linguistics & Phonetics, 25*(4), 321–334.

Burdin, L. G. (1940). A survey of speech defectives in the Indianapolis primary grades. *Journal of Speech Disorders, 5*, 247–258.

Burgess, S. R., & Lonigan, C. J. (1998). Bidirectional relations of phonological sensitivity and prereading abilities: Evidence from a preschool sample. *Journal of Experimental Child Psychology, 70*, 117–141.

Burgoyne, K., Lervåg, A., Malone, S., & Hulme, C. (2019). Speech difficulties at school entry are a significant risk factor for later reading difficulties. *Early Childhood Research Quarterly, 49*, 40–48.

Burns, F., Velleman, S., Green, L., & Roeper, T. (2010). New branches from old roots: Experts respond to questions about African American English development and language intervention. *Topics in Language Disorders, 30*, 253–264.

Burt, L., Holm, A., & Dodd, B. (1999). Phonological awareness skills of 4-year-old British children: An assessment and developmental data. *International Journal of Language & Communication Disorders, 34*(3), 311–335.

Cabbage, K. L., Farquharson, K., Iuzzini-Seigel, J., & Hogan, T. (2018). Exploring the overlap between dyslexia and speech sound production deficits. *Language, Speech, and Hearing Services in Schools, 49*(4), 774–786.

Calfee, R. C., Lindamood, P., & Lindamood, C. (1973). Acoustic-phonetic skills and reading: Kindergarten through twelfth grade. *Journal of Educational Psychology, 64*, 293–298.

Calnan, J. (1954). Submucous cleft palate. *British Journal of Plastic Surgery, 6*, 264–282.

Calvert, D. (1982). Articulation and hearing impairments. In L. Lass, J. Northern, D. Yoder, & L. McReynolds (Eds.), *Speech, language and hearing* (Vol. 2, pp. 638–651). Saunders.

Camarata, S. (1989). Final consonant repetition: A linguistic perspective. *Journal of Speech and Hearing Disorders, 54*, 159–162.

Camarata, S. (1993). The application of naturalistic conversation training to speech production in children with speech disabilities. *Journal of Applied Behavior Analysis, 26*, 173–182.

Camarata, S., & Gandour, J. (1985). Rule invention in the acquisition of morphology by a language-impaired child. *Journal of Speech and Hearing Disorders, 50*, 40–45.

Camarata, S., & Schwartz, R. (1985). Production of object words and action words: Evidence for a relationship between phonology and semantics. *Journal of Speech and Hearing Research, 26*, 50–53.

Camarata, S. M. (2021). Naturalistic recast intervention. In A. L. Williams, S. McLeod, & R. J. McCauley (Eds.), *Interventions for speech sound disorders in children* (2nd ed., pp. 337–361). Paul H. Brookes Publishing Co.

Camarata, S. M., Camarata, M., & Woodcock, R. (2019, November). *Word level assessment of speech production in children: Reliability & validity* [Seminar presentation]. ASHA 2019 Convention, Orlando, FL, United States.

Campbell, T. F., Dollaghan, C., Janosky, J., Rusiewicz, H. L., Small, S. L., Dick, F., Vick, J., & Adelson, P. D. (2013). Consonant accuracy after severe pediatric traumatic brain injury: A prospective cohort study. *Journal of Speech, Language, and Hearing Research, 56*, 1023–1034.

Campbell, T. F., Dollaghan, C., Needleman, H., & Janosky, J. (1997). Reducing bias in language assessment: Processing-dependent measures. *Journal of Speech, Language, and Hearing Research, 40*(3), 519–525.

Campbell, T. F., Dollaghan, C. A., Rockette, H. E., Paradise, J. L., Feldman, H. M., Shriberg, L. D., Sabo, D. L., & Kurs-Lasky, M. (2003). Risk factors for speech delay of unknown origin in 3-year-old children. *Child Development, 74*, 346–357.

Canning, B., & Rose, M. (1974). Clinical measurements of the speech, tongue and lip movements in British children with normal speech. *British Journal of Disorders of Communication, 9*, 45–50.

Canoy, D., Pekkanen, J., Elliott, P., Pouta, A., Laitinen, J., Hartikainen, A. L., Zitting, P., Patel, S., Little, M. P., & Jarvelin, M. R. (2007). Early growth and adult respiratory function in men and women followed from the fetal period to adulthood. *Thorax, 62*(5), 396–402.

Cantwell, D. P., & Baker, L. (1987). Clinical significance of childhood communication disorders: Perspectives from a longitudinal study. *Journal of Child Neurology, 2*, 257–264.

Carhart, R. (1939). A survey of speech defects in Illinois high schools. *Journal of Speech Disorders, 4*, 61–70.

Carlson, H. K., & McHenry, M. A. (2006). Effect of accent and dialect on employability. *Journal of Employment Counseling, 43*(2), 70–83.

Carrell, J., & Pendergast, K. (1954). An experimental study of the possible relation between errors of speech and spelling. *Journal of Speech and Hearing Disorders, 19*, 327–334.

Carrier, J. K. (1970). A program of articulation therapy administered by mothers. *Journal of Speech and Hearing Disorders, 33*, 344–353.

Carroll, J., Gillon, G. T., & McNeill, B. C. (2012). Explicit phonological knowledge of educational professionals. *Asia Pacific Journal of Speech, Language, and Hearing, 15*, 231–244.

Carroll, J. M., Snowling, M. J., Hulme, C., & Stevenson, J. (2003). The development of phonological awareness in preschool children. *Developmental Psychology, 39*, 913–923.

Carrow-Woolfolk, E. (2017). *CASL: Comprehensive assessment of spoken language* (2nd ed.). Western Psychological Services.

Carson, K., Boustead, T., & Gillon, G. T. (2014). Predicting reading outcomes in the classroom using a computer-based phonological awareness screening and monitoring assessment (Com-PASMA). *International Journal of Speech-Language Pathology, 16*, 552–561.

Carson, K., Gillon, G. T., & Boustead, T. (2013). Classroom phonological awareness instruction and literacy outcomes in the first year of school. *Language, Speech, and Hearing Services in Schools, 44*, 147–160.

Carter, E., & Buck, M. (1958). Prognostic testing for functional articulation disorders among children in the first grade. *Journal of Speech and Hearing Disorders, 23*, 124–133.

Carter, P., & Edwards, S. (2004). EPG therapy for children with long-standing speech disorders: Predictions and outcomes. *Clinical Linguistics & Phonetics, 18*, 359–372.

Catts, H. W. (1993). The relationship between speech-language impairments and reading disabilities. *Journal of Speech and Hearing Research, 36,* 948–958.

Catts, H. W., Fey, M. E., Zhang, X. Y., & Tomblin, J. B. (2001). Estimating the risk of future reading difficulties in kindergarten children: A research-based model and its clinical implementation. *Language, Speech, and Hearing Services in Schools, 32,* 38–50.

Catts, H., Petscher, W. Y., Schatschneider, C., Bridges, M. S., & Mendoza, K. (2009). Floor effects associated with universal screening and their impact on the early identification of reading disabilities. *Journal of Learning Disabilities, 42,* 163–176.

Cavagna, G. A., & Margaria, R. (1968). Airflow rates and efficiency changes during phonation: Sound production in man. *Annals of the New York Academy of Sciences, 155,* 152–164.

Celce-Murcia, M., Brinton, D. M., & Goodwin, J. M. (1996). *Teaching pronunciation: A reference for teachers of English to speakers of other languages.* Cambridge University Press.

Cenoz, J. (2000). Pauses and hesitation phenomena in second language production. *International Journal of Applied Linguistics, 127*(1), 53–69.

Chakraborty, R., Schwarz, A. L., & Chakraborty, P. (2017). Perception of nonnative accent: A cross-sectional perspective. *International Journal of Society, Culture, & Language, 5*(2), 26–36.

Chaney, C. (1992). Language development, metalinguistic skills, and print awareness in 3-year-old children. *Applied Psycholinguistics, 13,* 485–514.

Chaney, C., & Menyuk, P. (1975, November). *Production and identification of /w, l, r/ in normal and articulation-impaired children* [Paper presentation]. ASHA 1975 Convention, Washington, DC, United States.

Chappell, G. E. (1973). Childhood verbal apraxia and its treatment. *Journal of Speech and Hearing Disorders, 38*(3), 362–368.

Chenausky, K. V., Brignell, A., Morgan, A., Gagné, D., Norton, A., Tager-Flusberg, H., Schlaug, G., Shield, A., & Green, J. R. (2020). Factor analysis of signs of childhood apraxia of speech. *Journal of Communication Disorders, 87,* 106033.

Cheng, H. Y., Murdoch, B. E., & Goozee, J. V. (2007). Temporal features of articulation from childhood to adolescence: An electropalatographic investigation. *Clinical Linguistics & Phonetics, 21*(6), 481–499.

Cheng, H. Y., Murdoch, B. E., Goozee, J. V., & Scott, D. (2007a). Electropalatographic assessment of tongue-to-palate contact patterns and variability in children, adolescents, and adults. *Journal of Speech, Language, and Hearing Research, 50*(2), 375–392.

Cheng, H. Y., Murdoch, B. E., Goozee, J. V., & Scott, D. (2007b). Physiologic development of tongue-jaw coordination from childhood to adulthood. *Journal of Speech, Language, and Hearing Research, 50*(2), 352–360.

Cheng, L. R. L. (1987). *Assessing Asian language performance: Guidelines for evaluating limited-English-proficient students.* Aspen.

Cheng, L. R. L. (1993). Asian-American cultures. In D. Battle (Ed.), *Communication disorders in multicultural populations* (pp. 38–77). Andover Medical Publishers.

Cheng, L. R. L. (2001). Transcription of English influenced by selected Asian languages. *Communication Disorders Quarterly, 23*(1), 40–46.

Chervela, N. (1981). Medial consonant cluster acquisition by Telugu children. *Journal of Child Language, 8,* 63–73.

Cheung, P., & Abberton, E. (2000). Patterns of phonological disability in Cantonese-speaking children in Hong Kong. *International Journal of Language & Communication Disorders, 35,* 451–473.

Chiat, S. (1994). From lexical access to lexical output: What is the problem for children with impaired phonology? In M. Yavas (Ed.), *First and second language pathology* (pp. 107–133). Singular Publishing.

Chin, S. B. (1996). The role of the sonority hierarchy in delayed phonological systems. In T. Powell (Ed.), *Pathologies of speech and language: Contributions of clinical phonetics and linguistics* (pp. 109–117). International Clinical Phonetics and Linguistics Association.

Chin, S. B., & Pisoni, D. B. (2000). A phonological system at 2 years after cochlear implantation. *Clinical Linguistics & Phonetics, 14,* 53–73.

Ching, T. Y. C., Incerti, P., Hill, M., & van Wanrooy, E. (2006). An overview of binaural advantages for children and adults who use binaural/bimodal hearing devices. *Audiology and Neurotology, 11*(1), 6–11.

Chirlian, N. S., & Sharpley, C. F. (1982). Children's articulation development: Some regional differences. *Australian Journal of Human Communication Disorders, 10*, 23–30.

Chomsky, N., & Hallé, M. (1968). *The sound pattern of English.* Harper & Row.

Christian, D., Wolfram, W., & Nube, N. (1988). *Variation and change in geographically isolated communities: Appalachian English and Ozark English.* University of Alabama Press.

Christensen, M., & Hanson, M. (1981). An investigation of the efficacy of oral myofunctional therapy as a precursor to articulation therapy for pre–first grade children. *Journal of Speech and Hearing Disorders, 46*, 160–167.

Chumpelik, D. (1984). The prompt system of therapy: Theoretical framework and applications for developmental apraxia of speech. *Seminars in Speech and Language, 5*, 139–155.

Clark, R, (1959). Maturation and speech development. *Logos, 2*, 49–54.

Clarke-Klein, S., & Hodson, B. (1995). A phonologically based analysis of misspellings by third graders with disordered-phonology histories. *Journal of Speech and Hearing Research, 38*, 839–849.

Cleland, J., Timmins, C., Wood, S. E., Hardcastle, W. J., & Wishart, J. G. (2009). Electropalatographic therapy for children and young people with Down's syndrome. *Clinical Linguistics & Phonetics, 23*(12), 926–939.

Cleland, J., Wrench, A., Lloyd, S., & Sugden, E. (2018). ULTRAX2020: Ultrasound technology for optimizing the treatment of speech disorders: Clinicians' resource manual. https://strathprints.strath.ac.uk/63372/

Clements, G. N. (1990). The role of the sonority cycle in core syllabification. In J. Kingston & M. Beckman (Eds.), *Papers in laboratory phonology 1: Between the grammar and physics of speech* (pp. 283–333). Cambridge University Press.

Cohen, A., Collier, R., & t'Hart, J. (1982). Declination: Construct or intrinsic feature of speech pitch? *Phonetica, 39*, 254–273.

Cole, P., & Taylor, O. (1990). Performance of working class African-American children on three tests of articulation. *Language, Speech, and Hearing Services in Schools, 21*, 171–176.

Compton, A. J. (1983). *Compton phonological assessment of foreign accent.* Carousel House.

Connell, P., Elbert, M., & Dinnsen, D. (1991, June). *A syntax-delayed subgroup of phonologically delayed children* [Paper presentation]. Symposium on Research in Child Language Disorders, Madison, WI, United States.

Cooper, R. (1985). The method of meaningful minimal contrasts. In P. Newman, N. Creaghead, & W. Secord (Eds.), *Assessment and remediation of articulatory and phonological disorders* (pp. 369–382). Merrill.

Cooper, R. P., & Aslin, R. N. (1990). Preference for infant-directed speech in the first month after birth. *Child Development, 61*, 1584–1595.

Coplan, J., & Gleason, J. R. (1988). Unclear speech: Recognition and significance of unintelligible speech in preschool children. *Pediatrics, 82*, 447–452.

Cordeiro, P. G., & Chen, C. M. (2012). A 15-year review of midface reconstruction after total and subtotal maxillectomy: Part I. Algorithm and outcomes. *Plastic and Reconstructive Surgery, 129*, 124–136.

Corrales, C. E., & Oghalai, J. S. (2013). Cochlear implant consideration in children with additional disabilities. *Current Otolaryngology Reports, 1*, 61–68.

Costello, J., & Bosler, C. (1976). Generalization and articulation instruction. *Journal of Speech and Hearing Disorders, 41*, 359–373.

Couper, G. (2006). The short- and long-term effects of pronunciation instruction. *Prospect, 21*, 46–66.

Courchesne, E., Chisum, H. J., Townsend, J., Cowles, A., Covington, J., Egaas, B., Harwood, M., Hinds, S., & Press, G. A. (2000). Normal brain development and aging: Quantitative analysis at in vivo MR imaging in healthy volunteers. *Radiology, 216*, 672–682.

Craig, H., Thompson, C., Washington, J., & Potter, S. (2003). Phonological features of child African American English. *Journal of Speech, Language, and Hearing Research, 46*, 623–635.

Craig, H., & Washington, J. (2004). Grade-related changes in the production of African American English. *Journal of Speech, Language, and Hearing Research, 47*, 450–463.

Crosbie, S., Holm, A., & Dodd, B. (2005). Intervention for children with severe speech disorder: A comparison of two approaches. *International Journal of Language & Communication Disorders, 40*, 467–491.

Crosbie, S., Pine, C., Holm, A., & Dodd, B. (2006). Treating Jarrod: A core vocabulary approach. *Advances in Speech-Language Pathology, 8*(3), 316–321.

Crowe, K., & McLeod, S. (2020). Children's English consonant acquisition in the United States: A review. *American Journal of Speech-Language Pathology, 29*, 2155–2169.

Crowe-Hall, B. J. (1991). Attitudes of fourth and sixth graders toward peers with mild articulation disorders. *Language, Speech, and Hearing Services in Schools, 22*, 334–340.

Crystal, D. (1969). *Prosodic systems and intonation in English*. Cambridge University Press.

Crystal, D. (1973). Non-segmental phonology in language acquisition: A review of the issues. *Lingua, 32*, 1–45.

Crystal, D. (1986). Prosodic development. In P. J. Fletcher & M. Garman (Eds.), *Studies in first language development* (pp. 174–197). Cambridge University Press.

Crystal, D. (1987). Towards a "bucket" theory of language disability: Taking account of interaction between linguistic levels. *Clinical Linguistics & Phonetics, 1*, 7–22.

Crystal, D. (1997). *The Cambridge encyclopedia of language* (2nd ed.). Cambridge University Press.

Cumley, G. D., & Swanson, S. (1999). Augmentative and alternative communication options for children with developmental apraxia of speech: Three case studies. *Augmentative and Alternative Communication, 15*, 110–125.

Cummings, A. E., & Barlow, J. A. (2011). A comparison of word lexicality in the treatment of speech sound disorders. *Clinical Linguistics & Phonetics, 25*(4), 265–286.

Cunningham, A., & Carroll, J. (2011). Age and schooling effects on early literacy and phoneme awareness. *Journal of Experimental Child Psychology, 109*, 248–255.

Cunningham, I. (1992). *A syntactic analysis of Sea Island Creole*. University of Alabama Press.

Cunningham, U. (2010). *Quality, quantity and intelligibility of vowels in Vietnamese-accented English* (pp. 3–22). http://www.diva-portal.org/smash/get/diva2:520970/FULLTEXT01.pdf

Curtis, J., & Hardy, J. (1959). A phonetic study of misarticulations of /r/. *Journal of Speech and Hearing Research, 2*, 224–257.

Dagenais, P. A., Critz-Crosby, P., & Adams, J. B. (1994). Defining and remediating persistent lateral lisps in children using electropalatography: Preliminary findings. *American Journal of Speech-Language Pathology, 3*, 67–76.

Daggumati, S., Cohn, J. E., Brennan, M. J., Evarts, M., McKinnon, B. J., & Terk, A. R. (2019). Caregiver perception of speech quality in patients with ankyloglossia: Comparison between surgery and non-treatment. *International Journal of Pediatric Otorhinolaryngology, 119*, 70–74.

Dale, P. S., & Hayden, D. A. (2013). Treating speech subsystems in childhood apraxia of speech with tactual input: The PROMPT approach. *American Journal of Speech-Language Pathology, 22*, 644–661.

D'Antonio, L. L., Snyder, L. S., & Samadani, S. (1996). Tonsillectomy in children with or at risk for velopharyngeal insufficiency: Effects on speech. *Otolaryngology–Head and Neck Surgery, 115*, 319–323.

Daniloff, R. G., & Moll, K. L. (1968). Coarticulation of lip rounding. *Journal of Speech and Hearing Research, 11*, 707–721.

Darley, F., Aronson, A., & Brown, J. (1975). *Motor speech disorders*. Saunders.

Davis, B. L., Jakielski, K. J., & Marquardt, T. P. (1998). Developmental apraxia of speech: Determiners of differential diagnosis. *Clinical Linguistics & Phonetics, 12*, 25–45.

Davis, B. L., & MacNeilage, P. F. (1995). The articulatory basis of babbling. *Journal of Speech and Hearing Research, 38*, 1199–1211.

Davis, E. (1937). *The development of linguistic skills in twins, singletons with siblings, and only children from age five to ten years*. Institute of Child Welfare, monograph series 14. University of Minnesota Press.

Dawson, L. (1929). A study of the development of the rate of articulation. *Elementary School Journal, 29*, 610–615.

Dayton, N., & Schuele, C. (1997, November). *Effects of phonological awareness training on young children with specific language impairment* [Paper presentation]. ASHA 1997 Convention, Boston, MA, United States.

DeCasper, A. J., & Fifer, W. P. (1980). Of human bonding: Newborns prefer their mothers' voices. *Science, 208*, 1174–1176.

DeCasper, A. J., LeCanuet, J. P., Busnel, M. C., Granier-Deferre, C., & Maugeais, R. (1994). Fetal reactions to recurrent maternal speech. *Infant Behavior and Development, 17*, 159–164.

de Castro, M. M., & Wertzner, H. F. (2011). Speech inconsistency index in Brazilian Portuguese-speaking children. *Folio Phoniatrica et Logopaedica, 63*(5), 237–241.

De Jong, K. J. (1991). *The oral articulation of English stress accent* [Unpublished doctoral dissertation]. The Ohio State University.

De la Fuente, M. T. (1985). *The order of acquisition of Spanish consonant phonemes by monolingual Spanish speaking children between the ages of 2.0 and 6.5* [Unpublished doctoral dissertation]. Georgetown University.

De Letter, M., Criel, Y., Lind, A., Hartsuiker, R., & Santens, P. (2020). Articulation lost in space. The effects of local orobuccal anesthesia on articulation and intelligibility of phonemes. *Brain and Language, 207,* 1–7.

Denne, M., Langdown, N., Pring, T., & Roy, P. (2005). Treating children with expressive phonological disorders: Does phonological awareness therapy work in the clinic? *International Journal of Language & Communication Disorders, 40,* 493–504.

Derwing, T. M., & Munro, M. J. (2009). Putting accent in its place: Rethinking obstacles to communication. *Language Teaching, 42*(4), 476–490.

Derwing, T. M., Munro, M. J., & Wiebe, G. (1998). Evidence in favor of a broad framework for pronunciation instruction. *Language Learning, 48*(3), 393–410.

Derwing, T. M., Rossiter, M. J., & Munro, M. J. (2002). Teaching native speakers to listen to foreign-accented speech. *Journal of Multilingual and Multicultural Development, 23*(4), 245–259.

Dewey, G. (1923). *Relative frequency of English speech sounds.* Harvard University Press.

Diedrich, W. M. (1971). Procedures for counting and charting a target phoneme. *Language, Speech, and Hearing Services in Schools, 2,* 18–32.

Diedrich, W. M., & Bangert, J. (1976). *Training speech clinicians in recording and analysis of articulatory behavior.* Washington, DC: U.S. Office of Education. Grant nos. OEG-0-70-1689 and OEG-0-71-1689.

Dinnsen, D. A., Barlow, J. A., & Morrisette, M. L. (1997). Long-distance place assimilation with an interacting error pattern in phonological acquisition. *Clinical Linguistics & Phonetics, 11,* 319–338.

Dinnsen, D. A., Chin, S. B., Elbert, M., & Powell, T. (1990). Some constraints on functionally disordered phonologies: Phonetic inventories and phonotactics. *Journal of Speech and Hearing Research, 33,* 28–37.

Dinnsen, D., & Elbert, M. (1984). On the relationship between phonology and learning. In M. Elbert, D. Dinnsen, & G. Weismer (Eds.), *Phonological theory and the misarticulating child, ASHA monographs* (Vol. 22, pp. 59–68). ASHA.

Dodd, B. (1995a). Children's acquisition of phonology. In B. Dodd (Ed.), *Differential diagnosis and treatment of children with speech disorder* (pp. 21–48). Singular Publishing.

Dodd, B. (1995b). Procedures for classification of sub-groups of speech disorder. In B. Dodd (Ed.), *Differential diagnosis and treatment of children with speech disorder* (pp. 49–64). Singular Publishing.

Dodd, B. (2005). *Differential diagnosis and treatment of children with speech disorder* (2nd ed.). Whurr Publishers.

Dodd, B. (2011). Differentiating speech delay from disorder. Does it matter? *Topics in Language Disorders, 31,* 96–111.

Dodd, B. (2014). Differential diagnosis of pediatric speech sound disorder. *Current Developmental Disorders Reports, 1,* 189–196.

Dodd, B., & Barker, R. (1990). The efficacy of utilizing parents and teachers as agents of therapy for children with phonological disorders. *Australian Journal of Human Communication Disorders, 18*(1), 29–45.

Dodd, B., & Bradford, A. (2000). A comparison of three therapy methods for children with different types of developmental phonological disorder. *International Journal of Language & Communication Disorders, 35,* 189–209.

Dodd, B., Crosbie, S., & Holm, A. (2004). *Core vocabulary therapy: An intervention for children with inconsistent speech disorders.* Perinatal Research Centre, Royal Brisbane & Women's Hospital, University of Queensland.

Dodd, B., Crosbie, S., McIntosh, B., Holm, A., Harvey, C., Liddy, M., Fontyne, K., Pinchin, B., & Rigy, H. (2008). The impact of selecting different contrasts in phonological therapy. *International Journal of Speech-Language Pathology, 10,* 334–345.

Dodd, B., Crosbie, S., McIntosh, B., Teitzel, T., & Ozanne, A. (2003). *Pre-reading inventory of phonological awareness.* Harcourt.

Dodd, B., & Gillon, G. (2001). Exploring the relationship between phonological awareness, speech impairment, and literacy. *Advances in Speech-Language Pathology, 3*, 139–147.

Dodd, B., Holm, A., Crosbie, S., & McCormack, P. (2005). Differential diagnosis of phonological disorders. In B. Dodd (Ed.), *Differential diagnosis and treatment of children with speech disorder* (2nd ed., pp. 44–70). Whurr Publishers.

Dodd, B., Holm, A., Crosbie, S., & McIntosh, B. (2006). A core vocabulary approach for management of inconsistent speech disorder. *Advances in Speech-Language Pathology, 8*, 220–230.

Dodd, B., Holm, A., Hua, Z., & Crosbie, S. (2003). Phonological development: A normative study of British English–speaking children. *Clinical Linguistics & Phonetics, 17*, 617–643.

Dodd, B., Hua, Z., Crosbie, S., Holm, A., & Ozanne, A. (2002). *Diagnostic evaluation of articulation and phonology (DEAP)*. Psychological Corporation.

Dodd, B., Hua, Z., Crosbie, S., Holm, A., & Ozanne, A. (2006). *Diagnostic evaluation of articulation and phonology (DEAP)*. Harcourt Assessment.

Dodd, B., Leahy, J., & Hambly, G. (1989). Phonological disorders in children: Underlying cognitive deficits. *British Journal of Developmental Psychology, 7*, 55–71.

Dodd, B., Reilly, S., Eecen, K. T., & Morgan A. T. (2018). Articulation or phonology? Evidence from longitudinal error data. *Clinical Linguistics & Phonetics, 32*(11), 1027–1041.

Dodd, B., So., L., & Li, W. (1996). Symptoms of disorder without impairment: The written and spoken errors of bilinguals. In B. Dodd, R. Campbell, & L. Worrall (Eds.), *Evaluating theories of language: Evidence from disorder* (pp. 119–136). Whurr Publishers.

Dodd, B., Ttofari-Eecen, K., Brommeyer, K., Ng, K., Reilly, S., & Morgan, A. (2018). Delayed and disordered development of articulation and phonology between four and seven years. *Child Language Teaching and Therapy, 34*(2), 87–99.

Dollaghan, C. A. (2007). *The handbook for evidence-based practice in communication disorders*. Paul H. Brookes Publishing Co.

Dollberg, S., Manor, Y., Makai, E., & Botzer, E. (2011). Evaluation of speech intelligibility in children with tongue-tie. *Acta Pediatrica, 100*, e125–127.

Donegan, P. (2002). Normal vowel development. In M. J. Ball & F. E. Gibbon (Eds.), *Vowel disorders* (pp. 1–35). Butterworth-Heinemann.

Dore, J. (1975). Holophrases, speech acts and language universals. *Journal of Child Language, 2*(1), 21–40.

Dowker, A. (1989). Rhyme and alliteration in poems elicited from young children. *Journal of Child Language, 16*(1), 181–202.

Drake, M. (2002). *Easy does it for articulation: A phonological approach*. Pro-Ed.

Dubois, E., & Bernthal, J. (1978). A comparison of three methods for obtaining articulatory responses. *Journal of Speech and Hearing Disorders, 43*, 295–305.

Dubois, S., & Horvath, B. (2003). The English vernaculars of the creoles of Louisiana. *Language Variation and Change, 15*, 255–288.

Duff, M. C., Proctor, A., & Yairi, E. (2004). Prevalence of voice disorders in African American and European American preschoolers. *Journal of Voice, 18*, 348–353.

Duffy, J. R. (2005). *Motor speech disorders. Substrates, differential diagnosis, and management* (2nd ed.). Elsevier Mosby.

Duffy, J. R. (2020). *Motor speech disorders* (4th ed.). Elsevier Mosby.

Dunn, C., & Barron, C. (1982). A treatment program for disordered phonology: Phonetic and linguistic considerations. *Language, Speech, and Hearing Services in Schools, 13*, 100–109.

Dunn, C., & Newton, L. (1986). A comprehensive model for speech development in hearing-impaired children. *Topics in Language Disorders, 6*, 25–46.

Dunn, W. J., & Reeves, T. E. (2004). Tongue piercing: Case report and ethical overview. *General Dentistry, 52*(3), 244–247.

Dworkin, J. (1978). Protrusive lingual force and lingual diadochokinetic rates: A comparative analysis between normal and lisping speakers. *Language, Speech, and Hearing Services in Schools, 9*, 8–16.

Dworkin, J. P., & Culatta, R. A. (1985). Oral structural and neuromuscular characteristics in children with normal and disordered articulation. *Journal of Speech and Hearing Disorders, 50*, 150–156.

Dyson, A. T. (1986). Development of velar consonants among normal two-year-olds. *Journal of Speech and Hearing Research, 29*, 493–498.

Dyson, A. T. (1988). Phonetic inventories of 2- and 3-year-old children. *Journal of Speech and Hearing Disorders, 53,* 89–93.

Dyson, A. T., & Amayreh, M. (2000). Phonological errors and sound changes in Arabic-speaking children. *Clinical Linguistics & Phonetics, 14,* 79–109.

Dyson, A. T., & Paden, E. P. (1983). Some phonological acquisition strategies used by two-year-olds. *Journal of Childhood Communication Disorders, 7,* 6–18.

Eadie, P., Morgan, A., Ukoumunne, O. B., Eecen, K. T., Wake, M., & Reilly, S. (2015). Speech sound disorder at 4 years: Prevalence, comorbidities, and predictors in a community cohort of children. *Developmental Medicine & Child Neurology, 57*(6), 578–584.

Edeal, D. M., & Gildersleeve-Neumann, C. E. (2011). The importance of production frequency in therapy for childhood apraxia of speech. *American Journal of Speech-Language Pathology, 20,* 95–110.

Edwards, J., Fox, R. A., & Rogers, C. L. (2002). Final consonant discrimination in children: Effects of phonological disorder, vocabulary size and articulatory accuracy. *Journal of Speech, Language, and Hearing Research, 45,* 231–242.

Edwards, M. L. (1983). Issues in phonological assessment. *Seminars in Speech and Language, 4,* 351–374.

Edwards, M. L. (2007). Phonological theories. In B. W. Hodson (Ed.), *Evaluating and enhancing children's phonological systems* (pp. 145–170). Thinking Publications.

Ehri, L. C., Nunes, S. R., Willows, D. M, Schuster, B.V., Yaghoub-Zadeh, Z., & Shanahan, T. (2001). Phonemic awareness instruction helps children learn to read: Evidence from the National Reading Panel's meta-analysis. *Reading Research Quarterly, 36,* 250–287.

Eilers, R. E., & Oller, D. K. (1976). The role of speech discrimination in developmental sound substitutions. *Journal of Child Language, 3,* 319–329.

Eilers, R. E., Wilson, W. R., & Moore, J. M. (1977). Developmental changes in speech discrimination in infants. *Journal of Speech and Hearing Research, 20,* 766–780.

Eimas, P. (1974). Auditory and linguistic units of processing of cues for place of articulation by infants. *Perception and Psychophysics, 16,* 341–347.

Eimas, P., Siqueland, E., Jusczyk, P., & Vigorito, J. (1971). Speech perception in infants. *Science, 171,* 303–306.

Eising, E., Carrion-Castillo, A., Vino, A., Strand, E. A., Jakielski, K., Scerri, T. S., Hildebrand, M. S., Webster, R., Ma, A., Mazoyer, B., Francks, C., Bahlo, M., Scherrer, I. E., Morgan, A. T., Shriberg, L. D., & Fisher, S. E. (2019). A set of regulatory genes co-expressed in embryonic human brain is implicated in disrupted speech development. *Molecular Psychiatry, 24,* 1065–1078.

Elbers, L., & Ton, J. (1985). Play pen monologues: The interplay of words and babbles in the first words period. *Journal of Child Language, 12,* 551–565.

Elbert, M. (1967). *Dismissal criteria from therapy* [Unpublished manuscript].

Elbert, M., Dinnsen, D. A., Swartzlander, P., & Chin, S. B. (1990). Generalization to conversational speech. *Journal of Speech and Hearing Disorders, 55,* 694–699.

Elbert, M., & Gierut, J. (1986). *Handbook of clinical phonology: Approaches to assessment and treatment.* College-Hill Press.

Elbert, M., & McReynolds, L. V. (1975). Transfer of /r/ across contexts. *Journal of Speech and Hearing Disorders, 40,* 380–387.

Elbert, M., & McReynolds, L. V. (1978). An experimental analysis of misarticulating children's generalization. *Journal of Speech and Hearing Research, 21,* 136–149.

Elbert, M., Powell, T. W., & Swartzlander, P. (1991). Toward a technology of generalization: How many exemplars are sufficient? *Journal of Speech and Hearing Research, 34,* 81–87.

Elbert, M., Rockman, B., & Saltzman, D. (1980). *Contrasts: The use of minimal pairs in articulation training.* Exceptional Resources, Inc.

Elbert, M., Shelton, R. L., & Arndt, W. B. (1967). A task for education of articulation change. *Journal of Speech and Hearing Research, 10,* 281–288.

Ellis, R. (1997). *Second language acquisition.* Oxford University Press.

Engel, D. C., & Groth, L. R. (1976). Case studies of the effect on carry-over of reinforcing postarticulation responses based on feedback. *Language, Speech, and Hearing Services in Schools, 7,* 93–101.

Ertmer, D. J., & Maki, J. E. (2000). A comparison of speech training methods with deaf adolescents: Spectrographic versus noninstrumental instruction. *Journal of Speech, Language, and Hearing Research, 43,* 1509–1523.

Ertmer, D. J., Stark, R. E., & Karlan, G. R. (1996). Real-time spectrographic displays in vowel production training with children who have profound hearing loss. *American Journal of Speech-Language Pathology, 5*(4), 4–16.

Eski, M., Nisanci, M., Aktas, A., & Sengezer, M. (2007). Congenital double lip: Review of 5 cases. *British Journal of Oral and Maxillofacial Surgery, 45*, 68–70.

Everhart, R. (1953). The relationship between articulation and other developmental factors in children. *Journal of Speech and Hearing Disorders, 18*, 332–338.

Everhart, R. (1956). Paternal occupational classification and the maturation of articulation. *Speech Monographs, 23*, 75–77.

Everhart, R. (1960). Literature survey of growth and developmental factors in articulation maturation. *Journal of Speech and Hearing Disorders, 25*, 59–69.

Fabiano-Smith, L., & Goldstein, B. (2010). Phonological acquisition in bilingual Spanish-English speaking children. *Journal of Speech, Language, and Hearing Research, 53*, 160–178.

Fairbanks, G. (1954). Systematic research in experimental phonetics 1. A theory of the speech mechanism as a servosystem. *Journal of Speech and Hearing Disorders, 19*(2), 133–139.

Fairbanks, G., & Green, E. (1950). A study of minor organic deviations in "functional" disorders of articulation: 2. Dimension and relationships of the lips. *Journal of Speech and Hearing Disorders, 15*, 165–168.

Fairbanks, G., & Lintner, M. (1951). A study of minor organic deviations in functional disorders of articulation. *Journal of Speech and Hearing Disorders, 16*, 273–279.

Farquhar, M. S. (1961). Prognostic value of imitative and auditory discrimination tests. *Journal of Speech and Hearing Disorders, 26*, 342–347.

Farquharson, K. (2019). It might not be "Just Artic": The case for the single sound error. *Prospectives of the ASHA Special Interest Groups, SIG 1, 4*(1), 76–84.

Farquharson, K., & Boldini, L. (2018). Variability in interpreting "educational performance" for children with speech sound disorders. *Language, Speech, and Hearing Services in Schools, 49*(4), 938–949.

Fee, E. J. (1995). Segments and syllables in early language acquisition. In J. Archibald (Ed.), *Phonological acquisition and phonological theory* (pp. 43–61). Erlbaum.

Fee, J., & Ingram, D. (1982). Reproduction as a strategy of phonological development. *Journal of Child Language, 9*, 41–54.

Felsenfeld, S., McGue, M., & Broen, P. A. (1995). Familial aggregation of phonological disorders: Results from a 28-year follow-up. *Journal of Speech and Hearing Research, 38*, 1091–1107.

Ferguson, C. A. (1978). Learning to pronounce: The earliest stages of phonological development. In F. D. Minifie & L. L. Lloyd (Eds.), *Communicative and cognitive abilities: Early behavioral assessment* (pp. 273–297). University Park Press.

Ferguson, C. A., & Farwell, C. B. (1975). Words and sounds in early language acquisition. *Language, 51*, 419–439.

Ferguson, S. H., & Kewley-Port, D. (2002). Vowel intelligibility in clear and conversational speech for normal-hearing and hearing-impaired listeners. *Journal of the Acoustical Society of America, 112*(1), 259–271.

Ferguson, S. H., & Kewley-Port, D. (2007). Talker differences in clear and conversational speech: Acoustic characteristics of vowels. *Journal of Speech, Language, and Hearing Research, 50*, 1241–1255.

Fey, M. E. (1986). *Language intervention with young children.* College Hill Press.

Fey, M. E. (1991). *Language intervention with young children.* Allyn & Bacon.

Fey, M. E., Cleave, P. L., Ravida, A. I., Long, S. H., Dejmal, A. E., & Easton, D. L. (1994). Effects of grammar facilitation on the phonological performance of children with speech and language impairments. *Journal of Speech and Hearing Research, 37*, 594–607.

Fey, M. E., & Gandour, J. (1982). Rule discovery in phonological acquisition. *Journal of Child Language, 9*, 71–81.

Field, T. M., Woodson, R., Greenberg, R., & Cohen, D. (1982). Discrimination and imitation of facial expression by neonates. *Science, 218*(4568), 179–181.

Fields, D., & Polmanteer, K. (2002, November). *Effectiveness of oral motor techniques in articulation and phonology therapy* [Poster presentation]. ASHA 2002 Convention, Atlanta, GA, United States.

Fitch, W. T., & Giedd, J. (1999). Morphology and development of the human vocal tract: A study using magnetic resonance imaging. *Journal of the Acoustical Society of America, 106*(3), 1511–1522.

Fitzsimons, R. (1958). Developmental, psychosocial and educational factors in children with nonorganic articulation problems. *Child Development, 29,* 481–489.

Flege, J. E., Bohn, O.-S., & Jang, S. (1997). Effects of experience on non-native speakers' production and perception of English vowels. *Journal of Phonetics, 25,* 437–470.

Flege, J. E., Frieda, E. M., & Nozawa, T. (1997). Amount of native-language (L1) use affects the pronunciation of an L2. *Journal of Phonetics, 25*(2), 169–186.

Flege, J. E., Munro, M. J., & Fox, R. A. (1994). Auditory and categorical effects of cross-language vowel perception. *Journal of the Acoustical Society of America, 95*(6), 3623–3641.

Flege, J. E., Munro, M. J., & MacKay, J. R. (1995). Factors affecting strength of perceived foreign accent in a second language. *Journal of the Acoustical Society of America, 97*(5), 3125–3134.

Flege, J. E., Takagi, N., & Mann, V. (1995). Japanese adults can learn to produce English /r/ and /l/ accurately. *Language and Speech, 38*(1), 25–55.

Flege, J. E., Yeni-Komshian, G. H., & Liu, S. (1999). Age constraints on second-language acquisition. *Journal of Memory and Language, 41*(1), 78–104.

Fleming, K., & Hartman, J. (1989). Establishing cultural validity of the computer analysis of phonological processes. *Florida Educational Research Council Bulletin, 22,* 8–32.

Fletcher, S. (1972). Time-by-count measurement of diadochokinetic syllable rate. *Journal of Speech and Hearing Research, 15,* 763–780.

Fletcher, S. G. (1989). Palatometric specification of stop, affricate, and sibilant sounds. *Journal of Speech and Hearing Research, 32,* 736–748.

Fletcher, S. G. (1992). *Articulation: A physiological approach.* Singular Publishing.

Fletcher, S., Casteel, R., & Bradley, D. (1961). Tongue thrust swallow, speech articulation and age. *Journal of Speech and Hearing Disorders, 26,* 201–208.

Fletcher, S., & Meldrum, J. (1968). Lingual function and relative length of the lingual frenulum. *Journal of Speech and Hearing Research, 11,* 382–399.

Flipsen, P., Jr. (1995). Speaker-listener familiarity: Parents as judges of delayed speech intelligibility. *Journal of Communication Disorders, 28,* 3–19.

Flipsen, P., Jr. (2002a). Longitudinal changes in articulation rate and phonetic phrase length in children with speech delay. *Journal of Speech, Language, and Hearing Research, 45*(1), 100–110.

Flipsen, P., Jr. (2002b). *Causes and speech sound disorders. Why worry?* [Paper presentation]. Speech Pathology Australia National Conference, Alice Springs, Australia.

Flipsen, P., Jr. (2006a). Syllables per word in typical and delayed speech acquisition. *Clinical Linguistics & Phonetics, 20*(4), 293–301.

Flipsen, P., Jr. (2006b). Measuring the intelligibility of conversational speech in children. *Clinical Linguistics & Phonetics, 20*(4), 303–312.

Flipsen, P., Jr. (2007). Appalachian English speech acquisition. In S. McLeod (Ed.), *The international guide to speech acquisition* (pp. 161–168). Thomson Delmar Learning.

Flipsen, P., Jr. (2008). Intelligibility of spontaneous conversational speech produced by children with cochlear implants: A review. *International Journal of Pediatric Otorhinolaryngology, 72,* 559–564.

Flipsen, P., Jr. (2015). Emergence and prevalence of persistent and residual speech errors. *Seminars in Speech and Language, 36,* 217–223.

Flipsen, P., Jr., Hammer, J. B., & Yost, K. M. (2005). Measuring severity of involvement in speech delay: Segmental and whole-word measures. *American Journal of Speech-Language Pathology, 14,* 298–312.

Flipsen, P., Jr., & Ogiela, D. A. (2015). Psychometric characteristics of single-word tests of children's speech sound production. *Language, Speech, and Hearing Services in Schools, 46,* 166–178.

Flipsen, P., Jr., & Parker, R. G. (2008). Phonological patterns in the speech of children with cochlear implants. *Journal of Communication Disorders, 41,* 337–357.

Flipsen, P., Jr., & Sacks, S. (2015). Remediation of residual /r/ errors: A case study using the SATPAC approach. *Perspectives on School-Based Issues, 16,* 64–78.

Fluharty, N. (2001). *Fluharty preschool speech and language screening test* (2nd ed.). Pro-Ed.

Fokes, J., Bond, Z. S., & Steinberg, M. (1985). Acquisition of the English voicing contrast by Arab children. *Language and Speech, 28*(1), 81–92.

Forrest, K. (2002). Are oral-motor exercises useful in the treatment of phonological/articulatory disorders? *Seminars in Speech and Language, 23,* 15–25.

Forrest, K., Dinnsen, D. A., & Elbert, M. (1997). Impact of substitution patterns on phonological learning by misarticulating children. *Clinical Linguistics & Phonetics, 11*(1), 63–76.

Forrest, K., & Iuzzini, J. (2008). A comparison of oral motor and production training for children with speech sound disorders. *Seminars in Speech and Language, 29*(4), 304–311.

Fox, A. V., Dodd, B., & Howard, D. (2002). Risk factors for speech disorders in children. *International Journal of Language & Communication Disorders, 37*, 117–131.

Foy, J. G., & Mann, V. (2001). Does strength of phonological representations predict phonological awareness? *Applied Psycholinguistics, 22*, 301–325.

Francis, D. O., Krishnaswami, S., & McPheeters, M. (2015). Treatment of ankyloglossia and breastfeeding outcomes: A systematic review. *Pediatrics, 135*(6), e1458–1456.

Franklin, A., & McDaniel, L. (2016). Exploring a phonological process approach to adult pronunciation training. *American Journal of Speech-Language Pathology, 25*(2), 172–182.

French, A. (1989). The systematic acquisition of word forms by a child during the first fifty word stage. *Journal of Child Language, 16*, 69–90.

Frost, S. J., Landi, N., Mencl, W. E., Sandak, R., Fulbright, R. K., Tejada, E. T., Jacobsen, L., Grigorenko, E. L., Constable, R. T., & Pugh, K. R. (2009). Phonological awareness predicts activation patterns for print and speech. *Annals of Dyslexia, 59*, 78–97.

Fry, D. (1955). Duration and intensity as physical correlates of linguistic stress. *Journal of the Acoustical Society of America, 27*, 765–768.

Fucci, D. (1972). Oral vibrotactile sensation: An evaluation of normal and defective speakers. *Journal of Speech and Hearing Research, 15*, 179–184.

Fuchs, D., Fuchs, L. S., Thompson, A., Al Otaiba, S., Yen, L., Yang, N. J., Braun, M., & O'Connor, R. E. (2001). Is reading important in reading-readiness programs? A randomized field trial with teachers as program implementers. *Journal of Educational Psychology, 93*, 251–267.

Fudala, J. B., & Stegall, S. (2017). *Arizona articulation and phonology scale* (4th rev.). Western Psychological Services.

Furia, C. L. B., Kowalski, L. P., Latorre, M. R. D. O., Angelis, E. C., Mastins, N. M. S., Barros, A. P. B., & Ribeiro, K. C. B. (2001). Speech intelligibility after glossectomy and speech rehabilitation. *Archives of Otolaryngology: Head and Neck Surgery, 127*, 877–883.

Gable, T. O., Kummer, A. W., Lee, L., Creaghead, N. A., & Moore, L. J. (1995). Premature loss of the maxillary incisors: Effect on speech production. *Journal of Dentistry for Children, 62*, 173–179.

Galvin, K., Mok, M., & Dowell, R. (2007). *Sequential bilateral implants for young children: Subjective outcomes, left versus right localization and speech detection results* [Paper presentation]. 11th International Conference on Cochlear Implants in Children, Charlotte, NC, United States.

Gammon, S., Smith, P., Daniloff, R., & Kim, C. (1971). Articulation and stress juncture production under oral anesthetization and masking. *Journal of Speech and Hearing Research, 14*, 271–282.

Garmann, N. G., Kristoffersen, K. E., & Simonsen, H. (2018). Phonological patterns (templates) in 5p deletion syndrome. *Clinical Linguistics & Phonetics, 32*(2), 101–113.

Garrett, R. (1969). *A study of children's discrimination of phonetic variations of the /s/ phoneme* [Unpublished doctoral dissertation]. Ohio University.

Geers, A. E. (2002). Factors affecting the development of speech, language, and literacy in children with early cochlear implantation. *Language, Hearing, and Speech Services in Schools, 33*, 172–183.

Geers, A. E. (2006). Factors influencing spoken language outcomes in children following early cochlear implantation. *Advances in Otorhinolaryngology, 64*, 50–65.

Gerken, L., & McGregor, K. (1998). An overview of prosody and its role in normal and disordered child language. *American Journal of Speech-Language Pathology, 7*, 38–48.

Gibbon, F. (2013). Therapy for abnormal vowels in children with speech disorders. In M. J. Ball & F. E. Gibbon (Eds.), *Handbook of vowels and vowel disorders* (pp. 739–768). Psychology Press.

Gibbon, F. E. (1999). Undifferentiated lingual gestures in children with articulation/phonological disorders. *Journal of Speech, Language, and Hearing Research, 42*, 382–397.

Gibbon, F., Shockey, L., & Reid, J. (1992). Description and treatment of abnormal vowels in phonologically disordered child. *Child Language Teaching and Therapy, 8*(1), 30–59.

Gibbon, F. E., & Wood, S. E. (2010). Visual feedback therapy with electropalatography. In A. L. Williams, S. McLeod, & R. J. McCauley (Eds.), *Interventions for speech sound disorders* (pp. 509–536). Paul H. Brookes Publishing Co.

Gierut, J. (1989). Maximal opposition approach to phonological treatment. *Journal of Speech and Hearing Disorders, 54,* 9–19.

Gierut, J. A. (1990). Differential learning of phonological oppositions. *Journal of Speech and Hearing Research, 33,* 540–549.

Gierut, J. A. (1991). Homonymy in phonological changes. *Clinical Linguistics & Phonetics, 5,* 119–137.

Gierut, J. A. (1992). The conditions and courses of clinically-induced phonological changes. *Journal of Speech and Hearing Research, 35,* 1049–1063.

Gierut, J. A. (1998). Natural domains of cyclicity in phonological acquisition. *Clinical Linguistics & Phonetics, 12,* 481–499.

Gierut, J. A. (1999). Syllable onsets: Clusters and adjuncts in acquisition. *Journal of Speech, Language, and Hearing Research, 42,* 708–726.

Gierut, J. A. (2001). Complexity in phonological treatment: Clinical factors. *Language, Speech, and Hearing Services in Schools, 32,* 229–241.

Gierut, J. A. (2007). Phonological complexity and language learnability. *American Journal of Speech-Language Pathology, 16,* 6–17.

Gierut, J. A., & Champion, A. (2001). Syllable onsets: II. Three-element clusters in phonological treatment. *Journal of Speech, Language, and Hearing Research, 44,* 886–904.

Gierut, J. A., Elbert, M., & Dinnsen, D. A. (1987). A functional analysis of phonological knowledge and generalization learning in misarticulating children. *Journal of Speech and Hearing Research, 30,* 462–479.

Gierut, J. A., & Morrisette, M. L. (2012). Age of word acquisition effects in treatment of children with phonological delays. *Applied Psycholinguistics, 33*(1), 121–144.

Gierut, J. A., Morrisette, M. L., Hughes, M. T., & Rowland, S. (1996). Phonological treatment efficacy and developmental norms. *Language, Speech, and Hearing Services in Schools, 27,* 215–230.

Gierut, J. A., Morrisette, M. L., & Ziemer, S. M. (2010). Nonwords and generalization in children with phonological disorders. *American Journal of Speech-Language Pathology, 19,* 167–177.

Gildersleeve-Neumann, C., & Davis, B. (1998, November). *Learning English in a bilingual preschool environment: Change over time* [Paper presentation]. ASHA 1998 Convention, San Antonio, TX, United States.

Gildersleeve-Neumann, C. E., & Goldstein, B. (2012). Intervention for multilingual children with speech sound disorders. In S. McLeod & B. Goldstein (Eds.), *Multilingual aspects of speech sound disorders* (pp. 214–227). Multilingual Matters.

Gildersleeve-Neumann, C. E., Kester, E. S., Davis, B. L., & Peña, E. D. (2008). English speech sound development in preschool-aged children from bilingual English-Spanish environments. *Language, Speech, and Hearing Services in Schools, 39,* 314–328.

Gildersleeve-Neumann, C. E., & Wright, K. E. (2010). English phonological acquisition in 3- to 5-year-old children learning Russian and English. *Language, Speech, and Hearing Services in Schools, 41,* 429–444.

Giles, S. B. (1971). *A study of articulatory characteristics of /l/ allophones in English* [Unpublished doctoral dissertation]. University of Iowa.

Gillon, G. T. (2000a). The efficacy of phonological awareness intervention for children with spoken language impairment. *Language, Speech, and Hearing Services in Schools, 31,* 126–141.

Gillon, G. T. (2000b). *The Gillon phonological awareness training programme* (2nd ed.). Canterprise, University of Canterbury. https://www.canterbury.ac.nz/education-and-health/research/phonological-awareness-resources/

Gillon, G. T. (2002). Follow-up study investigating benefits of phonological awareness intervention for children with spoken language impairment. *International Journal of Language & Communication Disorders, 37,* 381–400.

Gillon, G. T. (2004). *Phonological awareness: From research to practice.* Guilford Press.

Gillon, G. T. (2005). Facilitating phoneme awareness development in 3- and 4-year-old children with speech impairment. *Language, Speech, and Hearing Services in Schools, 36,* 308–324.

Gillon, G. T. (2019). *Phonological awareness: From research to practice.* Guilford Press.

Gillon, G. T., & Dodd, B. (1995). The effects of training phonological, semantic, and syntactic processing skills in spoken language on reading ability. *Language, Speech, and Hearing Services in Schools, 26,* 58–68.

Gillon, G. T., & McNeill, B. C. (2007). An integrated phonological awareness programme for preschool children with speech disorder. https://www.canterbury.ac.nz/education-and-health/research/phonological-awareness-resources/

Gillon, G. T., McNeill, B. C., Denston, A., Scott, A., & Macfarlane, A. (2020). Evidence-based class literacy instruction for children with speech and language difficulties. *Topics in Language Disorders, 40*(4), 357–374.

Gillon, G. T., McNeill, B., Scott, A., Denston, A. Wilson, L., Cason, K., & Macfarlane, A. (2019). A better start to literacy learning: Findings from a teacher-implemented intervention in children's first year at school. *Reading and Writing, 32*(8), 1989–2012.

Gillon, G. T., & Moriarty, B. C. (2007). Childhood apraxia of speech: Children at risk for persistent reading and spelling disorder. *Seminars in Speech and Language, 28*(1), 48–57.

Gillon, G. T., & Schwarz, I. E. (2001). Screening New Zealand children's spoken language skills for academic success. In L. Wilson & S. Hewat (Eds.), *Proceedings of the 2001 Speech Pathology Australia National Conference* (pp. 207–214). Melbourne: Speech Pathology Australia.

Glaspey, A. M. (2012). Stimulability measures and dynamic assessment of speech adaptability, SIG 1. *Perspectives on Language, Learning, and Education, 19*, 12–18.

Glaspey, A. M. (2019). *Glaspey dynamic assessment of phonology.* ATP Assessments.

Glogowska, M., Roulstone, S., Peters, T. J., & Enderby, P. (2006). Early speech- and language-impaired children: Linguistic, literacy, and social outcomes. *Developmental Medicine & Child Neurology, 48*, 489–494.

Gold, T. (1980). Speech production in hearing-impaired children. *Journal of Communication Disorders, 13*, 397–418.

Goldman, R., & Fristoe, M. (2015). *Goldman-Fristoe test of articulation* (3rd ed.). NCS Pearson, Inc.

Goldman, R., Fristoe, M., & Woodcock, R. (1970). *The Goldman-Fristoe-Woodcock test of auditory discrimination.* American Guidance Service.

Goldsmith, J. (1979). *Autosegmental phonology* [Doctoral dissertation, Massachusetts Institute of Technology]. Garland Press.

Goldsmith, J. A. (1990). *Autosegmental and metrical phonology.* Blackwell.

Goldstein, B. (1988). *The evidence of phonological processes of 3- and 4-year-old Spanish speakers* [Unpublished master's thesis]. Temple University.

Goldstein, B. (1995). Spanish phonological development. In H. Kayser (Ed.), *Bilingual speech-language pathology: An Hispanic focus* (pp. 17–38). Singular Publishing.

Goldstein, B. (2000). *Cultural and linguistic diversity resource guide for speech-language pathology.* Singular Publishing.

Goldstein, B. (2001). Assessing phonological skills in Hispanic/Latino children. *Seminars in Speech and Language, 22*, 39–49.

Goldstein, B. (2004). Phonological development and disorders in bilingual children. In B. Goldstein (Ed.), *Bilingual language development and disorders in Spanish-English speakers* (pp. 257–286). Paul H. Brookes Publishing Co.

Goldstein, B. (2006). Clinical implications of research on language development and disorders in bilingual children. *Topics in Language Disorders, 26*, 318–334.

Goldstein, B. (2007a). Spanish speech acquisition. In S. McLeod (Ed.), *The international guide to speech acquisition* (pp. 539–553). Thomson Delmar Learning.

Goldstein, B. (2007b). Phonological skills in Puerto Rican and Mexican-Spanish speaking children with phonological disorders. *Clinical Linguistics & Phonetics, 21*, 93–109.

Goldstein, B. (2007c). Speech acquisition across the world: Spanish-influenced English. In S. McLeod (Ed.), *The international guide to speech acquisition* (pp. 345–356). Thomson Delmar Learning.

Goldstein, B., & Cintron, P. (2001). An investigation of phonological skills in Puerto Rican Spanish-speaking 2-year-olds. *Clinical Linguistics & Phonetics, 15*, 343–361.

Goldstein, B., Fabiano, L., & Washington, P. (2005). Phonological skills in predominantly English, predominantly Spanish, and Spanish-English bilingual children. *Language, Speech, and Hearing Services in Schools, 36*, 201–218.

Goldstein, B., & Gildersleeve-Neumann, C. (2012). Phonological development and disorders. In B. Goldstein (Ed.), *Bilingual language development and disorders in Spanish-English speakers* (2nd ed., pp. 285–309). Paul H. Brookes Publishing Co.

Goldstein, B., & Iglesias, A. (1996a). Phonological patterns in normally developing Spanish-speaking 3- and 4-year-olds of Puerto Rican descent. *Language, Speech, and Hearing Services in Schools, 27*, 82–90.

Goldstein, B., & Iglesias, A. (1996b). Phonological patterns in Puerto Rican Spanish-speaking children with phonological disorders. *Journal of Communication Disorders, 29*, 367–387.

Goldstein, B., & Iglesias, A. (1999). *Phonological patterns in bilingual (Spanish-English) children* [Seminar presentation]. Texas Research Symposium on Language Diversity, Austin.

Goldstein, B., & Iglesias, A. (2001). The effect of dialect on phonological analysis: Evidence from Spanish-speaking children. *American Journal of Speech-Language Pathology, 10*, 394–406.

Goldstein, B., & McLeod, S. (2012). Typical and atypical multilingual speech acquisition. In S. McLeod & B. Goldstein (Eds.), *Multilingual aspects of speech sound disorders* (pp. 84–100). Multilingual Matters.

Goldstein, B., & Pollock, K. (2000). Vowel errors in Spanish-speaking children with phonological disorders: A retrospective, comparative study. *Clinical Linguistics & Phonetics, 14*, 217–234.

Goldstein, B., & Washington, P. (2001). An initial investigation of phonological patterns in 4-year-old typically developing Spanish-English bilingual children. *Language, Speech, and Hearing Services in Schools, 10*, 153–164.

Good, R., & Kaminski, R. (2002). *Dynamic indicators of basic early literacy skills* (6th ed.). Institute for the Development of Educational Achievement.

Goodluck, H. (1991). *Language acquisition: A linguistic introduction*. Blackwell.

Goodman, R. (1997). The strengths and difficulties questionnaire: A research note. *The Journal of Child Psychology and Psychiatry, 38*(5), 581–586.

Gordon-Brannan, M. (1994). Assessing intelligibility: Children's expressive phonologies. *Topics in Language Disorders, 14*, 17–25.

Gordon-Brannan, M., Hodson, B., & Wynne, M (1992). Remediating unintelligible utterances of a child with a mild hearing loss. *American Journal of Speech-Language Pathology, 1*(4), 28–38.

Goswami, U., & Bryant, P. E. (1990). *Phonological skills and learning to read*. Psychology Press.

Gratier, M., & Devouche, E. (2011). Imitation and repetition of prosodic contour in vocal interaction at 3 months. *Developmental Psychology, 47*, 67–76.

Gray, B. (1974). A field study on programmed articulation therapy. *Language, Speech, and Hearing Services in Schools, 5*, 119–131.

Gray, B., & Ryan, B. (1973). *A language program for the nonlanguage child*. Research Press.

Gray, S. I., & Shelton, R. L. (1992). Self-monitoring effects on articulation carryover in school-age children. *Language, Speech, and Hearing Services in Schools, 23*, 334–342.

Grech, H., & Dodd, B. (2008). Phonological acquisition in Malta: A bilingual learning context. *International Journal of Bilingualism, 12*, 155–171.

Grech, H., & McLeod, S. (2012). Multilingual speech and language development and disorders. In D. Battle (Ed.), *Communication disorders and development in multicultural populations* (pp. 120–147). Academic Press.

Green, J. R., Moore, C. A., & Reilly, K. J. (2002). The sequential development of jaw and lip control for speech. *Journal of Speech, Language, and Hearing Research, 45*, 66–79.

Green, L. (2004). Research on African American English since 1998: Origins, description, theory, and practice. *Journal of English Linguistics, 32*, 210–229.

Greenlee, M. (1974). Interacting processes in the child's acquisition of stop-liquid clusters. *Papers and Reports on Child Language Disorders, Stanford University, 7*, 85–100.

Griffith, J., & Miner, L. E. (1979). *Phonetic context drillbook*. Prentice-Hall.

Grigos, M. I., Moss, A., & Lu, Y. (2015). Oral articulatory control in childhood apraxia of speech. *Journal of Speech, Language, and Hearing Research, 58*, 1103–1118.

Grimm, A., & Schulz, P. (2014). Specific language impairment and early second language acquisition: The risk of over- and under-diagnosis. *Child Indicators Report, 7*, 821–841.

Grogan, M. L., Barker, E. J., Dettman, S. J., & Blamey, P. J. (1995). Phonetic and phonologic changes in the connected speech of children using a cochlear implant. *Annals of Otology, Rhinology, and Laryngology, Suppl. 166*, 390–393.

Gruber, F. A., Lowery, S. D., Seung, H.-K., & Deal, R. E. (2003). Approaches to speech-language intervention and the true believer. *Journal of Medical Speech-Language Pathology, 11*, 95–104.

Grunwell, P. (1981). The development of phonology: A descriptive profile. *First Language, 3,* 61–191.

Grunwell, P. (1982). *Clinical phonology.* Aspen.

Grunwell, P. (1985). *Phonological assessment of child speech (PACS).* NFER-Nelson.

Grunwell, P. (1987). *Clinical phonology* (2nd ed.). Croom Helm.

Grunwell, P., & Yavas, M. (1988). Phonotactic restrictions in disordered child phonology: A case study. *Clinical Linguistics & Phonetics, 2,* 1–16.

Guadagnoli, M. A., & Lee, T. D. (2004). Challenge point: A framework for conceptualizing the effects of various practice conditions in motor learning. *Journal of Motor Behavior, 36,* 212–224.

Guenther, F. H. (1995). Speech sound acquisition, coarticulation, and rate effects in a neural network model of speech production. *Psychological Review, 102,* 594–621.

Guion, S. G., Flege, J. E., Liu, S. H., & Yeni-Komshian, G. H. (2000). Age of learning effects on the duration of sentences produced in a second language. *Applied Psycholinguistics, 21*(2), 205–228.

Guitart, J. (1978). Conservative versus radical dialects in American Spanish: Implications for language instruction. *Bilingual Review, 5,* 57–64.

Guitart, J. (1996). Spanish in contact with itself and the phonological characterization of conservative and radical styles. In A. Roca & J. Jensen (Eds.), *Spanish in contact: Issues in bilingualism* (pp. 151–157). Cascadilla Press.

Guyette, T., & Diedrich, W. (1981). A critical review of developmental apraxia of speech. In N. Lass (Ed.), *Speech and language: Advances in basic research and practice* (Vol. 5, pp. 1–49). Academic Press.

Haapanen, M.-L., Ignatious, J., Rihkanen, H., & Ertama, L. (1994). Velopharyngeal insufficiency following palatine tonsillectomy. *European Archives of Otorhinolaryngology, 251*(3), 186–189.

Hadlich, R., Holton, J., & Montes, M. (1968). *A drillbook of Spanish pronunciation.* Harper & Row.

Haelsig, P. C., & Madison, C. L. (1986). A study of phonological processes exhibited by 3-, 4-, and 5-year-old children. *Language, Speech, and Hearing Services in Schools, 17,* 107–114.

Hall, M. (1938). Auditory factors in functional articulatory speech defects. *Journal of Experimental Education, 7,* 110–132.

Hammond, R. (2001). *The sounds of Spanish: Analysis and application (with special reference to American English).* Cascadilla Press.

Hans, P. S., England, R., Prowse, S., Young, E., & Sheehan, P. Z. (2010). UK and Ireland experience of cochlear implants in children with Down syndrome. *International Journal of Pediatric Otorhinolaryngology, 74,* 260–264.

Hanson, M. L. (1988a). Orofacial myofunctional disorders: Guidelines for assessment and treatment. *International Journal of Orofacial Myology, 14,* 27–32.

Hanson, M. L. (1988b). Orofacial myofunctional therapy: Historical and philosophical considerations. *International Journal of Orofacial Myology, 14,* 3–10.

Hanson, M. L. (1994). Oral myofunctional disorders and articulatory patterns. In J. Bernthal & N. Bankson (Eds.), *Child phonology: Characteristics, assessment, and intervention with special populations* (pp. 29–53). Thieme Medical Publishers.

Hardcastle, W. J. (1976). *Physiology of speech production.* Academic Press.

Hardcastle, W. J., Morgan Berry, R. A., & Clark, C. J. (1987). An instrumental phonetic study of lingual activity in articulation-disordered children. *Journal of Speech and Hearing Research, 30,* 171–184.

Hardison, E. M., Bowers, L., & Huisingh, R. (2010). *LinguiSystems articulation test.* LinguiSystems.

Hargrove, P. M. (1982). Misarticulated vowels: A case study. *Language, Speech, and Hearing Services in Schools, 13*(2), 86–95.

Hargrove, P. M., Dauer, K. E., & Montelibano, M. (1989). Reducing vowel and final consonant prolongations in twin brothers. *Child Language Teaching and Therapy, 5*(1), 49–63.

Harrington, J., Lux, I., & Higgins, R. (1984, November). *Identification of error types as related to stimuli in articulation tests* [Paper presentation]. ASHA 1984 Convention, San Francisco, CA, United States.

Hart, T., Tsaousides, T., Zanca, J. M., Whyte, J., Packel, A., Ferraro, M., & Dijkers, M. P. (2014). Toward a theory-driven classification of rehabilitation treatments. *Archives of Physical Medicine and Rehabilitation: American Congress of Rehabilitation Medicine (ACRM), 95*(1), Supp., S33–S44.E2.

Haskill, A. M., & Tyler, A. A. (2007). A comparison of linguistic profiles in subgroups of children with specific language impairment. *American Journal of Speech-Language Pathology, 16,* 209–221.

Hassan, T., Naini, R. B., & Gill, D. S. (2007). The effects of orthognathic surgery on speech: A review. *Journal of Oral and Maxillofacial Surgery, 65,* 2536–2543.

Hassink, J. M., & Wendt, O. (2010). Remediation of phonological disorders in preschool age children: Evidence for the cycles approach. *EBP Briefs, 5*(2), 1–7.

Hauner, K. K. Y., Shriberg, L. D., Kwiatkowski, J., & Allen, C. T. (2005). A subtype of speech delay associated with developmental psychosocial involvement. *Journal of Speech, Language, and Hearing Research, 48,* 635–650.

Hayden, D. A., Namasivayam, A. K., Ward, R., Clark, A., & Eigen, J. (2021). The PROMPT approach. In A. L. Williams, S. McLeod, & R. J. McCauley (Eds.), *Interventions for Speech Sound Disorders in Children* (2nd edition), (pp. 477–504). Paul H. Brookes Publishing Co.

Hayiou-Tomas, M. E., Carroll, J. M., Leavett, R., Hulme, C., & Snowling, M. J. (2017). When does speech sound disorder matter for literacy? The role of disordered speech errors, co-occurring language impairment and family risk of dyslexia. *Journal of Child Psychology and Psychiatry, 58,* 197–205.

Haynes, W., & Moran, M. (1989). A cross-sectional developmental study of final consonant production in southern Black children from preschool through third grade. *Language, Speech, and Hearing Services in Schools, 20,* 400–406.

Hazan, V., & Barrett, S. (2000). The development of phonemic categorization in children aged 6–12. *Journal of Phonetics, 28,* 377–396.

Hearnshaw, S., Baker, E., & Munro, N. (2018). The speech perception skills of children with and without speech sound disorder. *Journal of Communication Disorders, 71*(1), 61–71.

Hearnshaw, S., Baker, E., & Munro, N. (2019). Speech perception skills of children with speech sound disorders: A systematic review and meta-analysis. *Journal of Speech, Language, and Hearing Research, 62*(10), 3771–3789.

Heggie, A. A. C., Vujcich, N. J., Portnof, J. E., & Morgan, A. T. (2013). Tongue reduction for macroglossia in Beckwith Wiedemann syndrome: Review and application of a new technique. *International Journal of Oral and Maxillofacial Surgery, 42,* 185–191.

Heinen, E., Birkholz, P., Willmes, K., & Neuschaefer-Rube, C. (2017). Do long-term tongue piercings affect speech quality? *Logopedics, Phoniatrics, Vocology, 42*(3), 126–132.

Heliövaara, A. (2011). Maxillary dental arch dimensions in 6-year-old children with articulatory speech disorders. *Folia Phoniatrica et Logopaedica, 63,* 242–246.

Heller, J., Gabbay, J., O'Hara, C., Heller, M., & Bradley, J. P. (2005). Improved ankyloglossia correction with four-flap z-frenuloplasty. *Annals of Plastic Surgery, 54,* 623–628.

Helmick, J. W. (1976). Effects of therapy on articulation skills in elementary-school children. *Language, Speech, and Hearing Services in Schools, 7*(3), 169–172.

Hempenstall, K. (1997). The role of phonemic awareness in beginning reading: A review. *Behaviour Change, 14,* 201–214.

Heng, Q., McCabe, P., Clarke, J., & Preston, J. L. (2016). Using ultrasound visual feedback to remediate velar fronting in preschool children: A pilot study. *Clinical Linguistics & Phonetics, 30*(3–5), 382–397.

Hepper, P. G., & Shahidullah, S. (1994). Development of fetal hearing. *Archives of Disease in Childhood, 71*(2), F81–F87.

Hesketh, A., Dima, E., & Nelson, V. (2007). Teaching phoneme awareness to pre-literate children with speech disorder: A randomized controlled trial. *International Journal of Language & Communication Disorders, 42,* 251–271.

Hetrick, R. D., & Sommers, R. K. (1988). Unisensory and bisensory processing skills of children having misarticulations and normally speaking peers. *Journal of Speech and Hearing Research, 31,* 575–581.

Hewlett, N. (1990). Processes of development and production. In P. Grunwell (Ed.), *Developmental speech disorders* (pp. 15–38). Churchill Livingstone.

Hewlett, N., Gibbon, F., & Cohen-McKenzie, W. (1998). When is a velar an alveolar? Evidence supporting a revised psycholinguistic model of speech production in children. *International Journal of Language & Communication Disorders, 33,* 161–176.

Higgs, J. A. W. (1968). The phonetic development of word initial /s/ plus stop clusters in a group of young children. *British Journal of Disorders of Communication, 3,* 130–138.

Hinton, L., & Pollock, K. (1999). *Regional variations in the phonological characteristics of African American Vernacular English (AAVE) speakers* [Paper presentation]. Texas Research Symposium on Language Diversity, Austin, TX, United States.

Hitchcock, E., Cabbage, K. L., Swartz, M. T., & Carrell, T. D. (2020). Measuring speech perception using the wide-range acoustic accuracy scale: Preliminary findings. *Perspectives of the ASHA Special Interest Groups, SIG 19, 5*(4), 1098–1112.

Hitchcock, E. R., & McAllister Byun, T. (2015a). Enhancing generalization in biofeedback intervention using the challenge point framework: A case study. *Clinical Linguistics & Phonetics, 29*, 59–75.

Hitchcock, E. R., & McAllister Byun, T. (2015b, November). *When should we treat residual speech errors? Survey data on social, emotional, and academic impacts* [Technical presentation]. ASHA 2015 Convention, Denver, CO, United States.

Hitchcock, E. R., McAllister Byun, T., Swartz, M., & Lazarus, R. (2017). Efficacy of electropalatography for treating misarticulation of /r/. *American Journal of Speech-Language Pathology, 26*, 1141–1158.

Hixon, T. J. (1971, November). *Mechanical aspects of speech production* [Paper presentation]. ASHA 1971 Convention, Chicago, IL, United States.

Hockett, C. F. (1955). A manual of phonology. *International Journal of American Linguistics (Memoir 11), 21*(4).

Hodson, B. (1985). *Hodson Computer analysis of phonological processes (CAPP)*. PhonoComp.

Hodson, B. (1989). Phonological remediation: A cycles approach. In N. Creaghead, P. Newman, & W. Secord (Eds.), *Assessment and remediation of articulatory and phonological disorders* (pp. 323–333). Merrill.

Hodson, B. W. (2003). *Computerized analysis of phonological patterns (HCAPP)*. PhonoComp Software. https://www.myphonocomp.com/

Hodson, B. W. (2004). *Hodson assessment of phonological patterns* (3rd ed.). Pro-Ed.

Hodson, B. W. (2010a). *Evaluating and enhancing children's phonological systems*. PhonoComp Publishing.

Hodson, B. W. (2010b). Overview of the diagnostic evaluation process for children with highly unintelligible speech. In B. W. Hodson (Ed.), *Evaluating and enhancing children's phonological systems* (pp. 45–64). PhonoComp Publishing.

Hodson, B. W., Chin, L., Redmond, B., & Simpson, R. (1983). Phonological evaluation and remediation of speech deviations of a child with a repaired cleft palate: A case study. *Journal of Speech and Hearing Disorders, 48*, 93–98.

Hodson, B. W., & Paden, E. P. (1991). *Targeting intelligible speech: A phonological approach to remediation* (2nd ed.). Pro-Ed.

Hoffman, P., Norris, J., & Monjure, J. (1990). Comparison of process targeting and whole language treatments of phonologically delayed children. *Language, Speech, and Hearing Services in Schools, 21*, 102–109.

Hoffman, P., & Schuckers, G. H. (1984). Articulation remediation treatment models. In R. G. Daniloff (Ed.), *Articulation assessment and treatment issues*. College-Hill Press.

Hoffman, P., Schuckers, G., & Daniloff, R. (1989). *Children's phonetic disorders: Theory and treatment*. Little, Brown.

Hoffman, P. R., & Norris, J. A. (1989). On the nature of phonological development: Evidence from normal children's spelling errors. *Journal of Speech and Hearing Research, 32*, 787–794.

Hoffman, P. R., & Norris, J. A. (2010). Dynamic systems and whole language intervention. In A. L. Williams, S. McLeod, & R. J. McCauley (Eds.), *Interventions for speech sound disorders in children* (pp. 333–354). Paul H. Brookes Publishing Co.

Hoffmann, B., Wendel, U., & Schweitzer-Kranz, S. (2011). Cross-sectional analysis of speech and cognitive performance in 32 patients with classic galactosemia. *Journal of Inherited Metabolic Disease, 34*, 421–427.

Hoffmann, K. A. (1982). *Speech sound acquisition and natural process occurrence in the continuous speech of three- to six-year-old children* [Unpublished master's thesis]. University of Wisconsin–Madison.

Hogan, T., Catts, H., & Little, T. (2005). The relationship between phonological awareness and reading: Implications for the assessment of phonological awareness. *Language, Speech, and Hearing Services in Schools, 36*, 285–293.

Holm, A., Crosbie, S., & Dodd, B. (2007). Differentiating normal variability from inconsistency in children's speech: Normative data. *International Journal of Language & Communication Disorders, 42*, 467–486.

Holm, A., & Dodd, B. (2000). A longitudinal study of the phonological development of two Cantonese-English bilingual children. *Applied Psycholinguistics, 20*, 349–376.

Holm, A., Dodd, B., & Ozanne, A. (1997). Efficacy of intervention for a bilingual child making articulation and phonological errors. *International Journal of Bilingualism, 1*, 55–69.

Holm, A., Farrier, F., & Dodd, B. (2007). Phonological awareness, reading accuracy and spelling ability of children with inconsistent phonological disorder. *International Journal of Language and Communication Disorders, 43*(3), 300–322.

Holm, J. (1988). *Pidgins and creoles: Volume I. Theory and structure.* Cambridge University Press.

Holm, J. (1989). *Pidgins and creoles: Volume II. Reference survey.* Cambridge University Press.

Hong, P., Lago, D., Seargeant, J., Pellman, L., Magit, A. E., & Pransky, S. M. (2010). Defining ankyloglossia: A case study of anterior and posterior tongue ties. *International Journal of Pediatric Otorhinolaryngology, 74*, 1003–1006.

Hori, Y., Koike, Y., Ohyama, G., Otsu, S.-Y., & Abe, K. (1996). Effects of tonsillectomy on articulation. *Acta Otolaryngologica, Supp. 523*, 248–251.

Horton-Ikard, R. (2010). Language sample analysis with children who speak nonmainstream dialects of English. *Perspectives on Language Learning and Education, 17*, 16–23.

Houde, J. F., & Nagarajan, S. S. (2011). Speech production as state feedback control. *Frontiers in Human Neuroscience, 5*(82), 1–14.

Howard, S. (2007). English speech acquisition. In S. McLeod (Ed.), *The international guide to speech acquisition* (pp. 188–203). Thomson Delmar Learning.

Howard, S. J., & Heselwood, B. C. (2002). The contribution of phonetics to the study of vowel development and disorders. In M. J. Ball & F. E. Gibbon (Eds.), *Vowel disorders* (pp. 37–82). Butterworth-Heinemann.

Howell, J., & Dean, E. (1991). *Treating phonological disorders in children: Metaphon. Theory to practice.* Singular Publishing.

Howland, C., Baker, E., Munro, N., & McLeod, S. (2019) Realisation of grammatical morphemes by children with phonological impairment. *Clinical Linguistics & Phonetics, 33*(1-2), 20–41.

Hua, Z. (2006). The normal and disordered phonology of Putonghua (modern standard Chinese)-speaking children. In Z. Hua & B. Dodd (Eds.), *Phonological development and disorders: A cross-linguistic perspective* (pp. 81–108). Multilingual Matters.

Hua, Z. (2007). Putonghua (modern standard Chinese) speech acquisition. In S. McLeod (Ed.), *The international guide to speech acquisition* (pp. 516–527). Thomson Delmar Learning.

Huckvale, M. (2016). SFS/WASP [software], version 1.6.

Huffman, M. J. F., Velleman, S. L., & Mervis, C. B. (2019, November). *Relations between articulatory accuracy and phonological processing* [Technical paper]. ASHA 2019 Convention, Orlando, FL, United States.

Hull, F., Mielke, P., Timmons, R., & Willeford, J. (1971). The national speech and hearing survey: Preliminary results. *ASHA, 13*, 501–509.

Hull, F. M., Mielke, Jr., P. W., Willeford, J. A., & Timmons, R. J. (1976). *National speech and hearing survey: Final report* (report 50978). Washington, DC: Bureau of Education for the Handicapped.

Hulme, C., Bowyer-Crane, C., Carroll, J., Duff, F., & Snowling, M. (2012). The causal role of phoneme awareness and letter-sound knowledge in learning to read combining intervention studies with mediation analyses. *Psychological Science, 23*, 572–577.

Hulme, C., Goetz, K., Gooch, D., Adams, J., & Snowling, M. J. (2007). Paired-associate learning, phoneme awareness, and learning to read. *Journal of Experimental Child Psychology, 96*, 150–166.

Humphreys, M. (1880). A contribution to infantile linguistics. *Transactions of the American Philological Association, 11*, 5–17.

Hustad, K. C., Oakes, A., & Allison, K. (2015). Variability and diagnostic accuracy of speech intelligibility scores in children. *Journal of Speech, Language, and Hearing Research, 58*(6), 1695–1707.

Hwa-Froelich, D., Hodson, B. W., & Edwards, H. T. (2002) Characteristics of Vietnamese phonology. *American Journal of Speech-Language Pathology, 11*(3), 264–273.

Hyde, J. S., & Linn, M. C. (1988). Sex differences in verbal ability: A meta-analysis. *Psychological Bulletin, 104*, 53–69.

Hyter, Y. (1996). Ties that bind: The sounds of African American English. *ASHA Special Interest Division 14 Newsletter, 2*, 3–6.

Individuals with Disabilities Education Act (IDEA). (2004). PL No. 108–446, 20 U.S.C. Section 1400 et seq.

Ingram, D. (1976). *Phonological disability in children.* Edward Arnold.

Ingram, D. (1989a). *Phonological disability in children* (2nd ed.). Cole and Whurr.

Ingram, D. (1989b). *First language acquisition: Method, description and explanation.* Cambridge University Press.

Ingram, D., Christensen, L., Veach, S., & Webster, B. (1980). The acquisition of word-initial fricatives and affricates in English by children between 2 and 6 years. In G. H. Yeni-Komshian, J. F. Kavanagh & C. A. Ferguson (Eds.), *Child phonology: Vol 1. Production* (pp. 169–192). Academic Press.

Ingram, J., Pittman, J., & Newman, D. (1985). Developmental and socio-linguistic variation in the speech of Brisbane school children. *Australian Journal of Linguistics, 5*, 233–246.

Invernizzi, M., & Meier, J. (2002–2003). *Phonological awareness literacy screening (PALS: 1–3).* The Virginia State Department of Education and The University of Virginia.

Invernizzi, M., Meier, J., Swank, L., & Juel, C. (2001). *Phonological awareness literacy screening (PALS: K).* The Virginia State Department of Education and The University of Virginia.

Irwin, J. V., & Wong, S. P. (Eds.). (1983). *Phonological development in children 18 to 72 months.* Southern Illinois University Press.

Irwin, R. B., West, J. F., & Trombetta, M. A. (1966). Effectiveness of speech therapy for second grade children with misarticulations: Predictive factors. *Exceptional Children, 32*, 471–479.

Iuzzini-Seigel, J., Hogan, T. P., Guarino, A. J., & Green, J. R. (2015). Reliance on auditory feedback in children with childhood apraxia of speech. *Journal of Communication Disorders, 54*, 32–42.

Iuzzini-Seigel, J., Hogan, T. P., & Green, J. R. (2017). Speech inconsistency in children with childhood apraxia of speech, language impairment, and speech delay: Depends on the stimuli. *Journal of Speech, Language, and Hearing Research, 60*(5), 1194–1210.

Jacks, A., Marquardt, T. P., & Davis, B. L. (2013). Vowel production in childhood and acquired apraxia of speech. In M. J. Ball & F. E. Gibbon (Eds.), *Handbook of vowels and vowel disorders* (pp. 566–600). Psychology Press.

Jakobson, R. (1968). *Child language aphasia and phonological universals.* Mouton.

James, D. (2001). The use of phonological processes in Australian children aged 2 to 7;11 years. *Advances in Speech-Language Pathology, 3*, 109–128.

James, D. (2007). *Hippopotamus is so hard to say: Children's acquisition of polysyllabic words* [Unpublished doctoral dissertation]. University of Sydney.

James, D., McCormack, P., & Butcher, A. (1999). Children's use of phonological processes in the age range of five to seven years. In S. McLeod & L. McAllister (Eds.), *Proceedings of the 1999 Speech Pathology Australia National Conference* (pp. 48–57). Speech Pathology Australia.

James, D., van Doorn, J., & McLeod, S. (2001). Vowel production in mono-, di- and poly-syllabic words in children 3;0 to 7;11 years. In L. Wilson & S. Hewat (Eds.), *Proceedings of the Speech Pathology Australia Conference* (pp. 127–136). Speech Pathology Australia.

James, D., van Doorn, J., & McLeod, S. (2002). Segment production in mono-, di- and polysyllabic words in children aged 3–7 years. In F. Windsor, L. Kelly, & N. Hewlett (Eds.), *Themes in clinical phonetics and linguistics* (pp. 287–298). Erlbaum.

James, D., van Doorn, J., & McLeod, S. (2008). The contribution of polysyllabic words in clinical decision making about children's speech. *Clinical Linguistics & Phonetics, 22*, 345–353.

James, D. G. H., Ferguson, W. A., & Butcher, A. (2016). Assessing children's speech using picture-naming: The influence of differing phonological variables on some speech outcomes. *International Journal of Speech-Language Pathology, 18*(4), 364–377.

Jann, G., Ward, M., & Jann, H. (1964). A longitudinal study of articulation, deglutition and malocclusion. *Journal of Speech and Hearing Disorders, 29*, 424–435.

Jesus, L. M. T., Martinez, M., Santos, J., Hall, A., & Joffe, V. (2019). Comparing traditional and tablet-based intervention for children with speech sound disorders: A randomized controlled trial. *Journal of Speech, Language, and Hearing Research, 62*(11), 4045–4061.

Jimenez, B. C. (1987). Acquisition of Spanish consonants in children aged 3–5 years, 7 months. *Language, Speech, and Hearing Services in Schools, 18*, 357–363.

Johns, D. F., Rohrich, R. J., & Awada, M. (2003). Velopharyngeal incompetence: A guide for clinical evaluation. *Plastic and Reconstructive Surgery, 112*, 1890–1898.

Johnson, C. A., Weston, A. D., & Bain, B. A. (2004). An objective and time efficient method for determining severity of childhood speech delay. *American Journal of Speech-Language Pathology, 13*, 55–65.

Johnson, C. J., Beitchman, J. H., & Brownlie, E. B. (2010). Twenty-year follow-up of children with and without speech-language impairments: Family, educational, occupational, and quality of life outcomes. *American Journal of Speech-Language Pathology, 19*, 51–65.

Johnson, E. P., Pennington, B. F., Lowenstein, J. H., & Nittrouer, S. (2011). Sensitivity to structure in the speech signal by children with speech sound disorder and reading disability. *Journal of Communication Disorders, 44*, 294–314.

Johnson, N. C. L., & Sandy, J. R. (1999). Tooth position and speech: Is there a relationship? *The Angle Orthodontist, 69*, 306–310.

Johnston, R. S., Anderson, M., & Holligan, C. (1996). Knowledge of the alphabet and explicit awareness of phonemes in pre-readers: The nature of the relationship. *Reading and Writing: An Interdisciplinary Journal, 8*, 217–234.

Jordan, L., Hardy, J., & Morris, H. (1978). Performance of children with good and poor articulation on tasks of tongue placement. *Journal of Speech and Hearing Research, 21*, 429–439.

Juel, C. (1988). Learning to read and write: A longitudinal study of 54 children from first through fourth grades. *Journal of Educational Psychology, 80*, 437–447.

Justice, L., Kaderavek, J. J., Bowles, R. J., & Grimm, K. (2005). Language impairment, parent-child shared reading, and phonological awareness: A feasibility study. *Topics in Early Childhood Special Education, 25*, 143–156.

Justice, L. M., & Ezell, H. K. (2004). Print referencing: An emergent literacy enhancement strategy and its clinical applications. *Language, Speech, and Hearing Services in Schools, 35*, 185–193.

Justice, L. M., McGinty, A. S., Cabell, S. Q., Kilday, C. R., Knighton, K., & Huffman, G. (2010). Language and literacy curriculum support for preschoolers who are academically at risk: A feasibility study. *Language, Speech, and Hearing Services in Schools, 41*, 161–178.

Justice, L. M., Pence, K., Bowles, R. B., & Wiggins, A. (2006). An investigation of four hypotheses concerning the order by which 4-year-old children learn the alphabet letters. *Early Childhood Research Quarterly, 21*, 374–389.

Kager, R. (1999). *Optimality theory.* Cambridge University Press.

Kaipa, R., & Peterson, A. M. (2016). A systematic review of treatment intensity in speech disorders. *International Journal of Speech-Language Pathology, 18*(6), 507–520.

Kaipa, R., Robb, M. P., O'Beirne, G. A., & Allison, R. S. (2012). Recovery of speech following total glossectomy: An acoustic and perceptual appraisal. *International Journal of Speech-Language Pathology, 14*(1), 24–34.

Kantner, C. E., & West, R. (1960). *Phonetics.* Harper & Row.

Kapoor, V., Douglas, P. S., Hill, P. S., Walsh, L. J., & Tennant, M. (2018). Frenotomy for tongue-tie in Australian children, 2006–2016: An increasing problem. *The Medical Journal of Australia, 208*(2), 88–89.

Karlsson, H. B., Shriberg, L. D., Flipsen, Jr., P., & McSweeny, J. L. (2002). Acoustic phenotypes for speech-genetics studies: Toward an acoustic marker for residual /s/ distortions. *Clinical Linguistics & Phonetics, 16*, 403–424.

Kaufman, N. (1995). *Kaufman speech praxis test for children.* Wayne State University Press.

Kaya, V., & Aytekin, A. (2017). Effects of pacifier use on transition to full breastfeeding and sucking skills in preterm infants: A randomized controlled trial. *Journal of Clinical Nursing, 26*, 2055–2063.

Kayser, H. (1995). Interpreters. In H. Kayser (Ed.), *Bilingual speech-language pathology: An Hispanic focus* (pp. 207–221). Singular Publishing.

Keating, D., Turrell, G., & Ozanne, A. (2001). Childhood speech disorders: Reported prevalence, comorbidity and socioeconomic profile. *Journal of Pediatric Child Health, 37*, 431–436.

Kehoe, M. (1997). Stress error patterns in English-speaking children's word productions. *Clinical Linguistics & Phonetics, 11*, 389–409.

Kehoe, M. M. (2001). Prosodic patterns in children's multisyllabic word productions. *Language, Speech, and Hearing Services in Schools, 32*, 284–294.

Kemaloglu, Y. K., Kobayashi, T., & Nakajima, T. (1999). Analysis of the craniofacial skeleton in cleft children with otitis media with effusion. *International Journal of Pediatric Otorhinolaryngology, 47*, 57–69.

Kenney, K., & Prather, E. (1986). Articulation in preschool children: Consistency of productions. *Journal of Speech and Hearing Research, 29,* 29–36.

Kent, R. D. (1976). Anatomical and neuromuscular maturation of the speech mechanism: Evidence from acoustic studies. *Journal of Speech and Hearing Research, 19,* 421–447.

Kent, R. D. (1982). Contextual facilitation of correct sound production. *Language, Speech, and Hearing Services in Schools, 13,* 66–76.

Kent, R. D., Martin, R. E., & Sufit, R. L. (1990). Oral sensation: A review and clinical prospective. In H. Winitz (Ed.), *Human communication and its disorders: A review* (pp. 135–191). Ablex.

Kent, R. D., & Minifie, F. D. (1977). Coarticulation in recent speech production models. *Journal of Phonetics, 5,* 115–133.

Kent, R. D., Miolo, G., & Bloedel, S. (1994). The intelligibility of children's speech: A review of evaluation procedures. *American Journal of Speech-Language Pathology, 3,* 81–95.

Kent, R. D., & Moll, K. L. (1972). Cinefluorographic analyses of selected lingual consonants. *Journal of Speech and Hearing Research, 15,* 453–473.

Kent, R. D., & Moll, K. L. (1975). Articulatory timing in selected consonant sequences. *Brain and Language, 2,* 304–323.

Kent, R. D., & Netsell, R. (1972). Effects of stress contrasts on certain articulatory parameters. *Phonetica, 24,* 23–44.

Kent, R. D., & Rountrey, C. (2020). What acoustic studies tell us about vowels in developing and disordered speech. *American Journal of Speech-Language Pathology, 29,* 1748–1778.

Kent, R. D., & Tilkens, C. (2007). Oromotor foundations of speech acquisition. In S. McLeod (Ed.), *International guide to speech acquisition* (pp. 8–13). Thomson Delmar Learning.

Kent, R. D., & Vorperian, H. K. (2013). Speech impairment in Down syndrome: A review. *Journal of Speech, Language, and Hearing Research, 56,* 178–210.

Khamis-Dakwar, R., & Khattab, G. (2014). Cultural and linguistic considerations in language assessment and intervention for Levantine Arabic speaking children. *Perspectives on Communication Disorders and Sciences in Culturally and Linguistically Diverse Populations, 21,* 78–88.

Khan, L. M. (1982). Major phonological processes. *Language, Speech, and Hearing Services in Schools, 13,* 77–85.

Khan, L. M. (1985). *Basics of phonological analysis: A programmed learning test.* College Hill Press.

Khan, L. M., & Lewis, N. P. (1986). *Khan-Lewis phonological analysis.* American Guidance Service.

Khan, L. M., & Lewis, N. P. (2002). *Khan-Lewis phonological analysis* (2nd ed.). American Guidance Service.

Khan, L. M., & Lewis, N. P. (2015). *Khan-Lewis phonological analysis* (3rd ed.). Psycorp.

Khattab, G. (2006). Phonological acquisition by Arabic-English bilingual children. In Z. Hua & B. J. Dodd (Eds.), *Phonological development and disorders in children: A multilingual perspective* (pp. 383–412). Multilingual Matters Ltd.

Khinda, V., & Grewal, N. (1999). Relationship of tongue-thrust swallowing and anterior open bite with articulation disorders: A clinical study. *Journal of the Indian Society of Pedodontia and Preventive Dentistry, 17,* 33–39.

Kilminster, M. G. E., & Laird, E. M. (1978). Articulation development in children aged three to nine years. *Australian Journal of Human Communication Disorders, 6,* 23–30.

Kim, M., & Pae, S. (2007). Korean speech acquisition. In S. McLeod (Ed.), *The international guide to speech acquisition* (pp. 472–482). Thomson Delmar Learning.

Kindler, A. (2001). *Survey of the states' LEP students 2000–2001 summary report.* National Clearinghouse for English Language Acquisition.

Kiparsky, P., & Menn, L. (1977). On the acquisition of phonology. In J. MacNamara (Ed.), *Language learning and thought* (pp. 47–78). Academic Press.

Kirk, C., & Gillon, G. T. (2007). Longitudinal effects of phonological awareness intervention on morphological awareness in children with speech impairment. *Language, Speech, and Hearing Services in Schools, 38,* 342–252.

Kirk, C., & Vigeland, L. (2014). A psychometric review of norm-referenced tests used to assess phonological error patterns. *Language, Speech, and Hearing Services in Schools, 45,* 365–377.

Kirk, C., & Vigeland, L. (2015). Content coverage of single-word tests used to assess common phonological error patterns. *Language, Speech, and Hearing Services in Schools, 46,* 14–29.

Kirtley, C., Bryant, P., MacLean, M., & Bradley, L. (1989). Rhyme, rime, and the onset of reading. *Journal of Experimental Child Psychology, 48,* 224–245.

Kisatsky, T. (1967). The prognostic value of Carter-Buck tests in measuring articulation skills in selected kindergarten children. *Exceptional Children, 34,* 81–85.

Klaiman, P., Witzel, M. A., Margar-Bacal, F., & Munro, I. R. (1988). Changes in aesthetic appearance and intelligibility of speech after partial glossectomy in patients with Down syndrome. *Plastic and Reconstructive Surgery, 82,* 403–408.

Kleffner, F. (1952). *A comparison of the reactions of a group of fourth grade children to recorded examples of defective and nondefective articulation* [Unpublished doctoral thesis]. University of Wisconsin–Madison.

Klein, E. S. (1996). Phonological/traditional approaches to articulation therapy: A retrospective group comparison. *Language, Speech, and Hearing Services in Schools, 27,* 314–323.

Klein, E. S., & Flint, C. B. (2006). Measurement of intelligibility in disordered speech. *Language, Speech, and Hearing Services in Schools, 37,* 191–199.

Klein, H. B., & Liu-Shea, M. (2009). Between word simplification patterns in the continuous speech of children with speech sound disorders. *Language, Speech, and Hearing Services in Schools, 40,* 17–30.

Koch, H. (1956). Sibling influence on children's speech. *Journal of Speech and Hearing Disorders, 21,* 322–329.

Koegel, L. K., Koegel, R. L., & Ingham, J. C. (1986). Programming rapid generalization of correct articulation through self-monitoring procedures. *Journal of Speech and Hearing Disorders, 51,* 24–32.

Koegel, R., Koegel, L., Van Voy, K., & Ingham, J. (1988). Within-clinic versus outside-of-clinic self-monitoring of articulation to promote generalization. *Journal of Speech and Hearing Disorders, 53,* 392–399.

Kohnert, K., & Derr, A. (2012). Language intervention with bilingual children. In B. Goldstein (Ed.), *Bilingual language development and disorders in Spanish-English speakers* (2nd ed., pp. 337–356). Paul H. Brookes Publishing Co.

Kohnert, K., Yim, D., Nett, K., Kan, P. F., & Duran, L. (2005). Intervention with linguistically diverse preschool children: A focus on developing home language(s). *Language, Speech, and Hearing Services in Schools, 36,* 251–263.

Koutsoftas, A., Harmon, M., & Gray, S. (2009). The effect of tier 2 intervention for phonemic awareness in a response-to-intervention model in low-income preschool classrooms. *Language, Speech, and Hearing Services in Schools, 40,* 116–130.

Kristoffersen, K. E., Garmann, N. G., & Simonsen, H. G. (2014). Consonant production and intelligibility in Cri du Chat syndrome. *Clinical Linguistics & Phonetics, 28*(10), 769–784.

Kronvall, E., & Diehl, C. (1954). The relationship of auditory discrimination to articulatory defects of children with no known organic impairment. *Journal of Speech and Hearing Disorders, 19,* 335–338.

Krueger, B. I. (2019). Eligibility and speech sound disorders: Assessment of social impact. *Perspectives of the ASHA Special Interest Groups, SIG 1, 4*(1), 85–90.

Kuhl, P. K. (2000). A new view of language acquisition. *Proceedings of the National Academy of Sciences, 97,* 11850–11857.

Kumin, L. (1994). Intelligibility of speech in children with Down syndrome in natural settings: Parents' perspective. *Perceptual and Motor Skills, 78,* 307–313.

Kumin, L., Council, C., & Goodman, M. (1994). A longitudinal study of emergence of phonemes in children with Down syndrome. *Journal of Communication Disorders, 27,* 293–303.

Kummer, A. (2009, November). *Ankyloglossia: An effect on speech . . . or not* [Paper presentation]. ASHA 2009 Convention, New Orleans, LA, United States.

Kummer, A. W. (2020). *Cleft palate and craniofacial conditions. A comprehensive guide to clinical management* (4th ed.). Jones & Bartlett Learning.

Kummer, A. W., Myer III, C. M., Smith, M. E., & Shott, S. R. (1993). Changes in nasal resonance secondary to adenotonsillectomy. *American Journal of Otolaryngology, 14*(4), 285–290.

Kwiatkowski, J., & Shriberg, L. D. (1993). Speech normalization in developmental phonological disorders: A retrospective study of capability-focus theory. *Language, Speech, and Hearing Services in Schools, 24,* 10–18.

Kwiatkowski, J., & Shriberg, L. D. (1998). The capability-focus treatment framework for child speech disorders. *American Journal of Speech-Language Pathology, 7,* 27–38.

Labov, W. (1969). The logic of non-standard English. In J. Alatis (Ed.), *Linguistics and the teaching of standard English to speakers of other languages and dialects: Georgetown University round table on languages and linguistics* (pp. 1–44). Georgetown University Press.

Labov, W. (1991). The three dialects of English. In P. Eckert (Ed.), *New ways of analyzing sound change* (pp. 1–44). Academic Press.

Ladefoged, P. (1971). *Preliminaries to linguistic phonetics.* University of Chicago Press.

Ladefoged, P. (1975). *A course in phonetics.* Harcourt Brace Jovanovich.

Ladefoged, P. (1993). *A course in phonetics* (3rd ed.). Harcourt Brace.

Ladefoged, P. (2005). *Vowels and consonants* (2nd ed.). Blackwell.

Laine, T., Jaroma, M., & Linnasalo, A. L. (1987). Relationships between interincisal occlusion and articulatory components of speech. *Folia Phoniatrica, 39,* 78–86.

Laitinen, J., Haapanen, M.-L., Paaso, M., Pulkkinen, J., Heltovaara, A., & Ranta, R. (1998). Occurrence of dental consonant misarticulations in different cleft types. *Folia Phoniatrica et Logopedica, 50,* 92–100.

Langdon, H., & Cheng, L. R. L. (2002). *Collaborating with interpreters and translators.* Thinking Publications.

Lanza, J. R., & Flahive, L. K. (2007). *Speech and language activities for young learners.* LinguiSystems.

Lapko, L., & Bankson, N. (1975). Relationship between auditory discrimination, articulation stimulability and consistency of misarticulation. *Perceptual and Motor Skills, 40,* 171–177.

Lapointe, L., & Wertz, R. (1974). Oral-movement abilities and articulatory characteristics of brain-injured adults. *Perceptual and Motor Skills, 39,* 39–46.

LaRiviere, C., Winitz, H., Reeds, J., & Herriman, E. (1974). The conceptual reality of selected distinctive features. *Journal of Speech and Hearing Research, 17,* 122–133.

Lasky, R. E., & Williams, A. L. (2005). The development of the auditory system from conception to term. *NeoReviews, 6*(3), e141–e152.

Lass, N. J., & Pannbacker, M. (2008). The application of evidence-based practice to nonspeech oral-motor treatments. *Language, Speech, and Hearing Services in Schools, 39,* 408–421.

Lau Remedies, Office of Civil Rights. (1975). Task force findings specifying remedies available for eliminating past educational practices rules unlawful under *Lau v. Nichols,* IX, pt. 5.

Lau v. Nichols. (1974). 414 U.S. S. Ct. 563.

Law, J., Boyle, J., Harris, F., Harkness, A., & Nye, C. (1998). Screening for speech and language delay: A systematic review of the literature. *Health Technology and Assessment, 2*(9), 1–183.

Law, J., Garrett, Z., & Nye, C. (2004). The efficacy of treatment for children with developmental speech and language delay disorders: A meta-analysis. *Journal of Speech and Hearing Research, 47,* 924–943.

Lawrence, K. (2014). Embedding a speech sound intervention in shared storybook reading. *Contemporary Issues in Communication Science and Disorders, 41,* 221–234.

Laws, G., & Hall, A. (2014). Early hearing loss and language abilities in children with Down syndrome. *International Journal of Language & Communication Disorders, 49*(3), 333–342.

Leap, W. (1981). American Indian languages. In C. Ferguson & S. Heath (Eds.), *Language in the USA* (pp. 116–144). Cambridge University Press.

Lebrun, Y. (1985). Tongue thrust, tongue tip position at rest, and stigmatism: A review. *Journal of Communication Disorders, 18,* 305–312.

Leder, S., & Lerman, J. W. (1985). Some acoustic evidence for vocal abuse in adult speakers with repaired cleft palate. *Laryngoscope, 95,* 837–840.

Leder, S., & Spitzer, J. (1990). A perceptual evaluation of the speech of adventitiously deaf adult males. *Ear and Hearing, 11,* 169–175.

Lee, A., Gibbon, F. E., Kearney, E., & Murphy, D. (2014). Tongue-palate contact during selected vowels in children with speech sound disorders. *International Journal of Speech-Language Pathology, 16*(6), 562–570.

Lee, A. S. Y., & Gibbon, F. E. (2015). Non-speech oral motor treatment for children with developmental speech sound disorders. *Cochrane Database of Systematic Reviews, 3*(CD009383). doi:10.1002/14651858.CD009383.pub2

Lee, S. A. S., & Sancibrian, S. (2013). Effectiveness of two different approaches to accent modification services for non-native English speakers of Korean background. *Perspectives on Communication Disorders and Sciences in Culturally and Linguistically Diverse Populations, 20*(3), 127–136.

Lehiste, I. (1970). *Suprasegmentals.* MIT Press.

Leitão, S., & Fletcher, J., (2004). Literacy outcomes for students with speech impairment: Long-term follow-up. *International Journal of Language & Communication Disorders, 39,* 245–256.

Lenden, J. M., & Flipsen, Jr., P. (2007). Prosody and voice characteristics of children with cochlear implants. *Journal of Communication Disorders, 40,* 66–81.

Leonard, L. (1973). The nature of deviant articulation. *Journal of Speech and Hearing Disorders, 38,* 156–161.

Leonard, L. B., & Leonard, J. S. (1985). The contribution of phonetic context to an unusual phonological pattern: A case study. *Language, Speech, and Hearing Services in Schools, 16,* 110–118.

Leonard, L. B., Rowan, L. E., Morris, B., & Fey, M. E. (1982). Intra-word phonological variability in young children. *Journal of Child Language, 9,* 55–69.

Leonard, R. J. (1994). Characteristics of speech in speakers with oral/oralpharyngeal ablation. In J. Bernthal & N. Bankson (Eds.), *Child phonology: Characteristics, assessment, and intervention with special populations* (pp. 54–78). Thieme Medical Publishers.

Leopold, W. (1939–1949). *Speech development of a bilingual child: A linguist's record. Vol. 1: Vocabulary growth in the first two years (1939), Vol. 2: Sound learning in the first two years (1947), Vol. 3: Grammar and general problems in the first two years (1949), Vol. 4: Diary from age two (1949).* Northwestern University Press.

Leopold, W. (1947). *Speech development of a bilingual child: A linguist's record. Vol. 2: Sound learning in the first two years.* Northwestern University Press.

Levitt, H., & Stromberg, H. (1983). Segmental characteristics of speech of hearing-impaired children: Factors affecting intelligibility. In I. Hochberg, H. Levitt, & M. Osberger (Eds.), *Speech of the hearing impaired* (pp. 53–73). University Park Press.

Lewis, B. A. (2009). Genetic influences on speech sound disorders. In R. Paul & P. Flipsen, Jr. (Eds.), *Speech sound disorders in children: In honor of Lawrence D. Shriberg* (pp. 51–70). Plural Publishing.

Lewis, B. A., Avrich, A. A., Freebairn, L. A., Taylor, H. G., Iyengar, S. K., & Stein, C. M. (2011). Subtyping children with speech sound disorders by endophenotypes. *Topics in Language Disorders, 31,* 112–127.

Lewis, B. A., Ekelman, B., & Aram, D. (1989). A familial study of severe phonological disorders. *Journal of Speech and Hearing Research, 32,* 713–724.

Lewis, B. A., Freebairn, L. A., Hansen, A. J., Iyengar, S. K., & Taylor, H. G. (2004). School-age follow-up of children with childhood apraxia of speech. *Language, Speech, and Hearing Services in Schools, 35*(2), 122–140.

Lewis, B. A., Freebairn, L. A., Hansen, A. J., Miscimarra, L., Iyengar, S. K., & Taylor, H. G. (2007). Speech and language skills of parents of children with speech sound disorders. *American Journal of Speech-Language Pathology, 16,* 108–118.

Lewis, B. A., Freebairn, L. A., Hansen, A. J., Stein, C. M., Shriberg, L. D., Iyengar, S. K., & Taylor, H. G. (2006a). Dimensions of early speech sound disorders: A factor analytic study. *Journal of Communication Disorders, 39,* 139–157.

Lewis, B. A., Freebairn, L. A., & Taylor, H. G. (2000). Follow-up of children with early expressive phonology disorders. *Journal of Learning Disabilities, 33,* 433–444.

Lewis, B. A., & Freebairn-Farr, L. (1991, November). *Preschool phonology disorders at school age, adolescence, and adulthood* [Paper presentation]. ASHA 1991 Convention, Atlanta, GA, United States.

Lewis, B. A., & Iyengar, S. (2018, November). *Genetics of speech sound disorders and co-morbid disorders: A new era of discovery* [Paper presentation]. ASHA 2018 Convention, Boston, MA, United States.

Li, C., & Thompson, S. (1977). The acquisition of tone in Mandarin-speaking children. *Journal of Child Language, 4,* 185–199.

Lieberman, P. (1967). *Intonation, perception and language.* MIT Press.

Lin, S., & Demuth, K. (2015). Children's acquisition of English onset and coda /l/: Articulatory evidence. *Journal of Speech, Language, and Hearing Research, 58,* 13–27.

Lindblom, B. (1963). Spectrographic study of vowel reduction. *Journal of the Acoustical Society of America, 35,* 1773–1781.

Lindblom, B. (1990). Explaining phonetic variation: A sketch of the H&H theory. In W. J. Hardcastle & A. Marchal (Eds.), *Speech production and speech modeling* (pp. 403–439). Kluwer.

Ling, D. (1989). *Foundations of spoken language for hearing-impaired children.* Washington, DC: Alexander Graham Bell Association for the Deaf.

Lippke, B. A., Dickey, S. E., Selmar, J. W., & Sodar, A.L. (1997). *Photo articulation test* (3rd ed.). Pro-Ed.

Lipski, J. (2008). *Varieties of Spanish in the United States.* Georgetown University Press.

Lively, S. E., Pisoni, D. B., Van Summers, W., & Bernacki, R. H. (1993). Effects of cognitive workload on speech production: Acoustic analysis and perceptual consequences. *Journal of the Acoustical Society of America, 93*(5), 2962–2973.

Lleó, C. (1990). Homonymy and reduplication: On the extended availability of two strategies in phonological acquisition. *Journal of Child Language, 17,* 267–278.

Lleó, C., & Kehoe, M. (2002). On the interaction of phonological systems in child bilingual acquisition. *International Journal of Bilingualism, 6,* 233–237.

Lleó, C., Kuchenbrandt, I., Kehoe, M., & Trujillo, C. (2003). Syllable final consonants in Spanish and German monolingual and bilingual acquisition. In N. Müller (Ed.), *(In)vulnerable domains in multilingualism* (pp. 191–220). John Benjamins Publishing.

Lleó, C., & Prinz, M. (1996). Consonant clusters in child phonology and the directionality of syllable structure assignment. *Journal of Child Language, 23,* 31–56.

Locke, J. (1980a). The inference of speech perception in the phonologically disordered child: Part I. A rationale, some criteria, the conventional tests. *Journal of Speech and Hearing Disorders, 45,* 431–444.

Locke, J. (1980b). The inference of speech perception in the phonologically disordered child: Part II. Some clinically novel procedures, their use, some findings. *Journal of Speech and Hearing Disorders, 45,* 445–468.

Locke, J. (2002). Vocal development in the human infant: Functions and phonetics. In F. Windsor, M. L. Kelly, & N. Hewlett (Eds.), *Investigations in clinical phonetics and linguistics* (pp. 243–256). Erlbaum.

Locke, J., & Kutz, K. (1975). Memory for speech and speech for memory. *Journal of Speech and Hearing Research, 18,* 179–191.

Locke, J., & Mather, P. (1987, November). *Genetic factors in phonology: Evidence from monozygotic and dizygotic twins* [Paper presentation]. ASHA 1987 Convention, New Orleans, LA, United States.

Lof, G., & Synan, S. (1997). Is there a speech discrimination/perception link to disordered articulation and phonology? A review of 80 years of literature. *Contemporary Issues in Communication Science and Disorders, 24,* 63–77.

Lof, G. L. (2010). Science-based practice and the speech-language pathologist. *International Journal of Speech-Language Pathology, 13,* 189–196.

Lof, G. L., & Watson, M. M. (2008). A nationwide survey of nonspeech oral motor exercise use: Implications for evidence-based practice. *Language, Speech, and Hearing Services in Schools, 39,* 392–407.

Lonigan, C. J., Anthony, J. L., Phillips, B. M., Purpura, D. J., Wilson, S. B., & McQueen, J. D. (2009). The nature of preschool phonological processing abilities and their relations to vocabulary, general cognitive abilities, and print knowledge. *Journal of Educational Psychology, 101,* 345–358.

Lonigan, C. J., Burgess, S. R., Anthony, J. L., & Barker, T. A. (1998). Development of phonological sensitivity in 2- to 5-year-old children. *Journal of Educational Psychology, 90,* 294–311.

Lonigan, C. J., Farver, J. M., Phillips, B. M., & Clancy-Menchetti, J. (2011). Promoting the development of preschool children's emergent literacy skills: A randomized evaluation of a literacy-focused curriculum and two professional development models. *Reading and Writing, 24,* 305–337.

Lonigan, C. J., & Vasey, M. W. (2009). Negative affectivity, effortful control, and attention to threat-relevant stimuli. *Journal of Abnormal Child Psychology, 37*(3), 387–399.

Long, S. (2001). About time: A comparison of computerized and manual procedures for grammatical and phonological analysis. *Clinical Linguistics & Phonetics, 15,* 399–426.

Long, S. H., Fey, M. E., & Channell, R. W. (2002). *Computerized profiling (version CP941.exe).* Case Western Reserve University.

Lorwatanapongsa, P., & Maroonroge, S. (2007). Thai speech acquisition. In S. McLeod (Ed.), *The international guide to speech acquisition* (pp. 554–565). Thomson Delmar Learning.

Louttit, C. M., & Halls, E. C. (1936). Survey of speech defects among public school children of Indiana. *Journal of Speech Disorders, 1*, 73–80.

Lowe, R. J., Knutson, P. J., & Monson, M. A. (1985). Incidence of fronting in preschool children. *Language, Speech, and Hearing Services in Schools, 16*, 119–123.

Lynch, E. (2004). Developing cross-cultural competence. In E. Lynch & M. Hanson (Eds.), *Developing cross-cultural competence: A guide for working with children and their families* (3rd ed., pp. 41–77). Paul H. Brookes Publishing Co.

Maas, E., Butalla, C. E., & Farinella, K. A. (2012). Feedback frequency in treatment for childhood apraxia of speech. *American Journal of Speech-Language Pathology, 21*, 239–257.

Maas, E., & Farinella, K. A. (2012). Random versus blocked practice in treatment for childhood apraxia of speech. *Journal of Speech, Language, and Hearing Research, 55*, 561–578.

Maas, E., Gildersleeve-Neumann, C. E., Jakielski, K. J., & Stoekel, R. (2014). Motor-based intervention protocols in treatment of childhood apraxia of speech (CAS). *Current Developmental Disorders Reports, 1*, 197–206.

Maas, E., Robin, D. A., Austermann Hula, S. N., Freedman, S. E., Wulf, G., Ballard, K. J., & Schmidt, R. A. (2008). Principles of motor learning in treatment of motor speech disorders. *American Journal of Speech-Language Pathology, 17*, 277–298.

Maassen, B., Nijland, L., & van der Meulen, S. (2001). Coarticulation within and between syllables by children with developmental apraxia of speech. *Clinical Linguistics & Phonetics, 15*(1 & 2), 145–150.

Macken, M. (1995). Phonological acquisition. In J. A. Goldsmith (Ed.), *The handbook of phonological theory* (pp. 671–696). Blackwell.

Macken, M. A. (1980a). The child's lexical representation: The "puzzle, puddle, pickle" evidence. *Journal of Linguistics, 16*, 1–17.

Macken, M. A. (1980b). Aspects of the acquisition of stop systems: A cross-linguistic perspective. In G. H. Yeni-Komshian, J. F. Kavanagh, & C. A. Ferguson (Eds.), *Child phonology: Volume 1. Production* (pp. 143–168). Academic Press.

Maclagan, M., & Gillon, G. T. (2007). New Zealand English speech acquisition. In S. McLeod (Ed.), *The international guide to speech acquisition* (pp. 257–268). Thomson Delmar Learning.

MacNeilage, P. F. (1972). Speech physiology. In H. H. Gilbert (Ed.), *Speech and cortical functioning* (pp. 1–72). Academic Press.

MacNeilage, P. F., & Davis, B. L. (1993). A motor learning perspective on speech and babbling. In B. Boysson-Bardies, S. Schoen, P. Jusczyk, P. MacNeilage, & J. Morton (Eds.), *Changes in speech and face processing in infancy: A glimpse at developmental mechanisms of cognition* (pp. 341–352). Kluwer.

Macrae, T., & Tyler, A. A. (2014). Speech abilities in preschool children with speech sound disorders with and without co-occurring language impairment. *Language, Speech, and Hearing Services in Schools, 45*, 302–313.

Maddieson, I., & Precoda, K. (1991). *The UCLA phonological segment inventory database, UPSID-PC.* http://phonetics.linguistics.ucla.edu/sales/software.htm

Madell, J. R., Sislian, N., & Hoffman, R. (2004). Speech perception for cochlear implant patients using hearing aids on the unimplanted ear. *International Congress Series, 1273*, 223–226.

Maez, L. (1981). *Spanish as a first language* [Unpublished doctoral dissertation]. University of California, Santa Barbara.

Majnemer, A., & Rosenblatt, B. (1994). Reliability of parental recall of developmental milestones. *Pediatric Neurology, 10*, 304–308.

Major, E. M., & Bernhardt, B. H. (1998). Metaphonological skills of children with phonological disorders before and after phonological and metaphonological intervention. *International Journal of Language & Communication Disorders, 33*, 413–444.

Mann, V. A., & Foy, J. G. (2007). Speech development patterns and phonological awareness in preschool children. *Annals of Dyslexia, 57*, 51–74.

Mantie-Kozlowski, A., & Pitt, K. (2014). Treating myofunctional disorders: A multiple baseline treatment using electropalatography. *American Journal of Speech-Language Pathology, 23*, 520–529.

Marchant, C. D., Shurin, P. A., Turczyk, V. A., Wasikowski, D. E., Tutihasi, M. A., & Kinney, S. E. (1984). Course and outcome of otitis media in early infancy: A prospective study. *Journal of Pediatrics, 104*, 826–831.

Marchesan, I. Q. (2012). Lingual frenulum protocol. *International Journal of Orofacial Myology, 38*, 89–103.

Marder, L., & Cholmain, C. N. (2006). Promoting language development for children with Down's syndrome. *Current Pediatrics, 16,* 495–500.

Margar-Bacal, F., Witzel, M. A., & Munro, I. (1987). Speech intelligibility after partial glossectomy in children with Down's syndrome. *Plastic and Reconstructive Surgery, 79,* 44–47.

Marquardt, T. P., Jacks, A., & Davis, B. L. (2004). Token-to-token variability in developmental apraxia of speech: Three longitudinal case studies. *Clinical Linguistics & Phonetics, 18,* 127–144.

Marquardt, T. P., Sussman, H. M., Snow, T., & Jacks, A. (2002). The integrity of the syllable in developmental apraxia of speech. *Journal of Communication Disorders, 35*(1), 31–49.

Martinelli, R. L. D. C., Marchesan, I. Q., & Berretin-Felix, G. (2012). Lingual frenulum protocol with scores for infants. *International Journal of Orofacial Myology, 38,* 104–112.

Martin Luther King Junior Elementary School Children et al. v. Ann Arbor School District Board, Civil Action No. 7-71861, 451 F. Supp. 1324 (E. D. Mich. 1978).

Marunick, M., & Tselios, N. (2004). The efficacy of palatal augmentation prostheses for speech and swallowing in patients undergoing glossectomy: A review of the literature. *Journal of Prosthetic Dentistry, 91,* 67–74.

Maryn, Y., Van Lierde, K., De Bodt, M., & Van Cauwenberge, P. (2004). The effects of adenoidectomy and tonsillectomy on speech and nasal resonance. *Folia Phoniatrica et Logopedica, 56,* 182–191.

Mase, D. (1946). Etiology of articulatory speech defects. *Teacher's College Contribution to Education, 921.* Columbia University.

Mason, R. (1988). Orthodontic perspectives on orofacial myofunctional therapy. *International Journal of Orofacial Myology, 14,* 49–55.

Mason, R., & Proffit, W. (1974). The tongue-thrust controversy: Background and recommendations. *Journal of Speech and Hearing Disorders, 39,* 115–132.

Mason, R., & Wickwire, N. (1978). Examining for orofacial variations. *Communiqué, 8,* 2–26.

Mason, R. M. (2011). Myths that persist about orofacial myology. *International Journal of Orofacial Myology, 37,* 26–38.

Masso, S., Baker E., McLeod S., & McCormack J. (2014). Identifying phonological awareness difficulties in preschool children with speech sound disorders. *Speech, Language and Hearing, 17,* 58–68.

Masso, S., Baker, E., McLeod, S., & Wang, C. (2017). Polysyllable speech accuracy and predictors of later literacy development in preschool children with speech sound disorders. *Journal of Speech, Language, and Hearing Research, 60*(7), 1877–1890.

Masso, S., McLeod, S., Baker, E., & McCormack, J. (2016). Polysyllable productions in preschool children with speech sound disorders: Error categories and the framework of polysyllable maturity. *International Journal of Speech-Language Pathology, 18*(3), 272–287.

Masso, S., McLeod, S., Wang, C., Baker, E., & McCormack, J. (2017). Longitudinal changes in polysyllable maturity in preschool children with phonologically-based speech sound disorders. *Clinical Linguistics & Phonetics, 31*(6), 424–439.

Masterson, J. (1993). Classroom-based phonological intervention. *American Journal of Speech-Language Pathology, 2,* 5–9.

Masterson, J. J., & Daniels, D. L. (1991). Motoric versus contrastive approaches to phonology therapy: A case study. *Child Language Teaching and Therapy, 7,* 127–140.

Masterson, J., Long, S., & Buder, E. (1998). Instrumentation in clinical phonology. In J. Bernthal & N. Bankson (Eds.), *Articulation and phonological disorders* (4th ed., pp. 378–406). Allyn & Bacon.

Matheny, A., & Bruggeman, C. (1973). Children's speech: Heredity components and sex differences. *Folia Phoniatrica, 25,* 442–449.

Matheny, N., & Panagos, J. (1978). Comparing the effects of articulation and syntax programs on syntax and articulation improvement. *Language, Speech, and Hearing Services in Schools, 9,* 57–61.

Matsune, S., Sando, I., & Takahashi, H. (1991). Insertion of the tensor veli palatini muscle into the Eustachian tube cartilage in cleft palate cases. *Annals of Otology, Rhinology, and Laryngology, 100,* 439–446.

Maxwell, E. M. (1984). On determining underlying phonological representations of children: A critique of the current theories. *Phonological theory and the misarticulating child, ASHA Monograph, 22,* 18–29.

Mayer, M. (1969). *Frog Where Are You?* Penguin Books.

Mayo, C., Scobbie, J. M., Hewlett, N., & Waters, D. (2003). The influence of phonemic awareness development on acoustic cue weighting strategies in children's speech perception. *Journal of Speech, Language, and Hearing Research, 46*, 1184–1196.

McAllister, A. (2003). Voice disorders in children with oral motor dysfunction: Perceptual evaluation pre and post oral motor therapy. *Logopedics, Phoniatrics, and Vocology, 28*, 117–125.

McAllister Byun, T., & Campbell, H. (2016). Differential effects of visual-acoustic biofeedback intervention for residual speech errors. *Frontiers in Human Neuroscience, 10*(567), 1–17.

McAllister Byun, T., & Hitchcock, E. R. (2012). Investigating the use of traditional and spectral biofeedback approaches to intervention for /r/ misarticulation. *American Journal of Speech-Language Pathology, 21*, 207–221.

McAllister Byun, T., Hitchcock, E. R., & Swartz, M. T. (2014). Retroflex versus bunched in treatment for rhotic misarticulation: Evidence from ultrasound biofeedback intervention. *Journal of Speech, Language, and Hearing Research, 57*, 2116–2130.

McAllister Byun, T., Swartz, M. T., Halpin, P. F., Szeredi, D., & Maas, E. (2016). Direction of attentional focus in biofeedback treatment for /r/ misarticulation. *International Journal of Language & Communication Disorders, 51*(4), 384–401.

McAuliffe, M. J., & Cornwell, P. L. (2008). Intervention for lateral /s/ using electropalatography (EPG) biofeedback and an intensive motor learning approach: A case report. *International Journal of Language & Communication Disorders, 43*, 219–229.

McCabe, P., Macdonald, A. G., van Rees, L. J., Ballard, K. J., & Arciuli, J. (2014). Orthographically sensitive treatment for dysprosody in children with childhood apraxia of speech using ReST intervention. *Developmental Neurorehabilitation, 17*(2), 137–146.

McCabe, P., Thomas, D. C., & Murray, E. (2020). Rapid syllable transition treatment–A treatment for childhood apraxia of speech and other pediatric motor speech disorders. *Perspectives of the ASHA Special Interest Groups, 5*, 821–830.

McCauley, R. J., & Strand, E. A. (2008). A review of standardized tests of nonverbal oral and speech motor performance in children. *American Journal of Speech-Language Pathology, 17*, 81–91.

McCauley, R. J., & Swisher, L. (1984). Use and misuse of norm-referenced tests in clinical assessment: A hypothetical case. *Journal of Speech and Hearing Disorders, 49*(4), 338–348.

McCormack, J., McLeod, S., McAllister, L., & Harrison, L. J. (2009). A systematic review of the association between childhood speech impairment and participation across the lifespan. *International Journal of Speech-Language Pathology, 11*(2), 155–170.

McCormack, P. (1997, Autumn). New approaches to the assessment of children's speech. *Australian Communication Quarterly*, 3–5.

McCormack, P. F., & Knighton, T. (1996). Gender differences in the speech patterns of two-and-a-half-year-old children. In P. McCormack & A. Russell (Eds.), *Speech science and technology: Sixth Australian international conference* (pp. 337–341). Australian Speech Science and Technology Association.

McDonald, E. T. (1964a). *Articulation testing and treatment: A sensory motor approach*. Stanwix House.

McDonald, E. T. (1964b). *A deep test of articulation*. Stanwix House.

McEnery, E., & Gaines, F. (1941). Tongue-tie in infants and children. *Journal of Pediatrics, 18*, 252–255.

McEwin, A., & Santow, E. (2018). The importance of the human right to communication. *International Journal of Speech-Language Pathology, 20*(1), 1–2.

McGlaughlin, A., & Grayson, A. (2003). A cross sectional and prospective study of crying in the first year of life. In S. P. Sohov (Ed.), *Advances in psychology research* (Vol. 22, pp. 37–58). Nova Science.

McGregor, K. K., & Schwartz, R. G. (1992). Converging evidence for underlying phonological representation in a child who misarticulates. *Journal of Speech and Hearing Research, 35*, 596–603.

McIntosh, B., & Dodd, B. (2013). *Toddler phonology test*. Pearson.

McKechnie, J., Ahmed, B., Gutierrez-Osuna, R., Murray, E., McCabe, P., & Ballard, K. J. (2020). The influence of type of feedback during tablet-based delivery of intensive treatment for childhood apraxia of speech. *Journal of Communication Disorders, 87*, 1–19.

McKercher, M., McFarlane, L., & Schneider, P. (1995). Phonological treatment dismissal: Optimal criteria. *Canadian Journal of Speech-Language Pathology and Audiology, 19*, 115–123.

McKinnon, D. H., McLeod, S., & Reilly, S. (2007). The prevalence of stuttering, voice and speech-sound disorders in primary school students in Australia. *Language, Speech, and Hearing Services in Schools, 38*(1), 5–15.

McLeod, S. (Ed.). (2007a). *The international guide to speech acquisition.* Thomson Delmar Learning.

McLeod, S. (2007b). Australian English speech acquisition. In S. McLeod (Ed.), *The international guide to speech acquisition* (pp. 241–256). Thomson Delmar Learning.

McLeod, S. (2015). Intelligibility in context scale. *Journal of Clinical Practice in Speech-Language Pathology, 17,* 7–12.

McLeod, S. (2020). Intelligibility in context scale: Cross-linguistic use, validity, and reliability. *Speech Language and Hearing, 23*(1), 9–16.

McLeod, S., & Arciuli, J. (2009). School-aged children's production of /s/ and /r/ consonant clusters. *Folia Phoniatrica et Logopaedica, 61,* 336–341.

McLeod, S., & Baker, E. (2014). Speech-language pathologists' practices regarding assessment, analysis, target selection, intervention, and service delivery for children with speech sound disorders. *Clinical Linguistics & Phonetics, 28*(7–8), 508–531.

McLeod, S., Baker, E., McCormack, J., Wren, Y., Roulstone, S., Crowe, K., Masso, S., White, P., & Howland, C. (2017). Cluster-randomized controlled trial evaluating the effectiveness of computer-assisted intervention delivered by educators for children with speech sound disorders. *Journal of Speech, Language, and Hearing Research, 60*(7), 1891–1910.

McLeod, S., & Crowe, K. (2018). Children's consonant acquisition in 27 languages: A cross-linguistic review. *American Journal of Speech-Language Pathology, 27,* 1546–1571.

McLeod, S., Crowe, K., & Shahaeian, A. (2015). Intelligibility in context scale: Normative and validation data for English-speaking preschoolers. *Language, Speech, and Hearing Services in Schools, 46,* 266–276.

McLeod, S., Harrison, L. J., & McCormack, J. (2012). The intelligibility in context scale: Validity and reliability of a subjective rating measure. *Journal of Speech, Language, and Hearing Research, 55,* 648–656.

McLeod, S., Harrison, L. J., & Wang, C. (2019). A longitudinal population study of literacy and numeracy outcomes for children identified with speech, language, and communication needs in early childhood. *Early Childhood Research Quarterly, 47,* 507–517.

McLeod, S., & Hewett, S. R. (2008). Variability in the production of words containing consonant clusters by typical two- and three-year-old children. *Folia Phoniatrica et Logopaedica, 60,* 163–172.

McLeod, S., van Doorn, J., & Reed, V. A. (1998). Homonyms in children's productions of consonant clusters. In W. Ziegler & K. Deger (Eds.), *Clinical phonetics and linguistics* (pp. 108–114). Whurr Publishers.

McLeod, S., van Doorn, J., & Reed, V. A. (2001a). Normal acquisition of consonant clusters. *American Journal of Speech-Language Pathology, 10,* 99–110.

McLeod, S., van Doorn, J., & Reed, V. A. (2001b). Consonant cluster development in two-year-olds: General trends and individual difference. *Journal of Speech, Language, and Hearing Research, 44,* 1144–1171.

McLeod, S., van Doorn, J., & Reed, V. A. (2002). Typological description of the normal acquisition of consonant clusters. In F. Windsor, L. Kelly, & N. Hewlett (Eds.), *Investigations in clinical phonetics and linguistics* (pp. 185–200). Erlbaum.

McNeill, B. (2007). *Advancing spoken and written language development in children with childhood apraxia of speech* [Unpublished doctoral dissertation]. University of Canterbury.

McNeill, B. C., & Gillon, G. T. (2021). Integrated phonological awareness intervention. In A. L. Williams, S. McLeod, & R. J. McCauley (Eds.), *Interventions for speech sound disorders in children* (2nd ed., pp. 111–139). Paul H. Brookes Publishing Co.

McNeill, B. C., Gillon, G. T., & Dodd, B. (2009). Phonological awareness and early reading development in childhood apraxia of speech (CAS). *International Journal of Language & Communication Disorders, 44,* 175–192.

McNeill, B. C., Wolter, J., & Gillon, G. T. (2017). A comparison of the metalinguistic performance and spelling development of children with inconsistent speech sound disorder and their age-matched and reading-matched peers. *American Journal of Speech-Language Pathology, 26*(2), 456–468.

McNutt, J. (1977). Oral sensory and motor behaviors of children with /s/ or /r/ misarticulations. *Journal of Speech and Hearing Research, 20,* 694–703.

McReynolds, L. V. (1972). Articulation generalization during articulation training. *Language and Speech, 15*, 149–155.

McReynolds, L. V., & Elbert, M. (1978). An experimental analysis of misarticulating children's generalization. *Journal of Speech and Hearing Research, 21*, 136–150.

Mekonnen, A. M. (2012). The effects of macroglossia on speech: A case study. *Clinical Linguistics & Phonetics, 26*, 39–50.

Melby-Lervåg, M., Lyster, S. A., & Hulme, C. (2012). Phonological skills and their role in learning to read: A meta-analytic review. *Psychological Bulletin, 138*, 322–352.

Menn, L. (1971). Phonotactic rules in beginning speech. *Lingua, 26*, 225–241.

Menn, L. (1978). Phonological units in beginning speech. In A. Bell & J. B. Hooper (Eds.), *Syllables and segments* (pp. 157–171). North Holland.

Menn, L. (1983). Development of articulatory, phonetic, and phonological capabilities. In B. Butterworth (Ed.), *Language production* (Vol. 2, pp. 3–50). Academic Press.

Menn, L. (1994). Perspective on research in first language developmental phonology. In M. Yavas (Ed.), *First and second language pathology* (pp. 3–8). Singular Publishing.

Menn, L., Markey, K., Mozer, M., & Lewis, C. (1993). Connectionist modeling and the microstructure of phonological development: A progress report. In B. de Boysson-Bardies, S. de Schonen, P. Jusczyk, P. McNeilage, & J. Morton (Eds.), *Developmental neurocognition: Speech and face processing in the first year of life* (pp. 421–433). Kluwer Academic.

Menn, L., & Matthei, E. (1992). The "two lexicon" account of child phonology: Looking back, looking ahead. In C. A. Ferguson, L. Menn, & C. Stoel-Gammon (Eds.), *Phonological development: Models, research, implications* (pp. 211–247). York.

Menn, L., & Stoel-Gammon, C. (1995). Phonological development. In P. Fletcher & B. MacWhinney (Eds.), *The handbook of child language* (pp. 335–359). Blackwell.

Messner, A. H., & Lalakea, M. L. (2002). The effect of ankyloglossia on speech in children. *Otolaryngology–Head and Neck Surgery, 127*, 539–545.

Mettias, B., O'Brien, R., Khatwa, M. M. A., Nasrallah, L., & Doddi, M. (2013). Division of tongue tie as an outpatient procedure: Technique, efficacy, and safety. *International Journal of Pediatric Otorhinolaryngology, 77*, 550–552.

Metz, D. E., Samar, V. J., Schiavetti, N., Sitler, R. W., & Whitehead, R. L. (1985). Acoustic dimensions of hearing-impaired speakers' intelligibility. *Journal of Speech and Hearing Research, 28*, 345–355.

Meza, P. (1983). *Phonological analysis of Spanish utterances of highly unintelligible Mexican-American children* [Unpublished master's thesis]. San Diego State University.

Miccio, A., & Elbert, M. (1996). Enhancing stimulability: A treatment program. *Journal of Communication Disorders, 29*, 335–363.

Miccio, A. W., Elbert, M., & Forrest, K. (1999). The relationship between stimulability and phonological acquisition in children with normally developing and disordered phonologies. *American Journal of Speech-Language Pathology, 8*, 347–363.

Mielke, J., Baker, A., & Archangeli, D. (2016). Individual-level contact limits phonological complexity: Evidence from bunched and retroflex /ɹ/. *Language, 92*(1), 101–140.

Miller, G. J., Lewis, B., Benchek, P., Freebairn, L., Tag, J., Budge, K., Iyengar, S. K., Voss-Hoynes, H., Taylor, H. G., & Stein, C. (2019). Reading outcomes for individuals with histories of suspected childhood apraxia of speech. *American Journal of Speech-Language Pathology, 28*, 1432–1447, 1–16.

Mills, A., & Streit, H. (1942). Report of a speech survey, Holyoke, Massachusetts. *Journal of Speech Disorders, 7*, 161–167.

Moats, L. (2000). *Speech to print*. Paul H. Brookes Publishing Co.

Moimaz, S. A. S., Garbin, A. J. I., Lima, A. M. C., Lolli, L. F., Saliba, O., & Garbin, C. A. S. (2014). Longitudinal study of habits leading to malocclusion development in childhood. *BMC Oral Health, 14*, 96.

Mojsin, L. (2016). *Mastering the American accent* (2nd ed.). Barrons.

Moll, K. L., & Daniloff, R. G. (1971). Investigation of the timing of velar movements during speech. *Journal of the Acoustical Society of America, 50*, 678–684.

Moon, S. J., & Lindblom, B. (1989). Formant undershoot in clear and citation-form speech: A second progress report. *Speech Transmission Laboratory, Quarterly Progress and Status Reports, 1*, 121–123. Stockholm: Royal Institute of Technology.

Moore, C. A., & Ruark, J. L. (1996). Does speech emerge from earlier appearing oral motor behaviors? *Journal of Speech and Hearing Research, 39*, 1034–1047.

Moore, P., & Kester, D. G. (1953). Historical notes on speech correction in the pre-association era. *Journal of Speech and Hearing Disorders, 18*, 48–53.

Moran, M. (1993). Final consonant deletion in African American English: A closer look. *Language, Speech, and Hearing Services in Schools, 24*, 161–166.

Morgan, A., Eecen, K. T., Pezic, A., Brommeyer, K., Mei, C., Eadie, P., Reilly, S., & Dodd, B. (2017). Who to refer speech therapy at 4 years of age versus who to "Watch and wait"? *The Journal of Pediatrics, 185*, 200–204.E1.

Morgan, R. (1959). Structural sketch of Saint Martin Creole. *Anthropological Linguistics, 1*(8), 20–24.

Moriarty, B. C., & Gillon, G. T. (2006). Phonological awareness intervention for children with childhood apraxia of speech. *International Journal of Language & Communication Disorders, 41*, 713–734.

Morley, D. (1952). A ten-year survey of speech disorders among university students. *Journal of Speech and Hearing Disorders, 17*, 25–31.

Morris, S. R. (2009). Test-retest reliability of independent measures of phonology in the assessment of toddler speech. *Language, Speech, and Hearing Services in Schools, 40*, 46–52.

Morris, S. R. (2010). Clinical application of the mean babbling level and syllable structure level. *Language, Speech, and Hearing Services in Schools, 41*, 223–230.

Morrisette, M. L. (2021). Complexity approach. In A. L. Williams, S. McLeod, & R. J. McCauley (Eds.), *Interventions for speech sound disorders in children* (2nd ed., pp. 91–110). Paul H. Brookes Publishing Co.

Morrison, G. S., & Assmann, P. F. (Eds.) (2012). *Vowel inherit spectral change.* Heidelberg: Springer Science & Business Media.

Morrison, J. A., & Shriberg, L. D. (1992). Articulation testing versus conversational speech sampling. *Journal of Speech and Hearing Research, 35*, 259–273.

Morrow, A., Goldstein, B., Gilhool, A., & Paradis, J. (2014). Phonological skills in English language learners. *Language, Speech, and Hearing in Schools, 45*, 26–39.

Mortimer, J., & Rvachew, S. (2010). A longitudinal investigation of morpho-syntax in children with speech sound disorders. *Journal of Communication Disorders, 43*, 61–76.

Mowrer, D., Baker, R., & Schutz, R. (1968). Operant procedures in the control of speech articulation. In H. Sloane & B. MacAulay (Eds.), *Operant procedures in remedial speech and language training* (pp. 296–321). Houghton Mifflin.

Mowrer, D. E. (1982). *Methods of modifying speech behaviors* (2nd ed.). Merrill.

Moyer, A. (1999). Ultimate attainment in L2 phonology: The critical factors of age, motivation, and instruction. *Studies in Second Language Acquisition, 21*(1), 81–108.

Mullen, R., & Schooling, T. (2010). The national outcomes measurement system for pediatric speech-language pathology. *Language, Speech, and Hearing Services in Schools, 41*, 44–60.

Munro, M. J. (1993). Productions of English vowels by native speakers of Arabic: Acoustic measurements and accentedness ratings. *Language and Speech, 36*, 39–66.

Munro, M. J., & Derwing, T. M. (1995). Foreign accent, comprehensibility, and intelligibility in the speech of second language learners. *Language Learning, 45*(1), 73–97.

Munro, M. J., & Derwing, T. M. (2008). Segmental acquisition in adult ESL learners: A longitudinal study of vowel production. *Language Learning, 58*(3), 479–502.

Munson, B., Bjorum, E. M., & Windsor, J. (2003). Acoustic and perceptual correlates of stress in nonwords produced by children with suspected developmental apraxia of speech and children with phonological disorder. *Journal of Speech, Language, and Hearing Research, 46*, 189–202.

Munson, B., Johnson, J. M., & Edwards, J. (2012). The role of experience in the perception of phonetic detail in children's speech: A comparison between speech-language pathologists and clinically untrained listeners. *American Journal of Speech-Language Pathology, 21*, 124–139.

Murdoch, B. E., Attard, M. D., Ozanne, A. E., & Stokes, P. D. (1995). Impaired tongue strength and endurance in developmental verbal dyspraxia: A physiological analysis. *European Journal of Disorders of Communication, 30*, 51–64.

Murray, E., McCabe, P., & Ballard, K. J. (2014). A systematic review of treatment outcomes for children with childhood apraxia of speech. *American Journal of Speech-Language Pathology, 23*, 486–504.

Murray, E., McCabe, P., & Ballard, K. J. (2015). A randomized controlled trial for children with childhood apraxia of speech comparing rapid syllable transition treatment and the Nuffield dyspraxia programme (3rd ed.). *Journal of Speech, Language, and Hearing Research, 58*, 669–686.

Murray, E., McCabe, P., Heard, R., & Ballard, K. J. (2015). Differential diagnosis of children with suspected childhood apraxia of speech. *Journal of Speech, Language, and Hearing Research, 58,* 43–60.

Murray, E., Thomas, D., & McKechnie, J. (2019). Comorbid morphological disorder apparent in some children aged 4–5 years with childhood apraxia of speech: Findings from standardised testing. *Clinical Linguistics & Phonetics, 33*(1–2), 42–59.

Muter, V., Hulme, C., Snowling, M. J., & Stevenson, J. (2004). Phonemes, rimes, vocabulary, and grammatical skills as foundations of early reading development: Evidence from a longitudinal study. *Developmental Psychology, 40,* 665–681.

Muyksen, P., & Smith, N. (1995). The study of pidgin and creole languages. In J. Arends, P. Muyksen, & N. Smith (Eds.), *Pidgins and Creoles: An introduction* (pp. 3–14). Amsterdam: John Benjamins Publishing.

Muyksen, P., & Veenstra, T. (1995). Haitian. In J. Arends, P. Muyksen, & N. Smith (Eds.), *Pidgins and Creoles: An introduction* (pp. 153–164). Amsterdam: John Benjamins Publishing.

Nagoda, T. M. (2013). *Pacifier use and speech development.* [Unpublished master's thesis]. Idaho State University.

Nagy, J. (1980). *5–6 éves gyermekeink iskolakészültsége (Preparedness for school of five- to six-year-old children).* Budapest: Akadémiai Kiadó.

Nakanishi, Y., Owada, K., & Fujita, N. (1972). Kōonkensa to sono kekka ni kansuru kōsatsu. *Tokyo Gakugei Daigaku Tokushu Kyoiku Shisetsu Hokoku, 1,* 1–19.

Namasivayam, A. K., Pukonen, M., Goshulak, D., Hard, J., Rudzicz, F., Rietveld, T., Maassen, B., Kroll, R., & van Lieshout, P. (2015). Treatment intensity and childhood apraxia of speech. *International Journal of Language & Communication Disorders, 50*(4), 529–546.

Namasivayam, A. K., Pukonen, M., Goshulak, D., Yu, V. Y., Kadis, D. S., Kroll, R., Pang, E. W., & De Nil, L. F. (2013). Relationship between speech motor control and speech intelligibility in children with speech sound disorders. *Journal of Communication Disorders, 46*(3), 264–280.

Nancollis, A., Lawrie, B. A., & Dodd, B. (2005). Phonological awareness intervention and the acquisition of literacy skills in children from deprived social backgrounds. *Language, Speech, and Hearing Services in Schools, 36*(4), 325–335.

Nathan, L., Stackhouse, J., Goulandris, N., & Snowling, M. (2004). The development of early literacy skills among children with speech difficulties: A test of the "critical age hypothesis." *Journal of Speech, Language, and Hearing Research, 47,* 377–391.

Nathani, S., Ertmer, D. J., & Stark, R. E. (2006). Assessing vocal development in infants and toddlers. *Clinical Linguistics & Phonetics, 20*(5), 351–369.

Neal, A. (2020). /r/ Therapy–Part 1. [Webinar]. Speechpathology.com. https://www.speechpathology.com/slp-ceus/course/r-therapy-part-1-9523

Neel, A. T., & Palmer, P. M. (2012). Is tongue strength an important influence on rate of articulation in diadochokinetic and reading tasks? *Journal of Speech, Language, and Hearing Research, 55,* 235–246.

Neils, J., & Aram, D. (1986). Family history of children with developmental language disorders. *Perceptual and Motor Skills, 63,* 655–658.

Nelson, H. D., Nygren, P., Walker, M., & Panoscha, R. (2006). Screening for speech and language delay in preschool children: Systematic evidence review for the US preventive services task force. *Pediatrics, 117,* e298–e319.

Nelson, L. (1995). Establishing production of speech sound contrasts using minimal "triads." *Clinical Connection, 8*(4), 16–19.

Netsell, R. (1986). *A neurobiologic view of speech production and the dysarthrias.* College-Hill Press.

Netsell, R., Lotz, W. K., Peters, J. E., & Schulte, L. (1994). Developmental patterns of laryngeal and respiratory function for speech production. *Journal of Voice, 8,* 123–131.

Newbold, E. J., Stackhouse, J., & Wells, B. (2013). Tracking change in children with severe and persisting speech difficulties. *Clinical Linguistics & Phonetics, 27*(6–7), 521–539.

Newcomer, P., & Barenbaum, E. (2003). *Test of phonological awareness skills.* Pro-Ed.

Newcomer, P. L., & Hammill, D. D. (2019). *Test of language development, primary* (5th ed.). Pro-Ed.

Newport, E. L. (1990). Maturational constraints on language learning. *Cognitive Science, 14*(1), 11–28.

New Zealand Speech-language Therapists' Association (NZSTA). (2012). Scope of practice. http://www.speechtherapy.org.nz/wp-content/uploads/2013/09/NZSTA-Scope-of-Practice-2012.pdf

Nichols, P. (1981). Creoles of the USA. In C. Ferguson & S. Heath (Eds.), *Language in the USA* (pp. 69–91). Cambridge University Press.

Niemi, M., Laaksonen, J. -P., Vahatalo, K., Tuomainen, J., Aaltonen, O., & Happonen, R. -P. (2002). Effects of transitory lingual nerve impairment on speech: An acoustic study of vowel sounds. *Journal of Oral and Maxillofacial Surgery, 60,* 647–652.

Nippold, M. A. (2002). Stuttering and phonology: Is there an interaction? *American Journal of Speech-Language, Pathology, 11,* 99–110.

Nittrouer, S. (1996). The relationship between speech perception and phonological awareness: Evidence from low SES children and children with chronic OM. *Journal of Speech and Hearing Research, 39,* 1059–1070.

Nittrouer, S. (2001). Challenging the notion of innate phonetic boundaries. *Journal of the Acoustical Society of America, 110*(3), 1598–1605.

Norris, J., & Hoffman, P. (1990). Language intervention within naturalistic environments. *Language, Speech, and Hearing Services in Schools, 2,* 72–84.

Norris, J. A., & Hoffman, P. R. (2005). Goals and targets: Facilitating the self-organizing nature of a neuro-network. In A. Kamhi & K. Pollack (Eds.), *Phonological disorders in children: Clinical decision making in assessment and intervention* (pp. 77–87). Paul H. Brookes Publishing Co.

North Dakota Department of Public Instruction. (2010). *Speech-language pathology public school guidelines: Section II. Eligibility criteria for speech-language impairment.* Bismark: North Dakota Department of Public Instruction.

Núñez-Cedeño, R., & Morales-Front, A. (1999). *Fonología generativa contemporánea de la lengua española (Contemporary generative phonology of the Spanish language).* Georgetown University Press.

O'Connor, M., Arnott, W., McIntosh, B., & Dodd, B. (2009). Phonological awareness and language intervention in preschoolers from low socio-economic backgrounds: A longitudinal investigation. *British Journal of Developmental Psychology, 27,* 767–782.

Oetting, J. (2007). Cajun English speech acquisition. In S. McLeod (Ed.), *The international guide to speech acquisition* (pp. 169–176). Thomson Delmar Learning.

Oetting, J., & Garrity, A. (2006). Variation within dialects: A case of Cajun/Creole influence within child SAAE and SWE. *Journal of Speech, Language, and Hearing Research, 49,* 16–26.

Oetting, J. B., Gregory, K. D., & Riviere, A. M. (2016). Changing how speech-language pathologists talk about language variation. *Perspectives of the ASHA Special Interest Groups, SIG 1,* Part 1, 28–37.

Oetting, J. B., Lee, R., & Porter, K. L. (2013). Evaluating the grammars of children who speak nonmainstream dialects of English. *Topics in Language Disorders, 33*(2), 140–151.

Oetting, J. B., & McDonald, J. L. (2002). Methods for characterizing participants' nonmainstream dialect use in child language research. *Journal of Speech, Language, and Hearing Research, 45,* 508–518.

Office of Special Education and Rehabilitative Services (OSERS). (2007, March 8). Letter to ASHA. https://www.asha.org/siteassets/uploadedfiles/advocacy/federal/idea/OSEPResponse LetterGuidance.pdf

O'Grady, W., Archibald, J., Aranoff, M., & Rees-Miller, J. (2010). *Contemporary linguistics: An introduction* (6th ed.). St. Martin's Press.

Ohala, D. (1999). The influence of sonority on children's cluster reductions. *Journal of Communication Disorders, 32,* 397–421.

Oller, D. K. (2000). *The emergence of the speech capacity.* Erlbaum.

Oller, D. K., & Eilers, R. (1982). Similarity of babbling in Spanish- and English-learning babies. *Journal of Child Language, 9,* 565–577.

Oller, D. K., & Eilers, R. E. (1988). The role of audition in infant babbling. *Child Development, 59*(2), 441–449.

Oller, D. K., Eilers, R. E., Neal, A. R., & Schwartz, H. K. (1999). Precursors to speech in infancy: The prediction of speech and language disorders. *Journal of Communication Disorders, 32,* 223–245.

Oller, Jr., J. W., Oller, S. D., & Badon, L. C. (2006). *Milestones: Normal speech and language development across the lifespan.* Plural Publishing.

Olmsted, D. (1971). *Out of the mouth of babes: Earliest stages in language learning.* The Hague: Mouton.

Olswang, L. B., & Bain, B. A. (1985). The natural occurrence of generalization during articulation treatment. *Journal of Communication Disorders, 18,* 109–129.

Olswang, L. B., & Bain, B. (1994). Data collection: Monitoring children's progress. *American Journal of Speech-Language Pathology, 3,* 55–66.

Onslow, M., & O'Brian, S. (2013). Management of childhood stuttering. *Journal of Pediatrics and Child Health, 49,* 112–115.

Osberger, M. J., Robbins, A. M., Todd, S. L., & Riley, A. I. (1994). Speech intelligibility of children with cochlear implants. *The Volta Review, 96*(5), 169–180.

O'Shea, J. E., Foster, J. P., O'Donnell, C. P. F., Breathnach, D., Jacobs, S. E., Todd, D. A., & Davis, P. G. (2017). Frenotomy for tongue-tie in newborn infants (Review). *Cochrane Database of Systematic Reviews, 3, cd011065,* 1–30.

Ota, M., & Ueda, I. (2007). Japanese speech acquisition. In S. McLeod (Ed.), *The international guide to speech acquisition* (pp. 457–471). Thomson Delmar Learning.

Otaiba, S., Puranik, C. S., Ziolkowski, R. A., & Montgomery, T. M. (2009). Effectiveness of early phonological awareness interventions for students with speech or language impairments. *Journal of Special Education, 43,* 107–128.

Otomo, K., & Stoel-Gammon, C. (1992). The acquisition of unrounded vowels in English. *Journal of Speech and Hearing Research, 35,* 604–616.

Overby, M. (2007). *Relationships among speech sound perception, speech sound production, and phonological spelling in second grade children* [Unpublished doctoral dissertation]. University of Nebraska–Lincoln.

Overby, M., Belardi, K., & Schreiber, J. (2020). A retrospective video analysis of canonical babbling and volubility in infants later diagnosed with childhood apraxia of speech. *Clinical Linguistics & Phonetics, 34*(7), 634–651.

Overby, M., Carrell, T., & Bernthal, J. (2007). Teachers' perceptions of students with speech sound disorders: A quantitative and qualitative analysis. *Language, Speech, and Hearing Services in Schools, 38,* 327–341.

Overby, M. S., Trainin, G., Bosma Smit, A., Bernthal, J. E., & Nelson, R. (2012). Preliteracy speech sound skills and later literacy outcomes: A study using the Templin archive. *Language, Speech, and Hearing Services in Schools, 43,* 97–115.

Overstake, C. P. (1976). Investigation of the efficacy of a treatment program for deviant swallowing and allied problems. *International Journal of Oral Myology, 2,* 1–6.

Owens, R. E. (1994). *Language development: An introduction* (4th ed.). Allyn & Bacon.

Oyama, S. (1978). The sensitive period and comprehension of speech. *NABE Journal of Research and Practive, 3*(1), 2540.

Ozanne, A. E. (1992). Normative data for sequenced oral movements and movements in context for children aged three to five years. *Australian Journal of Human Communication Disorders, 20,* 47–63.

Pagliarin, K. C., Mota, H. B., & Keske-Soares, M. (2009). Therapeutic efficacy analysis of three contrastive approach phonological models. *Pró-Fono Revista de Atualização Científica, 21*(4), 297–302.

Pahkala, R., Laine, T., & Lammi, S. (1991). Developmental stage of the dentition and speech sound production in a series of first-grade schoolchildren. *Journal of Craniofacial Genetics and Developmental Biology, 11,* 170–175.

Palin, M. (1992). *Contrast pairs for phonological training.* Pro-Ed.

Palmer, J. (1962). Tongue-thrusting: A clinical hypothesis. *Journal of Speech and Hearing Disorders, 27,* 323–333.

Pamplona, M. C., Ysunza, A., & Urióstegui, C. (1996). Linguistic interaction: The active role of parents in speech therapy for cleft palate patients. *International Journal of Pediatric Otorhinolaryngology, 37*(1), 17–27.

Panagos, J., & Prelock, P. (1982). Phonological constraints on the sentence productions of language disordered children. *Journal of Speech and Hearing Research, 25,* 171–176.

Panagos, J., Quine, M., & Klich, R. (1979). Syntactic and phonological influences on children's articulation. *Journal of Speech and Hearing Research, 22,* 841–848.

Pandolfi, A. M., & Herrera, M. O. (1990). Producción fonologica diastratica de niños menores de tres años (Phonological production in children less than three years old). *Revista Teorica, 28,* 101–122.

Parham, D. F., Buder, E. H., Oller, D. K., & Boliek, C. A. (2011, August 1). Syllable-related breathing in infants in the second year of life. *Journal of Speech, Language, and Hearing Research, 54*(4), 1039–1050.

Parker, F. (1976). Distinctive features in speech pathology: Phonology or phonemics? *Journal of Speech and Hearing Disorders, 41*, 23–39.

Parker, F., & Riley, K. (2000). *Linguistics for non-linguists: A primer with exercises* (3rd ed.). Allyn & Bacon.

Parker, R. G. (2005). *Phonological process use in the speech of children fitted with cochlear implants.* [Unpublished master's thesis]. University of Tennessee, Knoxville.

Parlour, S., & Broen, P. (1991, November). *Environmental factors in familial phonological disorders: Preliminary home scale results* [Paper presentation]. ASHA 1991 Convention, Atlanta, GA, United States.

Parsons, C. L., Iacono, T. A., & Rozner, L. (1987). Effect of tongue reduction on articulation in children with Down syndrome. *American Journal of Mental Deficiency, 91*, 328–332.

Pascoe, M., & Stackhouse, J. (2021). Psycholinguistic intervention. In A. L. Williams, S. McLeod, & R. J. McCauley (Eds.), *Interventions for speech sound disorders in children* (2nd ed., pp. 141–170). Paul H. Brookes Publishing Co.

Pascoe, M., Stackhouse, J., & Wells, B. (2005). Phonological therapy within a psycholinguistic framework: Promoting change in a child with persisting speech difficulties. *International Journal of Language & Communication Disorders, 40*, 189–220.

Pascoe, M., Wells, B., & Stackhouse, J. (2006). *Persisting speech difficulties in children: Children's speech and literacy difficulties, Book 3.* London: Wiley.

Paterson, M. (1994). Articulation and phonological disorders in hearing-impaired school-aged children with severe and profound sensorineural losses. In J. Bernthal & N. Bankson (Eds.), *Child phonology: Characteristics, assessment, and intervention with special populations* (pp. 199–224). Thieme Medical Publishers.

Paul, R., & Jennings, P. (1992). Phonological behavior in toddlers with slow expressive language development. *Journal of Speech and Hearing Research, 35*, 99–107.

Paul, R., & Shriberg, L. D. (1982). Associations between phonology and syntax in speech delayed children. *Journal of Speech and Hearing Research, 25*, 536–546.

Paul, R., & Shriberg, L. D. (1984). Reply to Panagos and Prelock [letter]. *Journal of Speech and Hearing Research, 27*, 319–320.

Pauloski, B. R., Logemann, J. A., Colangelo, L. A., Rademaker, A. W., McConnel, R. M. S., Heiser, M. A., Cardinale, S., Shedd, D., Stein, D., Beery, Q., Myers, E., Lewin, J., Haxer, M., & Esclamado, R. (1998). Surgical variables affecting speech in treated patients with oral and oropharyngeal cancer. *Laryngoscope, 108*, 908–916.

Paynter, E. T., & Petty, N. A. (1974). Articulatory sound acquisition of two-year-old children. *Perceptual and Motor Skills, 39*, 1079–1085.

Paynter, W., & Bumpas, T. (1977). Imitative and spontaneous articulatory assessment of three-year-old children. *Journal of Speech and Hearing Disorders, 42*, 119–125.

Pearson, B. Z., Velleman, S. L., Bryant, T. J., & Charko, T. (2009). Phonological milestones for African American speaking children learning mainstream American English as a second dialect. *Language, Speech, and Hearing Services in Schools, 40*, 229–244.

Peña, E. D., Spaulding, T. J., & Plante, E. (2006). The composition of normative groups and diagnostic decision making: Shooting ourselves in the foot. *American Journal of Speech-Language Pathology, 15*, 247–254.

Peña-Brooks, A., & Hegde, M. N. (2000). *Assessment and treatment of articulation and phonological disorders in children.* Pro-Ed.

Penney, G., Fee, E. J., & Dowdle, C. (1994). Vowel assessment and remediation: A case study. *Child Language Teaching and Therapy, 10*(1), 47–66.

Perez, E. (1994). Phonological differences among speakers of Spanish-influenced English. In J. Bernthal & N. Bankson (Eds.), *Child phonology: Characteristics, assessment, and intervention with special populations* (pp. 245–254). Thieme Medical Publishers.

Perfetti, C. A., Beck, I., Bell, L. C., & Hughes, C. (1987). Phonemic knowledge and learning to read are reciprocal: A longitudinal study of first grade children. *Merrill-Palmer Quarterly, 33*, 283–319.

Perkins, W. (1977). *Speech pathology: An applied behavioral science.* Mosby.

Peterson, R. L., Pennington, B. F., Shriberg, L. D., & Boada, R. (2009). What influences literacy outcome in children with speech disorder? *Journal of Speech, Language, and Hearing Research, 52*, 1175–1188.

Pew Research Center. (2018 July 3). *6 facts about English language learners in U.S. public schools.* https://www.pewresearch.org/fact-tank/2018/10/25/6-facts-about-english-language-learners-in-u-s-public-schools/

Pham, B., & McLeod, S. (2019). Vietnamese-speaking children's acquisition of consonants, semivowels, vowels, and tones in northern Viet Nam. *Journal of Speech, Language, and Hearing Research, 62,* 2645–2670.

Picheny, M. A., Durlach, N. I., & Braida, L. D. (1986). Speaking clearly for the hard of hearing: II. Acoustic characteristics of clear and conversational speech. *Journal of Speech and Hearing Research, 29,* 434–446.

Pigott, T., Barry, J., Hughes, B., Eastin, D., Titus, P., Stensil, H., Metcalf, K., & Porter, B. (1985). *Speech-ease screening inventory (K–1).* Pro-Ed.

Pinborough-Zimmerman, J., Satterfield, R., Miller, J., Bilder, D., Hossain, S., & McMahon, W. (2007). Communication disorders: Prevalence and comorbid intellectual disability, autism, and emotional/behavioral disorders. *American Journal of Speech-Language Pathology, 16,* 359–367.

Pinter, J. D., Eliez, S., Schmitt, J. E., Capone, G. T., & Reiss, A. L. (2001). Neuroanatomy of Down's syndrome: A high-resolution MRI study. *American Journal of Psychiatry, 158,* 1659–1665.

Piske, T., MacKay, I. R., & Flege, J. E. (2001). Factors affecting degree of foreign accent in an L2: A review. *Journal of Phonetics, 29*(2), 191–215.

Polka, L., & Bohn, O. (2003). Asymmetries in vowel perception. *Speech Communication, 41,* 221–231.

Pollock, K. (1991). The identification of vowel errors using transitional articulation or phonological process test stimuli. *Language, Speech, and Hearing Services in Schools, 22,* 39–50.

Pollock, K. (2002). Identification of vowel errors: Methodological issues and preliminary data from the Memphis Vowel Project. In M. J. Ball & F. E. Gibbon (Eds.), *Vowel disorders* (pp. 83–113). Butterworth Heinemann.

Pollock, K. E. (1994). Assessment and remediation of vowel misarticulation. *Clinics in Communication Disorders, 4*(1), 23–37.

Pollock, K., Bailey, G., Berni, M., Fletcher, D., Hinton, L., Johnson, I., & Weaver, R. (1998, November). *Phonological characteristics of African American English Vernacular (AAVE): An updated feature list* [Seminar presentation]. ASHA 1998 Convention, San Antonio, TX, United States.

Pollock, K., & Berni, M. C. (2003). Incidence of non-rhotic vowel errors in children: Data from the Memphis Vowel Project. *Clinical Linguistics & Phonetics, 17,* 393–401.

Poole, I. (1934). Genetic development of articulation of consonant sounds in speech. *Elementary English Review, 11,* 159–161.

Poplack, S. (1978). Dialect acquisition among Puerto Rican bilinguals. *Language in Society, 7,* 89–103.

Poplack, S. (2000). Introduction. In S. Poplack (Ed.), *The English history of African American English* (pp. 1–32). Blackwell.

Porter, J. H., & Hodson, B. W. (2001). Collaborating to obtain phonological acquisition data for local schools. *Language, Speech, and Hearing Services in Schools, 32,* 165–171.

Potter, N. L., Nievergelt, Y., & VanDam, M. (2019). Tongue strength in children with and without speech sound disorders. *American Journal of Speech-Language Pathology, 28*(2), 612–622.

Potter, N. L., & Short, R. (2009). Maximal tongue strength in typically developing children and adolescents. *Dysphagia, 24,* 391–397.

Potter, S. O. L. (1882). *Speech and its defects. Considered physiologically, pathologically, historically, and remedially.* P. Blakiston, Son & Co.

Powell, J., & McReynolds, L. (1969). A procedure for testing position generalization from articulation training. *Journal of Speech and Hearing Research, 12,* 625–645.

Powell, T. W., & Elbert, M. (1984). Generalization following the remediation of early- and later-developing consonant clusters. *Journal of Speech and Hearing Disorders, 49,* 211–218.

Powell, T. W., Elbert, M., & Dinnsen, D. A. (1991). Stimulability as a factor in the phonologic generalization of misarticulating preschool children. *Journal of Speech and Hearing Research, 34,* 1318–1328.

Powers, M. (1957, 1971). Functional disorders of articulation: Symptomatology and etiology. In L. Travis (Ed.), *Handbook of speech pathology and audiology.* Prentice-Hall.

Prather, E. M., Hedrick, D. L., & Kern, C. A. (1975). Articulation development in children aged two to four years. *Journal of Speech and Hearing Disorders, 60,* 179–191.

Preisser, D. A., Hodson, B. W., & Paden, E. P. (1988). Developmental phonology: 18–29 months. *Journal of Speech and Hearing Disorders, 53*, 125–130.

Preston, J., & Edwards, M. (2007). Phonological processing skills of adolescents with residual speech sound errors. *Language, Speech, and Hearing Services in Schools, 38*, 297–308.

Preston, J., & Edwards, M. (2010). Phonological awareness and types of sound errors in preschoolers with speech sound disorders. *Journal of Speech, Language, and Hearing Research, 53*, 44–60.

Preston, J., Hull, M., & Edwards, M. (2013). Preschool speech error patterns predict articulation and phonological awareness outcomes in children with histories of speech sound disorders. *American Journal of Speech-Language Pathology, 22*, 173–184.

Preston, J. L., Brick, N., & Landi, N. (2013). Ultrasound biofeedback treatment for persisting childhood apraxia of speech. *American Journal of Speech-Language Pathology, 22*, 627–643.

Preston, J. L., Holliman-Lopez, G., & Leece, M. C. (2018). Do participants report any undesired effects in ultrasound speech therapy? *American Journal of Speech-Language Pathology, 27*, 813–818.

Preston, J. L., & Leece, M. C. (2017). Intensive treatment for persisting rhotic distortions: A case series. *American Journal of Speech-Language Pathology, 26*, 1066–1079.

Preston, J. L., & Leece, M. C. (2021). Articulation interventions. In A. L. Williams, S. McLeod, & R. J. McCauley (Eds.), *Interventions for speech sound disorders in children* (2nd ed., pp. 419–445). Paul H. Brookes Publishing Co.

Preston, J. L., Leece, M. C., & Maas, E. (2016). Intensive treatment with ultrasound visual feedback for speech sound errors in childhood apraxia. *Frontiers in Human Neuroscience, 10*(440), 1–9.

Preston, J. L., Leece, M. C., & Maas, E. (2017). Motor-based treatment with and without ultrasound feedback for residual speech-sound errors. *International Journal of Language & Communication Disorders, 52*(1), 80–94.

Preston, J. L., Leece, M. C., McNamara, K., & Maas, E. (2017). Variable practice to enhance speech learning in ultrasound biofeedback treatment for childhood apraxia of speech: A single case experimental study. *American Journal of Speech-Language Pathology, 26*, 840–852.

Preston, J. L., Leece, M. C., & Storto, J. (2019). Tutorial: Speech motor chaining treatment for school-age children with speech sound disorders. *Language, Speech, and Hearing Services in Schools, 50*, 343–355.

Preston, J. L., Maas, E., Whittle, J., Leece, M. C., & McCabe, P. (2016). Limited acquisition and generalization of rhotics with ultrasound visual feedback in childhood apraxia. *Clinical Linguistics & Phonetics, 30*(3–5), 363–381.

Preston, J. L., McAllister, T., Phillips, E., Boyce, S., Tiede, M., Kim, J. S., & Whalen, D. H. (2019). Remediating residual rhotic errors with traditional and ultrasound-enhanced treatment: A single-case experimental study. *American Journal of Speech-Language Pathology, 28*, 1167–1183.

Preston, J. L., McCabe, P., Rivera-Campos, A., Whittle, J. L., Landry, E., & Maas, E. (2014). Ultrasound visual feedback treatment and practice variability for residual speech sound errors. *Journal of Speech, Language, and Hearing Research, 57*, 2102–2115.

Prezas, R., Hodson, B., & Schommer-Aikins, M. (2014). Phonological assessment and analysis of bilingual preschoolers' Spanish and English word productions. *American Journal of Speech-Language Pathology, 23*, 176–185.

Price, E., & Scarry-Larkin, M. (1999). *Phonology* [CD-ROM]. LocuTour Multimedia.

Prieto, P., & Esteve-Gibert, N. (Eds.). (2018). *The development of prosody in first language acquisition.* John Benjamins Publishing.

Prince, A. S., & Smolensky, P. (1993). *Optimality theory: Constraint interaction in generative grammar* [Technical report #2]. Rutgers University Center for Cognitive Science.

Prins, D. (1962a). Analysis of correlations among various articulatory deviations. *Journal of Speech and Hearing Research, 5*, 151–160.

Prins, D. (1962b). Motor and auditory abilities in different groups of children with articulatory deviations. *Journal of Speech and Hearing Research, 5*, 161–168.

Proffit, W. R. (1986). *Contemporary orthodontics.* Mosby.

Prosek, R., & House, A. (1975). Intraoral air pressure as a feedback cue in consonant production. *Journal of Speech and Hearing Research, 18*, 133–147.

Psaila, K., Foster, J. P., Pulbrook, N., & Jeffery, H. E. (2017). Infant pacifiers for reduction in risk of sudden infant death syndrome. *Cochrane Database of Systematic Reviews.* https://doi.org /10.1002/14651858.CD011147.pub2

Rabiner, L., Levitt, H., & Rosenberg, A. (1969). Investigation of stress patterns for speech synthesis by rule. *Journal of the Acoustical Society of America, 45,* 92–101.

Raitano, N. A., Penningtion, B. F., Tunick, R. A., Boada, R., & Shriberg, L. D. (2004). Pre-literacy skills of subgroups of children with speech sound disorders. *Journal of Child Psychology and Psychiatry, 45,* 821–835.

Ramirez, A., & Milk, R. (1986). Notions of grammaticality among teachers of bilingual pupils. *TESOL Quarterly, 20,* 495–513.

Read, C., & Schreiber, P. A. (1982). Why short subjects are harder to find than long ones. In E. Wanner & L. Gleitman (Eds.), *Language acquisition: The state of the art* (pp. 78–101). Cambridge University Press.

Reid, G. (1947a). The efficiency of speech re-education of functional articulatory defectives in elementary school. *Journal of Speech and Hearing Disorders, 12,* 301–313.

Reid, G. (1947b). The etiology and nature of functional articulatory defects in elementary school children. *Journal of Speech and Hearing Disorders, 12,* 143–150.

Reiter, R., Brosch, S., Wefel, H., Schlomer, G., & Hasse, S. (2011). The submucous cleft palate: Diagnosis and therapy. *International Journal of Pediatric Otorhinolaryngology, 75,* 85–88.

Rice, M. L., & Wexler, K. (1996). Toward tense as a clinical marker of specific language impairment in English-speaking children. *Journal of Speech and Hearing Research, 39,* 1239–1257.

Rickford, J. (1999). *African American vernacular English: Features, evolution, educational implications.* Blackwell.

Rieger, J., Wolfaardt, J., Seikaly, H., & Jha, N. (2002). Speech outcomes in patients rehabilitated with maxillary obturator prostheses after maxillectomy: A prospective study. *International Journal of Prosthodontics, 15,* 139–144.

Ringel, R., Burk, K., & Scott, C. (1970). Tactile perception: Form discrimination in the mouth. In J. Bosma (Ed.), *Second symposium on oral sensation and perception.* Charles Thomas.

Ringel, R., & Ewanowski, S. (1965). Oral perception: I. Two-point discrimination. *Journal of Speech and Hearing Research, 8,* 389–400.

Ringel, R., House, A., Burk, K., Dolinsky, J., & Scott, C. (1970). Some relations between orosensory discrimination and articulatory aspects of speech production. *Journal of Speech and Hearing Disorders, 35,* 3–11.

Riski, J. E., & DeLong, E. (1984). Articulation development in children with cleft lip/palate. *Cleft Palate Journal, 21,* 57–64.

Robb, M., Gilbert, H., Reed, V., & Bisson, A. (2003), Speech rates in young Australian English–speaking children: A preliminary study. *Contemporary Issues in Communication Science and Disorders, 30,* 84–91.

Robb, M. P., & Bleile, K. M. (1994). Consonant inventories of young children from 8 to 25 months. *Clinical Linguistics & Phonetics, 8,* 295–320.

Robb, M. P., & Gillon, G. T. (2007). Speech rates of New Zealand English– and American English–speaking children. *Advances in Speech-Language Pathology, 9*(2), 173–180.

Robbins, J., & Klee, T. (1987). Clinical assessment of oropharyngeal motor development in young children. *Journal of Speech and Hearing Disorders, 52,* 271–277.

Roberts, J., Long, S. H., Malkin, C., Barnes, E., Skinner, M., Hennon, E. A., & Anderson, K. (2005). A comparison of phonological skills of boys with fragile X syndrome and Down syndrome. *Journal of Speech, Language, and Hearing Research, 48,* 980–995.

Roberts, J. E., Burchinal, M., & Footo, M. M. (1990). Phonological process decline from 2;6 to 8 years. *Journal of Communication Disorders, 23,* 205–217.

Roberts, J. E., Rosenfeld, R. M., & Zeisel, S. A. (2004). Otitis media and speech and language: A meta-analysis of prospective studies. *Pediatrics, 113,* e238–e248.

Robertson, C., & Salter, W. (2007). *The phonological awareness test 2.* LinguiSystems.

Robin, D. A., Somodi, L. B., & Luschei, E. S. (1991). Measurement of tongue strength and endurance in normal and articulation disordered subjects. In C. A. Moore, K. M. Yorkston, & D. R. Beukelman (Eds.), *Dysarthria and apraxia of speech: Perspectives on management* (pp. 173–184). Paul H. Brookes Publishing Co.

Robinson, G., & Stockman, I. (2009). Cross-dialectal perceptual experiences of speech-language pathologists in predominantly Caucasian American school districts. *Language, Speech, and Hearing Services in Schools, 40,* 138–149.

Roca, I., & Johnson, W. (1999). *A course in phonology.* Blackwell.

Roe, V., & Milisen, R. (1942). The effect of maturation upon defective articulation in elementary grades. *Journal of Speech Disorders, 7,* 37–50.

Roepke, E., Bower, K, E., Miller, C. A., & Brosseau-Lapré, F. (2020). The speech "bamana": Using the syllable repetition task to identify underlying phonological deficits in children with speech and language impairments. *Journal of Speech, Language, and Hearing Research, 63*(7), 2229–2244.

Rogers, G. (2013). Hand-held tactile biofeedback as a cuing mechanism to elicit and generalize correct /R/: A case study. *eHearsay: Electronic Journal of the Ohio Speech-Language Hearing Association, 3*(2), 39–55.

Rogers, G., & Chesin, M. (2013, December). Examining the clinical application of intra-oral tactile biofeedback in short-duration therapy targeting misarticulated /s/. *PSHA Journal, 2013,* 5–18.

Rojare, C., Opdenakker, Y., Laborde, A., Nicot, R., Mention, K., & Ferri, J. (2019). The Smith-Lemi-Opitz syndrome and dentofacial anomalies diagnostic: Case reports and literature review. *International Orthodontics, 17,* 375–383.

Rosenfeld, J. A., Coppinger, J., Bejjani, B. A., Girirajan, S., Eichler, E. E., Shaffer, L. G., & Ballif, B. C. (2010). Speech delays and behavioral problems are the predominant features in individuals with developmental delays and 16p11,2 microdeletions and microduplications. *Journal of Neurodevelopmental Disorders, 2,* 26–38.

Rosin, M., Swift, E., Bless, D., & Vetter, D. K. (1988). Communication profiles of adolescents with Down's syndrome. *Journal of Childhood Communication Disorders, 12,* 49–62.

Roth, F. P., & Paul, D. R. (2006). Partnerships for literacy: Principles and practices. Foreword. *Topics in Language Disorders, 26,* 2–4.

Roulstone, S., Loader, S., Northstone, K., Beveridge, M., & the ALSPAC Team. (2002). The speech and language of children aged 25 months: Descriptive data from the Avon Longitudinal Study of Parents and Children. *Early Child Development and Care, 172*(3), 259–268.

Rovers, M. M., Numans, M. E., Langenback, E., Grobbee, D. E., Verheij, T. J. M., & Schilder, A. B. M. (2008). Is pacifier use a risk factor for acute otitis media? A dynamic cohort study. *Family Practice, 25*(4), 233–236.

Royal College of Speech and Language Therapists (RCSLT). (2006). Communicating quality 3: RCSLT's guidance on best practice in service organisation and provision. London: Royal College of Speech and Language Therapists.

Ruark, J. L., & Moore, C. A. (1997). Coordination of lip muscle activity by 2-year-old children during speech and nonspeech tasks. *Journal of Speech, Language, and Hearing Research, 40,* 1373–1385.

Ruben, R. J. (1997). A time frame of critical/sensitive periods of language development. *Acta Otolaryngology, 117,* 202–205.

Ruben, R. J. (2000). Redefining the survival of the fittest: Communication disorders in the 21st century. *The Laryngoscope, 110,* 241–245.

Rudolph, J. M., & Wendt, O. (2014). The efficacy of the cycles approach: A multiple baseline design. *Journal of Communication Disorders, 47,* 1–16.

Ruffoli, R., Giambellica, M. A., Scavuzzo, M. C., Bonfigli, D., Cristofani, R., Gabriele, M., Giuca, M. R., & Giannessi, F. (2005). Ankyloglossia: Amorphofunctional investigation in children. *Oral Diseases, 11,* 170–174.

Ruscello, D. (1972). *Articulation improvement and oral tactile changes in children* [Unpublished doctoral thesis]. University of West Virginia.

Ruscello, D. (1975). The importance of word position in articulation therapy. *Language, Speech, and Hearing Services in Schools, 6,* 190–196.

Ruscello, D. (1984). Motor learning as a model for articulation instruction. In J. Costello (Ed.), *Speech disorders in children* (pp. 129–156). College-Hill Press.

Ruscello, D. M., Cartwright, L. R., Haines, K. B., & Shuster, L. I. (1993). The use of different service delivery models for children with phonological disorders. *Journal of Communication Disorders, 26,* 193–203.

Ruscello, D. M., Shuster, L. I., & Sandwisch, A. (1991). Modification of context-specific nasal emission. *Journal of Speech and Hearing Research, 34,* 27–32.

Ruscello, D. M., St. Louis, K. O., & Mason, N. (1991). School-aged children with phonological disorders: Coexistence with other speech/language disorders. *Journal of Speech and Hearing Research, 34,* 236–242.

Ruscello, D. M., & Vallino, L. D. (2020). The use of nonspeech oral motor exercises in the treatment of children with cleft palate: A re-examination of available evidence. *American Journal of Speech-Language Pathology, 29*(4), 1811–1820.

Rvachew, S. (1994). Speech perception training can facilitate sound production learning. *Journal of Speech and Hearing Research, 37*, 347–357.

Rvachew, S. (2007a). Perceptual foundations of speech acquisition. In S. McLeod (Ed.), *The international guide to speech acquisition* (pp. 26–30). Thomson Delmar Learning.

Rvachew, S. (2007b). Phonological processing and reading in children with speech sound disorders. *American Journal of Speech-Language Pathology, 16*, 260–270.

Rvachew, S., & Brosseau-Lapré, F. (2010). Speech perception intervention. In A. L. Williams, S. McLeod, & R. J. McCauley (Eds.), *Interventions for speech sound disorders in children* (pp. 295–314), Paul H. Brookes Publishing Co.

Rvachew, S., & Brosseau-Lapré, F. (2012). *Developmental phonological disorders: Foundations of clinical practice.* Plural Publishing.

Rvachew, S., & Brosseau-Lapré, F. (2015). A randomized trial of 12-week interventions for the treatment of developmental phonological disorder in Francophone children. *American Journal of Speech-Language Pathology, 24*(4), 637–658.

Rvachew, S., Chiang, P., & Evans, N. (2007). Characteristics of speech errors produced by children with and without delayed phonological awareness skills. *Language, Speech, and Hearing Services in Schools, 38*, 60–71.

Rvachew, S., Gaines, B. R., Cloutier, G., & Blanchet, N. (2005). Productive morphology skills of children with speech delay. *Journal of Speech-Language Pathology and Audiology, 29*, 83–89.

Rvachew, S., & Grawburg, M. (2006). Correlates of phonological awareness in preschoolers with speech sound disorders. *Journal of Speech, Language, and Hearing Research, 49*, 74–87.

Rvachew, S., & Herbay, A. (2017). *Speech assessment and interactive learning system (SAILS),* Vol. 1.0. https://apps.apple.com/ca/app/sails/id1207583276

Rvachew, S., Matthews, T., Brosseau-Lapré, F., & Barbeau-Morrison, A. (2018, November). *How to apply the challenge point framework when treating severe speech disorders in children* [Seminar presentation]. ASHA 2018 Convention, Boston, MA, United States.

Rvachew, S., & Nowak, M. (2001). The effect of target-selection strategy on phonological learning. *Journal of Speech, Language, and Hearing Research, 44*, 610–623.

Rvachew, S., Nowak, M., & Cloutier, G. (2004). Effect of phonemic perception training on the speech production and phonological awareness skills of children with expressive phonological delay. *American Journal of Speech-Language Pathology, 13*, 250–263.

Rvachew, S., Ohberg, A., Grawburg, J., & Heyding, J. (2003). Phonological awareness and phonemic perception in 4-year-old children with delayed expressive phonology skills. *American Journal of Speech-Language Pathology, 12*, 463–471.

Rvachew, S., Rafaat, S., & Martin, M. (1999). Stimulability, speech perception skills, and the treatment of phonological disorders. *American Journal of Speech-Language Pathology, 8*, 33–43.

Sabri, M., & Fabiano-Smith, L. (2018). Phonological development in a bilingual Arabic-English-speaking child with bilateral cochlear implants. A longitudinal case study. *American Journal of Speech-Language Pathology, 27*, 1506–1522.

Sacks, S., Flipsen, Jr., P., & Neils-Strunjas, J. (2013). Effectiveness of systematic articulation training program accessing computers (SATPAC) approach to remediate dentalized and interdental /s,z/: A preliminary study. *Perceptual and Motor Skills: Perception, 117*, 559–577.

Sacks, S., & Shine, R. E. (2004). *SATPAC (systematic articulation training program accessing computers).* SATPAC Speech, LLC.

Salt, H., Claessen, M., Johnston, T., & Smart, S. (2020). Speech production in young children with tongue-tie. *International Journal of Pediatric Otorhinolaryngology, 134*, 1–6.

Salvago, P., Gorgone, E., Giaimo, S., Battaglia, E., Dispenza, F., Ferrara, S., & Martines, F. (2019). Is there an association between age at first words and speech sound disorders among 4- to 5-year-old children? An epidemiological cross-sectional study based on parental reports. *International Journal of Pediatric Otorhinolaryngology, 126*, 1–6.

Sander, E. K. (1972). When are speech sounds learned? *Journal of Speech and Hearing Disorders, 37*, 55–63.

Sayler, H. (1949). The effect of maturation upon defective articulation in grades seven through twelve. *Journal of Speech and Hearing Disorders, 14*, 202–207.

Schery, T. K. (1985). Correlates of language development in language-disordered children. *Journal of Speech and Hearing Disorders, 50*, 73–83.

Schiavettei, N. (1992). Scaling procedures for the measurement of speech intelligibility. In R. D. Kent (Ed.), *Intelligibility in speech disorders* (pp. 11–34). John Benjamin.

Schlanger, B. (1953). Speech examination of a group of institutionalized mentally handicapped children. *Journal of Speech and Hearing Disorders, 18*, 339–349.

Schlanger, B., & Gottsleben, R. (1957). Analysis of speech defects among the institutionalized mentally retarded. *Journal of Speech and Hearing Disorders, 22*, 98–103.

Schmauch, V., Panagos, J., & Klich, R. (1978). Syntax influences the accuracy of consonant production in language-disordered children. *Journal of Communication Disorders, 11*, 315–323.

Schmid, K. M., Kugler, R., Nalabothu, P., Bosch, C., & Verna, C. (2018). The effect of pacifier sucking on orofacial structures: A systematic literature review. *Progress in Orthodontics, 19*, 8.

Schmidt, A. (1997). Working with adult foreign accent: Strategies for intervention. *Contemporary Issues in Communication Science and Disorders, 24*(Spring), 47–56.

Schuele, C. M., & Dayton, N. D. (2000). *Intensive phonological awareness program.* Cleveland, OH: Authors.

Schuele, C. M., Justice, L., Cabell, S., Knighton, K., Kingery, B., & Lee, M. (2008). Field-based evaluation of two-tiered instruction for enhancing kindergarten phonological awareness. *Early Education and Development, 19*, 726–752.

Schwartz, A., & Goldman, R. (1974). Variables influencing performance on speech sound discrimination tests. *Journal of Speech and Hearing Research, 17*, 25–32.

Schwartz, R. G., & Leonard, L. B. (1982). "Do children pick and choose?" An examination of phonological selection and avoidance in early lexical acquisition. *Journal of Child Language, 9*, 319–336.

Schwartz, R. G., Leonard, L., Folger, M. K., & Wilcox, M. J. (1980). Evidence for a synergistic view of linguistic disorders: Early phonological behavior in normal and language disordered children. *Journal of Speech and Hearing Disorders, 45*, 357–377.

Schwartz, R. G., Leonard, L. B., Wilcox, M. J., & Folger, M. K. (1980). Again and again: Reduplication in child phonology. *Journal of Child Language, 7*, 75–87.

Scobbie, J. M., Gordeeva, O., & Matthews, B. (2007). Scottish English speech acquisition. In S. McLeod (Ed.), *The international guide to speech acquisition* (pp. 221–240). Thomson Delmar Learning.

Scott, C., & Ringel, R. (1971). Articulation without oral sensory control. *Journal of Speech and Hearing Research, 14*, 804–818.

Scripture, M. K., & Jackson, E. (1927). *A manual of exercises for the correction of speech disorders.* F. A. Davis.

Sealey, L. R., & Giddens, C. L. (2010). Aerodynamic indices of velopharyngeal function in childhood apraxia of speech. *Clinical Linguistics & Phonetics, 24*(6), 417–430.

Secord, W. (1989). The traditional approach to treatment. In N. Creaghead, P. Newman, & W. Secord (Eds.), *Assessment and remediation of articulatory and phonological disorders* (pp. 129–157). Merrill.

Secord, W., Boyce, S. E., Donahue, J. S., Fox, R. A., & Shine, R. E. (2007). *Eliciting sounds: Techniques and strategies for clinicians* (2nd ed.). Super Duper Publications.

Secord, W., & Donahue, J. S. (2014). *Clinical assessment of articulation and phonology* (2nd ed.). Super Duper Publications.

Secord, W., & Shine, R. (1997a). *Secord contextual articulation tests (S-CAT).* Red Rock Educational Publications.

Secord, W., & Shine, R. (1997b). *Target words for contextual training.* Red Rock Educational Publications.

Segal, L. M., Stephenson, R., Dawes, M., & Feldman, P. (2007). Prevalence, diagnosis, and treatment of ankyloglossia. *Canadian Family Physician, 53*, 1027–1033.

Selby, J. C., Robb, M. P., & Gilbert, H. R. (2000). Normal vowel articulations between 15 and 36 months of age. *Clinical Linguistics & Phonetics, 14*, 255–266.

Semel, E., Wiig, E., & Secord, W. (2013). *Clinical evaluation of language fundamentals–5.* Psychological Corporation.

Seymour, H., & Seymour, C. (1977). A therapeutic model for communicative disorders among children who speak Black English vernacular. *Journal of Speech and Hearing Disorders, 42*, 247–256.

Seymour, H., & Seymour, C. (1981). Black English and Standard American English contrasts in consonantal development of four- and five-year-old children. *Journal of Speech and Hearing Disorders, 46,* 274–280.

Shafer, V. L., Shucard, D. W., Shucard, J. L., & Gerken, L. (1998). An electrophysiological study of infants' sensitivity to the sound patterns of English speech. *Journal of Speech, Language, and Hearing Research, 41,* 874–886.

Shahidullah, S., & Hepper, P. G. (1992). Hearing in the fetus: Prenatal detection of deafness. *International Journal of Prenatal and Perinatal Studies, 4*(3/4), 235–240.

Shapiro, L. R., & Solity, J. (2008). Delivering phonological and phonics training within whole-class teaching. *British Journal of Educational Psychology, 78,* 597–620.

Sheahan, P., Miller, I., Sheahan, J. N., Earley, M. J., & Blayney, A. W. (2003). Incidence and outcome of middle ear disease in cleft lip and/or cleft palate. *International Journal of Pediatric Otorhinolaryngology, 67,* 758–793.

Shelton, R. (1978). Disorders of articulation. In P. Skinner & R. Shelton (Eds.), *Speech, language, and hearing* (pp. 170–211). Addison-Wesley.

Shelton, R., Johnson, A., & Arndt, W. (1977). Delayed judgment speech sound discrimination and /r/ or /s/ articulation status and improvement. *Journal of Speech and Hearing Research, 20,* 704–717.

Shelton, R., Johnson, A. F., & Arndt, W. B. (1972). Monitoring and reinforcement by parents as a means of automating articulatory responses. *Perceptual and Motor Skills, 35,* 759–767.

Shelton, R., Johnson, A. F., Willis, V., & Arndt, W. B. (1975). Monitoring and reinforcement by parents as a means of automating articulatory responses: II. Study of pre-school children. *Perceptual and Motor Skills, 40,* 599–610.

Shelton, R., Willis, V., Johnson, A. F., & Arndt, W. B. (1973). Oral form recognition training and articulation change. *Perceptual and Motor Skills, 36,* 523–531.

Sherman, D., & Geith, A. (1967). Speech sound discrimination and articulation skill. *Journal of Speech and Hearing Disorders, 10,* 277–280.

Shipster, C., Oliver, B., & Morgan, A. (2006). Speech and oral motor skills in children with Beckwith Wiedemann syndrome: Pre- and post-tongue reduction surgery. *Advances in Speech-Language Pathology, 8*(1), 45–55.

Shprintzen, R. J. (1997). *Genetics, syndromes, and communication disorders.* Singular Publishing.

Shprintzen, R. J., Sher, A. E., & Croft, C. B. (1987). Hypernasal speech caused by tonsillar hypertrophy. *International Journal of Pediatric Otorhinolaryngology, 14,* 45–56.

Shriberg, L. D. (1975). A response evocation program for /ɝ/. *Journal of Speech and Hearing Disorders, 40,* 92–105.

Shriberg, L. D. (1982). Toward classification of developmental phonological disorders. In N. J. Lass (Ed.), *Speech and language: Advances in basic research and practice* (Vol. 8, pp. 1–18). Saunders.

Shriberg, L. D. (1991). Directions for research in developmental phonological disorders. In J. Miller (Ed.), *Research on child language disorders: A decade of progress* (pp. 267–276). Pro-Ed.

Shriberg, L. D. (1993). Four new speech and prosody-voice measures for genetics research and other studies in developmental phonological disorders. *Journal of Speech and Hearing Research, 36,* 105–140.

Shriberg, L. D. (2010). Childhood speech sound disorders: From post-behaviorism to the post-genomic era. In R. Paul & P. Flipsen, Jr. (Eds.), *Speech sound disorders in children: In honor of Lawrence D. Shriberg* (pp. 1–34). Plural Publishing.

Shriberg, L. D. (2017, July). *Motor speech disorder–not otherwise specified: Prevalence and phenotype* [Paper presentation]. 7th International Conference on Speech Motor Control, Groningen, the Netherlands.

Shriberg, L. D. (2019). *PEPPER: Programs to examine phonetic and phonologic evaluation records* [Computer software]. University of Wisconsin–Madison. https://phonology.waisman.wisc.edu/

Shriberg, L. D., Aram, D. M., & Kwiatkowski, J. (1997a). Developmental apraxia of speech: I. Descriptive and theoretical perspectives. *Journal of Speech, Language, and Hearing Research, 40,* 273–285.

Shriberg, L. D., Aram, D. M., & Kwiatkowski, J. (1997b). Developmental apraxia of speech: II. Toward a diagnostic marker. *Journal of Speech, Language, and Hearing Research, 40,* 286–312.

Shriberg, L. D., & Austin, D. (1998). Comorbidity of speech-language disorder. Implications for a phenotype marker for speech delay. In R. Paul (Ed.), *Exploring the speech-language connection* (pp. 73–117). Paul H. Brookes Publishing Co.

Shriberg, L. D., Austin, D., Lewis, B. A., McSweeny, J. L., & Wilson, D. L. (1997). The percentage of consonants correct (PCC) metric: Extensions and reliability data. *Journal of Speech, Language, and Hearing Research, 40,* 708–722.

Shriberg, L. D., Flipsen, Jr., P., Karlsson, H. B., & McSweeny, J. L. (2001). Acoustic phenotypes for speech-genetics studies: An acoustic marker for residual /ɝ/ distortions. *Clinical Linguistics & Phonetics, 15,* 631–650.

Shriberg, L. D., Flipsen, Jr., P., Kwiatkowski, J., & McSweeny, J. L. (2003). A diagnostic marker for speech delay associated with otitis media with effusion: The intelligibility-speech gap. *Clinical Linguistics & Phonetics, 17,* 507–528.

Shriberg, L. D., Flipsen, Jr., P., Thielke, H., Kwiatkowski, J., Kertoy, M., Nellis, R., & Block, M. (2000). Risk for speech disorder associated with early recurrent otitis media with effusion: Two retrospective studies. *Journal of Speech, Language, and Hearing Research, 43,* 79–99.

Shriberg, L. D., Friel-Patti, S., Flipsen, Jr., P., & Brown, R. L. (2000). Otitis media, fluctuant hearing loss and speech-language delay: A preliminary structural equation model. *Journal of Speech, Language, and Hearing Research, 43,* 100–120.

Shriberg, L. D., Kent, R. D., Karlsson, H. B., Nadler, C. J., & Brown, R. L. (2003). A diagnostic marker for speech delay associated with otitis media with effusion: Backing of obstruents. *Clinical Linguistics & Phonetics, 17,* 529–547.

Shriberg, L. D., & Kwiatkowski, J. (1980). *Natural process analysis.* Wiley.

Shriberg, L. D., & Kwiatkowski, J. (1982a). Phonological disorders: III. A procedure for assessing severity of involvement. *Journal of Speech and Hearing Disorders, 42,* 256–270.

Shriberg, L. D., & Kwiatkowski, J. (1982b). Phonological disorders: II. A conceptual framework for management. *Journal of Speech and Hearing Disorders, 42,* 242–256.

Shriberg, L. D., & Kwiatkowski, J. (1982c). Phonological disorders: I. A diagnostic classification system. *Journal of Speech and Hearing Disorders, 42,* 226–241.

Shriberg, L. D., & Kwiatkowski, J. (1983). Computer-assisted natural process analysis (NPA): Recent issues and data. *Seminars in Speech and Language, 4,* 389–406.

Shriberg, L. D., & Kwiatkowski, J. (1987). A retrospective study of spontaneous generalization in speech-delayed children. *Language, Speech, and Hearing Services in Schools, 18,* 144–157.

Shriberg, L. D., & Kwiatkowski, J. (1990). Self-monitoring and generalization in preschool speech-delayed children. *Language, Speech, and Hearing Services in Schools, 21,* 157–170.

Shriberg, L. D., & Kwiatkowski, J. (1994). Developmental phonological disorders: I. A clinical profile. *Journal of Speech and Hearing Research, 37,* 1100–1126.

Shriberg, L. D., Kwiatkowski, J., Best, S., Hengst, J., & Terselic-Weber, B. (1986). Characteristics of children with phonologic disorders of unknown origin. *Journal of Speech and Hearing Disorders, 51,* 140–161.

Shriberg, L. D., Kwiatkowski, J., & Mabie, H. L. (2019). Estimates of the prevalence of motor speech disorders in children with idiopathic speech delay. *Clinical Linguistics & Phonetics, 33*(8), 679–706.

Shriberg, L. D., Kwiatkowski, J., & Rasmussen, C. (1990). *Prosody-voice screening profile.* Communication Skill Builders.

Shriberg, L. D., Kwiatkowski, J., Rasmussen, C., Lof, G. L., & Miller, J. F. (1992). *The prosody voice screening profile (PVSP): Psychometric data and reference information for children* [Phonology project technical report no. 1]. University of Wisconsin–Madison.

Shriberg, L. D., Kwiatkowski, J., & Snyder, T. (1989). Tabletop verses microcomputer-assisted speech management: Stabilization phase. *Journal of Speech and Hearing Disorders, 54*(2), 233–248.

Shriberg, L. D., Kwiatkowski, J., & Snyder, T. (1990). Tabletop versus microcomputer-assisted speech management: Response evocation phase. *Journal of Speech and Hearing Disorders, 55*(4), 635–655.

Shriberg, L. D., Lewis, B. A., Tomblin, J. B., McSweeny, J. L., Karlsson, H. B., & Scheer, A. R. (2005). Toward diagnostic and phenotype markers for genetically transmitted speech delay. *Journal of Speech, Language, and Hearing Research, 48,* 834–852.

Shriberg, L. D., & Lof, G. L. (1991). Reliability studies in broad and narrow phonetic transcription. *Clinical Linguistics & Phonetics, 5,* 225–279.

Shriberg, L. D., Lohmeier, H. L., Campbell, T. F., Dollaghan, C. A., Green, J. R., & Moore, C. A. (2009). A nonword repetition task for speakers with misarticulations: The syllable repetition task (SRT). *Journal of Speech, Language, and Hearing Research, 52*(5), 1189–1212.

Shriberg, L. D., Lohmeier, H. L., Strand, E. A., & Jakielski, K. J. (2012). Encoding, memory, and transcoding deficits in childhood apraxia of speech. *Clinical Linguistics & Phonetics, 26*, 445–482.

Shriberg, L. D., Paul, R., Black, L. M., & van Santen, J. P. (2011). The hypothesis of apraxia of speech in children with autism spectrum disorder. *Journal of Autism and Developmental Disorders, 41*, 405–426.

Shriberg, L. D., Potter, N. L., & Strand, E. A. (2011). Prevalence and phenotype of childhood apraxia of speech in youth with galactosemia. *Journal of Speech, Language, and Hearing Research, 54*, 487–519.

Shriberg, L. D., Strand, E. A., Fourakis, M., Jakielski, K. J., Hall, S. D., Karlsson, H. B., Mabie, H. L., McSweeny, J. L., Tilkens, C. M., & Wilson, D. L. (2017a). A diagnostic marker to discriminate childhood apraxia of speech from speech delay: Introduction [Supplement article]. *Journal of Speech, Language, and Hearing Research, 60*(4), S1094–S1095.

Shriberg, L. D., Strand, E. A., Fourakis, M., Jakielski, K. J., Hall, S. D., Karlsson, H. B., Mabie, H. L., McSweeny, J. L., Tilkens, C. M., & Wilson, D. L. (2017b). A diagnostic marker to childhood apraxia of speech (CAS): I. Development and description of the pause marker [Supplement article]. *Journal of Speech, Language, and Hearing Research, 60*(4), S1096–S1117.

Shriberg, L. D., Strand, E. A., Jakielski, K. J., & Mabie, H. L. (2019). Estimates of the prevalence of speech and motor speech disorders in persons with complex neurodevelopmental disorders. *Clinical Linguistics & Phonetics, 33*(8), 707–736.

Shriberg, L. D., Tomblin, J. B., & McSweeny, J. L. (1999). Prevalence of speech delay in 6-year-old children and comorbidity with language impairment. *Journal of Speech, Language, and Hearing Research, 42*, 1461–1481.

Shriberg, L. D., & Widder, C. (1990). Speech and prosody characteristics of adults with mental retardation. *Journal of Speech and Hearing Research, 33*, 627–653.

Shriner, T., Holloway, M., & Daniloff, R. (1969). The relationship between articulatory deficits and syntax in speech defective children. *Journal of Speech and Hearing Research, 12*, 319–325.

Shuster, L. I., Ruscello, D. M., & Smith, K. D. (1992). Evoking [r] using visual feedback. *American Journal of Speech-Language Pathology, 1*, 29–34.

Shuster, L. I., Ruscello, D. M., & Toth, A. R. (1995). The use of visual feedback to elicit correct /r/. *American Journal of Speech-Language Pathology, 4*, 37–44.

Shuy, R. (1972). Social dialect and employability: Some pitfalls of good intentions. In L. Davis (Ed.), *Studies in linguistics* (pp. 145–56). University of Alabama Press.

Siegel, R., Winitz, H., & Conkey, H. (1963). The influence of testing instruments on articulatory responses of children. *Journal of Speech and Hearing Disorders, 28*, 67–76.

Sikorski, L. (1991). *Proficiency in oral English communication.* Lorna D. Sikorski & Associates.

Sikorski, L. D. (2005). "Foreign accents": Suggested competencies for improving communication pronunciation. *Seminars in Speech and Language, 26*, 126–130.

Silverman, E. (1976). Listeners' impressions of speakers with lateral lisps. *Journal of Speech and Hearing Disorders, 41*, 547–552.

Silverman, F. H. (1989). *Communication for the speechless* (2nd ed.). Prentice-Hall.

Silverman, F. H., & Paulus, P. G. (1989). Peer reactions to teenagers who substitute /w/ for /r/. *Language, Speech, and Hearing Services in Schools, 20*, 219–221.

Siqueland, E. R., & Delucia, C. A. (1969). Visual reinforcement of non-nutritive sucking in human infants. *Science, 165*, 1144–1146.

Sjolie, G. M., Leece, M. C., & Preston, J. L. (2016). Acquisition, retention, and generalization of rhotics with and without ultrasound visual feedback. *Journal of Communication Disorders, 64*, 62–77.

Skebo, C., Lewis, B., Freebairn, L., Tag, J., Ciesla, A., & Stein, C. (2013). Reading skills of students with speech sound disorders at three stages of literacy development. *Language, Speech, and Hearing Services in Schools, 44*, 360–373.

Skelly, M., Spector, D., Donaldson, R., Brodeur, A., & Paletta, F. (1971). Compensatory physiologic phonetics for the glossectomee. *Journal of Speech and Hearing Disorders, 36*, 101–114.

Skelton, S. L. (2004). Concurrent task sequencing in single-phoneme phonologic treatment and generalization. *Journal of Communication Disorders, 37*, 131–155.

Skelton, S. L., & Funk, T. E. (2004). Teaching speech sounds to young children using randomly ordered, variably complex task sequences. *Perceptual and Motor Skills, 99*, 602–604.

Skelton, S. L., & Hagopian, A. L. (2014). Using randomized variable practice in the treatment of childhood apraxia of speech. *America Journal of Speech-Language Pathology, 23*, 599–611.

Skelton, S. L., & Price, J. R. (2006, November). *A preliminary comparison of concurrent & traditional speech-sound treatments* [Seminar presentation]. ASHA 2006 Convention, Miami, FL, United States.

Skelton, S. L., & Richard, J. T. (2016). Application of a motor learning treatment for speech sound disorders in small groups. *Perceptual and Motor Skills, 122*(3), 840–854.

Skinner, B. F. (1972). *Cumulative record: A selection of papers* (3rd ed.). Appleton-Century-Crofts.

Small, L. (2004). *Fundamentals of phonetics: A practical guide for students* (2nd ed.). Allyn & Bacon.

Smiljanic, R., & Bradlow, A. R. (2011). Bidirectional clear speech perception benefit for native and high-proficiency non-native talkers and listeners: Intelligibility and accentedness. *Journal of the Acoustical Society of America, 130*(6), 4020–4031.

Smit, A. B. (1986). Ages of speech sound acquisition: Comparisons and critiques of several normative studies. *Language, Speech, and Hearing Services in Schools, 17*, 175–186.

Smit, A. B. (1993a). Phonologic error distributions in the Iowa-Nebraska articulation norms project: Consonant singletons. *Journal of Speech and Hearing Research, 36*, 533–547.

Smit, A. B. (1993b). Phonologic error distributions in the Iowa-Nebraska articulation norms project: Word-initial consonant clusters. *Journal of Speech and Hearing Research, 36*, 931–947.

Smit, A. B. (2007). General American English speech acquisition. In S. McLeod (Ed.), *The international guide to speech acquisition* (pp. 128–147). Thomson Delmar Learning.

Smit, A. B., Hand, L., Freilinger, J. J., Bernthal, J. E., & Bird, A. (1990). The Iowa articulation norms project and its Nebraska replication. *Journal of Speech and Hearing Disorders, 55*, 779–798.

Smith, A., Goffman, L., Zelaznik, H. N., Ying, G., & McGillem, C. (1995). Spatiotemporal stability and patterning of speech movement sequences. *Experimental Brain Research, 104*, 493–501.

Smith, B. L., McGregor, K. K., & Demille, D. (2006). Phonological development in lexically precocious 2-year-olds. *Applied Psycholinguistics, 27*, 355–375.

Smith, B. L., & Stoel-Gammon, C. (1983). A longitudinal study of the development of stop consonant production in normal and Down's syndrome children. *Journal of Speech and Hearing Disorders, 48*, 114–118.

Smith, M. W., & Ainsworth, S. (1967). The effect of three types of stimulation on articulatory responses of speech defective children. *Journal of Speech and Hearing Research, 10*, 333–338.

Smith, N. V. (1973). *The acquisition of phonology: A case study.* Cambridge University Press.

Smith, N. V. (1978). Lexical representation and the acquisition of phonology. In B. B. Kachru (Ed.), *Linguistics in the seventies: Directions and prospects, 8*, 259–273.

Snow, D. (1994). Phrase-final syllable lengthening and intonation in early child speech. *Journal of Speech and Hearing Research, 37*, 831–840.

Snow, J., & Milisen, R. (1954). The influences of oral versus pictorial representation upon articulation testing results. *Journal of Speech and Hearing Disorders*, monograph supplement 4, 29–36.

Snow, K. (1961). Articulation proficiency in relation to certain dental abnormalities. *Journal of Speech and Hearing Disorders, 26*, 209–212.

So, L. K. H. (2006). Cantonese phonological development: Normal and disordered. In Z. Hua & B. Dodd (Eds.), *Phonological development and disorders: A cross-linguistic perspective* (pp. 109–134). Multilingual Matters.

So, L. K. H. (2007). Cantonese speech acquisition. In S. McLeod (Ed.), *The international guide to speech acquisition* (pp. 313–326). Thomson Delmar Learning.

So, L., & Dodd, B. (1994). Phonologically disordered Cantonese-speaking children. *Clinical Linguistics & Phonetics, 8*, 235–255.

So, L. K. H., & Dodd, B. J. (1995). The acquisition of phonology by Cantonese-speaking children. *Journal of Child Language, 22*, 473–495.

Sommers, R. K. (1962). Factors in the effectiveness of mothers trained to aid in speech correction. *Journal of Speech and Hearing Disorders, 27*, 178–186.

Sommers, R. K. (1969). The therapy program. In R. Van Hattum (Ed.), *Clinical speech in the schools* (pp. 277–334). Charles Thomas.

Sommers, R. K., Furlong, A. K., Rhodes, F. H., Fichter, G. R., Bowser, D. C., Copetas, F. H., & Saunders, Z. G. (1964). Effects of maternal attitudes upon improvement in articulation when mothers are trained to assist in speech correction. *Journal of Speech and Hearing Disorders, 29,* 126–132.

Sommers, R. K., Leiss, R., Delp, M., Gerber, A., Fundrella, D., Smith, R., Revucky, M., Ellis, D., & Haley, V. (1967). Factors related to the effectiveness of articulation therapy for kindergarten, first- and second-grade children. *Journal of Speech and Hearing Research, 10,* 428–437.

Sommers, R. K., Reinhart, R., & Sistrunk, D. (1988). Traditional articulation measures of Down's syndrome speakers, ages 13–22. *Journal of Childhood Communication Disorders, 12,* 93–108.

Sommers, R. K., Schaeffer, M. H., Leiss, R. H., Gerber, A. J., Bray, M. A., Fundrella, D., Olson, J. K., & Tomkins, E. R. (1966). The effectiveness of group and individual therapy. *Journal of Speech and Hearing Research, 9,* 219–225.

Sonderman, J. (1971, November). *An experimental study of clinical relationships between auditory discrimination and articulation skills* [Paper presentation]. ASHA 1971 Convention, San Francisco, CA, United States.

Sosa, A. V. (2015). Intraword variability in typical speech development. *American Journal of Speech-Language Pathology, 24,* 24–35.

Sowell, E. R., Thompson, P. M., Leonard, C. M., Welcome, S. E., Kan, E., & Toga, A. W. (2004). Longitudinal mapping of cortical thickness and brain growth in normal children. *Journal of Neuroscience, 24*(38), 8223–8231.

Sowell, E. R., Thompson, P. M., & Toga, A. W. (2004). Mapping changes in the human cortex throughout the span of life. *Neuroscientist, 10,* 372–392.

Spaulding, T. J., Szulga, M. S., & Figueroa, C. (2012). Using norm-referenced tests to determine severity of language impairment in children: Disconnect between U.S. policy makers and test developers. *Language, Speech, and Hearing Services in Schools, 43,* 176–190.

Spector, J., (1992). Predicting progress in beginning reading: Dynamic assessment of phonemic awareness. *Journal of Educational Psychology, 84,* 353–363.

Speech-Language and Audiology Canada. (2016). *Scope of practice for speech-language pathology.* http://www.sac-oac.ca › ca › files › scope_of_practice_speech-language_pathology_en

Speech Pathology Association of Australia (SPA). (2011). Scope of practice. http://www.speechpathologyaustralia.org.au/

Speirs, R. L., & Maktabi, M. A. (1990). Tongue skills and clearance of toffee in two age-groups and in children with problems of speech articulation. *Journal of Dentistry for Children, 57,* 356–360.

Spencer, A., (1986). Towards a theory of phonological development. *Lingua, 68,* 3–38.

Spencer, A. (1988). A phonological theory of phonological development. In M. J. Ball (Ed.), *Theoretical linguistics and disordered language* (pp. 115–151). Croom Helm.

Spencer, A. (1996). *Phonology.* Blackwell.

Stackhouse, J. (2000). Barriers to literacy development in children with speech and language difficulties. In D. Bishop & L. Leonard (Eds.), *Speech and language impairments in children: Causes, characteristics, intervention and outcome* (pp. 73–98). Psychology Press.

Stackhouse, J., Pascoe, M., & Gardner, H. (2006). Intervention for a child with persisting speech and literacy difficulties: A psycholinguistic approach. *Advances in Speech-Language Pathology, 8*(3), 231–244.

Stackhouse, J., Vance, M., Pascoe, M., & Wells, B. (2007). *Compendium of auditory and speech tasks: Children's speech and literacy difficulties, Book 4.* Wiley.

Stackhouse, J., & Wells, B. (1993). Psycholinguistic assessment of developmental speech disorders. *European Journal of Disorders of Communication, 28,* 331–348.

Stackhouse, J., & Wells, B. (1997). *Children's speech and literacy difficulties: A psycholinguistic framework.* Whurr Publishers.

Stackhouse, J., & Wells, B. (2001). *Children's speech and literacy difficulties: Identification and intervention.* Whurr Publishers.

Stahl, S. A., & Murray, B. A. (1994). Defining phonological awareness and its relationship to early reading. *Journal of Educational Psychology, 86*(2), 221–234.

Stampe, D. (1969). *The acquisition of phonetic representation* [Paper presentation]. Fifth Regional Meeting of the Chicago Linguistic Society, Chicago, IL, United States.

Stampe, D. (1979). *A dissertation on natural phonology.* Garland.

Stanovich, K. (1986). Matthew effects in reading: Some consequences of individual differences in the acquisition of literacy. *Reading Research Quarterly, 21*, 360–407.

Stanovich, K. (2000). *Progress in understanding reading: Scientific foundations and new frontiers.* Guilford Press.

Stark, R. E. (1971). The use of real-time visual displays of speech in the training of a profoundly deaf, nonspeaking child: A case report. *Journal of Speech and Hearing Disorders, 36*, 397–409.

Stark, R. E. (1972). Teaching /ba/ and /pa/ to deaf children using real-time spectral displays. *Language and Speech, 15*, 14–29.

Stark, R. E., Bernstein, L. E., & Demorest, M. E. (1983). Vocal communication in the first 18 months of life. *Journal of Speech and Hearing Research, 36*, 548–558.

Starr, C. (1972). Dental and occlusal hazards to normal speech production. In K. Bzoch (Ed.), *Communicative disorders related to cleft lip and palate* (pp. 66–76). Little, Brown.

Steeve, R. W., Moore, C. A., Green, J. R., Reilly, K. J., & Ruark McMurtrey, J. (2008). Babbling, chewing, and sucking: Oromandibular coordination at 9 months. *Journal of Speech, Language, and Hearing Research, 51*, 1390–1404.

Stelcik, J. (1972). *An investigation of internal versus external discrimination and general versus phoneme-specific discrimination* [Unpublished doctoral thesis]. University of Maryland.

Stemberger, J. P. (1988). Between-word processes in child phonology. *Journal of Child Language, 15*, 39–61.

Stemberger, J. P. (1989). Speech errors in early child language production. *Journal of Memory and Language, 28*, 164–188.

Stepanof, E. R. (1990). Procesos phonologicos de niños Puertorriqueños de 3 y 4 años evidenciado en la prueba APP-Spanish (Phonological processes evidenced on the APP-Spanish by 3- and 4-year-old Puerto Rican children). *Opphla, 8*(2), 15–20.

Stephens, N. S. (2011). *Implications of Beckwith-Wiedemann syndrome for the speech-language pathologist* [Unpublished master's thesis]. Idaho State University.

Steriade, D. (1990). *Greek prosodies and the nature of syllabification* [Unpublished doctoral dissertation]. Massachusetts Institute of Technology.

Stewart, S. R., & Weybright, G. (1980). Articulation norms used by practicing speech-language pathologists in Oregon: Results of a survey. *Journal of Speech and Hearing Disorders, 45*, 103–111.

Stewart, W. (1971). Continuity and change in American Negro dialects. In W. Wolfram & N. Clarke (Eds.), *Black-White speech relationships* (pp. 51–73). Washington, DC: Center for Applied Linguistics.

St. Louis, K., & Ruscello, D. (2000). *The oral speech mechanism screening examination.* University Park Press.

St. Louis, K. O., Ruscello, D. M., Grafton, S. J., & Hershman, K. T. (1994, November). *Coexistence of communication disorders in clinical populations over four decades* [Poster presentation]. ASHA 1994 Convention, New Orleans, LA, United States.

St. Louis, K. O., Ruscello, D. M., & Lundeen, C. (1992). Coexistence of communication disorders in schoolchildren. *ASHA Monographs, 27.*

Stockman, I. (1996a). Phonological development and disorders in African American children. In A. Kamhi, K. Pollock, & J. Harris (Eds.), *Communication development and disorders in African American children* (pp. 117–154). Paul H. Brookes Publishing Co.

Stockman, I. (1996b). The promises and pitfalls of language sample analysis as an assessment tool for linguistic minority children. *Language, Speech, and Hearing Services in Schools, 27*, 355–366.

Stockman, I. (2006a). Evidence for a minimal competence core of consonant sounds in the speech of African American children: A preliminary study. *Clinical Linguistics & Phonetics, 20*, 723–749.

Stockman, I. (2006b). Alveolar bias in the final consonant deletion patterns of African American children. *Language, Speech, and Hearing Services in Schools, 37*, 85–95.

Stockman, I. (2008). Toward a validation of a minimal competence phonetic core for African American children. *Journal of Speech, Language, and Hearing Research, 51*, 1244–1262.

Stockman, I. (2010). A review of developmental and applied language research on African American children: From a deficit to difference perspective on dialect differences. *Journal of Speech, Language, and Hearing Research, 41*, 123–138.

Stockman, I., Guillory, B., Seibert, M., & Boult, J. (2013). Toward validation of a minimal competence core of morphosyntax for African American children. *American Journal of Speech-Language Pathology, 22*, 40–56.

Stockman, I. J., & Stephenson, L. W. (1981). Children's articulation of medial consonant clusters: Implications for syllabification. *Language and Speech, 24*, 185–204.

Stoel-Gammon, C. (1985). Phonetic inventories, 15–24 months: A longitudinal study. *Journal of Speech and Hearing Research, 28*, 505–512.

Stoel-Gammon, C. (1987). Phonological skills of 2-year-olds. *Language, Speech, and Hearing Services in Schools, 18*, 323–329.

Stoel-Gammon, C. (1989). Prespeech and early speech development of two late talkers. *First Language, 9*, 207–224.

Stoel-Gammon, C. (1991). Normal and disordered phonology in two-year-olds. *Topics in Language Disorders, 11*, 21–32.

Stoel-Gammon, C. (1994). Normal and disordered phonology in two-year olds. In K. Butler (Ed.), *Early intervention: Working with infants and toddlers* (pp. 110–121). Aspen.

Stoel-Gammon, C. (2004). *Variability in the productions of young typically developing children* [Paper presentation]. International Clinical Linguistics & Phonetics Association Conference, Lafayette, LA, United States.

Stoel-Gammon, C. (2007). Variability in speech acquisition. In S. McLeod (Ed.), *The international guide to speech acquisition* (pp. 55–60). Thomson Delmar Learning.

Stoel-Gammon, C. (2011). Relationships between lexical and phonological development in young children. *Journal of Child Language, 38*, 1–34.

Stoel-Gammon, C., & Dunn, C. (1985). *Normal and disordered phonology in children.* University Park Press.

Stoel-Gammon, C., & Herrington, P. B. (1990). Vowel systems of normally developing and phonologically disordered children. *Clinical Linguistics & Phonetics, 4*, 145–160.

Stoel-Gammon, C., & Kehoe, M. (1994). Hearing impairment in infants and toddlers: Identification, vocal development, and intervention in child phonology. In J. Bernthal & N. Bankson (Eds.), *Child phonology: Characteristics, assessment, and intervention with special populations* (pp. 163–181). Thieme Medical Publishers.

Stoel-Gammon, C., & Otomo, K. (1986). Babbling development of hearing-impaired and normally hearing subjects. *Journal of Speech and Hearing Disorders, 51*(1), 33–41.

Stoel-Gammon, C., & Williams, A. L. (2013). Early phonological development: Creating an assessment test. *Clinical Linguistics & Phonetics, 27*(4), 278–286.

Stokes, S. F., Klee, T., Carson, C. P., & Carson, D. (2005). A phonemic implicational feature hierarchy of phonological contrasts for English-speaking children. *Journal of Speech, Language, and Hearing Research, 48*(4), 817–833.

Stokes, T. F., & Baer, D. M. (1977). An implicit technology of generalization. *Journal of Applied Behavior Analysis, 10*, 349–367.

Storkel, H. L. (2005). The emerging lexicon of children with phonological delays: Phonotactic constraints and probability in acquisition. *Journal of Speech, Language, and Hearing Research, 47*, 1194–1212.

Storkel, H. L. (2006). Do children still pick and choose? The relationship between phonological knowledge and lexical acquisition beyond 50 words. *Clinical Linguistics & Phonetics, 20*(7/8), 523–529.

Storkel, H. L. (2018a). The complexity approach to phonological treatment: How to select treatment targets. *Language, Speech, and Hearing Services in Schools, 49*, 463–481.

Storkel, H. L. (2018b). Implementing evidence-based practice: Selecting treatment words to boost phonological learning. *Language, Speech, and Hearing Services in Schools, 49*(3), 482–496.

Storkel, H. L. (2019). Using developmental norms for speech sounds as a means of determining treatment eligibility in schools. *Perspectives of the ASHA Special Interest Groups, SIG 1, 4*(1), 67–75.

Storkel, H. L., & Morrisette, M. L. (2002). The lexicon and phonology: Interactions in language acquisition. *Language, Speech, and Hearing Services in Schools, 33*(1), 24–37.

Strand, E., & Skinder, A. (1999). Treatment of developmental apraxia of speech: Integral stimulation methods. In A. Caruso & E. Strand (Eds.), *Clinical management of motor speech disorders in children* (pp. 109–148). Thieme Medical Publishers.

Strand, E. A. (2020). Dynamic temporal and tactile cueing: A treatment strategy for childhood apraxia of speech. *American Journal of Speech-Language Pathology, 29*, 30–48.

Strand, E. A., & Debertine, P. (2000). The efficacy of integral stimulation intervention with developmental apraxia of speech. *Journal of Medical Speech-Language Pathology, 8,* 295–300.

Strand, E. A., & McCauley, R. J. (2019). *Dynamic evaluation of motor speech skill (DEMSS).* Paul H. Brookes Publishing Co. https://products.brookespublishing.com/Dynamic-Evaluation-of-Motor-Speech-Skill-DEMSS-Manual-P1100.aspx

Strand, E. A., Stoeckel, R., & Baas, B. (2006). Treatment of severe childhood apraxia of speech: A treatment efficacy study. *Journal of Medical Speech-Language Pathology, 14,* 297–307.

Strang, T. M., & Piasta, S. B. (2016). Socioeconomic differences in code-focused emergent literacy skills. *Reading and Writing, 29,* 1337–1362.

Stringfellow, K., & McLeod, S. (1991). Using a facilitating phonetic context to reduce an unusual form of gliding. *Language, Speech, and Hearing Services in Schools, 25,* 191–193.

Subtelny, J. (1970). Malocclusions, orthodontic corrections and orofacial muscle adaptation. *Angle Orthodontist, 40,* 170.

Subtelny, J., Mestre, J., & Subtelny, J. (1964). Comparative study of normal and defective articulation of /s/ as related to malocclusion and deglutition. *Journal of Speech and Hearing Disorders, 29,* 269–285.

Subtelny, J., Worth, J., & Sakuda, M. (1966). Intraoral pressure and rate of flow during speech. *Journal of Speech and Hearing Research, 9,* 498–518.

Sugden, E., Baker, E., Munro, N., Williams, A. L., & Trivette, C. M. (2018a). Service delivery and intervention intensity for phonology-based speech sound disorders. *International Journal of Language & Communication Disorders, 53*(4), 718–734.

Sugden, E., Baker, E., Munro, N., Williams, A. L., & Trivette, C. M. (2018b). An Australian survey of parent involvement in intervention for childhood speech sound disorder. *International Journal of Speech-Language Pathology, 20*(7), 766–778.

Sugden, E., Baker, E., Williams, A. L., Munro, N., & Trivette, C. M. (2020). Evaluation of a parent- and speech-language pathologist-delivered multiple oppositions intervention for children with phonological impairment: A multiple-baseline design study. *American Journal of Speech-Language Pathology, 29,* 111–126.

Sugden, E., Lloyd, S., Lam, J., & Cleland, J. (2019). Systematic review of ultrasound visual feedback in intervention for speech sound disorders. *International Journal of Language & Communication Disorders, 54*(5), 705–728.

Suggate, S., Schaughency, E., McAnally, H., & Reese, E. (2018). From infancy to adolescence: The longitudinal links between vocabulary, early literacy skills, oral narrative, and reading comprehension. *Cognitive Development, 47,* 82–95.

Sullivan, M., Gaebler, C., Beukelman, D., Mahanna, G., Marshall, J., Lydiatt, D., & Lydiatt, W. (2002). Impact of palatal prosthodontic intervention on communication performance of patients' maxillectomy defects: A multi-level outcome study. *Head and Neck, 24*(6), 530–538.

Sun, J., Weng, Y., Li, J., Wang, G., & Zhang, Z. (2007). Analysis of determinants on speech function after glossectomy. *Journal of Oral and Maxillofacial Surgery, 65,* 1944–1950.

Surej, K. L. K., Kurien, N. M., & Sivan, M. P. (2010). Isolated congenital bifid tongue. *National Journal of Maxillofacial Surgery, 1*(2), 187–189.

Sutherland, D., & Gillon, G. T. (2005). Assessment of phonological representations in children with speech impairment. *Language, Speech, and Hearing Services in Schools, 36,* 294–307.

Sutherland, D., & Gillon, G. T. (2007). Development of phonological representations and phonological awareness in children with speech impairment. *International Journal of Language & Communication Disorders, 42*(2), 229–250.

Swanson, T. J., Hodson, B. W., & Schommer-Aikins, M. (2005). An examination of phonological awareness treatment outcomes for 7th grade poor readers from a bilingual community. *Language, Speech, and Hearing Services in Schools, 36,* 336–345.

Tambyraja, S. R. (2020). Facilitating parental involvement in speech therapy for children with speech sound disorders: A survey of speech-language pathologists' practices, perspectives and strategies. *American Journal of Speech-Language Pathology, 29*(4), 1987–1996.

Tambyraja, S. R., & Dunkle, J. T. (2014). Target selection in speech therapy: Is a nondevelopmental approach more efficient than a developmental approach? *EBP Briefs, 8*(5), 1–9.

Tambyraja, S. R., Farquharson, K., & Justice, L. (2020). Reading risk in children with speech sound disorder: Prevalence, persistence, and predictors. *Journal of Speech, Language, and Hearing Research, 63*(11), 1–13.

Tang, G., & Barlow, J. (2006). Characteristics of the sound systems of monolingual Vietnamese-speaking children with phonological impairment. *Clinical Linguistics & Phonetics, 20*, 423–445.

Taps, J. (2008). RTI services for children with mild articulation needs: Four years of data. *Perspectives of the ASHA Special Interest Groups, 9*(3), 104–110.

Tattersall, P. J., & Dawson, J. L. (2016). *The structured photographic articulation test featuring Dudsberry* (3rd ed.). Pro-Ed.

Taylor, O. (1986). Teaching standard English as a second dialect. In O. Taylor (Ed.), *Treatment of communication disorders in culturally and linguistically diverse populations* (pp. 153–178). College-Hill Press.

Taylor, O., Payne, K., & Anderson, N. (1987). Distinguishing between communication disorders and differences. *Seminars in Speech and Language, 8*, 415–427.

Templin, M. (1947). Spontaneous vs. imitated verbalization in testing pre-school children. *Journal of Speech and Hearing Disorders, 12*, 293–300.

Templin, M. (1957). Certain language skills in children. *Institute of child welfare, monograph series 26*. University of Minnesota.

Templin, M. (1963). Development of speech. *Journal of Pediatrics, 62*, 11–14.

Templin, M., & Glaman, G. (1976). *A longitudinal study of correlations of predictive measures obtained in prekindergarten and first grade with achievement measures through eleventh grade* [Unpublished report #101]. U.S. Department of Health, Education, and Welfare, Office of Education.

Tennessee Department of Education. (2009). *Speech and language impairments severity ratings scales*, ED–4070/Rev. 04.09.

Terai, H., & Shimahara, M. (2004). Evaluation of speech intelligibility after a secondary dehiscence operation using an artificial graft in patients with speech disorders after partial glossectomy. *British Journal of Oral and Maxillofacial Surgery, 42*, 190–194.

Terrell, S., & Terrell, F. (1983). Effects of speaking Black English upon employment opportunities. *ASHA, 25*, 27–29.

Tessel, C. A., & Luque, J. S. (2020). A comparison of phonological and articulation-based approaches to accent modification using small groups. *Speech, Language and Hearing*, 1–14. doi: 10.1080/2050571X.2020.1730544.

Thomas, D. C., McCabe, P., & Ballard, K. J. (2018). Combined clinician-parent delivery of rapid syllable transition (ReST) treatment for childhood apraxia of speech. *International Journal of Speech-Language Pathology, 20*(7), 683–698.

Thomas, J. L. (2016). Decoding eligibility under the IDEA: Interpretations of "Adversely Affect Educational Performance." *Campbell Law Review, 38*(1), Rev. 73, Article 3.

Thomas, R. M. (2000). *Comparing theories of child development* (5th ed.). Wadsworth.

Thomson, R. I. (2011). Computer assisted pronunciation training: Targeting second language vowel perception improves pronunciation. *CALICO Journal, 28*(3), 744–765.

Tiffany, W. (1980). Effects of syllable structure on diadochokinetic and reading rates. *Journal of Speech and Hearing Research, 23*, 894–908.

Tipton, G. (1975). Non-cognate consonants of Mandarin and Cantonese. *Journal of the Chinese Language Teachers Association, 10*(1), 1–13.

To, C. K.-S., Cheung, P. S.-P., & McLeod, S. (2013). A population study of children's acquisition of Hong Kong Cantonese consonants, vowels, and tones. *Journal of Speech, Language, and Hearing Research, 56*, 103–122.

Tomblin, J. B., Records, N. L., Buckwalter, P., Zhang, X., Smith, E., & O'Brien, M. (1997). Prevalence of specific language impairment in kindergarten children. *Journal of Speech, Language, and Hearing Research, 40*, 1245–1260.

Torgesen, J. (1999). Assessment and instruction for phonemic awareness and word recognition skills. In H. Catts & A. Kamhi (Eds.), *Language and reading disabilities* (pp. 128–153). Allyn & Bacon.

Torgesen, J., & Bryant, B. (2004). *Test of phonological awareness* (2nd ed.), *PLUS*. Pro-Ed.

Torgesen, J., & Mathes, P. (2000). *A basic guide to understanding, assessing, and teaching phonological awareness*. Pro-Ed.

Torgesen, J., Wagner, R., Rashotte, C., Alexander, A., & Conway, T. (1997). Preventative and remedial interventions for children with severe reading disabilities. *Learning Disabilities, 81*, 51–62.

Torrington Eaton, C., & Bernstein Ratner, N. (2016). An exploration of the role of executive functions in preschoolers' phonological development. *Clinical Linguistics & Phonetics, 30*(9), 679–695.

Travis, L., & Rasmus, B. (1931). The speech sound discrimination ability of cases with functional disorders of articulation. *Quarterly Journal of Speech, 17,* 217–226.

Treiman, R. (1983). The structure of spoken syllables: Evidence from novel word games. *Cognition, 15,* 49–74.

Tsao, F. M., Liu, H. M., & Kuhl, P. K. (2004). Speech perception in infancy predicts language development in the second year of life: A longitudinal study. *Child Development, 75,* 1067–1084.

Tse, J. (1978). Tone acquisition in Cantonese: A longitudinal case study. *Journal of Child Language, 5,* 191–204.

Tsukada, K., Birdsong, D., Bialystok, E., Mack, M., Sung, H., & Flege, J. (2005). A developmental study of English vowel production and perception by native Korean adults and children. *Journal of Phonetics, 33*(3), 263–290.

Ttofari-Eecen, K., Reilly, S., & Eadie, P. (2007). *Parent report of speech sound development at 12 months of age: Evidence from a cohort study* [Unpublished manuscript].

Tuan, L. T. (2011). Vietnamese EFL learners' difficulties with English consonants. *Studies in Literature and Language, 3*(2), 56–67.

Turner, J., & Gutierrez, A. (2013). Pronunciation training needs for Chinese and Korean interpreters-in-training. *Perspectives on Communication Disorders and Sciences in Culturally and Linguistically Diverse Populations, 20*(3), 90–100.

Tye-Murray, N. (2020). *Foundations of aural rehabilitation. Children, adults and their family members* (5th ed.). Plural Publishing.

Tyler, A. (2005). Planning and monitoring intervention programs. In K. E. Pollock & A. G. Kamhi (Eds.), *Phonological disorders in children: Clinical decision making in assessment and intervention* (pp. 123–138). Paul H. Brookes Publishing Co.

Tyler, A., Edwards, M. L., & Saxman, J. H. (1987). Clinical application of two phonologically based treatment procedures. *Journal of Speech and Hearing Disorders, 52,* 393–409.

Tyler, A., & Figurski, G. R. (1994). Phonetic inventory changes after treating distinctions along an implicational hierarchy. *Clinical Linguistics & Phonetics, 8,* 91–107.

Tyler, A., Gillon, G. T., Macrae, T., & Johnson, R. L. (2011). Direct and indirect effects of stimulating phoneme awareness versus other linguistic skills in preschoolers with co-occurring speech and language impairments. *Topics in Language Disorders, 31,* 128–144.

Tyler, A., Lewis, K. E., Haskill, A., & Tolbert, L. C. (2002). Efficacy of cross-domain effects of a morphosyntax and a phonologic intervention. *Language, Speech, and Hearing Services in Schools, 33,* 52–66.

Tyler, A., Lewis, K. E., Haskill, A., & Tolbert, L. C. (2003). Outcomes of different speech and language goal attack strategies. *Journal of Speech, Language, and Hearing Research, 46*(5), 1077–1094.

Tyler, A., Osterhouse, H., Wickham, K., McNutt, R., & Shao, Y. (2014). Effects of explicit teacher-implemented phoneme awareness instruction in 4-year-olds. *Clinical Linguistics & Phonetics, 28,* 493–507.

Tyler, A., & Theodore, R. (2015, November). *The phonology-morphology interface in children with SSD: Development, assessment and treatment considerations* [Seminar presentation]. ASHA 2015 Convention, Denver, CO, United States.

Tyler, A., & Watterson, K. (1991). Effects of phonological versus language intervention in preschoolers with both phonological and language impairment. *Child Language Teaching and Therapy, 7,* 141–160.

Ukrainetz, T. A., Cooney, M. H., Dyer, S. K., Kysar, A. J., & Harris, T. J. (2000). An investigation into teaching phonemic awareness through shared reading and writing. *Early Childhood Research Quarterly, 15,* 331–355.

Ukrainetz, T. A., Ross, C. L., & Harm, H. M. (2009). An investigation of treatment scheduling for phonemic awareness with kindergartners who are at risk for reading difficulties. *Language, Speech, and Hearing Services in Schools, 40,* 86–100.

Unicomb, R., Hewat, S., Spencer, E., & Harrison, E. (2017). Evidence for the treatment of co-occurring stuttering and speech sound disorder: A clinical case study. *International Journal of Speech-Language Pathology, 19*(3), 251–264.

Unicomb, R., Kefalianos, E., Reilly, S., Cook, F., & Morgan, A. (2020). Prevalence and features of comorbid stuttering and speech sound disorder at age 4 years. *Journal of Communication Disorders, 84,* 1–12.

U.S. Census Bureau. (2011). Language use in the United States. https://www.census.gov /library/publications/2013/acs/acs-22.html

U.S. Census Bureau. (2015a). Census Bureau reports at least 350 languages spoken in U.S. homes. https://www.census.gov/newsroom/press-releases/2015/cb15-185.html

U.S. Census Bureau. (2015b). Detailed language spoken at home and ability to speak English for the population 5 years and over: 2010–2013. https://www.census.gov/data/tables/2013 /demo/2009-2013-lang-tables.html

Vallino, L. D., Zuker, R., & Napoli, J. A. (2008). A study of speech, language, hearing and dentition in children with cleft lip only. *Cleft Palate-Craniofacial Journal, 45,* 485–494.

Van Beijsterveldt, C. E. M., Felsenfeld, S., & Boomsma, D. I. (2010). Bivariate genetic analyses of stuttering and nonfluency in a large sample of 5-year-old twins. *Journal of Speech, Language, and Hearing Research, 53,* 609–619.

Van Borsel, J., & Cornelis, C. (2009). Tongue piercing and speech. *Journal of Otolaryngology–Head and Neck Surgery, 38*(1), 11–15.

Van Borsel, J., Morlion, B., Van Snick, K., & Leroy, J. S. (2000). Articulation in Beckwith-Wiedemann syndrome: Two case studies. *American Journal of Speech-Language Pathology, 9,* 202–213.

Van Borsel, J., & Tetnowski, J. A. (2007). Fluency disorders in genetic syndromes. *Journal of Fluency Disorders, 32,* 279–296.

Van Borsel, J., Van Snick, K., & Leroy, J. (1999). Macroglossia and speech in Bechwith-Wiedemann syndrome: A sample survey study. *International Journal of Language & Communication Disorders, 34,* 209–221.

Vance, M., Rosen, S., & Coleman, M. (2009). Assessing speech perception in young children and relationships with language skills. *International Journal of Audiology, 48,* 708–717.

Vance, M., Stackhouse, J., & Wells, B. (2005). Speech production skills in children aged 3–7 years. *International Journal of Language & Communication Disorders, 40,* 29–48.

Vandervelden, M. C., & Siegel, L. S. (1995). Phonological recording and phoneme awareness in early literacy: A developmental approach. *Reading Research Quarterly, 30,* 854–875.

Van Hattum, R. J. (1969). Program scheduling. In R. Van Hattum (Ed.), *Clinical speech in the schools* (pp. 163–195). Charles Thomas.

van Kleeck, A. (1998). Preliteracy domains and stages: Laying the foundations for beginning reading. *Journal of Children's Communication Development, 20,* 33–51.

van Kleeck, A., Gillam, R., & McFadden, T. (1998). A study of classroom-based phonological awareness training for preschoolers with speech and/or language disorders. *American Journal of Speech-Language Pathology, 7*(3), 65–76.

Van Lierde, K. M., Mortier, G., Huysman, E., & Vermeersch, H. (2010). Long-term impact of tongue reduction on speech intelligibility, articulation and oromyofunctional behavior in a child with Beckwith-Wiedemann syndrome. *International Journal of Pediatric Otorhinolaryngology, 74,* 309–318.

Van Riper, C. (1939). *Speech correction: Principles and methods.* Prentice-Hall.

Van Riper, C. (1972). *Speech correction: Principles and methods* (5th ed.). Prentice-Hall.

Van Riper, C., & Emerick, L. (1984). *Speech correction: An introduction to speech pathology and audiology* (7th ed.). Prentice-Hall.

Van Riper, C., & Erickson, R. (1996). *Speech correction: An introduction to speech pathology and audiology* (9th ed.). Prentice-Hall.

Van Riper, C., & Irwin, J. V. (1958). *Voice and articulation.* Prentice-Hall.

Varni, J., Seid, M., & Rode, C. (1999). The PedsQL™: Measurement model for the pediatric quality of life inventory. *Medical Care, 37*(2), 126–139.

Veatch, J. (1970). *An experimental investigation of a motor theory of auditory discrimination* [Unpublished doctoral dissertation]. University of Idaho.

Velleman, S. (2003). *Childhood apraxia of speech, resource guide.* Thomson Delmar Learning.

Velleman, S., & Strand, K. (1994). Developmental verbal dyspraxia. In J. Bernthal & N. Bankson (Eds.), *Child phonology: Characteristics, assessment, and intervention with special populations* (pp. 110–139). Thieme Medical Publishers.

Velleman, S. L., & Pearson, B. Z. (2010). Differentiating speech sound disorders from phonological dialect differences: Implications for assessment and intervention. *Topics in Language Disorders, 30,* 176–188.

Velten, H. (1943). The growth of phonemic and lexical patterns in infant language. *Language*, *19*, 281–292.

Veltman, C. (1988). *The future of the Spanish language in the United States*. Washington, DC: Hispanic Policy Development Project.

Vihman, M. M. (1988). Early phonological development. In J. Bernthal & N. Bankson (Eds.), *Articulation and phonological disorders* (2nd ed., pp. 60–109). Williams and Wilkins.

Vihman, M. M. (1992). *Early syllables and the construction of phonology*. York.

Vihman, M. M. (1996). *Phonological development: The origins of language in the child*. Blackwell.

Vihman, M. M., & deBoysson-Bardies, B. (1994). The nature and origins of ambient language influence on infant vocal production and early words. *Phonetica*, *51*(1–3), 159–169.

Vihman, M. M., & Greenlee, M. (1987). Individual differences in phonological development: Ages one and three years. *Journal of Speech and Hearing Research*, *30*, 503–521.

Vogel, J. E., Mulliken, J. B., & Kaban, L. B. (1986). Macroglossia: A review of the condition and a new classification. *Plastic and Reconstructive Surgery*, *78*, 715–723.

Vogel Sosa, A., & Stoel-Gammon, C. (2006). Patterns of intra-word phonological variability during the second year of life. *Journal of Child Language*, *33*, 31–50.

Vorperian, H., Kent, R. D., Gentry, L. R., & Yandell, B. S. (1999). Magnetic resonance imaging procedures to study the concurrent anatomic development of vocal tract structures: Preliminary results. *International Journal of Pediatric Otorhinolaryngology*, *49*(3), 197–206.

Vorperian, H. K., Kent, R. D., Lindstrom, M. J., Kalina, C. M., Gentry, L. R., & Yandell, B. S. (2005). Development of vocal tract length during early childhood: A magnetic resonance imaging study. *Journal of the Acoustical Society of America*, *117*, 338–350.

Wachtel, J. M., Kuehn, D. P., & Weiss, K. S. (2000). Hypernasality after tonsillectomy without adenoidectomy in an adult. *Otolaryngology–Head and Neck Surgery*, *122*(1), 112–113.

Wadsworth, S. D., Maul, C. A., & Stevens, E. J. (1998). The prevalence of orofacial myofunctional disorders among children identified with speech and language disorders in grades kindergarten through six. *International Journal of Orofacial Myology*, *24*, 1–19.

Wagner, R., & Torgesen, J. K. (1987). The nature of phonological processing and its causal role in the acquisition of reading skills. *Psychological Bulletin*, *101*, 192–212.

Wagner, R., Torgesen, J., Rashotte, C., & Pearson, N. A. (2013). *Comprehensive test of phonological processing–2*. Pro-Ed.

Walker, J. F., & Archibald, L. M. D. (2006). Articulation rate in preschool children: A 3-year longitudinal study. *International Journal of Language & Communication Disorders*, *41*(5), 541–565.

Wallin, J. E. W. (1916). A census of speech defectives among 89,057 public-school pupils: A preliminary report. *School and Society*, *3*, 213–216.

Walls, A., Pierce, M., Wang, H., Steehler, A., Steehler, M., & Harley, Jr., E. H. (2014). Parental perception of speech and tongue mobility in three-year olds after neonatal frenotomy. *International Journal of Pediatric Otorhinolaryngology*, *78*, 128–131.

Walsh, B., & Smith, A. (2002). Articulatory movements in adolescents: Evidence for protracted development of speech motor control processes. *Journal of Speech, Language, and Hearing Research*, *45*(6), 1119–1133.

Walsh, H. (1974). On certain practical inadequacies of distinctive feature systems. *Journal of Speech and Hearing Disorders*, *39*, 32–43.

Walsh, J., Links, A., Boss, E., & Tunkel, D. (2017). Ankyloglossia and lingual frenotomy: National trends in inpatient diagnosis and management in the United States, 1997–2012. *Otolaryngology–Head and Neck Surgery*, *156*(4), 735–740.

Wang, W. (1989). *Languages and dialects of Chinese*. Stanford University Press.

Wang, W. (1990). Theoretical issues in studying Chinese dialects. *Journal of the Chinese Language Teachers Association*, *25*, 1–34.

Wang, X., & Munro, M. J. (2004). Computer-based training for learning English vowel contrasts. *System*, *32*(4), 539–552.

Waring, R., Eadie, P., Liow, S. R., & Dodd, B. (2017). Do children with phonological delay have phonological short-term and phonological working memory deficits? *Child Language, Teaching and Therapy*, *33*(1), 33–46.

Waring, R., Eadie, P., Liow, S. R., & Dodd, B. (2018). The phonological memory profile of preschool children who make atypical speech sound errors. *Clinical Linguistics & Phonetics*, *32*, 28–45.

Waring, R., Fisher, J., & Atkin, N. (2001). The articulation survey: Putting numbers to it. In L. Wilson & S. Hewat (Eds.), *Proceedings of the 2001 Speech Pathology Australia National Conference: Evidence and Innovation* (pp. 145–151). Speech Pathology Australia.

Waring, R., & Knight, R. (2013). How should children with speech sound disorders be classified? A review and critical evaluation of current classification systems. *International Journal of Language & Communication Disorders, 48,* 25–40.

Waring, R., Liow, R., Eadie, P., & Dodd, B. (2019). Speech development in preschool children: Evaluating the contribution of phonological short-term and phonological working memory. *Journal of Child Language, 46*(4), 632–652.

Warren, S. F., Fey, M. E., & Yoder, P. J. (2007). Differential treatment intensity research: A missing link to creating optimally effective communication interventions. *Mental Retardation and Developmental Disabilities Research Reviews, 13*(1), 70–77.

Washington, J., & Craig, H. (1992). Articulation test performances of low-income African American preschoolers with communication impairments. *Language, Speech, and Hearing Services in Schools, 23,* 201–207.

Washington, J., & Craig, H. (1998). Socioeconomic status and gender influences on children's dialectal variations. *Journal of Speech, Language, and Hearing Research, 41,* 618–626.

Washington, K. N., Fritz, K., Crowe, K., Kelly, B., & Wright Karem, R. (2019). Bilingual preschoolers' spontaneous productions: Considering Jamaican Creole and English. *Language, Speech, and Hearing Services in Schools, 50*(2), 179–195.

Watson, J. B. (1913/1994). Psychology as a behaviorist views it. *Psychological Review, 101,* 248–253.

Watson, M. M., & Scukanec, G. P. (1997a). Phonological changes in the speech of two-year olds: A longitudinal investigation. *Infant-Toddler Intervention, 7,* 67–77.

Watson, M. M., & Scukanec, G. P. (1997b). Profiling the phonological abilities of 2-year-olds: A longitudinal investigation. *Child Language Teaching and Therapy, 13,* 3–14.

Weaver, C., Furbee, C., & Everhart, R. (1960). Paternal occupational class and articulatory defects in children. *Journal of Speech and Hearing Disorders, 25,* 171–175.

Weber, J. (1970). Patterning of deviant articulation behavior. *Journal of Speech and Hearing Disorders, 35,* 135–141.

Weaver-Spurlock, S., & Brasseur, J. (1988). The effects of simultaneous sound-position training on the generalization of [s]. *Language, Speech, and Hearing Services in Schools, 19,* 259–271.

Weikum, W. M., Vouloumanos, A., Navarra, J., Soto-Faraco, S., Sebastián-Gallés, N., & Werker, J. F. (2007). Visual language discrimination in infancy. *Science, 316*(25), 1159.

Weinberg, B., Liss, G. M., & Hillis, J. (1970). A comparative study of visual, manual, and oral form identification in speech impaired and normal speaking children. In J. F. Bosma (Ed.), *Second symposium on oral sensation and perception* (pp. 350–356). Charles Thomas.

Weiner, F. (1979). *Phonological process analysis.* University Park Press.

Weiner, F. (1981a). Systematic sound preference as a characteristic of phonological disability. *Journal of Speech and Hearing Disorders, 46,* 281–286.

Weiner, F. (1981b). Treatment of phonological disability using the method of meaningful minimal contrast: Two case studies. *Journal of Speech and Hearing Disorders, 46,* 97–103.

Weismer, G. (2006). Philosophy of research in motor speech disorders. *Clinical Linguistics & Phonetics, 20,* 315–349.

Weiss, C. E., Gordon, M. E., & Lillywhite, H. S. (1987). *Clinical management of articulatory and phonologic disorders* (2nd ed.). Williams & Wilkins.

Wellman, B., Case, I., Mengert, I., & Bradbury, D. (1931). Speech sounds of young children. *University of Iowa Studies in Child Welfare, 5.*

Wells, B., & Peppé, S. (2003). Intonation abilities of children with speech and language impairments. *Journal of Speech, Language, and Hearing Research, 46,* 5–20.

Weston, A., & Irwin, J. (1985). Paired stimuli treatment. In P. Newman, N. Creaghead, & W. Secord (Eds.), *Assessment and remediation of articulatory and phonological disorders* (pp. 337–368). Merrill.

Whitehurst, G. J., & Lonigan, C. J. (1998). Child development and emergent literacy. *Child Development, 69,* 848–872.

Wiig, E., Semel, E., & Secord, W. (2020). *Clinical evaluation of language fundamentals preschool–3.* Psychological Corporation.

Wilcox, K., & Morris, S. (1995). Speech outcomes of the language-focused curriculum. In M. Rice & K. Wilcox (Eds.), *Building a language-focused curriculum for the preschool classroom: A foundation for lifelong communication* (pp. 73–79). Paul H. Brookes Publishing Co.

Wilcox, K., & Morris, S. (1999). *Children's speech intelligibility measure.* Psychological Corporation.

Wilcox, L., & Anderson, R. (1998). Distinguishing between phonological difference and disorder in children who speak African-American vernacular English: An experimental testing instrument. *Journal of Communication Disorders, 31*, 315–335.

Wilhelm, C. L. (1971). *The effects of oral form recognition training on articulation in children* [Unpublished doctoral dissertation]. University of Kansas.

Williams, A. L. (1991). Generalization patterns associated with training least phonological knowledge. *Journal of Speech and Hearing Research, 34*, 722–733.

Williams, A. L. (1993). Phonological reorganization: A qualitative measure of phonological improvement. *American Journal of Speech-Language Pathology, 2*, 44–51.

Williams, A. L. (1999). *A systemic approach to phonological assessment and intervention* [Workshop presentation]. The Speech and Hearing Association of Virginia.

Williams, A. L. (2000a). Multiple oppositions: Case studies of variables in phonological intervention. *American Journal of Speech-Language Pathology, 9*, 289–299.

Williams, A. L. (2000b). Multiple oppositions: Theoretical foundations for an alternative contrastive intervention approach. *American Journal of Speech-Language Pathology, 9*, 282–288.

Williams, A. L. (2001). Phonological assessment of child speech. In D. Ruscello (Ed.), *Tests and measurements in speech-language pathology* (pp. 31–76). Butterworth-Heinemann.

Williams, A. L. (2003). *Speech disorders resource guide for preschool children*. Singular Publishing.

Williams, A. L. (2005). Assessment, target selection, and intervention. Dynamic interactions within a systemic perspective. *Topics in Language Disorders, 25*(3), 231–242.

Williams, A. L. (2010). Multiple oppositions intervention. In A. L. Williams, S. McLeod, & R. J. McCauley (Eds.), *Interventions for speech sound disorders in children* (pp. 73–94). Paul H. Brookes Publishing Co.

Williams, A. L. (2012). Intensity in phonological intervention: Is there a prescribed amount? *International Journal of Speech-Language Pathology, 14*(5), 456–461.

Williams, A. L. (2016). *SCIP 2: Sound contrasts in phonology 2* (1.0) [Mobile application software]. http://itunes.apple.com

Williams, A. L., McLeod, S., & McCauley, R. J. (Eds.). (2021). *Interventions for speech sound disorders in children* (2nd ed.). Paul H. Brookes Publishing Co.

Williams, A. L., & Sugden, E. (2021). Multiple oppositions intervention. In A. L. Williams, S. McLeod, & R. J. McCauley (Eds.), *Interventions for speech sound disorders in children* (2nd ed., pp. 61–89). Paul H. Brookes Publishing Co.

Williams, F. (1972). *Language and speech: Introductory perspectives*. Prentice-Hall.

Williams, G., & McReynolds, L. (1975). The relationship between discrimination and articulation training in children with misarticulations. *Journal of Speech and Hearing Research, 18*, 401–412.

Williams, P. (2021). The Nuffield centre dyspraxia programme. In A. L. Williams, S. McLeod, & R. J. McCauley (Eds.), *Interventions for speech sound disorders in children* (2nd ed., pp. 447–475). Paul H. Brookes Publishing Co.

Williams, P., & Stackhouse, J. (1998). Diadochokinetic skills: Normal and atypical performance in children aged 3–5 years. *International Journal of Language & Communication Disorders, 33*, 481–486.

Williams, P., & Stackhouse, J. (2000). Rate, accuracy and consistency: Diadochokinetic performance of young, normally developing children. *Clinical Linguistics & Phonetics, 14*, 267–294.

Williams, P., & Stephens, H. (2004). *The Nuffield centre dyspraxia programme* (3rd ed.). The Miracle Factory.

Williams, P., & Stephens, H. (2010). The Nuffield centre dyspraxia programme. In A. L. Williams, S. McLeod, & R. J. McCauley (Eds.), *Interventions for speech sound disorders* (pp. 159–177). Paul H. Brookes Publishing Co.

Wilson, F. (1966). Efficacy of speech therapy with educable mentally retarded children. *Journal of Speech and Hearing Research, 9*, 423–433.

Wilson, L., McNeill, B. C., & Gillon, G. T. (2016). A comparison of inter-professional education programs in preparing prospective teachers and speech and language pathologists for collaborative language-literacy instruction. *Reading and Writing, 29*(6), 1179–1201.

Wilson, L., McNeill, B. C., & Gillon, G. T. (2017). Interprofessional education of prospective speech-language therapists and primary school teachers through shared professional practice placements. *International Journal of Language & Communication Disorders, 52*(4), 426–439.

Wing, K., & Flipsen, Jr., P. (2010, November). *Phonological disorders in Spanish-speaking children: Accounting for Mexican dialect* [Poster presentation]. ASHA 2010 Convention, Philadelphia, PA, United States.

Winitz, H. (1959a). Language skills of male and female kindergarten children. *Journal of Speech and Hearing Research, 2,* 377–386.

Winitz, H. (1959b). Relationship between language and nonlanguage measures of kindergarten children. *Journal of Speech and Hearing Research, 2,* 387–391.

Winitz, H. (1969). *Articulatory acquisition and behavior.* Prentice-Hall.

Winitz, H. (1975). *From syllable to conversation.* University Park Press.

Winitz, H. (1984). Auditory considerations in articulation training. In H. Winitz (Ed.), *Treating articulation disorders: For clinicians by clinicians* (pp. 21–49). University Park Press.

Wise, C. M. (1957a). *Introduction to phonetics.* Prentice-Hall.

Wise, C. M. (1957b). *Applied phonetics.* Prentice-Hall.

Witzel, M. A., Rich, R. H., Margar-Bacal, F., & Cox, C. (1986). Velopharyngeal insufficiency after adenoidectomy: An 8-year review. *International Journal of Pediatric Otorhinolaryngology, 11,* 15–20.

Wolfe, V., & Irwin, R. (1973). Sound discrimination ability of children with misarticulation of the /r/ sound. *Perceptual and Motor Skills, 37,* 415–420.

Wolfe, V., Presley, C., & Mesaris, J. (2003). The importance of sound identification training in phonological intervention. *American Journal of Speech-Language Pathology, 12,* 282–288.

Wolfram, W. (1974). *Sociolinguistic aspects of assimilation: Puerto Rican English in New York City.* Arlington, VA: Center for Applied Linguistics.

Wolfram, W. (1986). Language variation in the United States. In O. Taylor (Ed.), *Nature of communication disorders in culturally and linguistically diverse populations* (pp. 73–116). College-Hill Press.

Wolfram, W. (1994). The phonology of a sociocultural variety: The case of African American vernacular English. In J. Bernthal & N. Bankson (Eds.), *Child phonology: Characteristics, assessment, and intervention with special populations* (pp. 227–244). Thieme Medical Publishers.

Wolfram, W. (2004). Social varieties of American English. In E. Finnegan & J. Rickford (Eds.), *Language in the USA: Themes for the twenty-first century* (pp. 58–75). Cambridge University Press.

Wolfram, W., Adger, C. T., & Christian, D. (1999). *Dialects in schools and communities.* Erlbaum.

Wolfram, W., & Schilling-Estes, N. (1998). *American English: Dialects and variation.* Blackwell.

Woodcock, R. W., Camarata, S., & Camarata, M. (2019). *Woodcock-Camarata articulation battery (WCAB).* Schoolhouse Educational Services.

Woolf, G., & Pilberg, M. (1971). A comparison of three tests of auditory discrimination and their relationship to performance on a deep test of articulation. *Journal of Communication Disorders, 3,* 239–249.

Wren, Y., Miller, L. L., Peters, T. J., Edmond, A., & Roulstone, S. (2016). Prevalence and predictors of persistent speech sound disorder at eight years old: Findings from a population cohort study. *Journal of Speech, Language, and Hearing Research, 59,* 647–673.

Wren, Y., & Roulstone, S. (2008). A comparison between computer and tabletop delivery of phonology therapy. *International Journal of Speech-Language Pathology, 10*(5), 346–363.

Wright, V., Shelton, R., & Arndt, W. (1969). A task for evaluation of articulation change: III. Imitative task scores compared with scores for more spontaneous tasks. *Journal of Speech and Hearing Research, 12,* 875–884.

Wyllie-Smith, L., McLeod, S., & Ball, M. J. (2006). Typically developing and speech impaired children's adherence to the sonority hypothesis. *Clinical Linguistics & Phonetics, 20*(4–5), 271–291.

Yaruss, J. S., & Conture, E. G. (1996). Stuttering and phonological disorders in children: Examination of the covert repair hypothesis. *Journal of Speech and Hearing Research, 39,* 349–364.

Yavaş, M. (2000). *Sonority effects of vowel nuclei in onset duration* [Poster presentation]. The Eighth International Clinical Phonetics & Linguistics Association Conference, Edinburgh.

Yavaş, M. (2006). Sonority and the acquisition of #sC clusters. *Journal of Multilingual Communication Disorders, 4*(3), 159–168.

Yavaş, M., & Core, C. (2001). Phonemic awareness of coda consonants and sonority in bi-lingual children. *Clinical Linguistics & Phonetics, 15,* 35–39.

Yavaş, M., & Gogate, L. (1999). Phoneme awareness in children: A function of sonority. *Journal of Psycholinguistic Research, 28*, 245–260.

Yavaş, M., & Goldstein, B. (1998). Phonological assessment and treatment of bilingual speakers. *American Journal of Speech-Language Pathology, 7*, 49–60.

Yavaş, M., & McLeod, S. (2010). Acquisition of /s/ clusters in English-speaking children with phonological disorders. *Clinical Linguistics & Phonetics, 24*, 177–187.

Yin, R. (1989). *Case study research design and methods.* Sage.

Yoder, P., Camarata, S., & Gardner, E. (2005). Treatment effects on speech intelligibility and length of utterance in children with specific language and intelligibility impairments. *Journal of Early Intervention, 28*, 34–49.

Yoder, P. J., Camarata, S., & Woynaroski, T. (2016). Treating speech comprehensibility in students with Down syndrome. *Journal of Speech, Language, and Hearing Research, 59*, 446–459.

Yoon, A. J., Zaghi, S., Ha, S., Law, C. S., Guilleminault, C., & Liu, S. Y. (2017). Ankyloglossia as a risk factor for maxillary hypoplasia and soft palate elongation: A functional–morphological study. *Orthodontics & Craniofacial Research, 20*(4), 237–244.

Yoon, H.-K. (2012). Grammar errors in Korean EFL learners' TOEIC speaking test. *English Teaching, 67*(4), 287–309.

Yorkston, K. M., Beukelman, D. R., Strand, E. A., & Hakel, M. (2010). *Management of motor speech disorders in children and adults* (3rd ed.). Pro-Ed.

Yoss, K., & Darley, F. (1974). Developmental apraxia of speech in children with defective articulation. *Journal of Speech and Hearing Research, 17*, 399–416.

Young, E. C. (1987). The effects of treatment on consonant cluster and weak syllable reduction processes in misarticulating children. *Language, Speech, and Hearing Services in Schools, 18*, 23–33.

Young, E. H., & Hawk, S. S. (1955). *Motokinesthetic speech training.* Stanford University Press.

Yuzyuk, T., Viau, K., Andrews, A., Pasquali, M., & Longo, N. (2018). Biochemical changes and clinical outcomes in 34 patients with classic galactosemia. *Journal of Inherited Metabolic Disease, 41*, 197–208.

Zehel, Z., Shelton, R., Arndt, W., Wright, V., & Elbert, M. (1972). Item context and /s/ phone articulation results. *Journal of Speech and Hearing Research, 15*, 852–860.

Zhao, S., Koh, S. N., & Luke, K. K. (2012). *Accent reduction for computer-aided language learning.* 2012 Proceedings of the 20th European Signal Processing Conference (EUSIPCO), Bucharest, Romania, 335–339 IEEE.

Zhu, H., & Dodd, B. (2000a). The phonological acquisition of Putonghua (modern standard Chinese). *Journal of Child Language, 27*, 3–42.

Zhu, H., & Dodd, B. (2000b). Putonghua (modern standard Chinese)–speaking children with speech disorder. *Clinical Linguistics & Phonetics, 14*, 165–191.

Ziegler, J. C., & Goswami, U. (2005). Reading acquisition, developmental dyslexia, and skilled reading across languages: A psycholinguistic grain size theory. *Psychological Bulletin, 131*, 3–29.

Zimmerman, I., Steiner, V., & Pond, R. (2012). *Preschool language scale* (5th ed.). Merrill.

Index

Note: Page numbers followed by *f*, *b*, and *t* indicate figures, boxes, and tables, respectively.